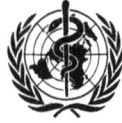

WORLD HEALTH ORGANIZATION

INTERNATIONAL AGENCY FOR RESEARCH ON CANCER

IARC MONOGRAPHS

ON THE

EVALUATION OF CARCINOGENIC

RISKS TO HUMANS

*Occupational Exposures of Hairdressers and Barbers
and Personal Use of Hair Colourants;
Some Hair Dyes, Cosmetic Colourants,
Industrial Dyestuffs and Aromatic Amines*

VOLUME 57

This publication represents the views and expert opinions
of an IARC Working Group on the
Evaluation of Carcinogenic Risks to Humans,
which met in Lyon,

6–13 October 1992

1993

IARC MONOGRAPHS

In 1969, the International Agency for Research on Cancer (IARC) initiated a programme on the evaluation of the carcinogenic risk of chemicals to humans involving the production of critically evaluated monographs on individual chemicals. In 1980 and 1986, the programme was expanded to include the evaluation of the carcinogenic risk associated with exposures to complex mixtures and other agents.

The objective of the programme is to elaborate and publish in the form of monographs critical reviews of data on carcinogenicity for agents to which humans are known to be exposed, and on specific exposure situations; to evaluate these data in terms of human risk with the help of international working groups of experts in chemical carcinogenesis and related fields; and to indicate where additional research efforts are needed.

This project is supported by PHS Grant No. 5-UO1 CA33193-11 awarded by the US National Cancer Institute, Department of Health and Human Services. Additional support has been provided since 1986 by the Commission of the European Communities.

©International Agency for Research on Cancer 1993

ISBN 92 832 1257 6

ISSN 0250-9555

Distributed for the International Agency for Research on Cancer
by the Secretariat of the World Health Organization, Geneva

PRINTED IN THE UNITED KINGDOM

CONTENTS

CONTENTS

NOTE TO THE READER

The term 'carcinogenic risk' in the *IARC Monographs* series is taken to mean the probability that exposure to an agent will lead to cancer in humans.

Inclusion of an agent in the *Monographs* does not imply that it is a carcinogen, only that the published data have been examined. Equally, the fact that an agent has not yet been evaluated in a monograph does not mean that it is not carcinogenic.

The evaluations of carcinogenic risk are made by international working groups of independent scientists and are qualitative in nature. No recommendation is given for regulation or legislation.

Anyone who is aware of published data that may alter the evaluation of the carcinogenic risk of an agent to humans is encouraged to make this information available to the Unit of Carcinogen Identification and Evaluation, International Agency for Research on Cancer, 150 cours Albert Thomas, 69372 Lyon Cedex 08, France, in order that the agent may be considered for re-evaluation by a future Working Group.

Although every effort is made to prepare the monographs as accurately as possible, mistakes may occur. Readers are requested to communicate any errors to the Unit of Carcinogen Identification and Evaluation, so that corrections can be reported in future volumes.

IARC WORKING GROUP ON THE EVALUATION OF CARCINOGENIC RISKS TO HUMANS: OCCUPATIONAL EXPOSURES OF HAIDRESSERS AND BARBERS AND PERSONAL USE OF HAIR COLOURANTS; SOME HAIR DYES, COSMETIC COLOURANTS, INDUSTRIAL DYESTUFFS AND AROMATIC AMINES

Lyon, 6–13 October 1992

LIST OF PARTICIPANTS

Members

M. Boeniger, National Institute for Occupational Safety and Health, Robert A. Taft Laboratories, 4676 Columbia Parkway, Cincinnati, OH 45226-1998, USA

R.D. Combes, LSU College of Higher Education, The Avenue, Southampton, Hants SO9 5HB, United Kingdom

T.A. Dragani, Division of Experimental Oncology A, Istituto Nazionale per lo Studio e la Cura dei Tumori, via Venezian 1, 20133 Milano, Italy

J. Fitzgerald, Public and Environmental Health Division, South Australian Health Commission, 11–13 Hindmarsh Square, Adelaide, SA 5000, Australia

B.D. Hardin, National Institute for Occupational Safety and Health, Hubert H. Humphrey Building, Room 714-B, 200 Independence Avenue SW, Washington DC 20201, USA

R.B. Hayes, Division of Cancer Etiology, National Cancer Institute, Executive Plaza North, Room 418, 6130 Executive Boulevard, North Bethesda, MD 20892, USA

F. Kadlubar, National Center for Toxicological Research, Jefferson, AR 72079-9502, USA

L.J. Kinlen, CRC Cancer Epidemiology Research Group, Department of Public Health & Primary Care, University of Oxford, The Radcliffe Infirmary, Oxford OX2 6HE, United Kingdom

E. Kriek, Division of Molecular Carcinogenesis, The Netherlands Cancer Institute, Plesmanlaan 121, 1066 CX Amsterdam, Netherlands

E. Lynge, Danish Cancer Registry, Rosenvængets Hovedvej 35, Box 839, 2100 Copenhagen Ø, Denmark

R.R. Maronpot, National Institute of Environmental Health Sciences, PO Box 12233, Research Triangle Park, NC 27709, USA

M.-J. Ghess, Unit of Carcinogen Identification and Evaluation
E. Heseltine, Lajarthe, 24290 St Léon-sur-Vézère, France
V. Krutovskikh, Unit of Multistage Carcinogenesis
J. Little, Unit of Analytical Epidemiology
D. McGregor, Unit of Carcinogen Identification and Evaluation
D. Mietton, Unit of Carcinogen Identification and Evaluation
H. Møller, Unit of Carcinogen Identification and Evaluation
R. Montesano, Unit of Mechanisms of Carcinogenesis
I. O'Neill, Unit of Environmental Carcinogens and Host Factors
C. Partensky, Unit of Carcinogen Identification and Evaluation
I. Peterschmitt, Unit of Carcinogen Identification and Evaluation, Geneva
D. Shuker, Unit of Environmental Carcinogens and Host Factors
L. Tomatis, Director
H. Vainio, Chief, Unit of Carcinogen Identification and Evaluation
J. Wilbourn, Unit of Carcinogen Identification and Evaluation
H. Yamasaki, Unit of Multistage Carcinogenesis

Secretarial assistance

M. Lézère
J. Mitchell
S. Reynaud

PREAMBLE

IARC MONOGRAPHS PROGRAMME ON THE EVALUATION OF CARCINOGENIC RISKS TO HUMANS[1]

PREAMBLE

1. BACKGROUND

In 1969, the International Agency for Research on Cancer (IARC) initiated a programme to evaluate the carcinogenic risk of chemicals to humans and to produce monographs on individual chemicals. The *Monographs* programme has since been expanded to include consideration of exposures to complex mixtures of chemicals (which occur, for example, in some occupations and as a result of human habits) and of exposures to other agents, such as radiation and viruses. With Supplement 6 (IARC, 1987a), the title of the series was modified from *IARC Monographs on the Evaluation of the Carcinogenic Risk of Chemicals to Humans* to *IARC Monographs on the Evaluation of Carcinogenic Risks to Humans*, in order to reflect the widened scope of the programme.

The criteria established in 1971 to evaluate carcinogenic risk to humans were adopted by the working groups whose deliberations resulted in the first 16 volumes of the *IARC Monographs* series. Those criteria were subsequently updated by further ad-hoc working groups (IARC, 1977, 1978, 1979, 1982, 1983, 1987b, 1988, 1991a; Vainio *et al.*, 1992).

2. OBJECTIVE AND SCOPE

The objective of the programme is to prepare, with the help of international working groups of experts, and to publish in the form of monographs, critical reviews and evaluations of evidence on the carcinogenicity of a wide range of human exposures. The *Monographs* may also indicate where additional research efforts are needed.

The *Monographs* represent the first step in carcinogenic risk assessment, which involves examination of all relevant information in order to assess the strength of the available evidence that certain exposures could alter the incidence of cancer in humans. The second step is quantitative risk estimation. Detailed, quantitative evaluations of epidemiological data may be made in the *Monographs*, but without extrapolation beyond the range of the data

[1]This project is supported by PHS Grant No. 5-UO1 CA33193-11 awarded by the US National Cancer Institute, Department of Health and Human Services. Since 1986, the programme has also been supported by the Commission of the European Communities.

available. Quantitative extrapolation from experimental data to the human situation is not undertaken.

The term 'carcinogen' is used in these monographs to denote an exposure that is capable of increasing the incidence of malignant neoplasms; the induction of benign neoplasms may in some circumstances (see p. 22) contribute to the judgement that the exposure is carcinogenic. The terms 'neoplasm' and 'tumour' are used interchangeably.

Some epidemiological and experimental studies indicate that different agents may act at different stages in the carcinogenic process, and several different mechanisms may be involved. The aim of the *Monographs* has been, from their inception, to evaluate evidence of carcinogenicity at any stage in the carcinogenesis process, independently of the underlying mechanisms. Information on mechanisms may, however, be used in making the overall evaluation (IARC, 1991a; Vainio *et al.*, 1992; see also pp. 28–30).

The *Monographs* may assist national and international authorities in making risk assessments and in formulating decisions concerning any necessary preventive measures. The evaluations of IARC working groups are scientific, qualitative judgements about the evidence for or against carcinogenicity provided by the available data. These evaluations represent only one part of the body of information on which regulatory measures may be based. Other components of regulatory decisions may vary from one situation to another and from country to country, responding to different socioeconomic and national priorities. **Therefore, no recommendation is given with regard to regulation or legislation, which are the responsibility of individual governments and/or other international organizations.**

The *IARC Monographs* are recognized as an authoritative source of information on the carcinogenicity of a wide range of human exposures. A users' survey, made in 1988, indicated that the *Monographs* are consulted by various agencies in 57 countries. Each volume is generally printed in 4000 copies for distribution to governments, regulatory bodies and interested scientists. The *Monographs* are also available *via* the Distribution and Sales Service of the World Health Organization.

3. SELECTION OF TOPICS FOR MONOGRAPHS

Topics are selected on the basis of two main criteria: (a) there is evidence of human exposure, and (b) there is some evidence or suspicion of carcinogenicity. The term 'agent' is used to include individual chemical compounds, groups of related chemical compounds, physical agents (such as radiation) and biological factors (such as viruses). Exposures to mixtures of agents may occur in occupational exposures and as a result of personal and cultural habits (like smoking and dietary practices). Chemical analogues and compounds with biological or physical characteristics similar to those of suspected carcinogens may also be considered, even in the absence of data on a possible carcinogenic effect in humans or experimental animals.

The scientific literature is surveyed for published data relevant to an assessment of carcinogenicity. The IARC surveys of chemicals being tested for carcinogenicity (IARC, 1973–1992) and directories of on-going research in cancer epidemiology (IARC, 1976–1992) often indicate those exposures that may be scheduled for future meetings. Ad-hoc working groups convened by IARC in 1984, 1989 and 1991 gave recommendations as to which agents should be evaluated in the *IARC Monographs* series (IARC, 1984, 1989, 1991b).

As significant new data on subjects on which monographs have already been prepared become available, re-evaluations are made at subsequent meetings, and revised monographs are published.

4.   DATA FOR MONOGRAPHS

The *Monographs* do not necessarily cite all the literature concerning the subject of an evaluation. Only those data considered by the Working Group to be relevant to making the evaluation are included.

With regard to biological and epidemiological data, only reports that have been published or accepted for publication in the openly available scientific literature are reviewed by the working groups. In certain instances, government agency reports that have undergone peer review and are widely available are considered. Exceptions may be made on an ad-hoc basis to include unpublished reports that are in their final form and publicly available, if their inclusion is considered pertinent to making a final evaluation (see pp. 26 *et seq.*). In the sections on chemical and physical properties, on analysis, on production and use and on occurrence, unpublished sources of information may be used.

5.   THE WORKING GROUP

Reviews and evaluations are formulated by a working group of experts. The tasks of the group are: (i) to ascertain that all appropriate data have been collected; (ii) to select the data relevant for the evaluation on the basis of scientific merit; (iii) to prepare accurate summaries of the data to enable the reader to follow the reasoning of the Working Group; (iv) to evaluate the results of epidemiological and experimental studies on cancer; (v) to evaluate data relevant to the understanding of mechanism of action; and (vi) to make an overall evaluation of the carcinogenicity of the exposure to humans.

Working Group participants who contributed to the considerations and evaluations within a particular volume are listed, with their addresses, at the beginning of each publication. Each participant who is a member of a working group serves as an individual scientist and not as a representative of any organization, government or industry. In addition, nominees of national and international agencies and industrial associations may be invited as observers.

6.   WORKING PROCEDURES

Approximately one year in advance of a meeting of a working group, the topics of the monographs are announced and participants are selected by IARC staff in consultation with other experts. Subsequently, relevant biological and epidemiological data are collected by IARC from recognized sources of information on carcinogenesis, including data storage and retrieval systems such as BIOSIS, Chemical Abstracts, CANCERLIT, MEDLINE and TOXLINE—including EMIC and ETIC for data on genetic and related effects and reproductive and developmental effects, respectively.

For chemicals and some complex mixtures, the major collection of data and the preparation of first drafts of the sections on chemical and physical properties, on analysis, on production and use and on occurrence are carried out under a separate contract funded by the US National Cancer Institute. Representatives from industrial associations may assist in the preparation of sections on production and use. Information on production and trade is obtained from governmental and trade publications and, in some cases, by direct contact with industries. Separate production data on some agents may not be available because their publication could disclose confidential information. Information on uses may be obtained from published sources but is often complemented by direct contact with manufacturers. Efforts are made to supplement this information with data from other national and international sources.

Six months before the meeting, the material obtained is sent to meeting participants, or is used by IARC staff, to prepare sections for the first drafts of monographs. The first drafts are compiled by IARC staff and sent, prior to the meeting, to all participants of the Working Group for review.

The Working Group meets in Lyon for seven to eight days to discuss and finalize the texts of the monographs and to formulate the evaluations. After the meeting, the master copy of each monograph is verified by consulting the original literature, edited and prepared for publication. The aim is to publish monographs within nine months of the Working Group meeting.

The available studies are summarized by the Working Group, with particular regard to the qualitative aspects discussed below. In general, numerical findings are indicated as they appear in the original report; units are converted when necessary for easier comparison. The Working Group may conduct additional analyses of the published data and use them in their assessment of the evidence; the results of such supplementary analyses are given in square brackets. When an important aspect of a study, directly impinging on its interpretation, should be brought to the attention of the reader, a comment is given in square brackets.

7. EXPOSURE DATA

Sections that indicate the extent of past and present human exposure, the sources of exposure, the people most likely to be exposed and the factors that contribute to the exposure are included at the beginning of each monograph.

Most monographs on individual chemicals, groups of chemicals or complex mixtures include sections on chemical and physical data, on analysis, on production and use and on occurrence. In monographs on, for example, physical agents, biological factors, occupational exposures and cultural habits, other sections may be included, such as: historical perspectives, description of an industry or habit, chemistry of the complex mixture or taxonomy.

For chemical exposures, the Chemical Abstracts Services Registry Number, the latest Chemical Abstracts Primary Name and the IUPAC Systematic Name are recorded; other synonyms are given, but the list is not necessarily comprehensive. For biological agents, taxonomy and structure are described, and the degree of variability is given, when applicable.

Information on chemical and physical properties and, in particular, data relevant to identification, occurrence and biological activity are included. For biological agents, mode of replication, life cycle, target cells, persistence and latency, host response and description of nonmalignant disease caused by them are given. A description of technical products of chemicals includes trades names, relevant specifications and available information on composition and impurities. Some of the trade names given may be those of mixtures in which the agent being evaluated is only one of the ingredients.

The purpose of the section on analysis is to give the reader an overview of current methods, with emphasis on those widely used for regulatory purposes. Methods for monitoring human exposure are also given, when available. No critical evaluation or recommendation of any of the methods is meant or implied. The IARC publishes a series of volumes, *Environmental Carcinogens: Methods of Analysis and Exposure Measurement* (IARC, 1978–92), that describe validated methods for analysing a wide variety of chemicals and mixtures. For biological agents, methods of detection and exposure assessment are described, including their sensitivity, specificity and reproducibility.

The dates of first synthesis and of first commercial production of a chemical or mixture are provided; for agents which do not occur naturally, this information may allow a reasonable estimate to be made of the date before which no human exposure to the agent could have occurred. The dates of first reported occurrence of an exposure are also provided. In addition, methods of synthesis used in past and present commercial production and different methods of production which may give rise to different impurities are described.

Data on production, international trade and uses are obtained for representative regions, which usually include Europe, Japan and the USA. It should not, however, be inferred that those areas or nations are necessarily the sole or major sources or users of the agent. Some identified uses may not be current or major applications, and the coverage is not necessarily comprehensive. In the case of drugs, mention of their therapeutic uses does not necessarily represent current practice nor does it imply judgement as to their therapeutic efficacy.

Information on the occurrence of an agent or mixture in the environment is obtained from data derived from the monitoring and surveillance of levels in occupational environments, air, water, soil, foods and animal and human tissues. When available, data on the generation, persistence and bioaccumulation of the agent are also included. In the case of mixtures, industries, occupations or processes, information is given about all agents present. For processes, industries and occupations, a historical description is also given, noting variations in chemical composition, physical properties and levels of occupational exposure with time and place. For biological agents, the epidemiology of infection is described.

Statements concerning regulations and guidelines (e.g., pesticide registrations, maximal levels permitted in foods, occupational exposure limits) are included for some countries as indications of potential exposures, but they may not reflect the most recent situation, since such limits are continuously reviewed and modified. The absence of information on regulatory status for a country should not be taken to imply that that country does not have regulations with regard to the exposure. For biological agents, legislation and control, including vaccines and therapy, are described.

8. STUDIES OF CANCER IN HUMANS

(a) Types of studies considered

Three types of epidemiological studies of cancer contribute to the assessment of carcinogenicity in humans—cohort studies, case–control studies and correlation (or ecological) studies. Rarely, results from randomized trials may be available. Case reports of cancer in humans may also be reviewed.

Cohort and case–control studies relate individual exposures under study to the occurrence of cancer in individuals and provide an estimate of relative risk (ratio of incidence in those exposed to incidence in those not exposed) as the main measure of association.

In correlation studies, the units of investigation are usually whole populations (e.g., in particular geographical areas or at particular times), and cancer frequency is related to a summary measure of the exposure of the population to the agent, mixture or exposure circumstance under study. Because individual exposure is not documented, however, a causal relationship is less easy to infer from correlation studies than from cohort and case–control studies. Case reports generally arise from a suspicion, based on clinical experience, that the concurrence of two events—that is, a particular exposure and occurrence of a cancer—has happened rather more frequently than would be expected by chance. Case reports usually lack complete ascertainment of cases in any population, definition or enumeration of the population at risk and estimation of the expected number of cases in the absence of exposure. The uncertainties surrounding interpretation of case reports and correlation studies make them inadequate, except in rare instances, to form the sole basis for inferring a causal relationship. When taken together with case–control and cohort studies, however, relevant case reports or correlation studies may add materially to the judgement that a causal relationship is present.

Epidemiological studies of benign neoplasms, presumed preneoplastic lesions and other end-points thought to be relevant to cancer are also reviewed by working groups. They may, in some instances, strengthen inferences drawn from studies of cancer itself.

(b) Quality of studies considered

The *Monographs* are not intended to summarize all published studies. Those that are judged to be inadequate or irrelevant to the evaluation are generally omitted. They may be mentioned briefly, particularly when the information is considered to be a useful supplement to that in other reports or when they provide the only data available. Their inclusion does not imply acceptance of the adequacy of the study design or of the analysis and interpretation of the results, and limitations are clearly outlined in square brackets at the end of the study description.

It is necessary to take into account the possible roles of bias, confounding and chance in the interpretation of epidemiological studies. By 'bias' is meant the operation of factors in study design or execution that lead erroneously to a stronger or weaker association than in fact exists between disease and an agent, mixture or exposure circumstance. By 'confounding' is meant a situation in which the relationship with disease is made to appear stronger or to appear weaker than it truly is as a result of an association between the apparent causal factor and another factor that is associated with either an increase or decrease in the incidence of the disease. In evaluating the extent to which these factors have been minimized in an individual study, working groups consider a number of aspects of design and analysis as described in the report of the study. Most of these considerations apply equally to case–control, cohort and correlation studies. Lack of clarity of any of these aspects in the reporting of a study can decrease its credibility and the weight given to it in the final evaluation of the exposure.

Firstly, the study population, disease (or diseases) and exposure should have been well defined by the authors. Cases of disease in the study population should have been identified in a way that was independent of the exposure of interest, and exposure should have been assessed in a way that was not related to disease status.

Secondly, the authors should have taken account in the study design and analysis of other variables that can influence the risk of disease and may have been related to the exposure of interest. Potential confounding by such variables should have been dealt with either in the design of the study, such as by matching, or in the analysis, by statistical adjustment. In cohort studies, comparisons with local rates of disease may be more appropriate than those with national rates. Internal comparisons of disease frequency among individuals at different levels of exposure should also have been made in the study.

Thirdly, the authors should have reported the basic data on which the conclusions are founded, even if sophisticated statistical analyses were employed. At the very least, they should have given the numbers of exposed and unexposed cases and controls in a case–control study and the numbers of cases observed and expected in a cohort study. Further tabulations by time since exposure began and other temporal factors are also important. In a cohort study, data on all cancer sites and all causes of death should have been given, to reveal the possibility of reporting bias. In a case–control study, the effects of investigated factors other than the exposure of interest should have been reported.

Finally, the statistical methods used to obtain estimates of relative risk, absolute rates of cancer, confidence intervals and significance tests, and to adjust for confounding should have been clearly stated by the authors. The methods used should preferably have been the generally accepted techniques that have been refined since the mid-1970s. These methods have been reviewed for case–control studies (Breslow & Day, 1980) and for cohort studies (Breslow & Day, 1987).

(c) Inferences about mechanism of action

Detailed analyses of both relative and absolute risks in relation to temporal variables, such as age at first exposure, time since first exposure, duration of exposure, cumulative exposure and time since exposure ceased, are reviewed and summarized when available. The analysis of temporal relationships can be useful in formulating models of carcinogenesis. In particular, such analyses may suggest whether a carcinogen acts early or late in the process of carcinogenesis, although at best they allow only indirect inferences about the mechanism of action. Special attention is given to measurements of biological markers of carcinogen exposure or action, such as DNA or protein adducts, as well as markers of early steps in the carcinogenic process, such as proto-oncogene mutation, when these are incorporated into epidemiological studies focused on cancer incidence or mortality. Such measurements may allow inferences to be made about putative mechanisms of action (IARC, 1991a; Vainio *et al.*, 1992).

(d) Criteria for causality

After the quality of individual epidemiological studies of cancer has been summarized and assessed, a judgement is made concerning the strength of evidence that the agent, mixture or exposure circumstance in question is carcinogenic for humans. In making their judgement, the Working Group considers several criteria for causality. A strong association (i.e., a large relative risk) is more likely to indicate causality than a weak association, although it is recognized that relative risks of small magnitude do not imply lack of causality and may be important if the disease is common. Associations that are replicated in several studies of the same design or using different epidemiological approaches or under different circumstances of exposure are more likely to represent a causal relationship than isolated observations from single studies. If there are inconsistent results among investigations, possible reasons are sought (such as differences in amount of exposure), and results of studies judged to be of high quality are given more weight than those from studies judged to be methodologically less sound. When suspicion of carcinogenicity arises largely from a single study, these data are not combined with those from later studies in any subsequent reassessment of the strength of the evidence.

If the risk of the disease in question increases with the amount of exposure, this is considered to be a strong indication of causality, although absence of a graded response is not necessarily evidence against a causal relationship. Demonstration of a decline in risk after cessation of or reduction in exposure in individuals or in whole populations also supports a causal interpretation of the findings.

Although a carcinogen may act upon more than one target, the specificity of an association (i.e., an increased occurrence of cancer at one anatomical site or of one morphological type) adds plausibility to a causal relationship, particularly when excess cancer occurrence is limited to one morphological type within the same organ.

Although rarely available, results from randomized trials showing different rates among exposed and unexposed individuals provide particularly strong evidence for causality.

When several epidemiological studies show little or no indication of an association between an exposure and cancer, the judgement may be made that, in the aggregate, they show evidence of lack of carcinogenicity. Such a judgement requires first of all that the studies giving rise to it meet, to a sufficient degree, the standards of design and analysis described above. Specifically, the possibility that bias, confounding or misclassification of exposure or outcome could explain the observed results should be considered and excluded with reasonable certainty. In addition, all studies that are judged to be methodologically sound should be consistent with a relative risk of unity for any observed level of exposure and, when considered together, should provide a pooled estimate of relative risk which is at or near unity and has a narrow confidence interval, due to sufficient population size. Moreover, no individual study nor the pooled results of all the studies should show any consistent tendency for relative risk of cancer to increase with increasing level of exposure. It is important to note that evidence of lack of carcinogenicity obtained in this way from several epidemiological studies can apply only to the type(s) of cancer studied and to dose levels and intervals between first exposure and observation of disease that are the same as or less than those observed in all the studies. Experience with human cancer indicates that, in some cases, the period from first exposure to the development of clinical cancer is seldom less than 20 years; latent periods substantially shorter than 30 years cannot provide evidence for lack of carcinogenicity.

9. STUDIES OF CANCER IN EXPERIMENTAL ANIMALS

All known human carcinogens that have been studied adequately in experimental animals have produced positive results in one or more animal species (Wilbourn *et al.*, 1986; Tomatis *et al.*, 1989). For several agents (aflatoxins, 4-aminobiphenyl, azathioprine, betel quid with tobacco, BCME and CMME (technical grade), chlorambucil, chlornaphazine, ciclosporin, coal-tar pitches, coal-tars, combined oral contraceptives, cyclophosphamide, diethylstilboestrol, melphalan, 8-methoxypsoralen plus UVA, mustard gas, myleran, 2-naphthylamine, nonsteroidal oestrogens, oestrogen replacement therapy/steroidal oestrogens, solar radiation, thiotepa and vinyl chloride), carcinogenicity in experimental animals was established or highly suspected before epidemiological studies confirmed the carcinogenicity in humans (Vainio *et al.*, 1993). Although this association cannot establish that all agents and mixtures that cause cancer in experimental animals also cause cancer in humans, nevertheless, **in the absence of adequate data on humans, it is biologically plausible and prudent to regard agents and mixtures for which there is sufficient evidence (see p. 27) of carcinogenicity in experimental animals as if they presented a carcinogenic risk to humans.** The possibility that a given agent may cause cancer through a species-specific mechanism which does not operate in humans, see p. 28, should also be taken into consideration.

The nature and extent of impurities or contaminants present in the chemical or mixture being evaluated are given when available. Animal strain, sex, numbers per group, age at start of treatment and survival are reported.

Other types of studies summarized include: experiments in which the agent or mixture was administered in conjunction with known carcinogens or factors that modify carcinogenic effects; studies in which the end-point was not cancer but a defined precancerous lesion; and experiments on the carcinogenicity of known metabolites and derivatives.

For experimental studies of mixtures, consideration is given to the possibility of changes in the physicochemical properties of the test substance during collection, storage, extraction, concentration and delivery. Chemical and toxicological interactions of the components of mixtures may result in nonlinear dose–response relationships.

An assessment is made as to the relevance to human exposure of samples tested in experimental animals, which may involve consideration of: (i) physical and chemical characteristics, (ii) constituent substances that indicate the presence of a class of substances, (iii) the results of tests for genetic and related effects, including genetic activity profiles, DNA adduct profiles, proto-oncogene mutation and expression and suppressor gene inactivation. The relevance of results obtained with viral strains analogous to that being evaluated in the monograph must also be considered.

(a) Qualitative aspects

An assessment of carcinogenicity involves several considerations of qualitative importance, including (i) the experimental conditions under which the test was performed, including route and schedule of exposure, species, strain, sex, age, duration of follow-up; (ii) the consistency of the results, for example, across species and target organ(s); (iii) the spectrum of neoplastic response, from preneoplastic lesions and benign tumours to malignant neoplasms; and (iv) the possible role of modifying factors.

As mentioned earlier (p. 15), the *Monographs* are not intended to summarize all published studies. Those studies in experimental animals that are inadequate (e.g., too short a duration, too few animals, poor survival; see below) or are judged irrelevant to the evaluation are generally omitted. Guidelines for conducting adequate long-term carcinogenicity experiments have been outlined (e.g., Montesano *et al.*, 1986).

Considerations of importance to the Working Group in the interpretation and evaluation of a particular study include: (i) how clearly the agent was defined and, in the case of mixtures, how adequately the sample characterization was reported; (ii) whether the dose was adequately monitored, particularly in inhalation experiments; (iii) whether the doses and duration of treatment were appropriate and whether the survival of treated animals was similar to that of controls; (iv) whether there were adequate numbers of animals per group; (v) whether animals of both sexes were used; (vi) whether animals were allocated randomly to groups; (vii) whether the duration of observation was adequate; and (viii) whether the data were adequately reported. If available, recent data on the incidence of specific tumours in historical controls, as well as in concurrent controls, should be taken into account in the evaluation of tumour response.

When benign tumours occur together with and originate from the same cell type in an organ or tissue as malignant tumours in a particular study and appear to represent a stage in the progression to malignancy, it may be valid to combine them in assessing tumour incidence (Huff *et al.*, 1989). The occurrence of lesions presumed to be preneoplastic may in certain instances aid in assessing the biological plausibility of any neoplastic response observed. If an agent or mixture induces only benign neoplasms that appear to be end-points that do not readily undergo transition to malignancy, it should nevertheless be suspected of being a carcinogen and it requires further investigation.

(b) Quantitative aspects

The probability that tumours will occur may depend on the species, sex, strain and age of the animal, the dose of the carcinogen and the route and length of exposure. Evidence of an increased incidence of neoplasms with increased level of exposure strengthens the inference of a causal association between the exposure and the development of neoplasms.

The form of the dose–response relationship can vary widely, depending on the particular agent under study and the target organ. Both DNA damage and increased cell division are important aspects of carcinogenesis, and cell proliferation is a strong determinant of dose–response relationships for some carcinogens (Cohen & Ellwein, 1990). Since many chemicals require metabolic activation before being converted into their reactive intermediates, both metabolic and pharmacokinetic aspects are important in determining the dose–response pattern. Saturation of steps such as absorption, activation, inactivation and elimination may produce nonlinearity in the dose–response relationship, as could saturation of processes such as DNA repair (Hoel *et al.*, 1983; Gart *et al.*, 1986).

(c) Statistical analysis of long-term experiments in animals

Factors considered by the Working Group include the adequacy of the information given for each treatment group: (i) the number of animals studied and the number examined histologically, (ii) the number of animals with a given tumour type and (iii) length of survival. The statistical methods used should be clearly stated and should be the generally accepted techniques refined for this purpose (Peto et al., 1980; Gart et al., 1986). When there is no difference in survival between control and treatment groups, the Working Group usually compares the proportions of animals developing each tumour type in each of the groups. Otherwise, consideration is given as to whether or not appropriate adjustments have been made for differences in survival. These adjustments can include: comparisons of the proportions of tumour-bearing animals among the effective number of animals (alive at the time the first tumour is discovered), in the case where most differences in survival occur before tumours appear; life-table methods, when tumours are visible or when they may be considered 'fatal' because mortality rapidly follows tumour development; and the Mantel-Haenszel test or logistic regression, when occult tumours do not affect the animals' risk of dying but are 'incidental' findings at autopsy.

In practice, classifying tumours as fatal or incidental may be difficult. Several survival-adjusted methods have been developed that do not require this distinction (Gart et al., 1986), although they have not been fully evaluated.

10. OTHER RELEVANT DATA

(a) Absorption, distribution, metabolism and excretion

Concise information is given on absorption, distribution (including placental transfer) and excretion in both humans and experimental animals. Kinetic factors that may affect the dose–response relationship, such as saturation of uptake, protein binding, metabolic activation, detoxification and DNA repair processes, are mentioned. Studies that indicate the metabolic fate of the agent in humans and in experimental animals are summarized briefly, and comparisons of data from humans and animals are made when possible. Comparative information on the relationship between exposure and the dose that reaches the target site may be of particular importance for extrapolation between species.

(b) Toxic effects

Data are given on acute and chronic toxic effects (other than cancer), such as organ toxicity, increased cell proliferation, immunotoxicity and endocrine effects. The presence and toxicological significance of cellular receptors is described.

(c) Reproductive and developmental effects

Effects on reproduction, teratogenicity, fetotoxicity and embryotoxicity are also summarized briefly.

(d) Genetic and related effects

Tests of genetic and related effects are described in view of the relevance of gene mutation and chromosomal damage to carcinogenesis (Vainio et al., 1992).

The adequacy of the reporting of sample characterization is considered and, where necessary, commented upon; with regard to complex mixtures, such comments are similar to those described for animal carcinogenicity tests on p. 21. The available data are interpreted critically by phylogenetic group according to the end-points detected, which may include DNA damage, gene mutation, sister chromatid exchange, micronucleus formation, chromosomal aberrations, aneuploidy and cell transformation. The concentrations employed are given, and mention is made of whether use of an exogenous metabolic system *in vitro* affected the test result. These data are given as listings of test systems, data and references; bar graphs (activity profiles) and corresponding summary tables with detailed information on the preparation of the profiles (Waters *et al.*, 1987) are given in appendices.

Positive results in tests using prokaryotes, lower eukaryotes, plants, insects and cultured mammalian cells suggest that genetic and related effects could occur in mammals. Results from such tests may also give information about the types of genetic effect produced and about the involvement of metabolic activation. Some end-points described are clearly genetic in nature (e.g., gene mutations and chromosomal aberrations), while others are to a greater or lesser degree associated with genetic effects (e.g., unscheduled DNA synthesis). In-vitro tests for tumour-promoting activity and for cell transformation may be sensitive to changes that are not necessarily the result of genetic alterations but that may have specific relevance to the process of carcinogenesis. A critical appraisal of these tests has been published (Montesano *et al.*, 1986).

Genetic or other activity manifest in experimental mammals and humans is regarded as being of greater relevance than that in other organisms. The demonstration that an agent or mixture can induce gene and chromosomal mutations in whole mammals indicates that it may have carcinogenic activity, although this activity may not be detectably expressed in any or all species. Relative potency in tests for mutagenicity and related effects is not a reliable indicator of carcinogenic potency. Negative results in tests for mutagenicity in selected tissues from animals treated *in vivo* provide less weight, partly because they do not exclude the possibility of an effect in tissues other than those examined. Moreover, negative results in short-term tests with genetic end-points cannot be considered to provide evidence to rule out carcinogenicity of agents or mixtures that act through other mechanisms (e.g., receptor-mediated effects, cellular toxicity with regenerative proliferation, peroxisome proliferation) (Vainio *et al.*, 1992). Factors that may lead to misleading results in short-term tests have been discussed in detail elsewhere (Montesano *et al.*, 1986).

When available, data relevant to mechanisms of carcinogenesis that do not involve structural changes at the level of the gene are also described.

The adequacy of epidemiological studies of reproductive outcome and genetic and related effects in humans is evaluated by the same criteria as are applied to epidemiological studies of cancer.

(e)   Structure–activity considerations

This section describes structure–activity relationships that may be relevant to an evaluation of the carcinogenicity of an agent.

11. SUMMARY OF DATA REPORTED

In this section, the relevant epidemiological and experimental data are summarized. Only reports, other than in abstract form, that meet the criteria outlined on p. 15 are considered for evaluating carcinogenicity. Inadequate studies are generally not summarized: such studies are usually identified by a square-bracketed comment in the preceding text.

(a) *Exposures*

Human exposure is summarized on the basis of elements such as production, use, occurrence in the environment and determinations in human tissues and body fluids. Quantitative data are given when available.

(b) *Carcinogenicity in humans*

Results of epidemiological studies that are considered to be pertinent to an assessment of human carcinogenicity are summarized. When relevant, case reports and correlation studies are also summarized.

(c) *Carcinogenicity in experimental animals*

Data relevant to an evaluation of carcinogenicity in animals are summarized. For each animal species and route of administration, it is stated whether an increased incidence of neoplasms or preneoplastic lesions was observed, and the tumour sites are indicated. If the agent or mixture produced tumours after prenatal exposure or in single-dose experiments, this is also indicated. Negative findings are also summarized. Dose–response and other quantitative data may be given when available.

(d) *Other data relevant to an evaluation of carcinogenicity and its mechanisms*

Data on biological effects in humans that are of particular relevance are summarized. These may include toxicological, kinetic and metabolic considerations and evidence of DNA binding, persistence of DNA lesions or genetic damage in exposed humans. Toxicological information, such as that on cytotoxicity and regeneration, receptor binding and hormonal and immunological effects, and data on kinetics and metabolism in experimental animals are given when considered relevant to the possible mechanism of the carcinogenic action of the agent. The results of tests for genetic and related effects are summarized for whole mammals, cultured mammalian cells and nonmammalian systems.

When available, comparisons of such data for humans and for animals, and particularly animals that have developed cancer, are described.

Structure–activity relationships are mentioned when relevant.

For the agent, mixture or exposure circumstance being evaluated, the available data on end-points or other phenomena relevant to mechanisms of carcinogenesis from studies in humans, experimental animals and tissue and cell test systems are summarized within one or more of the following descriptive dimensions:

(i) Evidence of genotoxicity (i.e., structural changes at the level of the gene): for example, structure–activity considerations, adduct formation, mutagenicity (effect on specific genes), chromosomal mutation/aneuploidy

(ii) Evidence of effects on the expression of relevant genes (i.e., functional changes at the intracellular level): for example, alterations to the structure or quantity of the product of a proto-oncogene or tumour suppressor gene, alterations to metabolic activation/-inactivation/DNA repair

(iii) Evidence of relevant effects on cell behaviour (i.e., morphological or behavioural changes at the cellular or tissue level): for example, induction of mitogenesis, compensatory cell proliferation, preneoplasia and hyperplasia, survival of premalignant or malignant cells (immortalization, immunosuppression), effects on metastatic potential

(iv)   Evidence from dose and time relationships of carcinogenic effects and interactions between agents: for example, early/late stage, as inferred from epidemiological studies; initiation/promotion/progression/malignant conversion, as defined in animal carcino-genicity experiments; toxicokinetics

These dimensions are not mutually exclusive, and an agent may fall within more than one of them. Thus, for example, the action of an agent on the expression of relevant genes could be summarized under both the first and second dimension, even if it were known with reasonable certainty that those effects resulted from genotoxicity.

12. EVALUATION

Evaluations of the strength of the evidence for carcinogenicity arising from human and experimental animal data are made, using standard terms.

It is recognized that the criteria for these evaluations, described below, cannot encompass all of the factors that may be relevant to an evaluation of carcinogenicity. In considering all of the relevant data, the Working Group may assign the agent, mixture or exposure circumstance to a higher or lower category than a strict interpretation of these criteria would indicate.

(a)   *Degrees of evidence for carcinogenicity in humans and in experimental animals and supporting evidence*

These categories refer only to the strength of the evidence that an exposure is carcinogenic and not to the extent of its carcinogenic activity (potency) nor to the mechanisms involved. A classification may change as new information becomes available.

An evaluation of degree of evidence, whether for a single agent or a mixture, is limited to the materials tested, as defined physically, chemically or biologically. When the agents evaluated are considered by the Working Group to be sufficiently closely related, they may be grouped together for the purpose of a single evaluation of degree of evidence.

(i)   *Carcinogenicity in humans*

The applicability of an evaluation of the carcinogenicity of a mixture, process, occupation or industry on the basis of evidence from epidemiological studies depends on the variability over time and place of the mixtures, processes, occupations and industries. The Working Group seeks to identify the specific exposure, process or activity which is considered most likely to be responsible for any excess risk. The evaluation is focused as narrowly as the available data on exposure and other aspects permit.

The evidence relevant to carcinogenicity from studies in humans is classified into one of the following categories:

Sufficient evidence of carcinogenicity: The Working Group considers that a causal relationship has been established between exposure to the agent, mixture or exposure circumstance and human cancer. That is, a positive relationship has been observed between the exposure and cancer in studies in which chance, bias and confounding could be ruled out with reasonable confidence.

Limited evidence of carcinogenicity: A positive association has been observed between exposure to the agent, mixture or exposure circumstance and cancer for which a causal interpretation is considered by the Working Group to be credible, but chance, bias or confounding could not be ruled out with reasonable confidence.

Inadequate evidence of carcinogenicity: The available studies are of insufficient quality, consistency or statistical power to permit a conclusion regarding the presence or absence of a causal association, or no data on cancer in humans are available.

Evidence suggesting lack of carcinogenicity: There are several adequate studies covering the full range of levels of exposure that human beings are known to encounter, which are mutually consistent in not showing a positive association between exposure to the agent, mixture or exposure circumstance and any studied cancer at any observed level of exposure. A conclusion of 'evidence suggesting lack of carcinogenicity' is inevitably limited to the cancer sites, conditions and levels of exposure and length of observation covered by the available studies. In addition, the possibility of a very small risk at the levels of exposure studied can never be excluded.

In some instances, the above categories may be used to classify the degree of evidence related to carcinogenicity in specific organs or tissues.

(ii)   *Carcinogenicity in experimental animals*

The evidence relevant to carcinogenicity in experimental animals is classified into one of the following categories:

Sufficient evidence of carcinogenicity: The Working Group considers that a causal relationship has been established between the agent or mixture and an increased incidence of malignant neoplasms or of an appropriate combination of benign and malignant neoplasms in (a) two or more species of animals or (b) in two or more independent studies in one species carried out at different times or in different laboratories or under different protocols.

Exceptionally, a single study in one species might be considered to provide sufficient evidence of carcinogenicity when malignant neoplasms occur to an unusual degree with regard to incidence, site, type of tumour or age at onset.

Limited evidence of carcinogenicity: The data suggest a carcinogenic effect but are limited for making a definitive evaluation because, e.g., (a) the evidence of carcinogenicity is restricted to a single experiment; or (b) there are unresolved questions regarding the adequacy of the design, conduct or interpretation of the study; or (c) the agent or mixture increases the incidence only of benign neoplasms or lesions of uncertain neoplastic potential, or of certain neoplasms which may occur spontaneously in high incidences in certain strains.

Inadequate evidence of carcinogenicity: The studies cannot be interpreted as showing either the presence or absence of a carcinogenic effect because of major qualitative or quantitative limitations, or no data on cancer in experimental animals are available.

Evidence suggesting lack of carcinogenicity: Adequate studies involving at least two species are available which show that, within the limits of the tests used, the agent or mixture is not carcinogenic. A conclusion of evidence suggesting lack of carcinogenicity is inevitably limited to the species, tumour sites and levels of exposure studied.

(b)   *Other data relevant to the evaluation of carcinogenicity*

Other evidence judged to be relevant to an evaluation of carcinogenicity and of sufficient importance to affect the overall evaluation is then described. This may include data on preneoplastic lesions, tumour pathology, genetic and related effects, structure–activity relationships, metabolism and pharmacokinetics, and physicochemical parameters.

Data relevant to mechanisms of the carcinogenic action are also evaluated. The strength of the evidence that any carcinogenic effect observed is due to a particular mechanism is assessed, using terms such as weak, moderate or strong. Then, the Working Group assesses if that particular mechanism is likely to be operative in humans. The strongest indications that a particular mechanism operates in humans come from data on humans or biological specimens obtained from exposed humans. The data may be considered to be especially relevant if they show that the agent in question has caused changes in exposed humans that are on the causal pathway to carcinogenesis. Such data may, however, never become available, because it is at least conceivable that certain compounds may be kept from human use solely on the basis of evidence of their toxicity and/or carcinogenicity in experimental systems.

For complex exposures, including occupational and industrial exposures, chemical composition and the potential contribution of carcinogens known to be present are considered by the Working Group in its overall evaluation of human carcinogenicity. The Working Group also determines the extent to which the materials tested in experimental systems are related to those to which humans are exposed.

(c) Overall evaluation

Finally, the body of evidence is considered as a whole, in order to reach an overall evaluation of the carcinogenicity to humans of an agent, mixture or circumstance of exposure.

An evaluation may be made for a group of chemical compounds that have been evaluated by the Working Group. In addition, when supporting data indicate that other, related compounds for which there is no direct evidence of capacity to induce cancer in humans or in animals may also be carcinogenic, a statement describing the rationale for this conclusion is added to the evaluation narrative; an additional evaluation may be made for this broader group of compounds if the strength of the evidence warrants it.

The agent, mixture or exposure circumstance is described according to the wording of one of the following categories, and the designated group is given. The categorization of an agent, mixture or exposure circumstance is a matter of scientific judgement, reflecting the strength of the evidence derived from studies in humans and in experimental animals and from other relevant data.

Group 1—The agent (mixture) is carcinogenic to humans.
The exposure circumstance entails exposures that are carcinogenic to humans.

This category is used when there is *sufficient evidence* of carcinogenicity in humans. Exceptionally, an agent (mixture) may be placed in this category when evidence in humans is less than sufficient but there is *sufficient evidence* of carcinogenicity in experimental animals and strong evidence in exposed humans that the agent (mixture) acts through a relevant mechanism of carcinogenicity.

Group 2

This category includes agents, mixtures and exposure circumstances for which, at one extreme, the degree of evidence of carcinogenicity in humans is almost sufficient, as well as those for which, at the other extreme, there are no human data but for which there is evidence of carcinogenicity in experimental animals. Agents, mixtures and exposure circumstances are assigned to either group 2A (probably carcinogenic to humans) or group 2B (possibly carcinogenic to humans) on the basis of epidemiological and experimental evidence of carcinogenicity and other relevant data.

Group 2A—The agent (mixture) is probably carcinogenic to humans.
The exposure circumstance entails exposures that are probably carcinogenic to humans.

This category is used when there is *limited evidence* of carcinogenicity in humans and *sufficient evidence* of carcinogenicity in experimental animals. In some cases, an agent (mixture) may be classified in this category when there is *inadequate evidence* of carcinogenicity in humans and *sufficient evidence* of carcinogenicity in experimental animals and strong evidence that the carcinogenesis is mediated by a mechanism that also operates in humans. Exceptionally, an agent, mixture or exposure circumstance may be classified in this category solely on the basis of *limited evidence* of carcinogenicity in humans.

Group 2B—The agent (mixture) is possibly carcinogenic to humans.
The exposure circumstance entails exposures that are possibly carcinogenic to humans.

This category is used for agents, mixtures and exposure circumstances for which there is *limited evidence* of carcinogenicity in humans and less than *sufficient evidence* of carcinogenicity in experimental animals. It may also be used when there is *inadequate evidence* of carcinogenicity in humans but there is *sufficient evidence* of carcinogenicity in experimental animals. In some instances, an agent, mixture or exposure circumstance for which there is *inadequate evidence* of carcinogenicity in humans but *limited evidence* of carcinogenicity in experimental animals together with supporting evidence from other relevant data may be placed in this group.

Group 3—The agent (mixture or exposure circumstance) is not classifiable as to its carcinogenicity to humans.

This category is used most commonly for agents, mixtures and exposure circumstances for which the evidence of carcinogenicity is inadequate in humans and inadequate or limited in experimental animals.

Exceptionally, agents (mixtures) for which the evidence of carcinogenicity is inadequate in humans but sufficient in experimental animals may be placed in this category when there is strong evidence that the mechanism of carcinogenicity in experimental animals does not operate in humans.

Agents, mixtures and exposure circumstances that do not fall into any other group are also placed in this category.

Group 4—The agent (mixture) is probably not carcinogenic to humans.

This category is used for agents or mixtures for which there is *evidence suggesting lack of carcinogenicity* in humans and in experimental animals. In some instances, agents or mixtures for which there is *inadequate evidence* of carcinogenicity in humans but *evidence suggesting lack of carcinogenicity* in experimental animals, consistently and strongly supported by a broad range of other relevant data, may be classified in this group.

References

Breslow, N.E. & Day, N.E. (1980) *Statistical Methods in Cancer Research*, Vol. 1, *The Analysis of Case-control Studies* (IARC Scientific Publications No. 32), Lyon, IARC

Breslow, N.E. & Day, N.E. (1987) *Statistical Methods in Cancer Research*, Vol. 2, *The Design and Analysis of Cohort Studies* (IARC Scientific Publications No. 82), Lyon, IARC

Cohen, S.M. & Ellwein, L.B. (1990) Cell proliferation in carcinogenesis. *Science, 249*, 1007–1011

Gart, J.J., Krewski, D., Lee, P.N., Tarone, R.E. & Wahrendorf, J. (1986) *Statistical Methods in Cancer Research*, Vol. 3, *The Design and Analysis of Long-term Animal Experiments* (IARC Scientific Publications No. 79), Lyon, IARC

Hoel, D.G., Kaplan, N.L. & Anderson, M.W. (1983) Implication of nonlinear kinetics on risk estimation in carcinogenesis. *Science, 219*, 1032–1037

Huff, J.E., Eustis, S.L. & Haseman, J.K. (1989) Occurrence and relevance of chemically induced benign neoplasms in long-term carcinogenicity studies. *Cancer Metastasis Rev., 8*, 1–21

IARC (1973–1992) *Information Bulletin on the Survey of Chemicals Being Tested for Carcinogenicity/- Directory of Agents Being Tested for Carcinogenicity*, Numbers 1–15, Lyon

Number 1 (1973)	52 pages
Number 2 (1973)	77 pages
Number 3 (1974)	67 pages
Number 4 (1974)	97 pages
Number 5 (1975)	88 pages
Number 6 (1976)	360 pages
Number 7 (1978)	460 pages
Number 8 (1979)	604 pages
Number 9 (1981)	294 pages
Number 10 (1983)	326 pages
Number 11 (1984)	370 pages
Number 12 (1986)	385 pages
Number 13 (1988)	404 pages
Number 14 (1990)	369 pages
Number 15 (1992)	317 pages

IARC (1976–1992)

  Directory of On-going Research in Cancer Epidemiology 1976. Edited by C.S. Muir & G. Wagner, Lyon

  Directory of On-going Research in Cancer Epidemiology 1977 (IARC Scientific Publications No. 17). Edited by C.S. Muir & G. Wagner, Lyon

  Directory of On-going Research in Cancer Epidemiology 1978 (IARC Scientific Publications No. 26). Edited by C.S. Muir & G. Wagner, Lyon

  Directory of On-going Research in Cancer Epidemiology 1979 (IARC Scientific Publications No. 28). Edited by C.S. Muir & G. Wagner, Lyon

  Directory of On-going Research in Cancer Epidemiology 1980 (IARC Scientific Publications No. 35). Edited by C.S. Muir & G. Wagner, Lyon

Directory of On-going Research in Cancer Epidemiology 1981 (IARC Scientific Publications No. 38). Edited by C.S. Muir & G. Wagner, Lyon

Directory of On-going Research in Cancer Epidemiology 1982 (IARC Scientific Publications No. 46). Edited by C.S. Muir & G. Wagner, Lyon

Directory of On-going Research in Cancer Epidemiology 1983 (IARC Scientific Publications No. 50). Edited by C.S. Muir & G. Wagner, Lyon

Directory of On-going Research in Cancer Epidemiology 1984 (IARC Scientific Publications No. 62). Edited by C.S. Muir & G. Wagner, Lyon

Directory of On-going Research in Cancer Epidemiology 1985 (IARC Scientific Publications No. 69). Edited by C.S. Muir & G. Wagner, Lyon

Directory of On-going Research in Cancer Epidemiology 1986 (IARC Scientific Publications No. 80). Edited by C.S. Muir & G. Wagner, Lyon

Directory of On-going Research in Cancer Epidemiology 1987 (IARC Scientific Publications No. 86). Edited by D.M. Parkin & J. Wahrendorf, Lyon

Directory of On-going Research in Cancer Epidemiology 1988 (IARC Scientific Publications No. 93). Edited by M. Coleman & J. Wahrendorf, Lyon

Directory of On-going Research in Cancer Epidemiology 1989/90 (IARC Scientific Publications No. 101). Edited by M. Coleman & J. Wahrendorf, Lyon

Directory of On-going Research in Cancer Epidemiology 1991 (IARC Scientific Publications No. 110). Edited by M. Coleman & J. Wahrendorf, Lyon

Directory of On-going Research in Cancer Epidemiology 1992 (IARC Scientific Publications No. 117). Edited by M. Coleman, J. Wahrendorf & E. Demaret, Lyon

IARC (1977) *IARC Monographs Programme on the Evaluation of the Carcinogenic Risk of Chemicals to Humans. Preamble* (IARC intern. tech. Rep. No. 77/002), Lyon

IARC (1978) *Chemicals with* Sufficient Evidence *of Carcinogenicity in Experimental Animals*—IARC Monographs *Volumes 1–17* (IARC intern. tech. Rep. No. 78/003), Lyon

IARC (1978–1993) *Environmental Carcinogens. Methods of Analysis and Exposure Measurement*:

Vol. 1. *Analysis of Volatile Nitrosamines in Food* (IARC Scientific Publications No. 18). Edited by R. Preussmann, M. Castegnaro, E.A. Walker & A.E. Wasserman (1978)

Vol. 2. *Methods for the Measurement of Vinyl Chloride in Poly(vinyl chloride), Air, Water and Foodstuffs* (IARC Scientific Publications No. 22). Edited by D.C.M. Squirrell & W. Thain (1978)

Vol. 3. *Analysis of Polycyclic Aromatic Hydrocarbons in Environmental Samples* (IARC Scientific Publications No. 29). Edited by M. Castegnaro, P. Bogovski, H. Kunte & E.A. Walker (1979)

Vol. 4. *Some Aromatic Amines and Azo Dyes in the General and Industrial Environment* (IARC Scientific Publications No. 40). Edited by L. Fishbein, M. Castegnaro, I.K. O'Neill & H. Bartsch (1981)

Vol. 5. *Some Mycotoxins* (IARC Scientific Publications No. 44). Edited by L. Stoloff, M. Castegnaro, P. Scott, I.K. O'Neill & H. Bartsch (1983)

Vol. 6. N-*Nitroso Compounds* (IARC Scientific Publications No. 45). Edited by R. Preussmann, I.K. O'Neill, G. Eisenbrand, B. Spiegelhalder & H. Bartsch (1983)

Vol. 7. *Some Volatile Halogenated Hydrocarbons* (IARC Scientific Publications No. 68). Edited by L. Fishbein & I.K. O'Neill (1985)

Vol. 8. *Some Metals: As, Be, Cd, Cr, Ni, Pb, Se, Zn* (IARC Scientific Publications No. 71). Edited by I.K. O'Neill, P. Schuller & L. Fishbein (1986)

Vol. 9. *Passive Smoking* (IARC Scientific Publications No. 81). Edited by I.K. O'Neill, K.D. Brunnemann, B. Dodet & D. Hoffmann (1987)

Vol. 10. *Benzene and Alkylated Benzenes* (IARC Scientific Publications No. 85). Edited by L. Fishbein & I.K. O'Neill (1988)

Vol. 11. *Polychlorinated Dioxins and Dibenzofurans* (IARC Scientific Publications No. 108). Edited by C. Rappe, H.R. Buser, B. Dodet & I.K. O'Neill (1991)

Vol. 12. *Indoor Air* (IARC Scientific Publications No. 109). Edited by B. Seifert, H. van de Wiel, B. Dodet & I.K. O'Neill (1993)

IARC (1979) *Criteria to Select Chemicals for* IARC Monographs (IARC intern. tech. Rep. No. 79/003), Lyon

IARC (1982) *IARC Monographs on the Evaluation of the Carcinogenic Risk of Chemicals to Humans, Supplement 4, Chemicals, Industrial Processes and Industries Associated with Cancer in Humans (IARC Monographs, Volumes 1 to 29)*, Lyon

IARC (1983) *Approaches to Classifying Chemical Carcinogens According to Mechanism of Action* (IARC intern. tech. Rep. No. 83/001), Lyon

IARC (1984) *Chemicals and Exposures to Complex Mixtures Recommended for Evaluation in IARC Monographs and Chemicals and Complex Mixtures Recommended for Long-term Carcinogenicity Testing* (IARC intern. tech. Rep. No. 84/002), Lyon

IARC (1987a) *IARC Monographs on the Evaluation of Carcinogenic Risks to Humans, Supplement 6, Genetic and Related Effects: An Updating of Selected* IARC Monographs *from Volumes 1 to 42*, Lyon

IARC (1987b) *IARC Monographs on the Evaluation of Carcinogenic Risks to Humans, Supplement 7, Overall Evaluations of Carcinogenicity: An Updating of* IARC Monographs *Volumes 1 to 42*, Lyon

IARC (1988) *Report of an IARC Working Group to Review the Approaches and Processes Used to Evaluate the Carcinogenicity of Mixtures and Groups of Chemicals* (IARC intern. tech. Rep. No. 88/002), Lyon

IARC (1989) *Chemicals, Groups of Chemicals, Mixtures and Exposure Circumstances to be Evaluated in Future IARC Monographs, Report of an ad hoc Working Group* (IARC intern. tech. Rep. No. 89/004), Lyon

IARC (1991a) *A Consensus Report of an* IARC Monographs *Working Group on the Use of Mechanims of Carcinogenesis in Risk Identification* (IARC intern. tech. Rep. No. 91/002), Lyon

IARC (1991b) *Report of an Ad-hoc* IARC Monographs *Advisory Group on Viruses and Other Biological Agents Such as Parasites* (IARC intern. tech. Rep. No. 91/001), Lyon

Montesano, R., Bartsch, H., Vainio, H., Wilbourn, J. & Yamasaki, H., eds (1986) *Long-term and Short-term Assays for Carcinogenesis—A Critical Appraisal* (IARC Scientific Publications No. 83), Lyon, IARC

Peto, R., Pike, M.C., Day, N.E., Gray, R.G., Lee, P.N., Parish, S., Peto, J., Richards, S. & Wahrendorf, J. (1980) Guidelines for simple, sensitive significance tests for carcinogenic effects in long-term animal experiments. In: *IARC Monographs on the Evaluation of the Carcinogenic Risk of Chemicals to Humans, Supplement 2, Long-term and Short-term Screening Assays for Carcinogens: A Critical Appraisal*, Lyon, pp. 311–426

Tomatis, L., Aitio, A., Wilbourn, J. & Shuker, L. (1989) Human carcinogens so far identified. *Jpn. J. Cancer Res., 80*, 795–807

Vainio, H., Magee, P., McGregor, D. & McMichael, A., eds (1992) *Mechanisms of Carcinogenesis in Risk Identification* (IARC Scientific Publications No. 116), Lyon, IARC

Vainio, H., Wilbourn, J. & Tomatis, L. (1993) Identification of environmental carcinogens: the first step in risk assessment. In: Mehlman, M.A. & Upton, A., eds, *The Identification and Control of Environmental and Occupational Diseases*, Princeton, Princeton Scientific Publishing Company (in press)

Waters, M.D., Stack, H.F., Brady, A.L., Lohman, P.H.M., Haroun, L. & Vainio, H. (1987) Appendix 1. Activity profiles for genetic and related tests. In: *IARC Monographs on the Evaluation of Carcinogenic Risks to Humans*, Suppl. 6, *Genetic and Related Effects: An Updating of Selected IARC Monographs from Volumes 1 to 42*, Lyon, IARC, pp. 687–696

Wilbourn, J., Haroun, L., Heseltine, E., Kaldor, J., Partensky, C. & Vainio, H. (1986) Response of experimental animals to human carcinogens: an analysis based upon the IARC Monographs Programme. *Carcinogenesis*, 7, 1853–1863

GENERAL REMARKS

This fifty-seventh volume of *IARC Monographs* contains 18 monographs in which the carcinogenicity of 17 chemicals is evaluated. The Working Group prepared a monograph on occupational exposure of hairdressers and barbers and the exposure of users of hair colourants. They also considered both nitro aromatic amines used in hair colouring formulations and benzidine congener-derived azo dyes used as industrial colourants. Four aromatic amines, three of which are used in dyestuff manufacture and have been found as pollutants in the general environment, are also included; the fourth is 4,4'-methylene bis(2-chloroaniline) (MOCA), used principally as a curing agent in certain castable poly-urethane products. Previous monographs on 1,4-diamino-2-nitrobenzene (IARC, 1978a), D&C Red No. 9 (IARC, 1975), magenta (IARC, 1974a, 1987a) and MOCA (IARC, 1974b, 1987b) were updated, because new data had become available. In 1982, a working group at IARC surveyed the epidemiological evidence relevant to hair dyes and cancer (IARC, 1982a) and included studies of hairdressers. Since that time, new epidemiological studies have become available, and a monograph was prepared.

The Group noted the lack of quantitative and detailed qualitative information on the potential exposures of hairdressers and barbers and of users of particular hair colouring products. Those groups are potentially exposed to many chemical products (estimated to be over 5000), both during hair treatments, such as shampooing, conditioning, styling and waving, and in the use of skin and nail products. The activities probably include frequent exposures to volatile solvents, propellants, formaldehyde (see IARC, 1982b), methacrylates (see IARC, 1979) and traces of nitrosamines (see IARC, 1978b). The composition of many of the products used by hairdressers has changed gradually with time. For example, some ingredients have been dropped from hair dyes for a variety of reasons, including regulatory activity, technical deficiencies and availability. New materials have been introduced to maintain the range of colours. Examples of this evolution are the declining use of 2-amino-4-nitrophenol and 2-amino-5-nitrophenol and the introduction of their *O*- and *N*-hydroxy-alkyl derivatives and certain isomers of the parent compounds.

As has been noted in previous *Monographs*, the present Working Group recognized the importance of data on the purity of the chemicals that were tested in carcinogenicity experiments in animals and in mutagenicity tests but were faced with the fact that many of the compounds considered were of technical grades, varying in purity from relatively high (> 95%) to indeterminate: Magenta, for example, is a mixture of various proportions of three or more components. The chemical analyses that were reported were often limited to identification of the major component of a dye mixture; minor contaminants were usually not addressed. Commercially available chemicals were often used as such, and no attempt was made to purify the compounds further. That the use of low-purity chemicals may lead to erroneous conclusions about the principal component is an obvious problem, which is commented upon in various parts of this volume.

Studies of experimental animals treated with commercially available hair dyes and laboratory mixtures of hair dyes were also considered. Because of the low levels of individual dyes in the mixtures, however, the results could not be used to evaluate the individual components. Furthermore, the lack of toxicity of the doses used in those studies made them inappropriate for evaluating the systemic toxicity or systemic carcinogenicity of the formulations.

Notes on the metabolism of aromatic amines and azo dyes

In order to be toxic, genotoxic or carcinogenic, aromatic amines usually require metabolic activation. The potential risk posed by structurally related compounds depends largely on their metabolic fate in the test sytem used and on the reactivity of the ultimate carcinogenic reactants. The Working Group noted the absence of pertinent data on the metabolism of a number of the compounds considered. Their metabolic activation and the subsequent formation of reactive metabolites capable of reacting with cellular macromolecules (e.g., nucleic acids and proteins) have not yet been adequately investigated.

Although specific information was not available on the absorption, distribution, metabolism and excretion of many of the aromatic amines in this volume, absorption may occur through the respiratory and gastrointestinal tracts and through the skin of humans. Aromatic amines and amides are readily metabolized enzymatically by oxidation of the ring carbon or of exocyclic nitrogen atoms in both experimental animals and in humans. The C-hydroxy metabolites are conjugated with glucuronide or sulfate and excreted in the urine. N-Oxidation is a necessary step in the formation of reactive intermediates that can form adducts with nucleic acid bases—mainly guanine and adenine.

Three of the hair dyes were studied within the US National Toxicology Program; these are HC Blue No. 1 (US National Toxicology Program, 1985a), HC Blue No. 2 (US National Toxicology Program, 1985b) and HC Red No. 3 (US National Toxicology Program, 1986), which were chosen because they are all derivatives of 1,4-diamino-2-nitrobenzene (2-nitro-*para*-phenylenediamine) (US National Cancer Institute, 1979) and structurally closely related. The N-hydroxyethyl groups on the nitrogens in positions 1 and 4 in HC Blue No. 2 may favour conjugation and urinary excretion, whereas the N-CH_3 group in position 4 of HC Blue No. 1 may favour N-oxidation and/or N-demethylation. In HC Red No. 3, the primary amino group in position 4 may undergo acetylation. These differences may affect the toxicological properties of the compounds. Comparisons of the results of experiments with HC Red No. 3 with those of the blue dyes are imbalanced, however, by the fact that the blue dyes were given in the diet but HC Red No. 3 was found to be unstable when mixed with feed and was administered by gavage in corn oil.

The route of administration of the dyes may have influenced the results of the studies. When they are administered orally, the dyes are exposed to the bacterial flora of the gastrointestinal tract and, since they are all nitro compounds, could undergo nitroreduction by the anaerobic flora, resulting in the formatiom of aromatic amines that might be absorbed and then subjected to N-acetylation and N-oxidation in the liver. HC Blue No. 1, for example, was not mutagenic *in vivo* in mice in the micronucleus test, in which compounds are administered by intraperitoneal injection. That route of administration limits the amount of chemical available for reduction to an aromatic amine by the intestinal flora, a process which may be more efficient than that occurring at other sites, such as the liver.

The industrial dyes CI Acid Red 114 (US National Toxicology Program, 1991), a 3,3′-dimethylbenzidine-derived dye, and CI Direct Blue 15 (US National Toxicology Program, 1992), which is a 3,3′-dimethoxybenzidine-derived dye, are among the five chemicals that were selected for studies of toxicity and carcinogenicity as part of the US National Toxicology Program's Benzidine Dye Initiative, designed to evaluate representative benzidine congeners, benzidine congener-derived dyes and benzidine-derived dyes. The compounds were selected for consideration in this volume of *Monographs* because of the potential for human exposure during the production of bis-azobiphenyl dyes and because benzidine (see IARC, 1972a, 1987c), benzidine-based dyes (see IARC, 1987d) and the benzidine congeners 3,3′-dimethylbenzidine (*ortho*-tolidine) (see IARC, 1972b) and 3,3′-dimethoxybenzidine (see IARC, 1974c, 1987e) are known carcinogens. CI Direct Blue 218 was initially considered by the Working Group, but no monograph was included because of lack of data.

The benzidine congener-based dyes are metabolized to their parent congeners or to their *N*-acetyl derivatives and excreted in the urine. Studies with benzidine congener-based dyes have shown that the ultimate reactive metabolite is an activated form of benzidine congener produced *via* azo reduction. Reductive cleavage of the benzidine congener azo dyes is thought to occur primarily by bacterial action in the intestinal tract (Cerniglia *et al.*, 1982; Bos *et al.*, 1986). Following reductive cleavage, the less polar metabolites are subject to intestinal absorption and further metabolism in the liver. After dogs and rats had been exposed to CI Acid Red 114, 3,3′-dimethylbenzidine was found in their urine (Lynn *et al.*, 1980). The US National Institute for Occupational Safety and Health (1981) reported the presence of 3,3′-dimethylbenzidine in the urine of workers employed in a dye manufacturing plant, who had been in contact with 3,3′-dimethylbenzidine-based dyes but not with 3,3′-dimethylbenzidine itself.

The sequence of benzidine metabolism proceeds along the general known pathways for aromatic amines; it begins with *N*-acetylation, followed by *N*-oxidation to form *N*′-hydroxy-*N*-acetylbenzidine, which can be further activated by *O*-esterification, resulting in electrophilic intermediates that bind to DNA, RNA and proteins (Beland & Kadlubar, 1990).

Postulated association between erythrocytic toxicity and splenic sarcomas in rats

Two aromatic amines and one azo dye considered in this volume were associated with the induction of splenic sarcomas in rats. For several years, it has been known that splenic sarcoma, a rare spontaneous neoplasm, occurs in rats treated with aniline and aniline-related aromatic amines. Since these chemical agents produce haemolytic anaemia with methaemoglobinaemia, a causal relationship has been proposed between the haematotoxicity and the ultimate appearance of splenic sarcomas. Inflammatory fibrosis in the red pulp and capsule occurs prior to the development of sarcomas, and the sarcomas are frequently seen to arise within areas of splenic fibrosis. While several morphological variants of sarcomas have been documented, most of the splenic tumours are well-differentiated fibrosarcomas. A proposed explanation for the pathogenesis of splenic sarcomas is that enhanced splenic haemosiderosis or splenic vascular congestion and haemorrhage promotes a cascade of events leading to the development of sarcoma. No time-course or mechanistic studies have been reported formally, and the definitive pathogenesis of these chemically induced splenic sarcomas remains unknown. The observed non-neoplastic and neoplastic splenic changes are typically dose-related, and female rats are more resistant than males, despite a similar degree of induced methaemoglobinaemia. Fischer 344 rats are more sensitive than other strains or stocks, and mice are relatively resistant to the development of splenic sarcomas. Furthermore, many of the chemicals that have been shown to produce sarcomas in the spleen of male Fischer 344 rats have also been shown to produce tumours in other organs, probably by other mechanisms (Ward *et al.*, 1980; Goodman *et al.*, 1984; Weinberger *et al.*, 1985; Bus & Popp, 1987; Chhabra *et al.*, 1990; Stefanski *et al.*, 1990; Chhabra *et al.*, 1991).

While the induction of splenic sarcomas by aniline and aniline-related aromatic amines may be a consequence of erythrocytic toxicity and may depend upon the strain of rat employed, this end-point is nevertheless considered to be a valid indicator of carcinogenic potential.

References

Beland, F.A. & Kadlubar, F.F. (1990) Metabolic activation and DNA adducts of aromatic amines. In: Cooper, C.S. & Grover, P.L., eds, *Chemical Carcinogenesis and Mutagenesis I*, Berlin, Springer Verlag, pp. 267–325

Bos, R.P., van der Krieken, W., Smeijsters, L., Koopman, J.P., de Jonge, H.R., Theuws, J.L.G. & Henderson, P.T. (1986) Internal exposure of rats to benzidine derived from orally administered benzidine-based dyes after intestinal azo reduction. *Toxicology*, **40**, 207–213

Bus, J.S. & Popp, J.A. (1987) Perspectives on the mechanism of action of the splenic toxicity of aniline and structurally-related compounds. *Food Chem. Toxicol.*, **25**, 619–626

Cerniglia, C.E., Freeman, J.P., Franklin, W. & Pack, L.D. (1982) Metabolism of azo dyes derived from benzidine, 3,3'-dimethylbenzidine and 3,3'-dimethoxybenzidine to potentially carcinogenic aromatic amines by intestinal bacteria. *Carcinogenesis*, **3**, 1255–1260

Chhabra, R.S., Thompson, M., Elwell, M.R. & Gerken, D.K. (1990) Toxicity of *p*-chloroaniline in rats and mice. *Food Chem. Toxicol.*, **28**, 717–722

Chhabra, R.S., Huff, J.E., Haseman, J.K., Elwell, M.R. & Peters, A.C. (1991) Carcinogenicity of *p*-chloroaniline in rats and mice. *Food Chem. Toxicol.*, **29**, 119–124

Goodman, D.G., Ward, J.M. & Reichardt, W.D. (1984) Splenic fibrosis and sarcomas in F344 rats fed diets containing aniline hydrochloride, *p*-chloroaniline, azobenzene, *o*-toluidine hydrochloride, 4,4'-sulfonyldianiline, or D & C Red No. 9. *J. natl Cancer Inst.*, **73**, 265–273

IARC (1972a) *IARC Monographs on the Evaluation of Carcinogenic Risk of Chemicals to Man*, Vol. 1, *Some Inorganic Substances, Chlorinated Hydrocarbons, Aromatic Amines, N-Nitroso Compounds and Natural Products*, Lyon, pp. 80–86

IARC (1972b) *IARC Monographs on the Evaluation of Carcinogenic Risk of Chemicals to Man*, Vol. 1, *Some Inorganic Substances, Chlorinated Hydrocarbons, Aromatic Amines, N-Nitroso Compounds and Natural Products*, Lyon, pp. 87–91

IARC (1974a) *IARC Monographs on the Evaluation of Carcinogenic Risk of Chemicals to Man*, Vol. 4, *Some Aromatic Amines, Hydrazine and Related Substances, N-Nitroso Compounds and Miscellaneous Alkylating Agents*, Lyon, pp. 57–64

IARC (1974b) *IARC Monographs on the Evaluation of Carcinogenic Risk of Chemicals to Man*, Vol. 4, *Some Aromatic Amines, Hydrazine and Related Substances*, N-*Nitroso Compounds and Miscellaneous Alkylating Agents*, Lyon, pp. 65–71

IARC (1974c) *IARC Monographs on the Evaluation of Carcinogenic Risk of Chemicals to Man*, Vol. 4, *Some Aromatic Amines, Hydrazine and Related Substances*, N-*Nitroso Compounds and Miscellaneous Alkylating Agents*, Lyon, pp. 41–47

IARC (1975) *IARC Monographs on the Evaluation of Carcinogenic Risk of Chemicals to Man*, Vol. 8, *Some Aromatic Azo Compounds*, Lyon, pp. 107–111

IARC (1978a) *IARC Monographs on the Evaluation of the Carcinogenic Risk of Chemicals to Man*, Vol. 16, *Some Aromatic Amines and Related Nitro Compounds—Hair Dyes, Colouring Agents and Miscellaneous Industrial Chemicals*, Lyon, pp. 27–37, 73–82

IARC (1978b) *IARC Monographs on the Evaluation of the Carcinogenic Risk of Chemicals to Humans*, Vol. 17, *Some N-Nitroso Compounds*, Lyon

IARC (1979) *IARC Monographs on the Evaluation of the Carcinogenic Risk of Chemicals to Humans*, Vol. 19, *Some Monomers, Plastics and Synthetic Elastomers, and Acrolein*, Lyon, pp. 187–211

IARC (1982a) *IARC Monographs on the Evaluation of the Carcinogenic Risk of Chemicals to Humans*, Vol. 27, *Some Aromatic Amines, Anthraquinones and Nitroso Compounds, and Inorganic Fluorides Used in Drinking-water and Dental Preparations*, Lyon, pp. 307–318

IARC (1982b) *IARC Monographs on the Evaluation of the Carcinogenic Risk of Chemicals to Humans*, Vol. 29, *Some Industrial Chemicals and Dyestuffs*, Lyon, pp. 345–389

IARC (1987a) *IARC Monographs on the Evaluation of Carcinogenic Risks to Humans*, Suppl. 7, *Overall Evaluations of Carcinogenicity: An Updating of* IARC Monographs *Volumes 1 to 42*, Lyon, pp. 238–239

IARC (1987b) *IARC Monographs on the Evaluation of Carcinogenic Risks to Humans*, Suppl. 7, *Overall Evaluations of Carcinogenicity: An Updating of* IARC Monographs *Volumes 1 to 42*, Lyon, pp. 246–247

IARC (1987c) *IARC Monographs on the Evaluation of Carcinogenic Risks to Humans*, Suppl. 7, *Overall Evaluations of Carcinogenicity: An Updating of* IARC Monographs *Volumes 1 to 42*, Lyon, pp. 123–125

IARC (1987d) *IARC Monographs on the Evaluation of Carcinogenic Risks to Humans*, Suppl. 7, *Overall Evaluations of Carcinogenicity: An Updating of* IARC Monographs *Volumes 1 to 42*, Lyon, pp. 125–126

IARC (1987e) *IARC Monographs on the Evaluation of Carcinogenic Risks to Humans*, Suppl. 7, *Overall Evaluations of Carcinogenicity: An Updating of* IARC Monographs *Volumes 1 to 42*, Lyon, pp. 198–199

Lynn, R.K., Donielson, D.W., Ilias, A.M., Kennish, J.M., Wong, K. & Matthews, H.B. (1980) Metabolism of bisazobiphenyl dyes derived from benzidine, 3,3'-dimethylbenzidine or 3,3'-dimethoxybenzidine to carcinogenic aromatic amines in the dog and rat. *Toxicol. appl. Pharmacol.*, **56**, 248–258

Stefanski, S.A., Elwell, M.R. & Stromberg, P.C. (1990) Spleen, lymph nodes, and thymus. In: Boorman, G.A., Eustis, S.L., Elwell, M.R., Montgomery, C.A., Jr & MacKenzie, W.F., eds, *Pathology of the Fischer Rat, Reference and Atlas*, New York, Academic Press, pp. 369–393

US National Cancer Institute (1979) *Bioassay of 2-Nitro-*p-*phenylenediamine for Possible Carcinogenicity (CAS No. 5307-14-2)* (Tech. Rep. Ser. No. 169; DHEW Publ. No. (NIH) 79-1725), Washington DC, US Government Printing Office

US National Institute of Occupational Safety and Health (1981) Health hazard alert. Benzidine-, *o*-toluidine, and *o*-dianisidine-based dyes. *Am. ind. Hyg. Assoc. J.*, **42**, A-36–A-60

US National Toxicology Program (1985a) *Toxicology and Carcinogenesis Studies of HC Blue No. 1 (CAS No. 2784-94-3) in F344/N Rats and B6C3F₁ Mice (Feed Studies)* (NTP Technical Report 271; NIH Publ. No. 85-2527), Research Triangle Park, NC

US National Toxicology Program (1985b) *Toxicology and Carcinogenesis Studies of HC Blue No. 2 (CAS No. 33229-34-4) in F344/N Rats and B6C3F₁ Mice (Feed Studies)* (NTP Technical Report 293; NIH Publ. No. 85-2549), Research Triangle Park, NC

US National Toxicology Program (1986) *Toxicology and Carcinogenesis Studies of HC Red No. 3 (CAS No. 2871-01-4) in F344/N Rats and B6C3F₁ Mice (Gavage Studies)* (NTP Technical Report 281; NIH Publ. No. 86-2537), Research Triangle Park, NC

US National Toxicology Program (1991) *Toxicology and Carcinogenesis Studies of C.I. Acid Red No. 114 (CAS No. 6459-94-5) in F344/N Rats (Drinking Water Studies)* (NTP Technical Report 405; NIH Publ. No. 92-3136), Research Triangle Park, NC

US National Toxicology Program (1992) *Toxicology and Carcinogenesis Studies of C.I. Direct Blue No. 15 (CAS No. 2429-74-5) in F344/N Rats (Drinking Water Studies)* (NTP Technical Report 397; NIH Publ. No. 92-2852), Research Triangle Park, NC

Ward, J.M., Reznik, G. & Garner, F.M. (1980) Proliferative lesions of the spleen in male F344 rats fed diets containing *p*-chloroaniline. *Vet. Pathol.*, **17**, 200–205

Weinberger, M.A., Albert, R.H. & Montgomery, S.B. (1985) Splenotoxicity associated with splenic sarcomas in rats fed high doses of D & C Red No. 9 or aniline hydrochloride. *J. natl Cancer Inst.*, **75**, 681–690

THE MONOGRAPHS

OCCUPATIONAL EXPOSURES OF HAIRDRESSERS AND BARBERS AND PERSONAL USE OF HAIR COLOURANTS

1. Exposure Data

1.1 Historical perspective

The history of the development and use of cosmetics has been reviewed (Zviak, 1986a,b). The dyeing of human hair can be traced back at least 4000 years: evidence from Egyptian tombs indicates the use of henna, from *Lawsonia inermis*, for dyeing hair, nails and skin, and there is evidence in other early eastern Mediterranean cultures of the use of henna and indigo for dyeing hair. During the time of the Roman civilization, a number of methods were used for colouring hair; one was the use of lead combs dipped in vinegar (presumably producing lead acetate), and another was the use of walnut stain. Pliny cited more than 100 recipes for colouring hair with vegetable and mineral materials.

In England, the Elizabethans treated hair with potash alum (aluminium potassium sulfate) followed by a concoction of rhubarb in order to produce a red tone, which was popular because of the colour of the Queen's hair. At the time of the French Revolution, 24 million pounds [11 000 tonnes] of starch were sold each year in France for use in colouring hair. In this technique, starch, a binder and, possibly, small amounts of colouring material were applied to the hair.

Bleaching of hair has also been popular for many centuries. In order to mimic the appearance of their Anglo slaves, Roman women devised a method of bleaching their hair using a mixture of tallow soap and the ashes of burnt beech wood. In sixteenth-century Venice, women treated their hair with a caustic soda solution and spent many hours sitting in the sun to decolorize the melanin. In 1867, the French chemist, Léon Hugot, and the British chemist, E.H. Thiellay, demonstrated the use of hydrogen peroxide for bleaching hair at the Paris Exhibition. Cora Pearl, mistress of Napoleon III, is reputed to have bleached her hair with hydrogen peroxide.

Of the hair colouring products currently on the market, only henna and lead acetate have a history of more than 100 years. The modern hair colouring industry was born in the nineteenth century with the development of organic chemistry. In 1863, Haussman observed that a mixture of *para*-phenylenediamine and an oxidizing agent produced a coloured material. In 1883, the first patent for the exploitation of this observation in hair dyeing was acquired by Monnet, who actually used 2,5-diaminotoluene and hydrogen peroxide. Shortly thereafter, patents were obtained by H. and E. Erdmann over the period 1888–97 for the use as hair dyes of a wide variety of *para*-phenylenediamines and aminophenols with hydrogen peroxide (Anon., 1966).

1.2 Characterization of the exposures of hairdressers, beauticians and users of hair colourants

Professional hairdressers and beauticians who work in beauty salons (parlours) and barber shops typically shampoo, cut and style hair and apply hair colourants, waving and straightening preparations and conditioners. They may also be manicurists, trimming finger and toe nails and applying nail care products. The term 'barber' has traditionally been applied to professionals who cut men's hair; they may also apply hair sprays and other styling preparations and may shave men's facial hair. The terms 'hairdresser', 'beautician' and 'cosmetologist' appear to be used interchangeably. In the USA, for example, the terms 'hairdresser' and 'beautician' apply to people involved in the care of hair, primarily women's hair, in beauty salons; they exclude barbers. In the United Kingdom, the term 'hairdresser' is more inclusive: it is used to denote ladies' hairdressers, and it may also mean barbers.

In the USA in 1937, there were about 60 000 to 70 000 salons and close to 200 000 professional hairdressers and beauticians (McDonough, 1937). Today, there are about 150 000 salons and between 500 000 and 750 000 professional hairdressers and beauticians, of whom approximately 80–85% are women (Cosmetic, Toiletry, and Fragrance Association, undated). In Europe, there are between 350 000 and 400 000 salons in which about 1 200 000 professional personnel work, not including manicurists.

Over 5000 different chemicals are currently used to make beauty products worldwide (Cosmetic, Toiletry, and Fragrance Association, 1991). Beauty products are manufactured by a few large companies, which make the majority of products used personally and professionally, and by many small companies which formulate products for professional trades. The various categories of products used by hairdressers are described in general terms below. The products are principally hair preparations but also include nail care products and, occasionally, skin care products. Although one of the focuses of this monograph is hair colourants, an enormous range of chemical substances may be present in beauty salons. Rather than attempting to list all of the chemicals that are or have been used in beauty products, this section gives the general composition of each type of product and examples of typical chemicals or chemical classes. Those compounds that have been evaluated in the *IARC Monographs* series are listed in Table 1.

Few actual measurements of the exposures of professional hairdressers are available. Use patterns provide a qualitative picture of the potential exposures of both hairdressers and clients. Information on skin penetration and inhalation is mentioned (see also section 4.1), although many hairdressers now use gloves for some operations, to reduce dermal exposure. In Finland, however, it was estimated that only about one-third of hairdressers currently use protective gloves when dyeing hair (Pukkala *et al.*, 1992). The method of dye application may affect exposures; for example, permanent cream dyes are commonly applied with a brush, whereas other dyes are more often worked into the hair by hand.

1.2.1 *Hair preparations*

The term 'hair preparations' covers all compounds used on the scalp and hair. The most important of these are hair colouring preparations (bleaches, dyes), cleansing and conditioning products (shampoos, conditioning agents), hair-styling preparations (setting

Table 1. Compounds used by hairdressers, beauticians and consumers that have been evaluated in the *IARC Monographs* series

Compound	Product in which found	Overall evaluation of carcinogenicity to humans[a]	IARC Monographs Volume	IARC Monographs Year
2-Amino-4-nitrophenol	Semi-permanent hair dyes	3	57	1993
2-Amino-5-nitrophenol	Semi-permanent hair dyes	3	57	1993
4-Amino-2-nitrophenol	Semi-permanent hair dyes	3	16	1978
Auramine	Brilliantines	2B	1	1972[b]
Butylated hydroxyanisole	Skin products	2B	40	1986
Carbon blacks	Nail products	3	33	1984[b]
Chlorodifluoromethane	Hair sprays	3	41	1986[b]
Chromium oxides	Nail products	1 or 3	49	1990
Chrysoidine	Brilliantines	3	8	1975[b]
CI Disperse Blue 1	Semi-permanent hair dyes	2B	48	1990
Coal-tars	Shampoos	1	35	1985[b]
Cobalt salts	Temporary hair dyes	2B	52	1991
D&C Red No. 9	Temporary hair dyes	3	57	1993
2,4-Diaminoanisole	Permanent hair dyes	2B	27	1982
2,4-Diaminotoluene	Permanent hair dyes	2B	16	1978
2,5-Diaminotoluene	Permanent hair dyes	3	16	1978
Dichloromethane	Hair sprays	2B	41	1986[b]
para-Dimethylaminoazobenzene	Brilliantines	2B	8	1975
1,4-Dioxane	Other exposures	2B	11	1976[b]
Ethanol	Setting lotions; hair sprays; nail products; skin products	Inadequate in experimental animals	44	1988
Formaldehyde	Shampoos; nail products	2A	29	1982[b]
HC Blue No.1	Semi-permanent hair dyes	2B	57	1993
HC Blue No. 2	Semi-permanent hair dyes	3	57	1993
HC Red No. 3	Semi-permanent hair dyes	3	57	1993
HC Yellow No. 4	Semi-permanent hair dyes	3	57	1993
Hydrogen peroxide	Bleaching agents; permanent-wave preparations	3	36	1985
Hydroquinone	Permanent hair dyes	3	15	1977
Iron oxide	Nail products	3	1	1972[b]

Table 1 (contd)

Compound	Product in which found	Overall evaluation of carcinogenicity to humans[a]	IARC Monographs Volume	Year
Isopropanol	Permanent hair dyes; nail products	3	15	1977[b]
Lead acetate	Temporary hair dyes	2B	23	1980[b]
Methyl methacrylate	Skin products	3	19	1979
Mineral oils	Conditioning treatments	1	33	1984[b]
Nickel salts	Temporary hair dyes	1	49	1990
2-Nitro-*para*-phenylenediamine	Permanent hair dyes; semi-permanent hair dyes	3	57	1993
N-Nitrosodiethanolamine	Other exposures	2B	17	1978
Phenacetin	Bleaching agents; permanent-wave preparations	2A	24	1980[b]
meta-Phenylenediamine	Permanent hair dyes	3	16	1978
para-Phenylenediamine	Permanent hair dyes	3	16	1978
Polyacrylic acid	Setting lotions	3	19	1979
Polyvinylpyrrolidone	Setting lotions; hair sprays	3	19	1979
Potassium bromate	Permanent-wave preparations	2B	40	1986
Resorcinol	Permanent hair dyes	3	15	1977
Selenium disulfide	Shampoos	3	9	1975
Sodium bisulfite	Permanent hair dyes	3	54	1992
Sodium sulfite	Permanent hair dyes	3	54	1992
Titanium oxide	Nail products; skin products	3	47	1989
Toluene	Nail products	3	47	1989
Vinyl chloride	Hair sprays	1	19	1979[b]
Xylene	Nail products	3	47	1989

[a]For definitions of the groups represented by numbers and letters, see Preamble, pp. 28–30.
[b]Also evaluated in Supplement 7 to the *Monographs* series

lotions, hair sprays), permanent-wave preparations and hair-straightening preparations. In recent years, fashion trends have spurred the development of new products, such as high-hold hair lacquers and styling gels and dyes that give brilliant colours. Toxicological considerations have also become increasingly important in product formulation (Lang, 1989a,b).

(a)   Hair colouring preparations

(i)   Bleaching

Bleaching has two objectives: to give hair a lighter look or, more often, to prepare it for application of a dye preparation, generally yielding a shade lighter than the natural one (Zviak, 1986a).

The chemistry of bleaching is described in detail by Zviak (1986a). All of the bleaching methods used currently are oxidation processes. Hydrogen peroxide is the commonest oxidant and is used usually as a 6 or 9% solution or, rarely, as a 12% solution. Solutions are normally preserved with phosphoric acid, quinine sulfate, pyrophosphates, acetanilide, phenacetin, ortho-oxyquinoline sulfate, ethylene diaminetetraacetic acid and certain stannates. Hydrogen peroxide can be used alone to bleach hair, but in hairdressing salons it is mixed with an alkaline solution, typically ammonia, before use, in order to accelerate the process.

Persulfates are often used in the formulation of bleaching powders that are mixed with hydrogen peroxide just before use, particularly as the sodium, potassium and ammonium salts; sodium percarbonate is used occasionally, diluted in water or hydrogen peroxide just before use; sodium perborate and magnesium perborate are rarely used; and magnesium dioxide and barium dioxide are sometimes present in bleaching powders. Bleaching formulations are available in several forms: hydrogen peroxide solutions and emulsions, creams, shampoos, powders, pastes and oils (Zviak, 1986a).

In order to remove permanent and semi-permanent hair colourings, hairdressers use reducing agents (sodium hydrosulfite or sodium or zinc formaldehyde sulfoxylate dissolved just before use in acidified water) or high-strength oxidants such as those mentioned above (Zviak, 1986a).

(ii)   Dyeing

The world market for hair colouring products is in excess of US$ 2500 million in factory sales. About one-third is bought by salon owners and the remainder by retail outlets for home use. The major markets are North America, Europe and Japan, each having US$ 300–900 million in factory sales. Retail sales represent 50–75% of the total business, being highest in North America and the United Kingdom and lowest in Italy, Spain and Australia.

The types of hair colourants are classified according to the permanence of the effect, i.e., temporary, semi-permanent or permanent, or to the type of ingredients that they contain. Only permanent and semi-permanent hair colourants are used to a significant extent in the hairdressing trade, whereas all three classes are used extensively by consumers.

In Europe and in North and South America, permanent dyes dominate the market, representing about 70% of the dollar volume of the retail market (Corbett, 1988) and 85% of the professional market. In Japan and parts of Asia, permanent dyes comprise an even greater share of the market. Semi-permanent dyes were introduced into Europe about 40 years ago and into the USA some 35 years ago. Temporary hair colourants are somewhat older but have rarely represented more than 5% of the market.

Permanent dyes (Zviak, 1986c): Permanent hair dyes, otherwise known as oxidation dyes, represent the major segment of the hair dye market. The hair is dyed by oxidation of dye precursors which penetrate the hair fibre, where they react with hydrogen peroxide to produce coloured indo dyes. Since hydrogen peroxide is an excellent decolorizing agent for melanin, the hair's natural colouring matter, manufacturers can balance the amounts of hydrogen peroxide and of dye precursors in such a way as to produce lightening, darkening or matching of the natural colour of the hair.

The dye precursors used in the permanent hair colour are of two types: 'primary intermediates', generally *para*-phenylenediamines or *para*-aminophenols, which undergo oxidation to produce highly reactive benzoquinoneimines; and compounds known as 'couplers' which react with these imines to produce a variety of indo dyes. Compounds used as couplers include resorcinol, *meta*-aminophenol, *meta*-phenylenediamine and certain other reactive intermediates such as 1-naphthol and phenylmethylpyrazolone. Permanent hair colouring preparations may contain as many as 15 different dyes and dye precursors so that they will produce the desired shade. Dye precursors are formulated in ammoniacal or detergent solutions. Two typical formulations of permanent hair colours are presented in Table 2, and oxidation dye precursors used in the USA and Europe are listed in Table 3.

Table 2. Ingredients of two typical hair colouring products

Light blond	Bronze (reddish)
Water	Water
Coconut acid diethanolamide	Oleic acid
Butoxyethanol	Isopropanol
Polyethyleneglycol-2 tallow amide	Nonoxynol-1
Ethanol	Propylene glycol
Polyglyceryl-4 oleyl ether	Ethoxydiglycol
Oleyl alcohol	Nonoxynol-4
Polyglyceryl-2 oleyl ether	Ammonium hydroxide
Propylene glycol	Linoleic acid diethanolamide
Oleic acid	Sodium lauryl sulfate
Sodium monodiethylaminopropyl cocoaspartamide	Sulfated castor oil
Ammonium hydroxide	Ethoxylated cetylalcohol-24
Pentasodium diethylenetriamine-pentaacetic acid	Ethoxylated cholesterol-24
Ammonium acetate	Fragrance
Sodium bisulfite	Sodium sulfite
Fragrance	Ethylene diaminetetraacetic acid
Phenylmethylpyrazolone	Erythorbic acid
Hydroquinone	N,N-Bis(2-hydroxyethyl)-*para*-phenylenediamine sulfate
para-Phenylenediamine	2-Methylresorcinol
Resorcinol	4-Amino-2-hydroxytoluene
	para-Aminophenol (4-aminophenol)

Table 2 (contd)

Light blond (contd)	Bronze (reddish) (contd)
para-Aminophenol (4-aminophenol)	para-Phenylenediamine (1,4-diaminobenzene)
meta-Aminophenol (3-aminophenol)	Resorcinol
2,4-Diaminophenoxyethanol HCl	1-Naphthol

From Cosmetic, Toiletry, and Fragrance Association (1992)

Table 3. Major oxidation dye precursors used in the USA and Europe

5-Amino-2-methylphenol
2-Aminophenol (ortho-Aminophenol)
3-Aminophenol (meta-Aminophenol)
4-Aminophenol (para-Aminophenol)
N,N-Bis(2-hydroxyethyl)-para-phenylenediamine
2-Chloro-para-phenylenediamine
4-Chlororesorcinol
1,3-Diaminobenzene (meta-Phenylenediamine)
1,4-Diaminobenzene (para-Phenylenediamine)
2,4-Diaminophenol
2,4-Diaminophenoxyethanol
2,5-Diaminotoluene
N,N-Dimethyl-para-phenylenediamine
3-N-Ethylamino-4-methylphenol
7-Hydroxybenzomorpholine
5-N-(2-Hydroxyethyl)amino-2-methylphenol
N-Methyl-4-aminophenol
2-Methylresorcinol
1-Phenyl-3-methylpyrazolone-5
N-Phenyl-para-phenylenediamine
2-Nitro-para-phenylenediamine
Resorcinol

From Cosmetic, Toiletry, and Fragrance Association (1992)

Most of the more important ingredients in permanent dyes have been in use for over 50 years, although a few new ones were introduced during the last 20 years. The use of some ingredients has been discontinued, usually simultaneously in North America, Europe and Japan, as a result of findings in assays of carcinogenicity in rodents. For example, use of 2,4-diaminotoluene (4-methyl-meta-phenylenediamine) was discontinued in 1970–71 and that of 2,4-diaminoanisole (4-methoxy-meta-phenylenediamine) some six years later. For other reasons, para-phenylenediamine was not used in France or Germany from about 1905 to 1980–85, during which time 2,5-diaminotoluene (2-methyl-para-phenylenediamine) was used in its place.

The usual conditions of use for permanent hair colours involve the mixing of equal volumes of the hair colouring lotion containing the dye precursors and a hydrogen peroxide solution with a strength of 3 or 9%. About 100 g of this mixture (containing 0.1–3 g of dye precursors and 2–4 g hydrogen peroxide) are then applied to the hair and left in contact for 20–40 min. During that time, the colour develops and the natural hair pigment is lightened. The residual product is then removed from the hair by rinsing.

Permanent colouring materials occur in a number of different forms: liquids, creams, gels, shampoos and powders. The first oxidation dyes were simple, aqueous solutions, but they were replaced by aqueous alcoholic dyes (15–20% alcohol), as the added alcohol enhanced penetration of dye precursors into the hair fibre. Liquid dyes have been replaced by cream- or gel-based formulae. Cream dyes are emulsions formed from self-emulsifying raw materials, such as fatty oxyethyleneated alcohols (partially sulfated or not), fatty amides and oxyethylated vegetable oils. Emollients such as lanolin derivatives, fatty alcohols and cation-active compounds may be added. Gel dyes (or, more properly, gelling dyes) offer the advantages of both liquids and creams. A number of formulations exist, but the following are typical: (i) soap solutions, generally ammonium oleate; (ii) solutions of low oxyethylated nonionic surfactants, most often polyoxyethylated alkylphenols; and (iii) anion–cation complexes in solution. 'Shampoo-in colours' are a simplified form of the usual permanent dye products, except that the vehicle is, or acts like, a shampoo. These materials colour and bleach less than other permanent dye products. Shampoo-in colours are the permanent dyes intended particularly for home use; they are also used in hairdressing salons, as fast-acting, permanent dye products, especially for producing dark shades or for 'tone-on-tone' shading. Powder dyes contain very stable oxidizing agents, such as sodium perborate, in powder form, and only non-lightening shades can be formulated. This type of product is offered for domestic use in countries where the people's natural hair colouring is very dark, e.g., for black Africans and Japanese (Zviak, 1986c; Clausen, 1989).

Owing to the rate of hair growth (about 1.25 cm per month), regrowth of undyed hair becomes evident after about four to six weeks. Permanent hair colouring products are therefore used about six to nine times per year in Europe and North America. More frequent applications, 'touch-ups' around the hair line and parting, are common in Asian countries.

Potential exposures to *para*-phenylenediamine by inhalation in some hairdressing parlours in Italy were assessed recently by air sampling; all samples contained less than the detection limit of 1 µg/m^3 (Gagliardi *et al.*, 1992). Measurements of skin penetration of some oxidation dye precursors are discussed in section 4.1 of this monograph.

Semi-permanent dyes: The term 'semi-permanent' is used to define hair colouring products that last through 6–12 washings and do not involve the use of an oxidizing agent in colour development. That level of wash fastness is achieved by using low-molecular-weight dyes capable of penetrating the hair cortex. Semi-permanent hair colours contain direct dyes, which are generally nitro derivatives of phenylenediamines or aminophenols, together with a selected number of azo dyes and aminoanthraquinone dyes. Because the dyes in semi-permanent hair colours are preformed and do not require added oxidant, such products cannot lighten the natural hair colour.

Some typical formulations are presented in Table 4; semi-permanent dyes used in the USA and Europe are listed in Table 5. Henna, an orange-red hair colouring derived from the powdered leaves and stems of *Lawsonia inermis*, a tropical shrub, has been used since antiquity and is still used, by both professional hairdressers and consumers (Feinland *et al.*, 1980). The active colouring matter in henna is 2-hydroxy-1,4-naphthoquinone (Farris, 1979).

Table 4. Ingredients of typical semi-permanent hair colouring products

Light blond

Water
Ethoxydiglycol
Polyethyleneglycol-50 tallow amide
Hydroxyethylcellulose
Lauric acid diethanolamide
Aminomethyl propanol
Erythorbic acid
Fragrance
Oleic acid
Triethanolammonium dodecylbenzenesulfonate
CI Disperse Black 9
CI Disperse Blue 3
CI Disperse Violet 1
FD&C Yellow No. 6
HC Blue No. 2
HC Orange No. 1
HC Red No. 3
HC Yellow No. 2
HC Yellow No. 4

Red

Water
Ethoxydiglycol
Polyethyleneglycol-50 tallow amide
Hydroxyethylcellulose
Lauric acid diethanolamide
Aminomethyl propanol
Erythorbic acid
Fragrance
Oleic acid
Triethanolammonium dodecylbenzenesulfonate
CI Disperse Black 9
HC Orange No. 1
HC Red No. 1
HC Red No. 3
HC Yellow No. 2

Reddish brown

Water
Butoxyethanol
Coconut acid diethanolamide
Hydroxyethylcellulose
Lauric acid
N-Methylaminoethanol
HC Blue No. 2
2-Nitro-5-glyceryl methylaniline
Fragrance
Butylparaben
Ethylparaben
Methylparaben
Propylparaben
3-Methylamino-4-nitrophenoxyethanol
3-Nitro-*para*-hydroxyethylaminophenol
HC Yellow No. 6
CI Disperse Violet 1
2-Amino-3-nitrophenol
4-Amino-3-nitrophenol
CI Disperse Blue 1

Dark brown

Water
Butoxyethanol
Polyglyceryl-2 oleyl ether
Coconut acid diethanolamide
Hydroxyethylcellulose
HC Blue No. 2
Lauric acid
N-Methylaminoethanol
2-Nitro-5-glyceryl methylaniline
Fragrance
HC Violet No. 2
CI Disperse Blue 1
Butylparaben
Ethylparaben
Methylparaben
Propylparaben
HC Yellow No. 7

Table 4 (contd)

Dark brown (contd)
3-Methylamino-4-nitrophenoxyethanol
CI Disperse Violet 1
3-Nitro-*para*-hydroxyethylaminophenol

From Cosmetic, Toiletry, and Fragrance Association (1992)

Table 5. Semi-permanent dyes used widely in the USA and Europe

2-Amino-3-nitrophenol
4-Amino-3-nitrophenol
CI Disperse Black 9
CI Disperse Blue 1
CI Disperse Blue 3
CI Disperse Violet 1
HC Blue No. 2
HC Orange No. 1
HC Red No. 1
HC Red No. 3
HC Red No. 7
HC Violet No. 2
HC Yellow No. 2
HC Yellow No. 4
HC Yellow No. 6
HC Yellow No. 7
HC Yellow No. 10
HC Yellow No. 11
2-(N-Hydroxyethylamino)-5-nitroanisole
4-β-Hydroxyethylamino-3-nitrophenol
3-Methylamino-4-nitrophenoxyethanol
3-Methylamino-4-nitrophenoxypropan-1,2-diol
2-Nitro-*para*-phenylenediamine
Sodium picramate

From Cosmetic, Toiletry, and Fragrance Association
(1992)

The dyes used in semi-permanent colourants have been used for 30 years or less, which is shorter than for permanent dyes, except for a few of the direct dyes that were used as toners in permanent colourants (the unsubstituted nitrophenylenediamines and nitroaminophenols). Use of HC Blue No. 1 (see monograph, p. 129) was discontinued in 1985 and that of 4-amino-2-nitrophenol somewhat earlier. 2-Amino-4-nitrophenol and 2-amino-5-nitrophenol were prohibited from use in cosmetic products, including hair dyes, in the countries of the European Economic Community in 1990 (Commission of the European Communities, 1990, 1991).

Semi-permanent colouring products come in several forms. Colour rinses are the simplest means for altering hair colour: The hair is rinsed with a dilute aqueous or aqueous alcoholic dye solution. The dyes are generally cationic and are adsorbed by the hair surface. Coloured or tint setting lotions are also used as rinses and usually contain cationic, disperse and/or nitro dyes. More pronounced colour changes are possible with tints, which are formulated with direct dyes; intense colours can be obtained, especially with nitro dyes. With foam tints, a surfactant solution is dispensed as a foam from an aerosol. Tints can be also thickened with cellulose derivatives, natural mucilage or synthetic polymers. Concentrated solutions with intense colouring action can be obtained by using co-solvents (e.g., alcohols and ethylene glycol ethers) and vehicles (e.g., urea derivatives and benzyl alcohol). In emulsion tints, the dye base consists of an emulsion (Clausen, 1989).

Semi-permanent colours are applied at 35–60 g to the hair for 10–30 min, followed by rinsing. The colouring lotion contains 0.1–5% of dye and generally less than 1% of any individual dyestuff. Users either apply such products at least monthly or use them only on special occasions, for example, three to four times a year. Measurements of skin penetration of some semi-permanent dyes are discussed in section 4.1 of this monograph.

Temporary dyes: Temporary hair colouring products, often referred to as 'colour rinses', are products that produce colour that is removed by a single shampoo. They are normally formulated with water-soluble acid or basic dyes of the type used in wool dyeing, which have a molecular size too great to penetrate the cortex of the hair. As a result, the dye is deposited on the surface, from which it is easily removed by washing. Temporary colourants may also comprise systems which produce insoluble complexes of an acid dye as a quaternary ammonium or metal salt. One of the compounds included in this volume, D&C Red No. 9 (see monograph, p. 203), is used in temporary hair dye formulations as a pigment in the form of its barium salt (Corbett, 1988). A commercial dye formulation may contain between 0.5 and 2.0% of the permitted colour, together with surface-active agents. Temporary dye formulations may also contain nitro aromatics as colourants, together with anionic detergents and urea to increase the solubility. Temporary colourants are occasionally used in the hairdressing trade but are more commonly used directly by consumers at home. While there are few data on skin absorption, very little of such materials will pass through the skin owing to the relatively high molecular weight of the dyes.

Virtually no metal salt (e.g., lead acetate) is used for hair colouring in the hairdressing trade, as coloration with such products occurs gradually and they must be applied daily. Furthermore, the selection of colours available is limited, and the shades look metallic and unnatural. Metal salts are also incompatible with permanent waving and bleaching of hair (Clausen, 1989).

(b) Hair cleansing and conditioning preparations

(i) Shampoos

Shampoos are cosmetic products for cleaning the hair and scalp. The word 'shampoo' is derived from a Hindi word meaning massage. Shampoos are the cosmetic products most often applied to the hair. Some of the characteristics considered in formulating modern shampoos are their ability to clean, to lather and to make the hair easy to comb, their capacity to condition the hair, mildness (compatibility with skin, eyes and mucosa; no burning on the scalp or in the eyes), colour, appearance and fragrance (Lang, 1989a).

The principal constituents and most important raw materials of shampoos are surfactants, and nearly all modern shampoos are aqueous surfactant preparations. Surfactants break the bonds between dirt and hair components and suspend the dirt in the aqueous medium (Lang, 1989a).

Bar soaps were probably used for washing hair from about 1800, when they first became available, until the 1930s and 1940s, when liquid soaps and cream shampoos were introduced. The first surfactants used for hair cleansing were fat soaps. In hard water, however, soaps create a deposit of calcium and magnesium fatty acid salts on the hair, so their use must be followed by treatment with an organic acid, such as citric or acetic acid. Another drawback is the alkaline pH of soap, which may increase the swelling of hair. In order to meet the requirements of high cleansing power, good lathering and safety (for the user and for the environment), modern shampoos are formulated mainly with anionic surfactants. Amphoteric surfactants are also used, whereas nonionic and cationic surfactants play only secondary roles in special-purpose formulations (Lang, 1989a).

The most important anionic surfactants used in shampoos are alkyl sulfates (ammonium lauryl sulfate), alkyl and alkylaryl sulfonates, olefin sulfonates, secondary alkyl sulfonates, alkyl ether sulfates, sulfosuccinates (disodium lauryl ether sulfosuccinate) and protein-fatty acid condensates (potassium coco-hydrolysed animal protein) (Lang, 1989a). Sulfonated oils, such as sulfonated castor, mineral and olive oils, were introduced for use in shampoos in the 1930s; their use continued into the 1950s, with declining popularity. Sulfated fatty alcohols were first introduced in Europe in the 1930s and in the USA late in the 1930s in salon products and some retail products. By 1957, 70% of the shampoos used in the USA were based on synthetic detergents such as sodium lauryl sulfate and triethanolamine lauryl sulfate, and those two detergents are still commonly found in salon shampoos (McDonough, 1937; Wall, 1954; Powers, 1972). The trend in the late 1950s was to increase the use of liquid shampoos over that of creams, and there was then a movement to use of ammonium lauryl sulfate, introduced in the early 1970s, and laurylether sulfates. Laurylether sulfates are the preferred detergents in Europe.

Amphoteric surfactants used in shampoos can be divided into two classes: betaines (coco-amidopropylbetaine) and alkyl amphoglycinates and alkyl amphopropionates (coco-amphocarboxyglycinates and coco-amphocarboxypropionates). Cationic surfactants have a positive charge and are strongly absorbed by the hair. Only a few special-purpose shampoos, especially those for the treatment of severely damaged hair, contain these compounds. The nonionic surfactants in use are polysorbates (Polysorbate 20, Polysorbate 80) and fatty alcohol ethoxylates and polyglycerides (Lang, 1989a).

Another important class of constituents of shampoos is foam builders, typified by the fatty acid mono- and dialkanolamides (Lang, 1989a) introduced in the late 1930s. By the mid 1950s, virtually all liquid shampoos based on lauryl sulfates contained alkanolamides. Two types of amides are used. Condensation of 1 mol of fatty acid with 1 mol of an alkanolamine such as diethanolamine gives a water-soluble product; condensation of 1 mol of fatty acid with 2 mol of diethanolamine gives a more water-soluble product. The 2:1 types of alkanolamides can have appreciable levels of free alkanolamine, fatty acid amide and free fatty acids. Some of the commonest examples of these constituents are the amides derived from reaction of diethanolamine with lauric acid and with coconut oil fatty acids (Kritchevsky, 1937; Barker, 1985).

Other constituents of shampoos include: refatting agents, conditioning additives (cationic polymers such as quaternary hydroxyalkyl celluloses), thickeners (salts such as sodium and ammonium chloride in combination with amphoteric surfactants), opacifiers (fatty acid alkanolamides in mixtures with ethylene glycol monostearate and distearate or cetyl alcohol and stearyl alcohol), colouring agents, fragrances and buffers (pH stabilizers, such as citric, tartaric, adipic and phosphoric acids and their salts). The preservatives added to shampoos today include formaldehyde and its donors and isothiazolinones, introduced in the 1980s. From the 1930s to the mid-1960s, the main preservatives were parabens and phenylmercuric acetate (Liem, 1977), which was banned in the late 1960s (Feinland et al., 1980; Lang, 1989a).

Shampoos may be clear, opaque or pearly liquids, gels or aerosols. Shampoos with special additives include those for frequent use and for babies, conditioning shampoos, antidandruff preparations, shampoos for oily hair, tinting shampoos and those containing insecticides. Shampoos for frequent use and for babies contain especially mild surfactants (e.g., sulfosuccinate esters, magnesium ethyl ether sulfates) or mixtures of anionic, amphoteric and sometimes nonionic surfactants. Conditioning shampoos are used to make the hair easy to comb in the wet state and glossy and soft when dry. These effects are provided chiefly through the addition of cationic polymers; addition of amphoteric surfactants or refatting agents can improve the conditioning qualities of anionic surfactant formulations. Antidandruff shampoos contain agents that reduce excessive scalp flaking to a normal level. The most important antidandruff ingredients are zinc pyrithione, Octopirox (1-hydroxy-4-methyl-6-[2,4,4-trimethylpentyl]-2[1H]-pyridone) and Climbazole (Baypival; 1-[4-chloro-phenoxy]-1-[1-imidazolyl]-3,3-dimethyl-2-butanone) (Lang, 1989a). Coal-tar formulations (Weinberg, 1980) and selenium disulfide have also been used extensively, but their use is regulated in some countries.

(ii) Conditioning agents and treatments

Hair can be damaged in a number of ways: by climatic effects such as humidity and temperature extremes (weathering); by exposure to sunlight; by washing with products containing surfactants; by cosmetic treatments, such as bleaching, dyeing, permanent waving and straightening; and by combing and brushing. These processes alter the physical, chemical and morphological properties of hair as well as its reaction to cosmetic treatments such as dyeing and permanent waving. They lead to perceptible roughening of the hair surface, difficulty in combing, tangling, increased static charge, formation of split ends and loss of natural lustre. Hair conditioning agents prevent, retard or mask such changes. Their action is restricted largely to modifying the surface qualities of the hair and making it glossy. Nearly all modern shampoos, permanent wave lotions, setting lotions and dyes contain conditioning additives that prevent excessive mechanical damage to the hair. This simple type of conditioning may not be sufficient for severely damaged or long hair, and special conditioning treatments are available for such cases (Lang, 1989a).

The earliest conditioning treatments were waxes and oils (vegetable and mineral oils, petrolatum), which provided lubrication and enhanced lustre, and acid rinses (lemon juice, vinegar), which counteracted the undesirable effects of soap shampoos. During the 1940s and 1950s, these ingredients were combined with surfactants in anionic emulsions as after-shampoo rinses. Alkaline rinses included water-softening ingredients such as borax and trisodium phosphate (Wall, 1954).

In the mid-1940s, the quaternary ammonium compound, stearyl dimethyl benzyl ammonium chloride, began to be investigated for use as an after-shampoo treatment. By the early 1960s, almost all after-shampoo conditioners contained quaternary ammonium compounds as cationic surfactants. Typical quaternary compounds in current use include cetyldimethylammonium chloride and cetyltrimethylammonium chloride, sometimes in formulations with fatty alcohols such as cetylstearyl alcohol or with simethicone (Lang, 1989a).

Cationic polymers can also be used in conditioning treatments, together with special ingredients such as antidandruff additives. The addition of special wax components yields pearly preparations; if water-insoluble components are omitted and cationic polymers are added, the formulae obtained are transparent and clear. Conditioning treatments are generally rinsed out after they have been allowed to work for a defined time; however, some newer products with a lower content of active ingredients can be left on the hair without rinsing (Lang, 1989a).

(c)   Hair-styling preparations

Styling preparations stabilize a hair-style during or after its creation with comb, brush or rollers, usually as a temporary set. Styling products may also make hair easier to manage, for example, by facilitating wet combing and brushing. The products are mainly setting lotions and hair sprays. Newer products developed in response to fashion changes are 'wet gels' and 'hair waxes', which were developed from the brilliantines, pomades and hair creams used formerly. Styling preparations are generally left on the hair and are not rinsed out. Their active ingredients are usually dissolved polymers, known as film-forming agents, which are deposited on the hair after evaporation of a solvent (Lang, 1989b).

(i)   Setting lotions

Setting lotions make a hair-style more durable and prevent hair from 'flying' away, reduce the amount of charge during combing and brushing, improve wet or dry combing and improve its feel and lustre. They may be applied before hair is wound on rollers and dried (wave sets) or before use of a hair dryer, brush or comb to style the hair (blow-dry sets) (Lang, 1989b).

The first preparations comparable to modern setting lotions were aqueous or aqueous alcoholic solutions and gels of natural substances, such as egg white, sugar solutions, plant mucilage (pectins, alginates, carrageenan, karaya gum, tragacanth) and beer. These products simply 'glued' the hairs together. They had the drawback of forming opaque, brittle residues which created dust during combing or brushing and became sticky in the presence of moisture. Modern setting lotions contain polymers (film-forming agents), solvents, agents to facilitate combing, plasticizers, fragrances, colouring agents, ultra-violet radiation stabilizers, preservatives (if necessary) and other special ingredients (Lang, 1989b).

Film-formers are nonionic, anionic or cationic polymers dissolved in water or water-alcohol mixtures. Nonionic film-forming polymers include polyvinylpyrrolidone, the first polymer used for this purpose, and vinylpyrrolidone-vinyl acetate copolymers. Anionic film formers are vinyl acetate-crotonic acid copolymers or copolymers of methyl vinyl ether and maleic acid semi-esters. Both types of polymer are usually neutralized with organic amines such as 2-amino-2-methyl-1,3-propanediol, 3-amino-2-methylpropanol or triisopropanol-amine. Other anionic polymers are terpolymers of vinyl acetate, crotonic acid and vinyl esters and graft polymers of vinyl acetate, crotonic acid and poly(ethylene oxide). Cationic polymers have an affinity for keratin, thus making the hair easier to untangle; they also prevent the accumulation of static charge during combing and brushing. The most important cationic film-forming polymers are quaternary vinylpyrrolidone–dimethylaminoethyl methacrylate copolymers (CTFA Polyquaternium 11), vinylpyrrolidone–vinylimidazole copolymers (CTFA Polyquaternium 16), cationic hydroxyethyl cellulose (CTFA Polyquaternium 10), poly(dimethyldiallylammonium chloride) (CTFA Polyquaternium 6), poly-(dimethyl–diallylammonium chloride) copolymers (CTFA Polyquaternium 7) and chitosan (obtained from chitin by alkali treatment) or its derivatives (Lang, 1989b).

The solvents used in setting lotions are water, ethanol, 2-propanol and their mixtures. Agents that facilitate combing include the cationic film-forming polymers listed above and cationic surfactants such as cetyltrimethylammonium chloride or bromide. Plasticizers enhance the flexibility of films formed on the hair. They include esters such as diethyl phthalate, diethyl citrate, adipates, silicones and polyglycols (Lang, 1989b).

Setting lotions are usually marketed as dilute, aqueous alcoholic solutions in single- or multiple-application packages. Depending on intended use, they contain 0.5–4% of polymers or polymer mixtures and up to 50% ethanol. Setting lotions for waving have a higher polymer content than those for blow-drying. Gels thickened by the addition of higher-molecular-mass polymers of the poly(acrylic acid) type are used far less frequently. Liquid lotions can also be packaged as aerosol sprays (propellant or pump spray). A novel form is the aerosol foam (mousse). Addition of adsorptive or penetrating dyes to setting lotions allows simultaneous hair colouring (Lang, 1989b).

(ii) Hair sprays

Aerosol spray-can products first came into widespread use in about 1948, on the basis of technology developed for insecticide applications during the Second World War. Hair sprays did not become practical until 'liquefied' gases with low vapour pressures became available. By virtue of the propellant liquid–gas equilibrium in the pressurized can, the pressure remains roughly constant during spraying. Pump sprays ('nonaerosol' sprays) do not use a propellant gas; the energy needed to swirl and atomize the concentrate is supplied by a manual pump. The ingredients of 'nonaerosol' hair sprays are generally the same as those of aerosol products, but the propellant content is replaced by additional solvent (Lang, 1989b).

The most important ingredients of hair sprays today are concentrates (film-forming agents, solvents, plasticizers, agents for lustre and fragrances) and propellants (Lang, 1989b). Hair spray products can be subdivided into six types on the basis of the hair fixative or film-forming component: polyvinylpyrrolidone, a copolymer of polyvinylpyrrolidone and polyvinyl acetate, shellac, dimethylhydantoin–formaldehyde resin, modified polyacrylic acid resin and lanolin (Draize *et al.*, 1959).

The first film-forming agent, shellac, was superseded in the 1950s by polyvinyl-pyrrolidone. Better results are obtained with vinylpyrrolidone–vinyl acetate copolymers, the harder, more hydrophobic types being used for hair sprays. Still harder films can be obtained with vinyl acetate–crotonic acid copolymers. Copolymers of methyl vinyl ether and ethyl or butyl maleate and polyvinyl methyl ether/maleic anhydride–ethyl half-ester copolymers are used most often in the USA. More recently, acrylate–acrylamide copolymers (such as *tert*-butylacrylamide–ethyl acrylate–acrylic acid copolymers and octylacrylamide–acrylate copolymers), vinyl acetate–crotonic acid–vinyl neodecanate copolymers and vinylcapro-lactam–vinylpyrrolidone–dimethylaminoethyl methacrylate copolymers have been used.

Ethanol, 2-propanol and acetone are the most important solvents in hair sprays. Dichloromethane has been used for many years (1965–89 in the USA) but is no longer used in some countries (including the USA) because of its toxicological properties (Lang, 1989b). Vinyl chloride was reportedly used to a limited extent as a solvent-propellant (US Consumer Product Safety Commission, 1974) before it was found to be a carcinogen (see IARC, 1979).

Until recently, the most common propellants in aerosol hair sprays were chlorofluoro-carbons. Those most frequently used were trichlorofluoromethane (F-11), trichloro-trifluoroethane (F-113), dichlorotetrafluoroethane (F-114) and chlorodifluoromethane (F-22). By 1979, controversy about the possible action of these compounds on the Earth's ozone layer led to a ban on their use as propellants in the USA. International agreements and national legislation have led to a gradual abandonment of chlorofluorocarbons as pro-pellants in Europe and elsewhere. Alternatives are the hydrocarbons propane, butane, iso-butane, pentane and their mixtures, although they are highly inflammable and poor solvents for most polymers (Lang, 1989b).

Exposures to hair spray components in beauty salons have been estimated on the basis of both use patterns and direct measurements. The average spray release time per application is 10 sec, and about 10 g of spray are emitted during a spray period (Gerkens *et al.*, 1989). About 65% of the unimpinged spray has a particle diameter less than or equal to 10 μm, making the aerosol highly respirable. Half of the particle weight is solvent. It was estimated that 0.03–0.4 mg were inhaled over a 5-min period following 10 sec of spraying (Draize *et al.*, 1959).

Concentrations of dichloromethane in the air of beauty salons were reported in three studies: 8-h time-weighted average exposures were in the range of 1–6 ppm (cm^3/m^3) (Hoffman, 1973 (USA); Sayad *et al.*, 1976 (USA); Gerkens *et al.*, 1989 (Italy)). Average exposure to dichloromethane while spraying from an aerosol can during one 219-min period was 18 ppm in the breathing zone (Sayad *et al.*, 1976). Peak exposure concentrations up to 130 ppm (Hoffman, 1973) and more (< 400 ppm) were measured (Sayad *et al.*, 1976). Total particulate levels in personal samples in beauty salons ranged from 0.3 to 0.6 mg/m^3 (Palmer *et al.*, 1979).

Trace quantities of airborne polyvinylpyrrolidone (< 7 μg/m^3 to 0.07 mg/m^3), ethanol (< 7 μg/m^3 to 3 mg/m^3) and trichlorofluoromethane (3–41 mg/m^3) were found to be associated with hair spray use in a beauty salon. Isobutane concentrations ranged from 373 to 1935 mg/m^3 (Gunter et al., 1976).

(iii)   *Other hair-styling preparations*

Brilliantine (pomade) is the oldest preparation for stabilizing styled hair. Colourants added to brilliantine in the past were reported to have included *N,N*-dimethyl-4-amino-azobenzene (*para*-dimethylaminoazobenzene; butter yellow), auramine and chrysoidine (Clemmesen, 1981; Gubéran et al., 1985). 2-Naphthylamine has been found as an impurity in yellow AB and yellow OB, which have been used in cosmetics (Conway & Lethco, 1960; Gubéran et al., 1985). Brilliantines consist mainly of vaseline and paraffin or other oils. The viscosity of the product and the hydrophobic layer with which it coats the hair are responsible for stabilization. These and similar formulations have reappeared on the market as hair waxes.

Setting gels are a new form of hair fixative. Fat-based gels are generally of the micro-emulsion type; aqueous gels are aqueous solutions thickened with poly(ethylene glycol), cellulose derivatives or polyacrylates and contain film-forming substances. They allow the creation of 'wet-look' hairstyles (Lang, 1989b).

Changes in fashion have meant that hair creams have lost much of their commercial importance. These products facilitate combing, add lustre and help to hold hair-styles. Creams include oil-in-water and water-in-oil types. Hair tonics refresh the scalp and serve as simple styling aids. They may also contain disinfectants, soothing, cooling or hair growth-promoting ingredients and anti-oil and antidandruff agents (Lang, 1989b).

(d)   *Permanent-wave preparations*

In permanent waving, intermolecular and intramolecular bonds in the hair are broken and then reformed after the hair has been shaped (curled). The strongest bonds that are broken and reformed are the disulfide bonds of cystine; approximately 25% of the cystine bridges are reduced to cysteine. After the hair has been reshaped, this reaction is reversed with an oxidant. Hydrogen bonds, salt bridges and hydrophobic and van der Waals inter-actions between individual amino acids are also involved but are of lesser importance (Kohler, 1989a).

Modern permanent waving traces its roots to a London hairdresser named Nessler who in 1906 introduced heat treatment of hair soaked in borax. The treatment required a whole day and often resulted in burns and hair loss. During the next 35 years, the use of heat, with and without alkaline solutions, was perfected. The image from the 1920s and 1930s of a person sitting under a salon hair dryer represents the classic picture of someone receiving a salon wave. Alkaline solutions in combination with heat were developed, and special pads with strong exothermic reactions when moistened were introduced. In the early 1940s, sulfides were tried but were discontinued because of toxicity (Winkel, 1936; Willat, 1939; Thomssen, 1947; Gershon et al., 1972; Zviak, 1986d).

It was also in the 1940s that thioglycolates were introduced. These preparations were called cold waves to differentiate them from earlier processes (Gershon et al., 1972). Since the 1950s, most waving preparations have involved salts of thioglycolic (mercaptoacetic) acid as the principal reducing agents. Ammonium thioglycolate (concentration, 6–11%) has been in constant use in salons since the late 1940s. In 1972, glyceryl or glycerol monothioglycolate was introduced in the USA and Canada. It was first used with heat (from a hair dryer), but by 1980 most such waves were processed without heat at a concentration of about 13%, expressed as thioglycolic acid (about 23% as glyceryl thioglycolate). Today glyceryl monothioglycolate waves account for about one-half of the 200 million waves done in salons in the USA each year. In Japan, cysteine is used in some waves, but the predominant waving material is still ammonium thioglycolate (concentrations up to 7%), as it is in Europe and elsewhere (Kohler, 1989a).

Ammonia and monoethanolamine are most commonly used for pH control (alkalinization) in waving preparations. Combinations of ammonium hydrogen carbonate and ammonium carbonate, or urea and the enzyme urease, are also used. Other additives include surfactants, fragrances, agents to facilitate combing (poly(dimethyldiallylammonium chloride), cetyltrimethylammonium chloride), thickeners (cellulose derivatives, polyacrylate salts), opacifiers (styrene–vinylpyrrolidone copolymers), colouring agents, carriers (urea, ethanol, 2-propanol) and complexing agents (Kohler, 1989a).

Waves must be 'neutralized' with an oxidizing agent. During 1940–70, potassium and sodium bromate were the chief agents used, at concentrations of 6–12%. Since then, hydrogen peroxide (at 0.5–3.0%) has been used in most parts of the world. In Asia, bromate-based neutralizers are used mainly, because they do not greatly lighten dark hair. Percarbamide (urea–hydrogen peroxide), sodium perborate and melamine peroxide hydrate have been used occasionally (Kohler, 1989a).

The most widely used preparations are those containing hydrogen peroxide, stabilized with inorganic phosphates, phenacetin, 4-acetaminophenol or α-bisabolol (a constituent of chamomile oil). The 'foam neutralizer' that is applied to curlers with a sponge and lathered into a foam is commonest; however, rinse and aerosol foam neutralizers are becoming increasingly popular (Kohler, 1989a).

A survey in the United Kingdom in 1992 of exposures of hairdressers during permanent waving showed ethanol at 2–30 mg/m^3, isopropanol at none detected to 9 mg/m^3 and ammonia at 5–25 mg/m^3. Dichloromethane was not detected (Rajan, 1992).

(e) Hair-straightening preparations

Preparations similar to those employed for permanent waving can be used to straighten naturally wavy or curly hair. Hair-straightening products are usually gels or creams rather than lotions. They contain strong bases such as alkali hydroxides (1.5–4.0 wt% lithium or sodium hydroxide) and other active ingredients such as guanidinium hydroxide and tetra-alkylammonium hydroxides. Lye-based products are so strong that they do not require oxidative post-treatment; however, improper use can easily make the hair brittle, and skin burns may even occur. In order to reduce such hazards, formulations have a high content of mineral oil (Kohler, 1989b).

1.2.2 Nail products

Nail-care products fall into three categories: coloured products; colourless products that include base coats, top coats and strengthener/hardener coats; and lacquer/enamel removers. The main ingredients of coloured and colourless nail-care products are:

nitrocellulose (10–15%), resins (5–15%), solvents (30–40%), diluents (20–30%), plasticizers (1–6%), suspending agents for colourants (0.7–3%) and colourants (3–5%). Nitrocellulose is used as a film-former in conjunction with a plasticizer to avoid shrinkage and brittleness; it is usually wetted with isopropanol for safety reasons. The function of resins is to produce adhesion to the nail and a glossy surface. Those most commonly used are toluene-sulfonamide/formaldehyde resin, polyester, polyamide (e.g., nylon) and acrylates and acrylics. The most commonly used solvents are ethyl acetate, butyl acetate, isopropanol and ethanol. Diluents help stabilize the viscosity of the formula. Those most commonly used are alcohols (ethyl, isopropyl, butyl), aromatic hydrocarbons (toluene, xylene) and aliphatic hydrocarbons (heptane). Plasticizers are used to achieve flexibility in the nitrocellulose film; the commonest are dibutyl phthalate and camphor. Dispersing agents help to keep colourants suspended; the commonest is stearalkonium hectorite. Colourants may be organic or inorganic and may include natural or synthetic pearl. The pigments used in nail lacquer formulations are carbon black, iron oxides, chromium oxides, ultramarines, metallic powders (gold, bronze, aluminium, copper), aluminium and calcium lakes of FD&C and D&C blue, red, yellow and orange, and titanium oxide. Transparent systems require the use of solvent-soluble colourants such as D&C red, green, yellow and violet. A typical nail lacquer formulation contains (% by weight): toluene, 30.5; *n*-butyl acetate, 12.8; *n*-amyl acetate, 11.1; ethyl acetate, 11.1; nitrocellulose, 10.0; aryl sulfonamide–formaldehyde resin, 10.0; isopropanol, 5.0; bentonite, 3.0; camphor, 2.5; dibutyl phthalate, 2.5; and ethanol, 1.5 (Isacoff, 1979). Nail hardeners usually contain an 'active' ingredient to strengthen the nail plate and include isobutyraldehyde, glutaraldehyde and sometimes formaldehyde.

A typical nail treatment, at home or in a salon, includes application of a base coat, two coats of lacquer (coloured product) and then a top coat. For added durability, an additional layer of each coat might be added. Typical drying time for a single layer is about 7 min; more time is needed between successive layers, because barriers to evaporation are created. A total nail treatment takes 1 h or more.

Lacquer/enamel removers may be made from any number of solvents, including any of those used in the formulation of the enamels. The fastest acting is acetone, but ethyl acetate is also used. Various oils and emollient compounds added to lacquer removers include castor oil, lanolins and lanolin derivatives. The formula of a typical nail polish remover is (% by weight): ethyl acetate, 40; acetone, 30; carbitol, 19; dibutyl phthalate, 10; sesame oil, 1; and a small amount of perfume. Cuticle removers and cuticle softeners usually consist of a dilute solution of alkali in water with some glycerol or other humectant added to keep the water from evaporating too rapidly. Potassium hydroxide, trisodium phosphate, triethanolamine and some quaternary ammonium salts have been used (Isacoff, 1979).

A quantitative evaluation of the exposure of manicurists during the production of synthetic fingernails showed 8-h time-weighted average exposures of 5.3 ppm methyl methacrylate, 7.3 ppm ethyl methacrylate and 1.6 ppm isobutyl methacrylate. Intermittent exposure to 9–48 ppm (average, 20 ppm) methyl methacrylate was measured during application, with peak exposures to up to 137 ppm (average peak, 54 ppm); intermittent exposure to ethyl methacrylate was 7–18 ppm (average, 13 ppm) and that to isobutyl methacrylate, 5–8 ppm (average, 6 ppm). The average time to create a full set of artificial nails was 40 min (Froines & Garabrant, 1986). In another investigation of artificial nail application, personal exposures to methyl methacrylate were 15–25 ppm (Kronoveter, 1977).

1.2.3 *Skin products*

Skin preparations used in beauty salons comprise various lotions, creams, perfumes, colours, powders and soaps intended to beautify and improve the complexion of the skin, including colouring foundation creams, concealers/blemish-covering creams and solids, eyeliners, eyeshadows, face powders, facial colouring products (blush, powders, liquid make-up), facial masks and beauty packs, hair removers (depilatories), lipstick, mascara, moisturizing creams and lotions, skin cleansing creams and lotions and skin fresheners/-toners.

The typical chemical content of a clay mask is (%): water, 50–80; fillers (bentonite clay, kaolin, titanium oxide), 10–40; thickeners (algin, potassium alginate, magnesium aluminium silicate, carbomers), 0–10; humectants (glycerol, propylene glycol, lanolin, polyethylene glycol, sorbitol), 5–10; astringents and healing agents (zinc oxide, witch hazel extract), 0–5; emulsifiers (beeswax, magnesium aluminium silicate, polysorbates), 0–5; preservatives (citric acid, methyl and propyl parabens), 0–1.5; fragrance (essential oils), 0–1; and colourants, 0–0.1. The typical chemical content of paste and peel-off facial masks is (%): water, 50–75; film formers (hydroxyethylcellulose, polyvinylpyrrolidone–vinyl acetate, gums), 10–25; ethanol, 5–12; humectants and emollients (glyceryl stearate, polyethylene glycol stearate, glycerol, sorbitol, polysorbates, cetyl alcohol, stearyl alcohol, lanolin, beeswax), 0–5; clay (bentonite, kaolin), 0–5; preservatives (butylated hydroxyanisole, citric acid, methyl and propyl parabens), 0–0.1; fragrance (essential oils), 0–1; aloe plant gel; and colourants.

1.2.4 *Other exposures in beauty salons*

Nitrosamines have been found in a wide variety of cosmetic and toiletry products, including hair dyes, shampoos, rinses, conditioners and fragrance preparations. The use of 2-bromo-2-nitropropane-1,3-diol as an antibacterial and antifungal agent was associated with the highest concentrations, since it may act as a source of nitrosation of amines or amides (Fan *et al.*, 1977; US Food and Drug Administration, 1991). The commonest nitrosamine found is *N*-nitrosodiethanolamine. Between 1978 and 1980, the US Food and Drug Administration analysed more than 300 cosmetic samples for this compound and found concentrations of < 30 ppb in 7% of the samples, 30 ppb to 2 ppm in 26% and 2–150 ppm in 7% (US Food and Drug Administration, 1991). In 1986, 40% of samples of cosmetics and shampoos in Germany were found to be contaminated with *N*-nitrosodiethanolamine (up to 275 μg/kg) and *N*-nitrosobis(2-hydroxy-propyl)amine (20–30 μg/kg). The introduction of official recommendations by the German Federal Health Office in 1987 to stop use of secondary amines in cosmetic products led to a reduction in such contamination; only 15% of the products were contaminated in a 1987–88 survey (Eisenbrand *et al.*, 1991). These nitrosamines may be absorbed appreciably through human skin (US Food and Drug Administration, 1979; Marzulli *et al.*, 1981).

Formaldehyde is added to many cosmetic products, particularly shampoos, as an antibacterial agent and preservative. It is also used in processes for hair setting that employ urea– or melamine–formaldehyde condensation products (Walker, 1975). Formaldehyde can also form during storage as a degradation product of materials containing polyethylene glycol (Fregert, 1986). Formaldehyde and formaldehyde donors, such as 1-hydroxymethyl-5,5-dimethylhydantoin, were found at levels of up to 0.5% in cosmetics (Liem, 1977). Concentrations of formaldehyde found in some specific products were: shampoo, up to 0.03%; hair rinse, 0.41%; bubble bath, 0.61%; and nail hardener, 7% (Wilson, 1974). Although formaldehyde is known to penetrate the skin and is volatile, no study was found that reported levels of exposure during the use of cosmetic products (Lodén, 1986a,b).

Paraformaldehyde may be used as a fumigant in towel cabinets, equipment drawers and cosmetic kits in beauty parlours and barber shops. Such use was found at one site to contribute to general air concentrations of formaldehyde of between 0.01 and 0.03 ppm [0.012 and 0.037 mg/m^3] (Almaguer & Blade, 1990). In area air samples in a high-school cosmetology laboratory, levels of 0.01–0.9 ppm [0.012–1.1 mg/m^3] formaldehyde were detected over a 6-h period (Almaguer & Klein, 1991). Short-term exposure to several parts per million of formaldehyde may be experienced when opening cabinets containing paraformaldehyde.

1,4-Dioxane is a common trace component of cosmetic products containing polyethoxylated surfactants, such as some shampoos and conditioners, hair dyes and skin conditioners. Of the cosmetic products tested, including shampoos, hair and body gels, liquid soaps, balms and foam preparations, 82% contained 1,4-dioxane in the range of 0.3–96 ppm [mg/kg or l] (Rastogi, 1990). In other evaluations, 48% of commercially available cosmetic products containing polyethoxylated surfactants contained 7–86 ppm [mg/kg] 1,4-dioxane (Scalia & Menegatti, 1991), and up to 613 ppm [mg/kg] was found in shampoo (Beernaert *et al.*, 1987). 1,4-Dioxane penetrates the skin (Marzulli *et al.*, 1981).

1.3 Consumer use of hair dyes

While permanent hair colours have been in use since the late nineteenth century, they were first applied only by professionals; retail consumer use became significant in the years following 1945. Subsequently, total use of hair colourings increased, until by about 1965 35–40% of women in the USA and Europe aged 18–60 were using them, and that prevalence has remained stable. Permanent hair colouring constituted > 90% of use until the introduction of semi-permanent dyes in the late 1950s. In Europe and the USA, semi-permanent dyes now represent about 20% of use, permanent dyes about 75% and temporary dyes about 5%. In Japan, mainly permanent colourants are used; the prevalence of use among women is similar to that in Europe and the USA.

In the USA and Europe, use of hair colourants among men is almost completely for grey coverage and is mainly among men over 40 years of age. No published data are available, but it is unlikely that more than 10% of men aged 35–60 use hair colourants. Progressive colourants (see below) have been used by about 80% of male users (Zahm *et al.*, 1992). Use of hair colouring materials is believed to be greater among Japanese men than among US and European men.

The products used by hairdressers and beauticians are, with few exceptions, similar to the retail products sold for home use. Thus, consumers are exposed potentially either in beauty salons or during home use of the products to a similar range of chemical substances as are hairdressers and beauticians. The frequency and duration of exposure, however, may be quite different for consumers and professionals.

As noted above, one class of hair colouring products that is not used in beauty salons is the metal salts used as temporary hair colourants. This practice is as ancient as the use of vegetable dyes, but metal salts are rarely used today except by people who do 'progressive' colouring, involving daily applications of the product. Metal salts used as temporary hair colourants are, for the most part, lead and silver salts; occasionally, copper, nickel, bismuth, cobalt and manganese salts are added to solutions to vary shades. While there is still some uncertainty about how these dyes work, it is thought that the hair shaft is coloured by reaction of the metallic salt with keratin sulfur, depositing a metallic sulfide. In addition, it is thought that some of the colour is attributable to slow formation of metallic oxide. Lead salts commonly used for this purpose are the acetate and the nitrate. Sometimes, finely divided sulfur is added to formulations. Silver nitrate, used since the beginning of the nineteenth century, has a dual mode of action, in that the silver salts darken when exposed to light, and silver combines with protein, yielding a dark-coloured proteinate. A rapid colouring process has also been used (e.g., on eyelashes and eyebrows) in which a solution of trihydroxybenzene is applied, followed by ammoniacal silver nitrate (Zviak, 1986b).

1.4 Regulatory aspects

A detailed discussion of the laws and regulations related to toiletry and cosmetic products is presented by Zviak and Camp (1986). In order to authorize, restrict or ban the use of substances in cosmetic products, some countries have set up negative and positive lists or derogatory and restrictive lists. A negative list comprises substances that cannot be part of a cosmetic composition; a positive list includes only substances authorized for a definite purpose. When a positive list is adopted, any other substance is banned for the said purpose. A derogatory and restrictive list covers substances outside the scope of negative lists for certain types of use and/or within certain concentration limits, or a list of substances the use of which is permitted only under certain conditions (e.g., ingredient warning labelling).

General provisions for cosmetic products, including hair-care products, are compiled in the Council Directive of the European Economic Community (EEC) of 27 July 1976 on the Approximation of the Laws of the Member States Relating to Cosmetic Products (Commission of the European Communities, 1976), which is amended constantly. Hair-care products include hair tints and bleaches; products for waving, straightening and fixing; setting products; cleansing products (lotions, powders, shampoos); conditioning products (lotions, creams, oils); and hairdressing products (lotions, lacquers, brilliantines). The Directives include: lists of substances that must not form part of the composition of cosmetic products; lists of substances which cosmetic products must not contain except subject to the restrictions and conditions laid down; lists of colouring agents allowed for use in cosmetic products; lists of colouring agents provisionally allowed for use in cosmetic products; lists of preservatives which cosmetic products may contain; and lists of ultraviolet radiation filters which cosmetic products may contain. Oxalic acid, its esters and alkaline products, hydrogen peroxide, 1,3-bis(hydroxymethyl)imidazolidine-2-thione, quinolin-8-ol, bis(2-hydroxyquinolium) sulfate and etidronic acid and its salts are permitted in hair-care products with restrictions on concentrations (Commission of the European Communities, 1990). Some countries of the EEC, however, such as France, Denmark and Italy, depart from the EEC Directive regarding restrictions and labelling requirements. In Greece, cosmetics must be registered. Spain requires government notification before a product is marketed. In Germany, hair preparations are classified as cosmetics and subject to legal provisions (Liebscher & Spengler, 1989). Under the EEC Cosmetics Directive, cosmetics must not be liable to endanger human health when applied under normal conditions of use (Commission of the European Communities, 1990, 1991, 1992). The cosmetic regulations in Norway, Finland and Turkey are closely modelled on the EEC Directive (Liebscher & Spengler, 1989).

In the USA, certain cosmetics are subject to registration as over-the-counter drugs. The list of cosmetic colour additives is very limited, and stringent purity standards must be observed. In preparations sold directly to the consumer, all ingredients must currently be listed on the label. Registration is required for cosmetics in Canada and in most countries of Latin America and Southeast Asia. In Japan, cosmetics are classified as quasi-drugs or cosmetics. New raw materials must be registered and extensive toxicological data submitted; human tests from other countries are not recognized (Liebscher & Spengler, 1989).

1.4.1 *Hair dyes*

2,4-Diaminoanisole and 2,5-diaminoanisole, 1,2-diaminobenzene (*ortho*-phenylene-diamine) and 2,4-diaminotoluene (4-methyl-*meta*-phenylenediamine) and their salts, 2-amino-4-nitrophenol and 2-amino-5-nitrophenol, are banned in the EEC. Other diaminobenzenes and diaminotoluenes, as well as their *N*-substituted derivatives and their salts, diaminophenols, hydroquinone, α-naphthol and resorcinol are permitted, with restrictions on concentrations. With the exception of α-naphthol, these substances may be used for dyeing eyelashes and eyebrows by professionals only. Lead acetate is permitted for hair dyeing only at a concentration of 0.6% calculated as lead; it is not allowed for dyeing eyelashes, eyebrows or moustaches. Warning labels are also prescribed (Commission of the European Communities, 1990, 1992). In addition to the EEC provisions, 1,4-diamino-2-nitrobenzene and 1,2-diamino-4-nitrobenzene are banned in Italy and Denmark, and 1,3-diaminobenzene is also banned in Denmark. The USA requires a special warning label; with the label, any hair dye can be used without restriction. In Japan, a list of permissible hair dyes is issued; new dyes must be registered (Liebscher & Spengler, 1989).

1.4.2 *Shampoos*

The general provisions stated above apply to shampoos in the EEC countries. Furthermore, phenol and its alkali salts, quinine and its salts and selenium disulfide are permitted with restriction on concentrations (Commission of the European Communities, 1990). Antidandruff shampoos are classified as over-the-counter drugs in the USA and as quasi-drugs in Japan (Liebscher & Spengler, 1989). Quinine and its salts are permitted in hair lotions at a concentration of 0.2% calculated as quinine base in the finished product (Commission of the European Communities, 1990).

1.4.3 *Bleaching preparations*

In the EEC, persulfates can be used without restriction. Argentina and Thailand limit their concentration, and in Finland a warning label is required for ammonium persulfate. The USA does not have any specific regulations for this group (Liebscher & Spengler, 1989).

1.4.4 *Permanent-wave preparations*

The EEC Directive restricts the pH range of permanent-wave preparations and hair straighteners based on thioglycolic acid, its salts and esters (pH 7–9.5 or 7–12.7 for the acid and salts, 6–9.5 for esters). The maximal concentration (calculated as thioglycolic acid) is 8% by weight for general use, and 11% by weight at pH 7–9.5, 5% at pH 7–12.7 for the acid and salts and 11% at pH 6–9.5 for esters for professional use. A special warning label is required. Potassium and sodium hydroxide are permitted with a restriction on concentration in hair straighteners (Commission of the European Communities, 1990). France further restricts permanent-wave and straightening preparations made from thioglycolic acid, its salts and esters to professional use only. In the USA, no legal restriction is known. Because of self-imposed industry restrictions, however, the thioglycolic acid content does not exceed 14% by weight at a pH of not more than 9.5. In Japan, permanent-wave products are classified as quasi-drugs. Thioglycolic acid and its salts are permitted, as is cysteine, with restrictions on concentration and pH. Thioglycolate esters are not allowed. Concentration limits also apply to neutralizers (Liebscher & Spengler, 1989).

1.4.5 *Hair sprays*

In the EEC, dichloromethane is allowed as a solvent up to a concentration of 35% by weight in the finished product. When dichloromethane is mixed with 1,1,1-trichloroethane, a total concentration of both is limited to a maximum of 35% by weight (Commission of the European Communities, 1990). Chlorofluorocarbons are now being phased out in most parts of the world in accordance with the 'Montreal Protocol', as amended in London in 1990 and in Copenhagen in 1992 (see US Environmental Protection Agency, 1993).

1.4.6 *Nail hardeners*

Formaldehyde is permitted at a concentration of 5% in the finished product. Potassium and sodium hydroxide are permitted in nail cuticle solvent at the same concentration (Commission of the European Communities, 1990).

2. Studies of Cancer in Humans

The available studies relate to exposures that occurred at different times over the last 30 years or more, during which period there were changes in both the types and quantities of products used by hairdressers and barbers and by the consumer (Wall, 1972).

2.1 Occupational exposure

2.1.1 *Descriptive studies*

Cancer mortality among men and single women in England and Wales was examined for the period 1949–53 (Registrar General, 1958). For male barbers and hairdressers, the sites examined were all sites, stomach, lung and leukaemia. Lung cancer occurred in excess (standardized mortality ratio [SMR], 1.15; 114 observed, 99 expected); for cancers at all sites, there were 257 observed and 273 expected. For single female hairdressers and manicurists, the numbers of observed deaths exceeded those expected for cancers at all sites combined (43 observed, 37 expected) and for cancers of the lung and bronchus (4 and 2), breast (13 and 9) and cervix uteri (4 and 1).

Similar data from the Registrar General (1971) for the period 1959–63 showed no significant excess mortality from cancers at all sites or from lung or stomach cancers or leukaemia among male hairdressers and barbers. Among single female hairdressers and manicurists, there were 21 observed deaths from breast cancer, with 12 expected ($p < 0.05$); for cancers of the cervix uteri and other parts of the uterus the ratios of observed to expected deaths were 3:2 and 4:2, respectively. A further report from England and Wales (Office of Population Censuses and Surveys, 1978), in which occupational mortality for the period 1970–72 was analysed, did not indicate a significant excess of any of the above cancers in men or in women in those occupations, including breast cancer among single female hairdressers and manicurists (eight observed, seven expected).

In the latest report in this series (Office of Population Censuses and Surveys, 1986), covering the years 1979–80 and 1982–83, male barbers in England and Wales were reported to have had increased mortality from cancers at all sites at ages 15–64 (45 deaths, 21.6 expected) and from lung cancer (21 deaths, 7.9 expected). Nonsignificant increases were seen for cancers of the lip, oesophagus, stomach, colorectum, prostate and bladder and for Hodgkin's disease and leukaemia, all based on five cases or fewer. Single female hairdressers also showed a significant excess of cancers at all sites at ages 15–64 (22 observed, 9.2 expected; $p < 0.01$) and of cancer of the breast (7 observed, 1.6 expected; $p < 0.05$). Nonsignificant excesses were seen for cancers of the stomach, colorectum, cervix, ovary and brain and for malignant melanoma, which were based on few cases.

Clemmesen (1977) studied the incidence of malignant neoplasms in the period 1943–72 among hairdressers in Denmark on the basis of the numbers recorded with this occupation in successive censuses. Among male hairdressers, 447 malignant neoplasms were observed, with 517.4 expected (Clemmesen, 1981). There was no excess in any of 13 groupings of cancer sites. In women, there was a large overall excess, with 872 malignant neoplasms observed and only 475.4 expected, which appeared in each five-year period and for each of 14 site groups. [The Working Group noted that the consistent excess of cancers at markedly different sites in women in this study suggests use of different criteria for reporting women's occupation as hairdresser at the census and in hospital records.]

Garfinkel *et al.* (1977) analysed a series of death certificates with mention of cancer covering Alameda County, California, USA, in the period 1958–62. Of 3460 such deaths in females, 24 occurred in beauticians, at the following sites: lung (6), breast (5), cervix (4), ovary (3), brain (1), bladder (1), stomach (1), synovium (1) and unspecified (2). An expected number of 21.8 cancers was calculated for beauticians on the basis of 1000 death certificates for women of similar age and race which had no mention of cancer (24 observed; $p = 0.43$). When women who had died from causes other than cancer were matched to those who had died from lung cancer by age, race, date of death and county of residence, of 176 lung cancer cases, six were in beauticians, compared with one among the 176 controls. The relative risk (RR) was 6.0, with a one-tailed $p = 0.06$.

Menck *et al*. (1977) used data on 15 230 men and 22 792 women, aged 20–64, white and with non-Spanish names, from the Los Angeles County (USA) Cancer Surveillance Program in 1972–75 to investigate the association of cancer with occupation reported at hospital admission. Of 135 cases of cancer found in female beauticians, 20 were of the lung. Proportionate incidence ratios (PIR) and standardized incidence ratios (SIR) were computed, the latter being derived from the sex-specific populations at risk by occupation as ascertained in a 2% sample census of Los Angeles County. Both the PIRs and SIRs for lung cancer among beauticians were significantly increased (about two-fold; $p < 0.05$). No data on smoking habits were available. The authors mentioned parenthetically, without giving details, that a case–control study of 199 lung cancer cases and 187 controls had shown a RR of 0.94 for beauticians, on the basis of six cases.

In a study of cancers registered in the Los Angeles (USA) Tumor Registry, in 1972–78, which partially overlaps with the above study, Guidotti *et al*. (1982) noted an excess of multiple myeloma in the category of cosmetologists, hairdressers and manicurists. The PIR was 4.67 in women, on the basis of eight cases, and 3.47 in men, on the basis of one case.

Milham (1983) studied the occupations of 429 926 men in Washington State, USA, who had died during 1950–79 and of 25 066 women who had died during 1974–79. Among male barbers (3014 deaths), the proportionate mortality ratio (PMR) was elevated for multiple myeloma. Among female hairdressers and cosmetologists (409 deaths), the PMRs were elevated for stomach cancer, other lymphomas, multiple myeloma, acute leukaemias and neoplasms at other and unspecified sites. [The Working Group noted that detailed figures were not given.]

Dubrow and Wegman (1982, 1983, 1984) analysed mortality by occupation among 34 879 white men in Massachusetts, USA, who had died during 1971–73. Overall, there were 179 deaths among barbers. Nonsignificantly elevated odds ratios (ORs) were found for cancers of the pancreas (1.46) and lung (1.34), on the basis of six and 29 deaths, respectively. For hairdressers and cosmetologists, an elevated OR was found for bladder cancer (11.56; four deaths).

Baxter and McDowall (1986) conducted a study of death certificates analysed as a case–control study of bladder cancer among men in six boroughs of London (United Kingdom), in the period 1968–78, using as controls all other causes of death, including cancer. There were four deaths in hairdressers, giving a RR of 2.0.

Pearce and Howard (1986) examined male cancer mortality by occupation in New Zealand in the period 1974–78 in relation to census-based estimates of the relevant populations. The RR for bladder cancer, adjusted for social class, was 12.94 (95% confidence interval [CI], 1.45–46.7; two cases). The adjusted RR for 'other urinary' cancers was 12.85 (1.44–46.4; two cases) and that for lung cancer was 2.54, on the basis of five cases (0.82–5.93).

Gallagher *et al*. (1989) analysed the death certificates of 320 423 male residents of British Columbia, Canada, who had died during 1950–84. There were 1209 deaths among barbers: cancer mortality was slightly reduced from that expected (PMR, 0.95; 95% CI, 0.82–1.08; 224 deaths), and PMRs were not elevated for any cancer site. The PMRs were 1.34

for bladder cancer, 1.33 for all non-Hodgkin's lymphomas and 0.58 for multiple myeloma, on the basis of 12, 8 and 2 deaths, respectively. In a similar analysis of mortality among female cosmetologists and hairdressers in 1950–78 in British Columbia, a significantly increased PMR was found for multiple myeloma (6.19; 95% CI, 1.27–18.11; three deaths) (Spinelli *et al.*, 1984). A nonsignificant excess of ovarian cancer was also noted (PMR, 2.04; 95% CI, 0.88–4.03; eight deaths), which reached statistical significance ($p < 0.05$) in the age group 20–65 years.

Neuberger *et al.* (1991) examined 375 industries and occupations that were associated with five or more deaths from brain cancer in Missouri, USA, between January 1983 and October 1984. Seven deaths were observed in the beauty shop industry against 1.49 expected (standardized proportionate mortality ratio, 4.7; $p < 0.005$). Among hairdressers and cosmetologists, there were eight deaths with 1.50 expected (5.3; $p < 0.005$).

2.1.2 Cohort studies

The studies summarized below are also presented in Table 6, with the results for the sites at which cancer occurred most commonly. Bias may have been introduced in the case of certain malignancies (other than bladder and breast cancers), owing to failure to present relevant results in some of the studies.

Alderson (1980) followed a sample of 1831 male hairdressers identified at the 1961 census of England and Wales until 1978. Mortality from all cancers was similar to that expected (134 observed, 126.1 expected), and no specific cancer showed a significant excess: oesophagus, 5 observed, 3.4 expected; lung, 52 and 50.8; bladder, 7 and 5.6; and leukaemia, 3 and 2.7.

Kono *et al.* (1983) followed the mortality of a cohort of 7736 registered female beauticians from 1948 to 1960 in Fukuoka Prefecture, Japan, for an average of 22.5 years. Among the site-specific cancers examined, only stomach cancer occurred in significant excess (61 observed, 45.59 expected; 95% CI, 1.02–1.72). They found no case of bladder cancer (1.01 expected), five cases of breast cancer (8.5 expected) and nine cases of lung cancer (7.4 expected).

Teta *et al.* (1984) examined cancer incidence in 1935–78 in 11 845 female and 1805 male cosmetologists in Connecticut (USA) who had held licences for five years or more and had begun hairdressing school prior to 1 January 1966. A significant excess of lung cancer (SIR, 1.41) and excesses of brain (SIR, 1.68) and ovarian cancer (SIR, 1.34) of borderline significance were observed among women; the SIR for bladder cancer was 1.36 (95% CI, 0.74–2.27), on the basis of 14 cases. No significant cancer risk was evident for female cosmetologists licensed since 1935, even for those with 35 years or more of follow-up, although the SIRs for brain cancer, lymphoma and leukaemia were elevated. Female cosmetologists who had entered the profession between 1925 and 1934, however, experienced a significant overall increase in cancer incidence (SIR, 1.29) and significant excesses of respiratory, breast, corpus uterine and ovarian cancers. Among the men in the cohort, there was no excess of cancers at all sites (77 observed, 73.4 expected), but cancers of the brain occurred more frequently than expected (4 observed, 1.9 expected). [The Working Group noted that no other numbers were given for cancers at specific sites in men.]

Gubéran et al. (1985) studied cancer mortality in the period 1942–82 and incidence in the years 1970–80 in a cohort of 703 male and 677 female hairdressers in Geneva, Switzerland. Increased mortality from bladder cancer was observed among men (10 observed, 3.9 expected; $p < 0.01$) and women (2 observed, 1.0 expected). The corresponding values for incident cases were 11 and 5.3 for men ($p < 0.01$) and 2 and 1.5 for women. Significant ($p < 0.05$) excesses of incident cases of cancer of the buccal cavity and pharynx (6 observed, 2.5 expected) and of prostatic cancer (12 observed, 6.1 expected) were seen in men in the period 1970–80. No case of cancer of the buccal cavity and pharynx was seen in women (0.8 expected); for neither of these sites, however, was there an excess in the longer period covered by the mortality analysis (1942–82). A nested case–control study of 18 cases of bladder cancer among men in this cohort (10 deceased, six incident cases that occurred during 1970–80 and two incident cases that occurred in 1981) showed a non-significantly greater duration of exposure (measured from the start of apprenticeship) among those who dressed men's hair but not among those who dressed women's hair. Enquiries indicated that the great majority of male hairdressers in this study never dyed men's hair. In the period 1900–50, application of brilliantines to men's scalps after haircuts was widespread in Geneva. The authors stated that those preparations may have contained colouring agents that are bladder carcinogens, such as para-dimethylaminoazobenzene, chrysoidine and auramine, which have been found in brilliantines in other countries. They also mentioned that 2-naphthylamine has been found as an impurity in Yellow AB and Yellow OB, which have been used in cosmetics.

In a study linking 1960 census and 1961–79 cancer incidence in Sweden, 11 cases of multiple myeloma were found in people classified as beauticians (SIR, 1.3; $p > 0.05$) (McLaughlin et al., 1988).

In a brief note, Shibata et al. (1989) reported three deaths from leukaemia (3.84 expected) and two from lymphoma (3.01 expected) in a cohort of 8316 male and female barbers surveyed in 1976–87 in Aichi Prefecture, Japan.

An analysis of the incidence of bladder cancer and lung cancer in men and women employed as hairdressers and beauticians in 1960 in Norway and Sweden and as hairdressers and barbers in 1970 in Denmark and Finland was reported by Skov et al. (1990). Lynge and Thygesen (1988) found an increased risk for bladder cancer in hairdressers in Denmark: the RR was 2.05 for men, on the basis of 41 cases (95% CI, 1.51–2.78), and 1.76 for women, on the basis of seven cases (95% CI, 0.71–3.63). No corresponding increase in lung cancer was observed. In Finland, Norway and Denmark, the expected numbers of cancer cases were calculated by multiplying the person-years at risk for each of the five-year birth cohorts of hairdressers by the sex-specific incidence rate for the equivalent five-year birth cohort of all people who were economically active at the time of the census. In Sweden, the expected number of cancer cases was calculated by multiplying the number of hairdressers in a given region of Sweden in each five-year birth cohort at the time of the census by the sex-specific estimated cancer probability for the equivalent five-year birth cohort of all people in the region. National figures were obtained by aggregating the observed and the expected numbers across the 27 Swedish regions. The pattern of excess bladder cancer incidence without a corresponding increase in lung cancer incidence was not found in any of the other Nordic countries (Skov et al., 1990). In Sweden (Malker et al., 1987; Skov et al., 1990), the incidence of lung cancer was increased in male (98 cases; RR, 1.5; 95% CI, 1.2–1.8) and female (31 cases; 1.6; 1.1–2.2) hairdressers, and bladder cancer incidence was increased in men (54 cases; 1.5; 1.1–1.9) but not in women (six cases; 0.4; 0.2–1.0). The authors noted that a national survey of smoking in Sweden carried out in 1963 had found that 74% of male barbers and beauticians aged 50–69 were regular smokers, compared to 46% of all men aged 50–69 years. In Norway, the incidences of bladder cancer and lung cancer were increased in hairdressers (RR, 1.4–1.6), but the increase was significant only for lung cancer in men. In the data from Finland, no case of bladder cancer was recorded among male hairdressers in the period 1971–80 (expected, 0.3), but three cases occurred in women (1.8 expected). The incidence of lung cancer was not increased: 3 observed, 2.0 expected in men and 2 observed, 4.4 expected in women (Skov et al., 1990). The incidence of non-Hodgkin's lymphoma was examined in Denmark (1970–80) by occupational category by Skov and Lynge (1991) using a similar method. No significant excess was observed in female hairdressers (RR, 1.98; 95% CI, 0.24–7.15; two cases); no case was recorded among male hairdressers. When all groups of hairdressers were included (self-employed/barber, work in beauty shops and hairdresser), the RRs were 1.3 (0.48–2.83; six cases) for men and 2.0 (0.81–4.14; seven cases) for women.

In a study not entirely independent of the study of Skov et al. (1990), a cohort of 3637 female and 168 male hairdressers, born in or before 1946 and who were members of the Finnish Hairdressers' Association between 1970 and 1982, were followed up for cancer incidence through the national cancer registry between 1970 and 1987 (Pukkala et al., 1992). Expected numbers of cases were calculated by multiplying the number of person-years in each age group by the corresponding overall cancer incidence in Finland during the period of observation. Among women, there were 247 cases of cancer and 195.0 expected. Non-significant excesses were seen for breast cancer (70 cases, 56.3 expected), cervical cancer (11 cases, 7.1 expected), lung cancer (13 cases, 7.6 expected) and ovarian cancer (21 cases, 12.8 expected). Risks were not elevated for cancers at other sites, including the bladder (1 and 2.5), leukaemia (4 and 4.2) and multiple myeloma (1 and 2.4). The risk for all cancers was higher during the period 1970–75 ($p < 0.05$) than during 1976–81 ($p > 0.05$) or 1982–87 ($p > 0.05$). Among men, 25 cases of cancer were observed (17.9 expected; 95% CI, 0.90–2.06); nonsignificantly elevated risks were found for cancers of the lung and pancreas, on the basis of seven and three cases, respectively.

In a cohort study of 248 046 US male veterans who served during 1917–40 and were interviewed during 1954 or 1957 on smoking habits and occupations, Hrubec et al. (1992) analysed the mortality pattern of 740 barbers through 1980. Smoking-adjusted RRs were 1.2 for all cancers (110 deaths; 95% CI, 1.06–1.45), 1.6 for respiratory cancers (31; 1.22–2.20), 1.5 for prostatic cancer (20; 1.03–2.15) and 2.5 for multiple myeloma (4; 1.08–5.63). No excess was found for bladder cancer (3 deaths; OR, 0.7).

2.1.3 Case–control studies (Table 7)

The Working Group systematically reviewed studies dealing with occupational risk factors for cancer of the urinary bladder and breast (sites that have been studied extensively), lymphatic and haematopoietic neoplasms and childhood cancer. No systematic review was made of studies of other cancer sites. Many of the case–control studies that have been published did not present results for all of the occupational categories covered in the

Table 6. Occupational exposure: results of cohort studies on cancers at selected sites

Reference	Study population	Sex	Breast cancer			Bladder cancer			Lung cancer			Ovarian cancer			Lymphatic and haematopoietic neoplasms				Notes
			O	E	RR	O	E	RR	O	E	RR	O	E	RR	Type	O	E	RR	
Alderson (1980)	1831 male hairdressers at 1961 census, England and Wales, follow-up (M), 1961–78	M				7	5.6	1.25	52	50.8	1.02				Leu	3	2.7	1.1	
Kono et al. (1983)	7736 female beauticians, Fukuoka, Japan, registered, 1948–60, follow-up (M), 1953–77	F	5	8.46	0.59	0	1.01	–	9	7.41	1.21	5	3.69	1.36	Leu	6	4.38	1.37	Excess of stomach cancer (RR, 1.34*)
Teta et al. (1984)	11 845 female cosmetologists, Connecticut, USA licensed, 1925–74, follow-up (I), 1935–78	F	204	199.59	1.02	14	10.33	1.36	49[a]	34.83	1.41*	48	35.83	1.34	Leu	14	11.62	1.20	Higher RRs for women licensed during 1925–34 than among those licensed since 1935.
															MM	3	4.33	0.69	
															Lym	22	17.07	1.29	
Gubéran et al. (1985)	677 female and 703 male hairdressers, Geneva, Switzerland, employed 1900–64, follow-up (I), 1970–80	F	7	12.5	[0.6]	2	1.5	[1.3]	3	1.6	[1.9]	1	2.0	[0.5]	All	4	2.0	[2.0]	The only excess in a parallel analysis of 1942–82 mortality was bladder cancer among males (10 observed [RR, 2.6*])
		M				11	5.3	[2.1*]	8	10.3	[0.78]				All	0	2.3	–	
McLaughlin et al. (1988)	3067 male MM cases, Swedish Cancer Registry, 1961–79, employed at 1960 census as beautician	M													MM	11		1.3	
Shibata et al. (1989)	3701 female and 4615 male barbers, Aichi Prefecture, Japan, employed in 1976, follow-up (M), 1976–87	F													Leu	0	1.26	–	
															Lym	1	0.73	1.37	
		M													Leu	3	2.58	1.16	
															Lym	1	2.29	0.44	
Skov et al. (1990)	4356 female and 2149 male hairdressers and beauticians, Norway, employed at 1960 census, follow-up (I), 1961–84	F				11	7.2	1.5	16	11.1	1.4								
		M				23	15.1	1.5	47	29.2	1.6*								
Malker et al. (1987); Skov et al. (1990)	16 942 female and 6522 male hairdressers and beauticians, Sweden, employed at 1960 census, follow-up (I), 1961–79	F				6	13.5	0.4	31	20.0	1.6*								
		M				54	36.6	1.5*	98	67.2	1.5*								

Table 6 (contd)

Reference	Study population	Sex	Breast cancer			Bladder cancer			Lung cancer			Ovarian cancer			Lymphatic and haematopoietic neoplasms				Notes
			O	E	RR	O	E	RR	O	E	RR	O	E	RR	Type	O	E	RR	
Skov et al. (1990)	9138 female and 428 male hairdressers and barbers, Finland, employed at 1970 census, follow-up (I), 1971-80	F M				3 0	1.8 0.3	1.7 –	2 3	4.4 2.0	0.5 1.5								Partially overlapping with the study of Pukkala et al. (1992)
Lynge & Thygesen (1988; Skov et al. (1990); Skov & Lynge (1991)	9497 female and 4874 male hairdressers and barbers, Denmark, employed at 1970 census, follow-up (I), 1970-80	F M				7 41	4.0 20.0	1.8 2.1*	12 56	11.0 50.5	1.1 1.1				NHL NHL	7 6		2.01 1.30	For all hairdressers and barbers. For hairdressers only, RR, 1.98 in women
Pukkala et al. (1992)	3637 female hairdressers, Finland, employed 1970-82, follow-up (I), 1970-87	F	70	56.3	1.24	1	2.5	0.40	13	7.6	1.72	21	12.8	1.64*	Leu MM	4 1	4.2 2.4	0.96 0.42	Higher RRs during 1970-75 than in subsequent periods. Excess incidence of all cancers (1.27*). Partially overlapping with the study of Skov et al. (1990).
Hrubec et al. (1992)	740 male barbers, beauticians and manicurists, serving in the US Army during 1917-40, follow-up (M), 1954-80	M				3	[4.3]	0.7	31	[19.4]	1.6*				NHL HD MM Leu	4 1 4 5	[3.1] [0.7] [1.6] [4.6]	1.3 1.4 2.5* 1.1	Smoking-adjusted RRs. Excess mortality from all cancers (RR, 1.2*)

O, observed cases/deaths; E, expected cases/deaths; RR, relative risk; M, mortality; I, incidence; Leu, leukaemias; Lym, lymphomas; MM, multiple myeloma; NHL, non-Hodgkin's lymphoma; HD, Hodgkin's disease. Numbers in square brackets, calculated by the Working Group.

aRespiratory and intrathoracic neoplasms

*, $p < 0.05$

analysis, including barbers, hairdressers and cosmetologists. A possible reporting bias derives from the fact that occupations associated with an elevated cancer risk are more likely to be reported than those that are not.

(a) Bladder cancer

Wynder *et al*. (1963) carried out a case–control study of smoking habits and occupations among 300 male patients with bladder carcinoma and 300 hospital controls in New York City, USA, during the period 1957–61; 93% of cases and 82% of controls were smokers. Four of the patients (all smokers) and none of the controls had worked as hairdressers.

Dunham *et al*. (1968) compared the most recent occupations of 265 white, male patients with bladder cancer (mostly transitional-cell carcinomas) with those of 272 comparable controls in New Orleans, Louisiana, USA, during 1958–64. They found four barbers in the case group, while 1.45 were expected (OR, 2.76).

Anthony and Thomas (1970) interviewed 812 men and 218 women with bladder papillomas and carcinomas in Leeds, United Kingdom, in the period 1959–67; 47% had known smoking histories. Of several alternative analyses presented by the authors, the most reliable appears to be based upon a comparison of the male cases with a control group comprising cases of non-malignant surgical disease matched by sex, age and number of cigarettes smoked. Among the cases, four were hairdressers, of whom three had worked more than 20 years in the occupation; one control was a hairdresser. The ORs for bladder cancer among hairdressers were 4.1 (predominant occupation), 4.0 (occupation ever undertaken) and 3.0 (20 or more years in the occupation). None of the female cases was in a hairdresser (0.6 expected). None of the differences was significant.

Cole *et al*. (1972) studied occupation in a systematic sample of patients (356 men, 105 women) aged 20–89 with transitional- or squamous-cell carcinoma of the lower urinary tract in a defined population in Boston, Massachusetts, USA, during an 18-month period in 1967–68 (Cole *et al*., 1971). Controls were comparable with respect to age and sex. There was no increased risk for barbers (men: 4 observed cases, 7.2 expected; women: 1 observed case, 0.9 expected).

A hospital-based study of many types of cancer in males was conducted in Buffalo, New York, in the period 1956–65 (Viadana *et al*., 1976). In an unspecified number of cases of bladder cancer and controls out of a total of 11 591 white men, the RR for bladder cancer associated with occupation as a barber was 1.49 (five cases; $p > 0.05$). Restriction to those with five or more years of exposure (still five cases) increased the RR to 1.77 ($p > 0.05$).

Howe *et al*. (1980) reported a population-based study of all 480 men and 152 women with bladder cancer diagnosed in 1974–76 in three Canadian provinces and of individually matched controls. Among men, three cases but no control were barbers; and among women, two cases but no control were hairdressers.

Vineis and Magnani (1985) conducted a case–control study of 512 male cases of bladder cancer in northern Italy in the period 1978–83. An OR of 0.9 was recorded for barbers and hairdressers on the basis of nine cases (95% CI, 0.4–2.3).

Morrison *et al*. (1985) conducted case–control studies in 1976–78 of cancer of the lower urinary tract among men in Boston, USA, Manchester, United Kingdom, and Nagoya, Japan.

No increased risk was recorded among barbers in Boston (OR, 1.00; 90% CI, 0.4–2.6; seven cases); only two cases were recorded in Manchester and one in Nagoya.

Jensen *et al*. (1988) reported a case–control study on incident cases of renal pelvis and ureter cancer. Cases were identified from hospitals in the eastern part of Denmark in 1979–82, and a total of 97 patients were included, corresponding to some 80% of those eligible. Three matched hospital controls were selected for each case, excluding patients with urinary tract and smoking-related diseases. A personal interview was obtained for 94% of cases and controls. A total of 36 female cases and 108 controls were interviewed, of whom two in each group reported occupation as a hairdresser (OR, 3.0; 95% CI, 0.3–33.0). Data were not reported on occupation as a hairdresser among men.

Risch *et al*. (1988) carried out a case–control study of 826 male and female cases of bladder cancer in Canada in 1979–82. The OR among barbers or hairdressers was not increased (men, 0.66, 11 cases; women, 1.00, nine cases). No significant trend was noted with increasing duration of employment.

The US National Bladder Cancer study is a population-based case–control study carried out in 10 areas of the USA during 1977–78. In 2100 white male cases and 3874 population controls, an OR of 1.3 (95% CI, 0.8–2.3; 28 exposed cases) was found for hairdressers and barbers and an OR of 2.8 (95% CI, 0.7–11.6; seven exposed cases) was found for hairdressers alone (Silverman *et al*., 1989). For 652 white female bladder cancer patients and 1266 controls, an OR of 1.4 (95% CI, 0.7–2.9; 17 exposed cases) was found for hairdressers (Silverman *et al*., 1990).

(b) Lymphatic and haematopoietic cancers

In a case–control study in Sweden, Persson *et al*. (1989) recorded crude ORs in hairdressers of 2.6 (one case) for Hodgkin's disease and 1.3 (one case) for other lymphomas. The logistic odds ratios were 2.7 and 2.2, respectively. [The Working Group noted that the two sexes cannot be distinguished.]

A case–control study of 622 white male cases of non-Hodgkin's lymphoma and 1245 controls was carried out in Iowa and Minnesota, USA. Case identification was population based; for living cases, living population-based controls were selected, while for the deceased, dead controls were identified from state vital records. Employment in a barber-shop was associated with a 2.7-fold risk (95% CI, 0.9–8.7; six exposed cases). The occupation of barber/cosmetologist showed an OR of 2.1 (95% CI, 0.7–5.9; seven exposed cases) (Blair *et al*., 1993).

Four case–control studies on multiple myeloma analysed the risk among hairdressers or barbers. In a study from Sweden, cases diagnosed between 1973 and 1983 were collected as survivors into the period 1981–83; one case and one control were employed as hairdresssers (OR, 3.3; 95% CI, 0.24–45.7) (Flodin *et al*., 1987). In a study nested in a large American Cancer Society cohort, no case and four controls were classified as beauticians, cosmetologists or barbers (Boffetta *et al*., 1989). In another study from Sweden, of 256 cases and 256 population controls, two cases and three controls were employed as hairdressers or cosmetologists (OR, 0.67; 90% CI, 0.15–2.71) (Eriksson & Karlsson, 1992). Finally, in a study on the incidence of multiple melanoma among women in the Danish Cancer Registry, one case and six controls were classified as hairdressers (OR, 0.7; 95% CI, 0.0–5.8) (Pottern *et al.*, 1992).

A case–control study conducted in Tasmania, Australia, included 51 female cases of acute nonlymphoblastic leukaemia, 27 of chronic lymphoblastic leukaemia, 32 of Hodgkin's disease, 116 of non-Hodgkin's lymphoma and 59 of multiple myeloma diagnosed during 1972–80, as well as population controls. Five cases of non-Hodgkin's lymphoma and no control were employed as hairdressers (*p* < 0.05); all five cases had been employed for more than five years. For none of the remaining neoplasms was there a significant difference between cases and controls for employment as a hairdressr (Giles *et al.*, 1984).

(c) *Cancers at other sites*

Viadana *et al.* (1976) reported an increase in the incidence of laryngeal cancer among barbers in the study described on p. 74. Barbers had an age-adjusted OR of 2.83 for laryngeal cancer (10 cases); this excess persisted in men who had been barbers for five or more years (OR, 2.49; eight cases). The overall OR after adjustment for tobacco use was 3.39 (*p* < 0.05).

Osorio *et al.* (1986) noted a PIR of 1.44 for lung cancer among female cosmetologists aged 20–65 in the Los Angeles (USA) Tumor Registry in 1972–82, on the basis of 81 cases. In a case–control study of 50 cases and 56 non-pulmonary cancer controls, no occupational exposure factor was identified that could explain the lung cancer excess.

Koenig *et al.* (1991) carried out a case–control study of 398 women with breast cancer and 790 controls identified from the records of a multiphasic screening clinic in New York City, USA. They noted a three-fold excess (95% CI, 1.1–7.9) among beauticians with five or more years of exposure, on the basis of 12 cases.

(d) *Childhood cancer*

Kuijten *et al.* (1992) carried out a case–control study of astrocytoma diagnosed in children under 15 in the period 1980–86 in Pennsylvania, New Jersey and Delaware, USA. Controls were recruited by random-digit dialling and pair-matched with cases on age, race and telephone exchange. Mothers and fathers of cases and controls were interviewed separately by telephone. A total of 217 eligible cases were identified; a maternal occupational history was obtained for 163 case–control pairs (75%) and a paternal one for 158 pairs (73%). Of the 163 controls, 115 (71%) were the first eligible control identified. A complete occupational history was obtained for each parent. Maternal employment as a hairdresser in the period before conception was associated with an OR of 2.5 (95% CI, 0.4–26.2, seven discordant pairs), employment during pregnancy with an OR of 1.5 (95% CI, 0.2–18.0, five discordant pairs) and employment postnatally with an OR of 3.0 (95% CI, 0.2–157.7, four discordant pairs). [The Working Group noted that cases and controls could have been exposed during more than one period.]

Table 7. Occupational exposure: results of case-control studies on cancers at selected sites

Reference	Study population	Controls	Exposure	Control for smoking (when relevant)	Sex	Type of cancer	Exposed cases	Odds ratio	Comments
Bladder cancer									
Wynder et al. (1963)	300 male cases, 2 hospitals, New York, USA, 1957-61	Hospital controls	Ever employed as hairdresser	No	M		4	NR	No exposed control
Dunham et al. (1968)	265 male cases, hospital in New Orleans, USA, 1958-64	272 hospital controls	Employed as barber	No	M		4	2.76	NS
Anthony & Thomas (1970)	812 male, 218 female cases, Leeds, UK, 1959-67	Non-malignant surgical diseases (340 men, 50 women)	Hairdresser as predominant occupation	No	M		4	4.1	
Cole et al. (1972)	356 male, 105 female cases, Boston, USA, 1967-68	485 population controls	Ever employed as barber or hairdresser	No	M F		4 1	0.56	0.9 expected cases
Viadana et al. (1976)	Male cases, Buffalo, USA, 1956-65	Non-neoplastic hospital controls	Ever employed as barber	No	M		5	1.49	RR 1.77 for ≥ 5 years of employment
Howe et al. (1980)	480 male, 152 female cases, 3 Canadian provinces, 1974-76	480 male, 152 female neighbourhood controls	Ever employed as barber or hairdresser	No	M F		3 2		No exposed control of either sex
Gubéran et al. (1985)	18 male cases nested in a cohort of hairdressers in Geneva, Switzerland, 1970-80	54 cohort members	Duration of employment						Nonsignificant association with men's hairdressing, no association with women's hairdressing
Vineis & Magnani (1985)	512 male cases, Turin, Italy, 1978-83	596 hospital controls	Ever employed as barber or hairdresser	No	M		9	0.9	
Morrison et al. (1985)	430 male cases, Boston, USA, 1976-78	397 population controls	Employed as barber	Yes	M		7	1.00	
Morrison et al. (1985)	399 male cases, Manchester, UK, 1976-78	493 population controls	Employed as barber	No	M		2	[1.3]	
Morrison et al. (1985)	226 male cases, Nagoya, Japan, 1976-78	443 population controls	Employed as barber	No	M		1	[1.0]	

Table 7 (contd)

Reference	Study population	Controls	Exposure	Control for smoking (when relevant)	Sex	Type of cancer	Exposed cases	Odds ratio	Comments
Bladder cancer (contd)									
Risch et al. (1988)	826 male and female cases, Canada, 1979–82	792 population controls	Ever employed as barber or hairdresser	Yes	M F		11 9	0.66 1.00	No trend with duration of exposure in either sex
Silverman et al. (1989)	2100 white male cases, 10 US areas, 1977–78	3874 population controls	Ever employed as barber or hairdresser Ever employed as hairdresser	Yes	M M		28 7	1.3 2.8	
Silverman et al. (1990)	652 white female cases, 10 US areas, 1977–78	1266 population controls	Ever employed as hairdresser	Yes	F		17	1.4	
Lymphatic and haematopoietic neoplasms									
Persson et al. (1989)	54 HD and 106 NHL cases, hospital in Sweden, 1964–86	275 population controls	Employed as hairdresser		Both	HD NHL	1 1	2.7 2.2	Logistic odds ratio
Blair et al. (1993)	622 white male NHL cases, Iowa and Minnesota, USA 1980–83	1245 population controls	Ever employed in barbershop Ever employed as barber/cosmetologist		M M	NHL NHL	6 7	2.7 2.1	
Flodin et al. (1987)	131 MM cases, 6 hospitals in Sweden, 1981–83	431 population controls	Employed as hairdresser		Both	MM	1	3.3	Surviving cases included
Boffetta et al. (1989)	128 MM incident cases, American Cancer Society cohort, 1982–86	512 controls from the cohort	Employed as beautician, cosmetologist or barber		Both	MM	0	–	Four exposed controls
Eriksson & Karlsson (1992)	256 MM cases, northern Sweden, 1982–86	256 population controls	Employed as hairdresser or cosmetologist		Both	MM	2	0.7	
Potterm et al. (1992)	607 female MM cases, Denmark, 1970–84	2596 population controls	Most recent employment as hairdresser		F	MM	1	0.7	
Giles et al. (1984)	116 female NHL cases, Tasmania, Australia, 1972–80	Population controls	Employed as hairdresser		F	NHL	5	*	No exposed control
Giles et al. (1984)	32 female HD cases, Tasmania, Australia, 1972–80	Population controls	Employed as hairdresser		F	HD	2		No exposed control

Table 7 (contd)

Lymphatic and haematopoietic neoplasms (contd)

Reference	Study population	Controls	Exposure	Control for smoking (when relevant)	Sex	Type of cancer	Exposed cases	Odds ratio	Comments
Giles et al. (1984)	51 female ANLL cases, Tasmania, Australia, 1972–80	Population controls	Employed as hair-dresser		F	ANLL	1		No exposed control
Giles et al. (1984)	27 female CLL cases, Tasmania, Australia, 1972–80	Population controls	Employed as hair-dresser		F	CLL	0	–	No exposed control
Giles et al. (1984)	59 female MM cases, Tasmania, Australia, 1972–80	Population controls	Employed as hair-dresser		F	MM	0	–	One exposed control

NR, not reported; NS, not significant; RR, relative risk; HD, Hodgkin's disease; NHL, non-Hodgkin's lymphoma; MM, multiple myeloma; ANLL, acute nonlymphocytic leukaemias; CLL, chronic lymphocytic leukaemias. Numbers in square brackets, calculated by the Working Group

$*p < 0.05$

2.2 Use of hair colourants

2.2.1 *Cohort studies* (Table 8)

Hennekens *et al.* (1979) carried out a cross-sectional postal questionnaire survey in 1976 on 172 413 married female nurses, aged 30–55, in 11 US states whose names appeared in the 1972 register of the American Nurses' Association. Of the 120 557 responders, 38 459 reported some use of permanent hair dyes; of these, 773 had been diagnosed as having a cancer. The risk ratio for the association of cancers at all sites with hair-dye use (at any time) was 1.10 ($p = 0.02$). When 16 cancer sites were examined separately, significant associations with permanent hair-dye use were found for cancer of the cervix uteri (RR, 1.44; $p < 0.001$) and for cancer of the vagina and vulva (RR, 2.58; $p = 0.02$). These associations were reduced but remained significant after adjustment for smoking habits. There was no consistent trend of cancer risk with increasing interval from first use of hair dyes, although women who had used permanent dyes 21 years or more before the onset of cancer had a significant increase in risk for cancers at all sites combined (RR, 1.38 adjusted for smoking; $p = 0.02$), largely because of an excess of breast cancers (RR, 1.48), which, however, was balanced by a decrease of similar magnitude 16–20 years before the onset of cancer. Analyses of cases of cancer that had occurred only after 1972 (the year the study population was defined from the nurses' register) and were reported by surviving cases in 1976 yielded essentially the same results, thus indicating that self-selection for the study, early retirement and loss from the professional register were not sources of bias in the study. [The Working Group noted the low response rate and the fact that information on both cancer and exposure to hair dyes was derived from participants.]

Green *et al.* (1987) examined hair dye use in relation to breast cancer in a follow-up study of a subgroup of the population described above, comprising 118 404 nurses who had no cancer in 1976 and were followed up to 1982. No relationship was detected: the rate ratio for ever use was 1.1 (95% CI, 0.9–1.2), on the basis of 353 cases, compared to 505 for never use. The risk for breast cancer did not increase with frequency or duration of use.

2.2.2 *Case–control studies* (Table 9)

The Working Group systematically reviewed studies dealing with exposures of cases of cancer of the urinary bladder and breast (sites that have been studied extensively), lymphatic and haematopoietic neoplasms and childhood cancer. No systematic review was made of studies of other cancer sites.

(*a*) *Cancers of the urinary bladder and renal pelvis*

Lockwood (1961) performed a case–control study of bladder tumours in Copenhagen, Denmark. All patients diagnosed with bladder tumours from 1942 until 1 March 1956 and able to be interviewed in 1956–57 were eligible for inclusion. Of the 428 patients, 369 (282 men) were interviewed, together with 369 population controls (282 men) selected from the electoral rolls and matched for sex, age, marital status, occupation and residence and interviewed in 1956–59. Later in the study, a question on use of brilliantine was added, and this question was answered by 51% of the male and female patients and by 93% of male and 80% of female controls. The crude OR for brilliantine use, relative to those reporting no use,

Table 8. Hair dye users: Results of cohort studies on cancers at selected sites

Reference	Study population	Sex	Breast cancer			Bladder cancer			Lymphatic and haema-topoietic neoplasms				Comments
			O	E	RR	O	E	RR	Type	O	E	RR	
Hennekens et al. (1979)	120 557 female nurses, aged 30–55, 11 US states, active in 1972, follow-up (I), 1972–76	F	270	258.2	1.06	5	7.4	0.62	Lym	10	15.7	0.59	30% non-respondents; similar results after adjustment for smoking; excess of breast cancer for hair dye use ≥ 21 years before cancer; excess for all cancer sites (1.10*), cervix (1.44*) and lower genital tract (2.58*)
Green et al. (1987)	1976–82 follow-up (M) of 118 404 nurses enrolled in the study above	F	353		1.1								No trend with duration of use

M, mortality; I, cancer incidence; Lym, lymphomas
*, $p < 0.05$

was [1.7] for men (51 exposed patients [95% CI, 1.1–2.6]) and [1.1] for women (two exposed patients [95% CI, 0.2–6.6]). [The Working Group noted that the reported data do not allow control for age or tobacco smoking and that the cases were surviving patients.]

In the study reported on p. 74, Dunham et al. (1968) compared 132 cases of bladder cancer with 136 controls for history of 'use of tonics, lotions and other preparations for the hair and scalp'. The percentage of cases who used such preparations (32%) was slightly lower than that of controls (36%).

Jain et al. (1977) reported (in a letter) data on hair-dye use among 107 patients with bladder cancer and an equal number of sex- and age-matched controls in Canada. All male controls had benign prostatic hypertrophy, and all female controls had stress incontinence. The OR for bladder cancer in association with any exposure to hair dyes (based on 19 pairs discordant for use of hair dye) was 1.1 (95% CI, 0.41–3.03). [The Working Group noted that the choice of controls was unusually limited.]

Neutel et al. (1978) reported (in a letter) data on hair-dye use in a subset of 50 case–control pairs (matched by sex and 10-year age group) re-interviewed after a previous, larger case–control study of bladder cancer in Canada. Use of hair dyes was reported by 18 cases and 19 controls. Frequent use of hair dyes and hairdressing as an occupation, however, were said to show protective effects (the former being significant, $p < 0.01$) against bladder cancer, although the numbers on which these statements were based are not given in the report.

In the study described on p. 74, Howe et al. (1980) found that eight male cases (including two of the barbers) and no male control had a history of personal use of hair dyes ($p = 0.004$, one-tailed test); only one of them had used hair dyes for more than six years before diagnosis of bladder cancer. There was no evidence in women of an increased risk for bladder cancer associated with personal use of hair dyes (OR, 0.7; 95% CI, 0.3–1.4 for ever versus never use).

Hartge et al. (1982) examined hair dye use among participants in the US National Bladder Cancer Study (see p. 75) in a case–control study of bladder cancer involving 2982 incident cases and 5782 controls, of which 615 cases and 1164 controls had ever dyed their hair. The overall ORs for hair dye users were 1.1 (95% CI 0.9–1.4) among men and 0.9 (0.8–1.1) among women. No trend with frequency or duration of use was seen in people of either sex. Use of black hair dye was associated with elevated ORs in both men and women; the OR was of borderline significance for the two sexes combined (1.4; 95% CI, 1.0–1.9; 68 exposed cases).

Ohno et al. (1985) conducted a case–control study of 65 female bladder cancer patients in Nagoya, Japan, in the period 1976–78. Hair dye use was associated with an increased RR among those who smoked but not among non-smokers. There was a positive relationship between smoking and hair dye use more than once a month; after adjustment for smoking, no significant effect of hair dyes remained (RR, 1.7; 95% CI, 0.82–3.52; 22 exposed cases).

A matched case–control study was carried out by Claude et al. (1986) of 340 men and 91 women with bladder cancer in Lower Saxony, Germany, in the period 1977–82. It was stated that no association with hair dye use was found, but details were not provided.

Nomura et al. (1989) carried out a case–control study among 137 Caucasian and 124 Japanese cases of cancer of the lower urinary tract in Hawaii (USA) and two population-based controls for each case, in the period 1977–86. A weak, nonsignificant association with hair dye use was found for both men and women, but there was no positive trend with increasing duration of use.

(b)   Breast cancer

Shafer and Shafer (1976) reported that, of 100 consecutive breast cancer patients seen in a clinical practice in New York, USA, 87% had been long-term users of hair colouring agents, compared with 26% of age-comparable controls, who were regular users of permanent hair dyes over prolonged periods. [The Working Group noted the dissimilarity of the exposure definitions for the two groups and that no information was provided on the number of controls nor the manner of eliciting information on use of hair dyes.]

Kinlen et al. (1977) reported a study of 191 breast cancer patients interviewed in hospital in 1975 and 1976 in Oxford, United Kingdom, and 561 controls without cancer, matched to the patients by age (within three years), marital status and social class. Seventy-three cases and 213 controls had used permanent or semi-permanent hair dyes, giving an OR of 1.01. There was no evidence of an increasing risk for breast cancer with increasing duration of use of hair dyes or with use beginning more than four or more than nine years before diagnosis. Stratification by age at first pregnancy showed a deficit of cases in which hair-dye use was reported among women whose first pregnancy occurred at ages 15–19 (33.3% of cases used hair dyes, compared with 64.7% of controls) and an excess of cases with use of hair dyes among women whose first pregnancy had occurred at 30 years of age or older (38.3% of cases and 25.5% of controls). There were two hairdressers among cases (1.0%) and 10 among controls (1.8%).

Shore et al. (1979) compared the hair-dye use of 129 breast cancer patients and 193 control subjects aged 25 and over identified from the records of a multiphasic screening clinic in New York City, USA. Adjusted ORs for use of permanent hair dyes for 0, 5, 10 and 15 years were, respectively, 1.08, 1.31, 1.58 and 1.44 (none significantly different from 1.0). A significant relationship ($p = 0.01$) was noted between a measure of cumulative hair-dye use (number of years times frequency per year) and breast cancer. This relationship also held if the analysis was limited to cases in which the patient herself had responded to the telephone interview. Among women who had used hair dyes 10 years before developing breast cancer, the relationship held only for women at 'low risk' (as assessed from the distribution of a multivariate confounder score) and for those 50–79 years old. [The Working Group noted that use of a multivariate confounder score for the control of confounding may produce misleading results.]

In order to follow up these findings, Koenig et al. (1991) carried out a case–control study of 398 women with breast cancer and 790 controls identified at the same screening centre. For ever use, the adjusted OR was 0.8 (95% CI, 0.6–1.1), and there was no trend with increased use.

Stavraky et al. (1979) compared 50 breast cancer cases at a cancer treatment centre with 100 hospitalized controls in London, Ontario, and 35 breast cancer cases with 70 neighbourhood controls in Toronto, Ontario, with respect to hair-dye use. The ORs for breast cancer from use of permanent hair dyes (at any time) were 1.3 (95% CI, 0.6–2.5) in London and 1.1 (0.5–2.4) in Toronto. Further statistical analyses, allowing for smoking habits, family history of cancer and age at first birth, showed no significant relationship between hair-dye use and breast cancer incidence.

Nasca et al. (1980) reported a study of 118 patients with breast cancer and 233 controls matched to the patients by age and county of residence (115 matched triplets and three matched pairs) in Upper State New York, USA. In the study overall, there was no significant association between breast cancer and use of permanent or semi-permanent dyes (OR, 1.11), nor was an increase in risk seen with increasing numbers of times hair dyes were used or increasing time since first use. The authors commented that women who dyed their hair to change its colour, as distinct from those who dyed their hair to mask greyness, had a significantly increased risk for breast cancer (OR, 3.13; 95% CI, 1.50–6.54). In this group, there was a significant trend towards increasing risk with increasing numbers of exposures to hair dyes. Examination of risk for hair-dye use in subgroups of women defined by other risk factors for breast cancer showed an OR of 4.5 (95% CI, 1.20–16.78) for women with a past history of benign breast disease, an OR of 1.75 ($p = 0.03$, one-tailed test) for 12 or more years of schooling and an OR of 3.33 (95% CI, 1.10–10.85) for women aged 40–49 years; the OR was near unity for all other age groups. These effects appeared to be independent of one another and were not explained by confounding by past pregnancy, age at first pregnancy, history of artificial menopause or age at menarche. The authors stressed that the associations observed in the subgroups should be considered newly generated hypotheses requiring further testing. In a larger, subsequent study (Nasca et al., 1990) (reported as an abstract) of 1617 cases of breast cancer in New York State and 1617 controls, they found no relationship with hair-dye use (OR, 1.04; 95% CI, 0.90–1.21), no significant difference in the ORs for women with a history of benign breast disease (1.15; 95% CI, 0.86–1.53) and those without (0.98; 95% CI, 0.83–1.16) and no association with duration of hair-dye use.

Wynder and Goodman (1983) carried out a hospital-based case–control study of 401 cases of breast cancer in New York City in 1979–81. No association was found with hair-dye use (OR, 1.02; 95% CI, 0.78–1.32) and there was no dose–response relationship.

(c)   Lymphatic and haematopoietic cancers

In a further report of the study of Stavraky et al. (1979) in Canada, p. 83, Stavraky et al. (1981) found no significant increase in risk for leukaemia or lymphoma (70 cases). [The Working Group noted that it was not possible to distinguish different haematopoietic malignancies.]

In a hospital-based case–control study (101 matched pairs) of acute non-lymphocytic leukaemia in the Baltimore (USA) area, published only as an abstract, Markowitz et al. (1985) found a significant positive association with hair-dye use (OR, 3.1). There was, however, no difference between regular use (at least once a year) (OR, 2.7) and less frequent use (OR, 2.2) [95% confidence intervals not presented].

Cantor et al. (1988) carried out a population-based case–control study of hair-dye use among 578 men with leukaemia, 622 with non-Hodgkin's lymphoma and 1245 population controls in Iowa and Minnesota, USA, in 1980–83. Significantly raised ORs were found for leukaemia (1.8; 95% CI, 1.1–2.7) and for non-Hodgkin's lymphoma (2.0; 1.3–3.0) in association with personal use or other potential exposure to hair tints, any hair colouring product or hair dyes. The authors stated that the ORs were not substantially changed after exclusion of the 10 men with other potential exposure to hair colouring products (e.g., occupational exposure), but detailed results were not presented. [The Working Group noted that, although the authors suggested an increased risk with increasing extent of hair dye use, an examination of the paper could not verify this.]

A population-based case–control study carried out in eastern Nebraska, USA, during 1983–86 investigated use of hair colouring products among a total of 201 male and 184 female cases of non-Hodgkin's lymphoma, 35 male and 35 female cases of Hodgkin's disease, 32 male and 40 female cases of multiple myeloma, 37 male and 19 female cases of chronic lymphocytic leukaemia and 725 male and 707 female residential controls who could be interviewed (Zahm *et al.*, 1992). Telephone interviews were conducted with cases, controls or their next of kin; response rates were 81–96% for cases and 84% for controls. Among women, use of any hair colouring product was associated with an increased risk for non-Hodgkin's lymphoma (OR, 1.5; 95% CI, 1.1–2.2), Hodgkin's disease (1.7; 0.7–4.0) and multiple myeloma (1.8; 0.9–3.7), and women who used permanent hair dyes had high ORs for all three neoplasms (non-Hodgkin's lymphoma, 1.7, 1.1–2.8; Hodgkin's disease, 3.0, 1.1–7.9; and multiple myeloma, 2.8, 1.1–7.1; all $p < 0.05$). For non-Hodgkin's lymphoma and multiple myeloma, the risks were highest among women who used dark permanent dyes. Long duration and early age at first use tended to increase the risk, but the patterns were not consistent. Among men, use of any hair colouring product was associated with nonsignificantly increased ORs for Hodgkin's disease (1.7) and multiple myeloma (1.8), on the basis of three and four exposed cases, respectively; no increase was found for non-Hodgkin's lymphoma (0.8). Use of any hair dye was not associated with chronic lymphocytic leukaemia in either women or men (1.0).

A population-based case–control study of 173 white men with multiple myeloma and 650 controls was carried out in Iowa, USA. The risk for multiple myeloma was significantly elevated (OR, 1.9; 95% CI, 1.0–3.6; 14 exposed cases) among users of hair dyes. For men who had used hair dyes for one year or more at a frequency or one or more times per month, the OR was 4.3 (95% CI, 0.9–19.7; four exposed cases) (Brown *et al.*, 1992).

(d)   Cancers at other sites

Stavraky *et al.* (1981) (see p. 84) found no significant increase in crude or adjusted risks for cancer of the cervix (38 cases), cancer of the ovary (58 cases), cancer of the lung (70 cases), cancers of the kidney and bladder (35 cases) or endometrial cancers (36 cases) among ever users of hair colouring agents in either Toronto or London, Ontario.

Holman and Armstrong (1983) examined hair dye use in a population-based case–control study of 511 patients with malignant melanoma and individually matched controls in Western Australia in 1980–81. No relationship was found with ever use of permanent hair dyes. The ORs obtained from a conditional logistic regression analysis with adjustment for solar exposure, reaction to sunlight and hair colour (Armstrong & Holman, 1985), for 86 cases of Hutchinson's melanotic freckle associated with use of semi-permanent and temporary dyes were: never used, 1.00; used 1–9 times, 1.5 (95% CI, 0.3–6.8); used ≥ 10 times, 3.3 (1.0–11.5; *p* for trend, 0.05). The OR for Hutchinson's melanotic freckle in relation to use of permanent dyes was not elevated. [The Working Group noted that the number of exposed subjects was not reported.]

Østerlind et al. (1988a,b) found a negative association with use of permanent or semi-permanent hair dyes among women with malignant melanoma in Denmark in 1982–85 (OR for hair dye use, 0.6; 95% CI, 0.5–0.9; 136 exposed cases). Cases of Hutchinson's melanotic freckle were not included in this population-based study.

Ahlbom et al. (1986) carried out a case–control study in Stockholm and Uppsala, Sweden, of 78 patients with astrocytoma diagnosed in 1980–81, 197 hospital controls (with meningioma, pituitary adenoma or cerebral aneurysm) and 92 population controls. The ORs for the 23 astrocytoma patients who had dyed their hair were 0.8 (95% CI, 0.4–1.8) in relation to 83 hospital controls and 1.5 (0.6–3.7) when compared with 46 population controls who had dyed their hair.

Burch et al. (1987) found that significantly more adults with brain cancer diagnosed in Canada in 1977–81 than hospital controls reported having used hair dye or hair spray (OR, 1.96; $p = 0.013$; 43/22 discordant pairs).

Spitz et al. (1990) examined hair-dye use in a case–control study of 37 male and 27 female patients with salivary gland cancer in Texas, USA, in the period 1985–89. Controls were patients with other malignancies. Among ever users of hair dyes, an increased OR was found for women (OR, 4.1; 95% CI, 1.5–11.5; 14 cases). There was no difference between female cases and controls with respect to frequency of use, except that the OR for use for more than 15 years (OR, 3.5; 95% CI, 0.9–12.8) was higher than that for shorter duration of use (2.3; 0.9–6.2).

(e)   Childhood cancer

Kramer et al. (1987) reported a matched case–control study of maternal exposures during pregnancy and neuroblastoma diagnosed during the period 1970–79 in the Greater Delaware Valley, USA. Of the 181 cases identified, 139 met the eligibility criteria, and interviews were completed with 104 case families (75%). Control subjects were selected by random-digit dialling and were matched with cases on age, race and the first five digits of their telephone number at the time of diagnosis; the response rate among those eligible was 57% (101 of 177). In addition, the authors compared 86 patients who had at least one sibling with a randomly selected sibling. Mothers were asked about six main exposures, specified for hypothesis testing, and about a variety of other exposures, including the use of hair colouring products. The OR associated with maternal exposure to hair dye was 3.00 (90% CI, 1.64–5.48; one-sided p value 0.002; 36 discordant pairs) in comparison with controls selected by telephone and 2.20 (90% CI, 0.93–5.22; one-sided p value 0.07; 16 discordant pairs) in comparison with siblings.

Bunin et al. (1987) did a case–control study of Wilms' tumour diagnosed in children under 15 during the period 1970–83 in the Greater Philadelphia (USA) area in relation to use of hair dyes by their mothers during pregnancy. Of 152 white cases, 28 were ineligible for a variety of reasons. Interviews were completed with the parents of 88 (71%) of the 124 eligible cases and 88 of 159 (55%) controls, on average 10 years after the relevant pregnancy. For Wilms' tumour overall, the OR associated with maternal hair dye use was 3.6 (95% CI, 1.4–10.2, based on 32 discordant pairs). A total of 68 cases could be classified as 'genetic' (26 cases) (if they were bilateral or had nephroblastomatosis) or 'nongenetic' (42 cases) (if they were unilateral without nephroblastomatosis or a Wilms' tumour-associated congenital anomaly). The OR associated with maternal use of hair colouring agents was 5.5 (95% CI, 1.0–71.9; on the basis of 13 discordant pairs out of 42) for nongenetic cases and 3.3 (0.7–22.1; on the basis of 13 out of 26 discordant pairs) for genetic cases. The ORs associated with exposure to hair dyes were similar for an interval of 2–10 years and an interval of 11–24 years between pregnancy and interview.

Kuijten et al. (1990), in an earlier report of the study of Kuitjen et al. (1992) (p. 76), found no association between astrocytoma and maternal use of hair-colouring products during pregnancy (OR, 0.9; 95% 0.4–1.8; 37 discordant pairs).

3. Studies of Cancer in Experimental Animals

3.1 Skin application

3.1.1 *Mouse*

Groups of 50 male and 50 female Swiss Webster mice, six to eight weeks old, received applications of one of three oxidation (permanent) hair dye formulations, PP-7588, PP-7586 or PP-7585 (all three formulations contained 2,5-toluenediamine sulfate, *para*-phenylene-diamine and resorcinol; PP-7586 also contained 2,4-diaminoanisole sulfate, PP-7585 con-tained *meta*-phenylenediamine and PP-7588 contained 2,4-toluenediamine), mixed with an equal volume of 6% hydrogen peroxide just prior to use; 0.05 ml of the mixture in acetone was applied to the shaved skin of the mid-scapular region. Controls were given acetone or were left untreated. For each formulation and for the vehicle control, one group was treated once weekly and another group once every other week for 18 months. Survival at 18 months varied from 58 to 80%. No sign of systemic toxicity was found in any of the dye-treated groups. Average body weights were comparable in all groups throughout the study. The incidence of lung tumours was not statistically different between treated and control groups. No skin tumour was observed at the site of application (Burnett et al., 1975).

Groups of 26 male and 22 female DBAf and 26 male and 26 female strain A mice, six to seven weeks old, received skin applications of 0.4 ml (reduced to 0.2 ml at 24 weeks for DBAf mice) of a 10% solution of a commercially available semi-permanent hair dye ('GS'), containing, among other constituents, 1,4-diamino-2-nitrobenzene (2-nitro-*para*-phenylene-diamine) and 1,2-diamino-4-nitrobenzene (4-nitro-*ortho*-phenylenediamine), in 50% aqueous acetone twice a week on the clipped dorsal skin. Groups of 16 male and 16 female control mice of each strain received applications of acetone alone. When the experiment was terminated at 80 weeks, four lymphomas and six tumours of the reproductive tract (four ovarian cystadenomas and two uterine fibrosarcomas) had developed in the 22 treated female DBAf mice within 37–80 weeks and one lymphoma at week 26 among the 26 treated males. In control DBAf mice, one lymphoma and one lung adenoma were found in females and one hepatoma in males. No difference was observed in the incidence of lymphomas or liver or lung tumours between treated and control strain A mice. No skin tumour at the site of application was observed in either strain. Of the treated animals, 27 DBAf mice and 32 strain A mice survived 60–80 weeks without tumours (Searle & Jones, 1977). [The Working Group noted the small number of animals used in the study.]

Table 9. Hair colourant users: results of case–control studies on cancers at selected sites

Reference	Study population	Controls (case: control ratio)	Exposure	Sex	Type of cancer	Exposed cases	Odds ratio	Comments
Bladder cancer								
Lockwood (1961)	282 male and 87 female cases, Copenhagen, Denmark, 1942–56	Population controls (1:1)	Use of brilliantine	M F		51 2	[1.7*] [1.1]	
Dunham et al. (1968)	132 male cases, hospital in New Orleans, USA, 1958–64	136 hospital controls	Use of tonics, lotions and other preparations for hair and scalp	M		42	[0.9]	
Howe et al. (1980)	480 male, 152 female cases, 3 Canadian provinces, 1974–76	Neighbourhood controls (1:1)	Use of hair dye	F M		NR 8	0.7 *	No exposed male control
Hartge et al. (1982)	2249 male and 733 female cases, 10 US areas, 1977–78	4282 male and 1500 female population controls	Use of hair dye	M F		172 443	1.1 0.9	No trend with frequency or duration in either sex
Ohno et al. (1985)	65 female cases, Nagoya, Japan, 1976–78	143 population controls	Use of hair dye	F		[42]	[1.6]	RRs higher among smokers Crude 10.0* for < 1/month, 25.0* for ≥ 1/month Adjusted for smoking 1.3 for < 1/month 1.7 for ≥ 1/month
Claude et al. (1986)	340 male cases, 91 female cases, northern Germany, 1977–82	Hospital controls (1:1)	Use of hair dye	Both				No association
Nomura et al. (1989)	195 male, 66 female cases, Hawaii, USA, 1977–86	Population controls (2:1)	Use of hair dye	M F		15 41	1.3 1.5	No trend with duration of exposure for either sex
Breast cancer								
Shafer & Shafer (1976)	100 cases, New York, USA	No information	Use of hair dye	F		87	[19]	Limited reporting
Kinlen et al. (1977)	191 cases, Oxford, UK, 1975–76	561 hospital controls	Use of permanent or semi-permanent hair dye	F		73	1.01	No trend with duration of use

Table 9 (contd)

Reference	Study population	Controls (case: control ratio)	Exposure	Sex	Type of cancer	Exposed cases	Odds ratio	Comments
Breast cancer (contd)								
Shore et al. (1979)	129 cases, New York, USA, screening centre, 1964–76	193 clinic controls	Use of permanent hair dye	F		[43]	1.08	Higher RRs for use ≥ 5 years (1.31), ≥ 10 years (1.58) or ≥ 15 years (1.44) before diagnosis. Signifi-cant association with cumu-lative hair dye exposure
Stavraky et al. (1979)	50 cases, London, Canada, 1976–< 1979	Hospital controls (2:1)	Use of permanent hair dye	F		28	1.3	
	35 cases, Toronto, Canada, 1976–< 1979	Neighbourhood controls (2:1)	Use of permanent hair dye	F		16	1.1	
Nasca et al. (1980)	118 cases, 3 counties in New York State, USA, 1975–76	233 random-digit dialling controls	Use of permanent or semi-permanent hair dye	F		NR	1.11	No trend with frequency of use or latency. Excess for use of hair dye to change colour (3.1*).
Wynder & Goodman (1983)	401 cases, New York, USA, 1979–81	625 cancer controls	Use of hair dye	F		267	1.02	No dose–response relation-ship
Koenig et al. (1991)	398 cases, New York, USA, screening centre, 1977–81	790 screening centre controls	Use of hair dye	F		294	0.8	No trend with number of uses
Lymphatic and haematopoietic neoplasms								
Stavraky et al. (1981)	45 female cases, Toronto, Canada, 1976–< 1979	Neighbourhood controls (2:1)	Use of permanent or semi-permanent dye	F	All		0.7	
	25 female cases, London, Canada, 1976–< 1979	Hospital controls (2:1)	Use of permanent or semi-permanent dye	F	All		1.2	
Cantor et al. (1988)	578 male cases of leukemia and 622 male NHL cases, Iowa and Minnesota, USA, 1980–83	1245 population controls	Use of hair tints, colouring products or dyes	M M	Leu NHL	43 53	1.8* 2.0*	
Zahm et al. (1992)	201 male and 184 female NHL cases, Nebraska, USA, 1983–86	725 male and 707 female population controls	Use of any hair dye	F M	NHL NHL	106 11	1.5* 0.8	ORs higher among women using permanent dark hair dye. No trend with dura-tion or frequency of use of permanent hair dye
			Use of permanent hair dye	F	NHL	41	1.7*	

Table 9 (contd)

Lymphatic and haematopoietic neoplasms (contd)

Reference	Study population	Controls (case: control ratio)	Exposure	Sex	Type of cancer	Exposed cases	Odds ratio	Comments
Zahm *et al.* (1992) (contd)	35 male and 35 female HD cases, Nebraska, USA, 1983–86	725 male and 707 female population controls	Use of any hair dye Use of permanent hair dye	F M F	HD HD HD	16 3 12	1.7* 1.7 3.0*	Trend with duration and not with frequency of use of permanent hair dye
	32 male and 40 female MM cases, Nebraska, USA, 1983–86	725 male and 707 female population controls	Use of any hair dye Use of permanent hair dye	F M F	MM MM MM	24 4 11	1.8 1.8 2.8*	ORs higher among women using permanent dark hair dye. Trend with duration and frequency of use of permanent hair dye
	37 male and 19 female CLL cases, Nebraska, USA, 1983–86	725 male and 707 female population controls	Use of any hair dye Use of permanent hair dye	F M F	CLL CLL CLL	9 3 2	1.0 1.0 0.8	
Brown *et al.* (1992)	173 white male MM cases, Iowa, USA, 1981–84	650 population controls	Use of hair dye	M	MM	14	1.9	Higher OR for high frequency

NR, not reported; RR, relative risk; Leu, leukaemia; NHL, non-Hodgkin's lymphoma; OR, odds ratio; HD, Hodgkin's disease; MM, multiple myeloma; CLL, chronic lymphocytic leukaemia. Numbers in square brackets, calculated by the Working Group

*$p < 0.05$

In the same study, groups of 17 male and 15 female DBAf and 16 male and 16 female strain A mice, six to seven weeks old, received skin aplications of 0.4 ml (reduced to 0.2 ml at 24 weeks for DBAf mice) of a 10% solution of a commercially available semi-permanent hair dye ('RB'), containing, among other constituents, 4-amino-2-nitrophenol and CI Acid Black 107, in 50% aqueous acetone twice a week on the clipped dorsal skin. The experiment was terminated at 80 weeks. No significant difference was observed in the incidence of tumours at any site between treated and control animals of either strain, and no skin tumour at the site of application was observed in either strain (Searle & Jones, 1977). [The Working Group noted the small number of animals used in the study.]

Groups of 60 male and 60 female Swiss Webster mice, eight weeks of age, received topical applications of a semi-permanent hair dye formulation (7611) containing 0.15% 2-amino-5-nitrophenol, 0.11% 4-amino-2-nitrophenol, 0.85% 2-nitro-*para*-phenylene-diamine, 0.30% CI Solvent Blue 6, 0.95% CI Solvent Blue 7, 0.06% CI Solvent Blue 16, 0.45% CI Solvent Blue 18, 0.35% CI Solvent Orange 9, 0.15% CI Solvent Red 26, 0.11% CI Solvent Green 3, 0.76% CI Basic Orange 1, 0.50% CI Basic Blue 3, 0.15% CI Basic Blue 47, 0.12% CI Basic Red 2, 0.10% CI Basic Violet 1, 0.10% CI Basic Violet 2, 0.10% CI Basic Violet 13, 0.15% CI Basic Violet 14, 2.76% hydroxyethyl cellulose, 7.78% phenoxyethanol, 5.00% ethoxydiglycol, 4.60% Amphoteric 1, 4.60% Polysorbate 20, 4.12% propylene glycol, 2.70% methacrylamide, 0.42% Quarternium 4 and 0.41% tetrasodium EDTA in water. The formulation was applied at 0.05 ml/mouse three times a week for 20 months to a 1-cm^2 area of clipped shaved skin. Control animals were shaved only and received no treatment. Body weights of treated animals were depressed by no more than 10% of those of controls; all mice survived until termination of the experiment. The incidences of liver haemangiomas, lung adenomas and malignant lymphomas, which occur spontaneously in this strain of mice, were no greater than in controls. No skin tumour was observed at the site of application (Jacob *et al.*, 1984).

3.1.2 *Rat*

Groups of 50 male and 50 female Sprague-Dawley rats, about 14 weeks of age, received topical applications of 0.5 ml of permanent hair dye mixtures containing either 4% *para*-toluenediamine or 3% *para*-toluenediamine, 0.75% resorcinol and 0.75% *meta*-diamino-anisole in vehicle solution (4% Tylose HT, 0.5% sodium sulfite, 8.5–13% ammonia (25%), 3.7% ammonium sulfate or as formed by neutralization and deionized water to 100.0%), with 6% hydrogen peroxide added, immediately before use, on a 3-cm^2 area of shaved dorsal skin twice a week for two years. The animals were then observed for a further six months. Control groups of 25 males and 25 females of the same strain and age received topical applications of 0.5 ml vehicle alone, to which 6% hydrogen peroxide was added immediately before use. Another group of 50 males and 50 females of the same strain served as untreated controls. No difference in survival was observed between treated, vehicle and untreated control groups. Skin at the application site, liver, kidney, lung and gross lesions were studied histologically. No skin tumour was observed at the site of application, and there was no significant difference in the incidence of tumours, including those of the skin, between treated, vehicle control and untreated control groups (Kinkel & Holzmann, 1973). [The Working Group noted the limited histopathology undertaken in the study.]

Groups of 10 male and 10 female Wistar rats, weighing 120–140 g, received topical applications of 0.5 ml oxidized *para*-phenylenediamine (1:1 mixture of 5% *para*-phenylene-diamine in 2% ammonium hydroxide) and 6% hydrogen peroxide on shaved dorsal skin once a week for 18 months. Control rats were shaved and treated with the vehicle. Treated and control groups did not differ significantly in body weight gain or survival. All surviving rats were killed after 21 months. Treated rats had a significantly increased incidence of mammary tumours (5/10; $p < 0.05$ [incidental tumour test]) in comparison with female vehicle controls (0/9). The first mammary tumour observed was a fibrosarcoma, which occurred at week 47; the others were three adenomas and one fibroadenoma. No skin tumour was observed at the site of application (Rojanapo *et al.*, 1986). [The Working Group noted the small number of animals used in this study and the fact that only selected organs were examined histo-logically.]

Groups of 60 male and 60 female Sprague-Dawley rats, six to eight weeks of age, received topical applications of an oxidative hair dye formulation (7406) containing 0.5% 2-amino-5-nitrophenol, 4.0% *para*-phenylenediamine, 0.7% *para*-aminophenol, 2.0% 4-chlororesorcinol, 5.0% oleic acid, 15.0% isopropanol, 0.2% sodium sulfite, 6.0% ammonia and water to 100%. The formulation was diluted in an equal volume of 6% hydrogen peroxide before application, and 0.5 ml were applied to a shaved area of the back (approximately 2.5 cm in diameter) twice a week up to week 117. Three separate, similarly treated, concurrent control groups of 60 rats received applications of vehicle alone. Mean body weights and survival were similar in treated and control groups. No skin tumour was observed. The incidence of pituitary adenomas was increased in females in comparison with all three control groups (45/51 *versus* 34/50, 36/51 and 35/50; $p < 0.05$, χ^2 test) (Burnett & Goldenthal, 1988).

In the same study, groups of 60 male and female Sprague-Dawley rats, six to eight weeks of age, received topical applications of an oxidative hair dye formulation (7405) containing 0.4% 2-amino-4-nitrophenol, 6.0% 2,5-diaminoanisole sulfate, 2.0% resorcinol, 0.3% *ortho*-aminophenol, 5.0% oleic acid, 3.0% isopropanol, 0.2% sodium sulfite, 6.0% ammonia (29%) and water to 100%. The formulation was diluted in an equal volume of 6% hydrogen peroxide, and 0.5 ml were applied to a shaved area of the back (approximately 2.5 cm in diameter) twice a week up to week 117. Mean body weights and survival were similar in treated and control groups. No skin tumour was observed, and no increase in the incidence of tumours at any site was observed in treated as compared with control animals (Burnett & Goldenthal, 1988).

In the same study, groups of 60 male and female Sprague-Dawley rats, six to eight weeks of age, received topical applications of an oxidative hair dye formulation (7401) containing 1.1% 1,4-diamino-2-nitrobenzene (2-nitro-*para*-phenylenediamine), 3.0% *para*-phenylene-diamine, 2.0% 2,4-diaminoanisole sulfate, 1.7% resorcinol, 5.0% oleic acid, 3.0% iso-propanol, 0.2% sodium sulfite, 6.0% ammonia (29%) and water to 100%. The formulation was diluted in an equal volume of 6% hydrogen peroxide before application, and 0.5 ml were applied to a shaved area of the back (approximately 2.5 cm in diameter) twice a week up until week 117. Mean body weights and survival were similar in treated and control groups. There was no significant increase in the incidence of tumours at any site, and no skin tumour was observed (Burnett & Goldenthal, 1988).

3.2 Subcutaneous injection

Rat

Groups of 10 male and 10 female rats, weighing 120–140 g, received subcutaneous injections of 0.5 ml oxidized *para*-phenylenediamine (5% *para*-phenylenediamine in 2% ammonium hydroxide and 1.8% sodium chloride) in an equal volume of 6% hydrogen peroxide in the hip area every other week for 18 months. Controls were injected similarly with vehicle only. There was no significant difference between treated and control groups in body weight gain or survival. All survivors were killed after 21 months. The incidence of mammary lesions [duct ectasia or adenosis] was significantly increased (4/7; $p < 0.05$ incidental tumour test) in females in comparison with vehicle controls (0/10). Two uterine tumours, an adenocarcinoma and an endometrial polyp, were observed in females; no such tumour was observed in controls. Two sarcomas [not otherwise classified] at the injection site and two lipomas were also observed in treated animals (Rojanapo *et al.*, 1986). [The Working Group noted the small number of animals used in this study and the fact that only selected organs were examined histologically.]

4. Other Relevant Data

4.1 Absorption, distribution, metabolism and excretion

Many factors influence skin absorption. The upper layer of the epidermis (stratum corneum) is the primary barrier, but this protective layer can be affected by changes in humidity, temperature and pH. Skin damage, irritation and inflammation can also influence permeability. Many hair colouring formulations contain detergents and organic solvents, which at low concentrations may damage the skin barrier and thus facilitate uptake by the skin (Malkinson & Gehlmann, 1977). The absorption of different substances varies between species; generally, the skin of humans is less permeable than that of experimental animals (Bartek *et al.*, 1972), although the permeability of the skin of the back of rats is similar to that of the human scalp (Ammenheuser & Warren, 1979). [The Working Group noted that very little information was available on absorption by men and women following exposure to hair dyes.]

4.1.1 *Occupational exposure*

2,4-Toluenediamine, one possible diamino constituent of permanent hair dyes, was detected in five of 30 urine samples from professional hairdressers who had been exposed professionally for four to five years and who reportedly did not usually wear gloves when applying hair dyes. The range of detectable concentrations was 16–67 μg/l (Şardaş *et al.*, 1986).

Differences in the mutagenicity of the urine of cosmetologists exposed to hair dyes and of those without exposure (Babish *et al.*, 1991; see pp. 102–103) suggest that the exposed cosmetologists absorbed hair-dye components systemically.

4.1.2 *User exposure*

Kiese and Rauscher (1968) studied the absorption of 2,5-diaminotoluene (*para*-toluene-diamine) through human scalp skin, applying a formulation containing the dye, resorcinol and hydrogen peroxide for 40 min and then washing. Urinary excretion was followed in aliquots over the next 48 h. The highest rate of excretion occurred 5–8 h after dyeing, and traces were found 36 h later. The average total amount of metabolite excreted after application of 2.5 g of the sulfate was 3.7 mg N,N'-diacetyl-2,5-diaminotoluene (0.09%), equivalent to 2.17 mg 2,5-diaminotoluene. Other metabolites were not identified.

Scalp penetration of four semi-permanent dyes (HC Blue No. 1, HC Blue No. 2 (see monographs, pp. 129 and 143), 1,4-diamino-2-nitrobenzene [2-nitro-para-phenylenedi-amine] and 4-amino-2-nitrophenol) and of three ingredients of oxidative dyes (1,4-di-aminobenzene [para-phenylenediamine], resorcinol and 4-amino-2-hydroxytoluene), under conditions similar to those of use of oxidative hair dyes, was studied in humans and rhesus monkeys. The absorption of [ring-^{14}C]-labelled compounds [radiochemical purity not specified] was quantified in urinary assays. The two species showed a similar pattern of dye absorption. Slightly more of the semi-permanent dyes penetrated the scalp, but in neither case did penetration exceed 1% of the applied dose. Metabolites were not identified in the urine (Maibach & Wolfram, 1981; Wolfram & Maibach, 1985).

Marzulli et al. (1981) investigated skin penetration of 2,4-diaminoanisole in humans and rhesus monkeys. [Ring-^{14}C]-labelled 2,4-diaminoanisole [radiochemical purity not specified] in acetone solution was applied to the abdomens of monkeys and to the ventral forearms of male subjects. The remaining substance was removed after 24 h by washing with soap and water. Urine was collected over a five-day period and analysed for radiolabel. Men absorbed 3.9% and monkeys 4.7% of the applied dose. Metabolites were not identified in the urine.

Application of a commercial hair colouring formulation containing 2% lead acetate to the hair of the head of nine men for 90 days led to increasing lead concentrations in axillary, pubic and capillary hair, indicating systemic uptake of lead (Marzulli et al., 1978). Two hair dye formulations containing lead acetate were spiked with lead-203 acetate and applied to the foreheads of eight men for 12 h. Absorption was estimated by measuring lead-203 activity in blood, urine and the whole body. Absorption through the skin was low: 0–0.3% of the dose (Moore et al., 1980). [The Working Group noted that such small increments cannot be measured by conventional methods such as those used in other studies.] In a study of 53 adult volunteers and 13 controls, the hair of the head was treated 63 times over a six-month period with preparations containing 0.6 or 1.8% lead acetate. No difference in lead concentration in whole blood or in urine was found between exposed and control volunteers, nor in a number of other blood parameters (Ippen et al., 1981).

4.2 Toxic effects

4.2.1 General exposures of hairdressers

The principal occupational hazards for hairdressers are irritant and allergic contact dermatitis. The irritants used include soap, detergents, shampoos, rinse solutions, bleaches and water. Two predisposing risk factors for the development of irritant contact dermatitis in hairdressers and beauticians are atopic status (defined as allergies, hay fever, asthma or atopic eczema) and nickel allergy (Cronin & Kullavanijaya, 1979; Landthaler et al., 1981; Lindemayr, 1984; Holness & Nethercott, 1990). The various agents and their uses that induce allergic contact dermatitis in hairdressers have been described (Marks, 1986), and a number of reviews on the chemistry and toxicology of hair dyeing are available (Corbett, 1976; Iyer *et al.*, 1985; Corbett, 1988). The most important group of sensitizers are synthetic organic dyes (Lynde & Mitchell, 1982; Stovall *et al.*, 1983; Nethercott *et al.*, 1986; Matsunaga *et al.*, 1988), which contain dyes, couplers and an oxidizing agent—usually a hydrogen peroxide solution. Ammonium persulfate, which is used for bleaching, has been reported to cause asthma (Pepys *et al.*, 1976; Blainey *et al.*, 1986; Schwaiblmair *et al.*, 1990), contact dermatitis and urticaria (Fisher & Dooms-Goossens, 1976; Kleinhans & Rannederg, 1988).

Application of henna has also been associated with the development of asthma in hairdressers (Pepys *et al.*, 1976; Starr *et al.*, 1982).

4.2.2 *Personal use of hair dyes*

[The Working Group noted that very little information was available on toxic effects associated with the use of hair dyes.]

Hair dyeing was the procedure associated with the highest risk of sensitization in a group of patients with contact dermatitis who were hairdresser clients. *para*-Phenylenediamine dihydrochloride was the most frequent sensitizer (Guerra *et al.*, 1992).

Case reports linking the use of hair dyes with bone-marrow suppression and aplastic anaemia (which occurs in about four people per million population) have appeared occasionally in the medical literature (Hopkins & Manoharan, 1985). The postulated etiological agent, a hair dye, contained 2,5-diaminotoluene, which is suspected of causing aplastic anaemia (Cavignaux, 1962).

A case–control study (Freni-Titulaer *et al.*, 1989) of 44 cases of connective tissue disease, comprising 23 cases of systemic lupus erythematosus, 10 of scleroderma, two of polymyositis and nine cases of undifferentiated disease, and of 88 controls selected by random-digit dialling, was carried out in Georgia, USA. Significant associations were found between the occurrence of connective tissue disease and use of hair dyes (crude OR, 6.5; 95% CI, 2.4–17.4; 21 exposed cases).

A US study involved 218 cases of systemic lupus erythematosus; 178 first- and second-degree relatives and 186 friends were identified by the patients as being close to them in age, race and sex and served as controls. No excess risk was found for hair dye use during the five years prior to diagnosis (OR compared to friends, 0.92; 95% CI, 0.59–1.45; OR compared to relatives, 1.33; 95% CI, 0.83–2.12) (Petri & Allbritton, 1992). [The Working Group noted that the choice of controls may have biased the frequency of hair dye use.]

4.2.3 *Hair lacquers and pulmonary disease*

Ameille *et al.* (1985) reviewed the evidence for possible associations between respiratory lesions of various types and inhalation of hair lacquers. The link was first suggested by Bergmann *et al.* (1958), who considered that the pulmonary findings in two cases were secondary to thesaurosis, which involves storage of nonbiodegradable macromolecules in the reticuloendothelial system. A further 15 case reports on about 30 individuals showed similar associations, with pulmonary radiological anomalies and associated symptoms regressing six months on average after cessation of exposure. McLaughlin *et al.* (1963)

observed that in a case of interstitial pulmonary disease in a hairdresser, clinical and radiological signs resolved after cessation of exposure to shellac-based hair spray but reappeared after recommencement of exposure. Valeyre *et al.* (1983) reported a case of diffuse interstitial pulmonary disease in a woman aged 66, which regressed after cessation of use of hair lacquer. The presence of the lacquer was demonstrated in a lung biopsy. No case of thesaurosis, however, was diagnosed in more than 1500 hairdressers surveyed in a number of countries (Ameille *et al.* (1985).

Palmer *et al.* (1979) compared the prevalence of respiratory disease in 213 licensed, practising beauticians, 262 student cosmetologists and 569 women who were not exposed to hair sprays as part of their occupation, in Utah, USA, using a respiratory symptom questionnaire, chest x ray and forced expiratory spirogram. The prevalences of radiological abnormality and/or reduced forced vital capacity, which were considered to be signs of possible thesaurosis or sarcoidosis, were 6.1% in practising beauticians, 1.1% in student cosmetologists and 2.8% in controls. The prevalences of a third sign, reduced diffusing capacity of the lung, which was assessed only in every tenth person, were 16.2, 10.5 and 11.4%, respectively. Some 12% of cosmetologists and 8% of controls reported 'abnormal' respiratory symptoms, the percentages being adjusted for smoking habits and geographical area. None of the differences was significant, but the authors reported that the difference was significant when the two categories of symptoms were combined. Among cosmetologists, particulate concentrations (as determined by personal samplers) were 0.48 mg/m^3 for those considered to have 'abnormal' symptoms on the basis of a questionnaire and 0.51 mg/m^3 for those with 'borderline' symptoms; each of those levels is significantly higher than the 0.36 mg/m^3 for cosmetologists who had 'normal' respiratory function. No difference in the prevalence of abnormal chest x rays was found between cosmetologists and controls, and there was no substantial difference between the groups in the frequency of restrictive or large-airway obstructive disease. Employees working in small salons, however, which the investigators found had more limited ventilation than large salons, had significantly reduced forced expiratory flow rates, suggesting some obstructive effect in the small airways. For all cosmetologists, the forced expiratory flow rate decreased with increasing number of years worked in cosmetology. In the subsamples for which lung closing volume measurements were obtained, a higher prevalence of abnormality was observed among beauticians, but none of the differences was significant. In the 40% of subjects from whom sputum samples were obtained, 42% of the cosmetologists had atypia, which is significantly higher than the 22% in control subjects. The major contribution to the difference was employees working in small salons. Particulate concentrations were similar in cosmetologists with normal and abnormal sputum cytology.

The cosmetologists in the study of Palmer *et al.* (1979) who were suspected to have thesaurosis were re-examined two years later (Renzetti *et al.*, 1980). The radiological anomalies and anomalies of pulmonary function had regressed in the majority of subjects (5% compared to 4% in controls), all but one of whom had continued working as a cosmetologist.

4.2.4 *Experimental data*

Pulmonary granulomas were found in albino rats after prolonged inhalation of various types of hair lacquers (Vivoli, 1966). Thesaurosis was not induced in rabbits (Draize *et al.*,

1959), rats (Brunner *et al.*, 1963; Lowsma *et al.*, 1966; Ameille *et al.*, 1984), guinea-pigs (Calendra & Kay, 1958; Brunner *et al.*, 1963) or dogs (Giovacchini *et al.*, 1965) after repeated inhalation of hair sprays. Chronic exposure of mice, rats, rabbits and dogs to hair dye formulations by various routes gave no indication of adverse effects on haematopoiesis or other systemic effects (Kinkel & Holzmann, 1973; Burnett *et al.*, 1975, 1977, 1980; Burnett & Goldenthal, 1988).

In a chronic feeding study, a composite test material containing 0.24% Acid Orange 3, 1.63% HC Blue No. 2, 0.64% Celliton Fast Navy Blue BRA (mixture of Disperse Yellow 1, Disperse Blue 1, Disperse Violet 4, Disperse Red 17), 0.24% 2-nitro-*para*-phenylene-diamine, 0.16% 4-nitro-*ortho*-phenylenediamine, 0.05% 2-amino-4-nitrophenol, 0.31% HC Yellow No. 4, 0.4% Disperse Violet 11, 0.61% Disperse Blue 1, 0.13% Disperse Black 9, 1.54% HC Blue No. 1, 0.02% HC Red No. 3, 0.65% HC Yellow No. 3, 0.28% HC Yellow No. 2 plus base, representative of commercial semi-permanent hair dyes, was incorporated into the diets of male and female beagle dogs (Wernick *et al.*, 1975). Groups of six dogs of each sex were fed the composite at doses of 0, 19.5 or 97.5 mg/kg bw per day for two years. Physical examinations and clinical analyses of blood and urine were performed after 3, 6, 12, 18 and 24 months of the study. One dog of each sex was necropsied at 6, 12 and 18 months, and all survivors were necropsied at 24 months. All dogs fed the composite material excreted blue–brown urine, indicating systemic absorption of the dyes. The weight gain and physical, clinical and histological indices were normal.

In 13-week dermal toxicity studies, nine oxidative and three semi-permanent composite test materials, representative of commercial hair dye formulations, were applied twice weekly to the shaved dorsolateral skin of six male and six female New Zealand rabbits (Burnett *et al.*, 1976). The semi-permanent formulations were applied without dilution, while the oxidative formulations were mixed 1:1 with 6% hydrogen peroxide immediately prior to application. The applied dose in each case was 1 ml/kg bw. Application sites were abraded on three rabbits of each sex; all rabbits were restrained for 1 h after treatment, then were shampooed, rinsed and dried. Haematological and clinical chemical tests were performed at weeks 0, 3, 7 and 13: no toxic sign was noted, and there was no meaningful change in haematological or clinical parameters. Slight epidermal hyperplasia associated with some of the oxidative formulations was seen in 25 tissues collected at necroscopy for microscopic examination.

One commercial non-oxidative colouring formulation, containing 0.3% HC Blue No. 1, several other colouring agents and 23% of 40% active sodium lauryl sulfate, was applied at 50 µl to the skin of random-bred Swiss Webster mice of each sex three times a week for 20 months. Survival and mean body weights were similar in dosed and control animals. Haematological analyses (haemoglobin, haematocrit, red blood cells, total or differential white blood cells) and urinary tests indicated no toxic effect, but significant increases in the degree of chronic inflammation of the skin were observed in all treated animals in comparison with controls (Jacobs *et al.*, 1984).

4.3 Reproductive toxicity and developmental effects

4.3.1 *Humans*

Vaughan *et al.* (1984) noted a small excess of spontaneous abortions among hairdressers from the 1980–81 birth records of Washington State, USA (RR, 1.4; 95% CI, 1.2–1.7).

In the 1980 US National Natality and National Fetal Mortality Survey, no difference in the prevalence of malformations (1.9%) or of fetal deaths (1.6%) was found among offspring of women employed in beauty and barber shops from that in the whole sample. A nonsignificant difference was noted in the prevalence of low-birth-weight infants (2.5%) (Shilling & Lalich, 1984).

A total of 40 346 congenital malformations routinely notified during 1980–82 in England and Wales were analysed with regard to parental occupation (McDowall, 1985). Paternal occupation was reported for 62% and maternal occupation for 28%: 298 mothers and 49 fathers were categorized as hairdressers, barbers and hairdressing supervisors, managers and proprietors. The rates of all malformations and of specific malformations were not significantly different from those in the overall group.

A survey was carried out of spontaneous abortion and maternal occupation during pregnancy in Montréal, Canada (McDonald *et al.*, 1986), in maternity units in which 90% of births in the city are estimated to occur. Interviews were done with 51 885 hospitalized women who delivered at term (participation rate, 90%) and 4127 hospitalized women who were undergoing a spontaneous abortion (participation rate, < 75%). The interviews identified 48 608 previous pregnancies, 10 910 of which had terminated spontaneously in abortion whether in hospital or elsewhere. The expected numbers of abortions were adjusted for maternal age, parity, history of previous abortion, smoking habits and educational level reached. Hairdressers were represented by 458 current pregnancies, of which 34 ended in spontaneous abortion, and 417 previous pregnancies, of which 102 ended in spontaneous abortion; the observed:expected ratios were 1.05 and 1.08 (p > 0.1), respectively. A subsequent analysis for spontaneous abortion, low birth weight and congenital defects among women who had worked at least 30 h per week at the beginning of their pregnancies showed no excess risk among 688 hairdressers (McDonald *et al.*, 1987).

In another analysis (McDonald *et al.*, 1988a), the 22 613 previous pregnancies in which the woman had been employed for at least 30 h a week at the time of conception were evaluated with regard to the period of pregnancy at which fetal death occurred. Of 354 pregnancies among hairdressers, 83 had terminated in fetal death, 76 before the 16th week, six between the 16th and the 27th week and one after the 27th week; the corresponding observed: expected ratios were 1.1, 0.6 and 0.3 (none was significant). Similar ORs were estimated in a separate case–control analysis of the same study (Goulet & Thériault, 1991), which included 227 fetal deaths of 20 weeks' gestation or more without major malformations and a similar number of live-born controls matched on maternal age and gravidity. The OR associated with maternal employment in hairdressing was 0.3 (95% CI, 0.1–1.7; 2/6 discordant pairs) for fetal deaths at 20–27 weeks' gestation and 0.1 (95% CI, 0.0–1.4; 1/6 discordant pairs) for fetal deaths at ≥ 28 weeks' gestation. The combined OR was 0.1 (95% CI, 0.0–0.3).

In the same data base, the association between congenital defects in index and previous births and maternal occupation for at least 15 h per week at the time of conception was investigated. Of 714 pregnancies among hairdressers, 17 resulted in offspring with congenital malformations, comprising three chromosomal errors, seven 'developmental defects probably arising in the first few weeks of gestation' and seven 'musculoskeletal defects and hernias perhaps related to influences after the first trimester'. The corresponding observed:expected ratios were, respectively, 2.3, 0.9 and 0.8; none was statistically significant (McDonald *et al.*, 1988b).

Tikkanen *et al.* (1988) analysed data on cardiovascular anomalies for the period 1980–81 from the Finnish Register of Congenital Malformations; 160 infants with specific anomalies confirmed by a paediatric cardiologist were compared with 160 controls. 'Substantial' exposure to 'hairdresser's chemicals' was reported for no case and six controls. A previous analysis of the same data base identified 34 children with hypoplastic left ventricle; regular maternal use of aerosols (deodorant or hair sprays) was reported for 44.1% of case mothers and 23.9% of 752 control mothers (Tikkanen, 1986).

A report on all 6166 naturally terminated pregnancies in the district of Gottwaldov in Czechoslovakia in 1981–83 described an increased proportion of reproductive losses, but not premature births, in an unspecified number of hairdressers (Mareš & Baran, 1989).

4.3.2 *Experimental systems*

No evidence of teratogenicity was seen when hair dye formulations were applied to the skin of pregnant rats and rabbits (Wernick *et al.*, 1975; Burnett *et al.*, 1976) or when individual hair dye components were administered by gavage or subcutaneous injection to pregnant rats and mice (Marks *et al.*, 1981; DiNardo *et al.*, 1985). Similarly, topical application of hair dye formulations produced no adverse reproductive effect in rats in a multigeneration study (Burnett & Goldenthal, 1988) or in a test for heritable translocation (Burnett *et al.*, 1981; see p. 104 for a detailed description).

(*a*) *Reproduction*

In a study of fertility and reproductive performance, a composite test material, representative of commercial semi-permanent hair dye formulations (see p. 97), was incorporated into the diets of Sprague-Dawley rats at 0, 1950 or 7800 ppm (Wernick *et al.*, 1975). Groups of 10 male rats fed the test diet for eight weeks prior to and throughout the mating period were mated with groups of 20 females fed the basal diet. Groups of 10 male rats fed the basal diet were mated with groups of 20 females fed the test diet for eight weeks prior to mating and throughout mating, gestation and lactation. One female made pregnant by each male was killed in mid-pregnancy in order to evaluate the status of the uterine contents. The remaining dams were allowed to deliver litters normally and to maintain pups until 21 days of age. Systemic absorption of dyes was indicated by the production of blue–brown urine by all animals receiving the treated diet, but no reduction in food consumption or body weight gain was associated with exposure. Similarly, there was no evidence of an adverse effect on fertility or other reproductive parameters in exposed male or female rats.

Six composite test materials, representative of commercial oxidative hair dye formulations, were evaluated in rats in a two-generation study of reproduction (Burnett & Goldenthal, 1988). Test materials were mixed 1:1 with 6% hydrogen peroxide and then applied at 0.5 ml twice weekly to the clipped backs of 20 male and 20 female Sprague-Dawley rats. The F_0 rats began treatment at six to eight weeks of age, and rats of the second litter (F_{1b}) began treatment at weaning. Breeding for both generations began at 100 days of age, and skin applications continued throughout mating, gestation and lactation periods. Occasional mild dermatitis was the only adverse effect noted. Body weight gain, food consumption, survival and reproductive indices (fertility, gestation, live birth and survival, weaning weight) in F_{1a}, F_{1b}, F_{2a} and F_{2b} litters were unaffected by the treatments.

(b)   Teratogenesis

A composite test material, representative of commercial semi-permanent hair dye formulations (see p. 97), was evaluated for teratogenic potential in rats and rabbits (Wernick *et al.*, 1975). Groups of 20 pregnant CFE-S rats were fed diets containing 0, 1950 or 7800 ppm of the material on gestation days 6–15, and groups of 12 pregnant New Zealand rabbits were dosed by gavage on gestation days 6–18 with 0, 19.5 or 97.5 mg/kg bw. All animals receiving the composite produced blue–brown urine, indicating systemic absorption of dyes, but food consumption and body weight gain were unaffected in both species. Similarly, there was no evidence in rats or rabbits of an adverse effect on intrauterine growth or development or of treatment-related gross, visceral or skeletal malformation.

The teratogenicity of nine oxidative and three semi-permanent composite test materials, representative of commercial hair dye formulations, was tested by Burnett *et al.* (1976). The materials were applied to the shaved dorsoscapular area of pregnant Charles River CD rats in groups of 20 on every third day of gestation (days 1, 4, 7, 10, 13, 16 and 19). The semi-permanent formulations were applied without dilution, while the oxidative formulations were mixed 1:1 with 6% hydrogen peroxide immediately prior to application. The applied dose in each case was 2 ml/kg bw per day. No maternal toxicity was observed, there was no effect of treatment on implantation or untrauterine growth or survival, and there was no evidence of external, visceral or skeletal malformation.

Five oxidative dyes (12.5, 25 or 50 mg/kg bw 4,4'-diaminodiphenylene sulfate, 50, 100 or 200 mg/kg bw N'-(2-hydroxyethyl)-4-nitro-*ortho*-phenylenediamine, 110, 220 or 450 mg/kg bw 2,3-dihydroxynaphthalene, 50, 100 or 150 mg/kg bw N,N-dimethyl-*para*-phenylene-diamine and 125, 250 or 500 mg/kg bw resorcinol) used in hair colouring formulations were evaluated for teratogenicity in Sprague-Dawley rats (DiNardo *et al.*, 1985). Groups of 10–13 pregnant rats were administered the low, intermediate or high doses by gavage on days 6–15 of gestation. Significant reductions in maternal body weight gain during days 6–16 of gestation were seen in rats treated with the high doses of 4,4'-diaminodiphenylene sulfate, N'-(2-hydroxyethyl)-4-nitro-*ortho*-phenylenediamine and 2,3-dihydroxynaphthalene; the high doses of N,N-dimethyl-*para*-phenylenediamine and resorcinol reduced maternal body weight gain during treatment, but not significantly. There was a significant compensatory increase in maternal body weight gain after treatment (on days 16–20) with the high doses of 4,4'-diaminodiphenylene sulfate and N'-(2-hydroxyethyl)-4-nitro-*ortho*-phenylenediamine. None of the dyes impaired implantation, intrauterine growth or survival or external, visceral or skeletal malformation. [The Working Group noted the small number of animals used in the study.]

4.4 Genetic and related effects

4.4.1 *Humans*

Chromosomal aberrations in peripheral lymphocytes were examined in a study of 60 professional hair colourists (28 men, 28.4 ± 9.4 years old; 32 women, 23.3 ± 5.1 years old) and 36 control subjects matched for age and sex (17 men, 28.1 ± 7.3 years old; 19 women, 25.3 ± 6.5 years old) (Kirkland *et al.*, 1978a,b) in the United Kingdom. Information was recorded on smoking habits, alcohol consumption, use of medicinal drugs and drugs of abuse, infections, vaccinations and exposure to x rays; details of occupational exposure to hair dyes were collected: women had done an average of 11 000 permanent and 5000 semi-permanent tinting operations and men, 15 000 permanent and 6000 semi-permanent operations, over periods ranging from 1 to 15 years. Blood samples were taken at the time of interview, but the time since last hair tint application (to themselves or clients) was not recorded. More gaps were found per cell among female tinters than controls (0.065 *versus* 0.048; $p < 0.02$) but not among male tinters (0.064 *versus* 0.063). The number of breaks per cell (assumed from the observed aberrations) was not altered among women (0.028 *versus* 0.031) but was lower among men (0.034 *versus* 0.047; $p < 0.05$). Exclusion of subjects exposed to high doses of diagnostic x rays or who had recently had viral infections removed these differences (breaks in tinters *versus* controls: women, 0.023 *versus* 0.027; men, 0.036 *versus* 0.038). Reallocation of this smaller set of subjects according to whether or not their own hair was dyed revealed that the number of breaks per cell was higher among women who dyed their hair (dyed *versus* not dyed, 0.031 *versus* 0.018; $p < 0.02$) and lower among men who dyed their hair (0.023 *versus* 0.044; $p < 0.01$). The women had given themselves an average of 90 permanent and 10 semi-permanent tints and the men an average of 30 permanent tints [semi-permanent tints not stated] over a period similar to their occupational exposure. The authors stated that there was no association between chromosomal damage and the duration and/or frequency of hair dyeing in the women. [The Working Group noted the absence of data to substantiate this statement.] They record that 20/23 female and 11/18 male tinters wore protective gloves for all applications of permanent and semi-permanent tints and deduced that most of the subjects would receive greater exposure to hair-dye components when their own hair was treated. [The Working Group noted that most aberrations were of the chromatid type and were, therefore, likely to have occurred recently; the absence of information on the actual dyes used recently by the subjects is regrettable, since some components are relatively potent clastogens while others are not.] The finding that the number of breaks per cell was lower among men who dyed their hair was explained by the age difference between the group with tinted hair (22.7 ± 5.1 years, n = 10) and the group with non-tinted hair (31.8 ± 10.1, n = 17). Kirkland *et al.* (1978a) based their argument on the observation of Court Brown *et al.* (1966) that there was much less chromosomal damage of all types in 48-h blood cultures from men aged 15–24 than from men aged 25–34, whereas there was no difference among women in these age ranges. [The

Working Group noted that the results of subsequent studies, by Hedner *et al.* (1982) and Ivanov *et al.* (1978), do not confirm the latter observations.]

Hofer *et al.* (1983) studied chromosomal aberrations in lymphocytes from six women and four men who volunteered to have their hair dyed and a similar group of 10 controls matched for age (men: hair-dyed, 35.7 ± 67; controls, 30.8 ± 6.4; women: hair-dyed, 30.3 ± 5.7; controls, 35.0 ± 5.8). Records were taken of smoking habits, alcohol consumption and medical drug use and, during the experiment, exposure to x rays, illness and vaccinations. There were more smokers in the test group. None of the volunteers had used hair dyes or shades for at least one year before entering the study, and the control group did not use hair colourants during the study. The treated group had their hair dyed 13 times at intervals of three to six weeks with commercial preparations containing mixtures of aminotoluenes, aminophenols and hydroxybenzenes and, in some cases, naphthol, as active ingredients; the colouring product used was chosen according to each subject's hair colour, and the same material was used throughout the study. The colouring preparations were mixed (1:1) with 3–6% hydrogen peroxide. Nine blood samples were taken: three weeks before the first treatment, 24 h after a sham dyeing (no dye or hydrogen peroxide) and 24 h after each of the first three and last four dyeing procedures. No difference was observed between the control and treated groups in the percentage of cells with one or more structural aberration (excluding gaps) before treatment, after sham dyeing or after treatment. Subdivision of the groups according to sex revealed no difference. A significant increase in aberration rate with age was observed among the male but not the female subjects. Neither smoking nor x-ray exposure had an effect.

In conjunction with this study, sister chromatid exchange was examined in peripheral lymphocytes; no evidence was found of an effect on the frequency (Turanitz *et al.*, 1983).

Sister chromatid exchange was studied in the peripheral lymphocytes of a small group of volunteers comprising 13 women and one man immediately before and 6 h and seven days after one normal application of a four semi-permanent and 10 permanent hair dyes, all of which were mutagenic to *Salmonella typhimurium* TA1538 and TA98. There was no consistent increase in the number of sister chromatid exchanges per cell (Kirkland *et al.*, 1981).

In a study in the USA involving 30 women aged 45–60 years, mutagenicity was determined in urine specimens collected prior to and during a 24-h period immediately after application of dark shades of several hair colouring products containing high levels of dyes and dye intermediates (Burnett *et al.*, 1979). Many of the women had used hair dyes regularly for over 20 years. Concentrated (XAD-2 resin) urine samples did not increase the number of reverse mutations in *S. typhimurium* TA1538 in the presence of an exogenous metabolic system from rat liver (S9). [The Working Group noted the inadequate reporting of the results.]

A study was conducted in New York State, USA, on cosmetologists (91 women, 7 men) who were occupationally exposed to a wide range of chemicals, including hair dyes, and who had reported a prevalence of skin rashes twice that of a control group of 87 female dental personnel (29% *versus* 15%) (Babish *et al.*, 1991). The two groups were matched for median age, smoking status and proportion of subjects (13–16%) who had had their hair permanent-waved or dyed within seven days of the study. At the end of a normal working day, subjects from each group provided a urine sample, which was later concentrated and tested for mutagenicity in *S. typhimurium* TA100 in the presence and absence of S9. In the presence of S9, there was no difference between the groups, but in tests conducted without S9 the frequency of mutagenic urine samples was 15% higher among cosmetologists (39%) than dental personnel (24%). Multivariate analysis, with adjustment for age and smoking habits, revealed an OR of 2.0 (95% CI, 1.1–3.8) for the presence of urinary mutagens in cosmetologists compared to dental personnel. [The Working Group noted the inadequate reporting of the results.]

4.4.2 *Experimental systems*

Of 25 commercial permanent hair dye formulations containing *para*-phenylenediamine, resorcinol and aminophenols incubated with hydrogen peroxide, 12 were mutagenic to *S. typhimurium* TA98 only in the presence of S9. Without the addition of hydrogen peroxide, mutagenicity was reduced for three dyes and eliminated for three others. Four of six formulations, with degrees of mutagenicity varying from zero to high, administered topically with 3% hydrogen peroxide to male rats induced urine that was mutagenic to *S. typhimurium* TA98 in the presence of S9 (Albano *et al.*, 1982).

Forty products chosen from among 12 brands of commercially available hair colourants used in New Zealand were tested for mutagenicity in *S. typhimurium* TA98 and TA100 without S9; activators were added when recommended (Ferguson *et al.*, 1990). Twenty-three were mutagenic in one or both strains. When 10 mutagenic hair dye preparations were tested in the presence of the drug verapamil, used for treating cardiac conditions (Ferguson & Baguley, 1988), the mutagenic activity of four was decreased and that of two was increased (Ferguson *et al.*, 1990).

Two of four commercial hair dye formulations containing phenylenediamines and aminophenols (two of which also contained 2,5-diaminophenol) and oxidized with 6% hydrogen peroxide were mutagenic to *S. typhimurium* TA98 in the presence of Kanechlor 500-induced S9. When toxicity was reduced by adsorbing bactericidal products on blue rayon, peroxide treatment increased the mutagenicity of all preparations to different extents; in the two preparations with markedly increased mutagenicity, activity was attributed to the oxidation of *meta*-phenylenediamine to 2,7-diaminophenazine, itself a potent mutagen (Watanabe *et al.*, 1990).

Two commercial oxidative hair colouring products were applied at 10–30 ml, both with (10–30 ml) and without hydrogen peroxide, to the backs of male Sprague-Dawley rats [number unspecified]. Both colourants contained 1,4-diamino-2-nitrobenzene (see monograph, p. 185) and 1,2-diamino-4-nitrobenzene (4-nitro-*ortho*-phenylenediamine). The solutions were left on the hair for 20 min and then removed by shampooing and rinsing. Urine was collected before and every 24 h after product application for four days and tested in *S. typhimurium* TA1538, the volumes of urine applied to each plate varying from 3.4 to 11.5% of the total volume. Urine samples collected during the first 24 h from rats treated with either of the preparations were mutagenic (two to three times background); no significant mutagenicity was observed in urine samples collected two to four days after application. Prior reaction with hydrogen peroxide had little or no effect on the mutagenicity of the urine (Ammenheuser & Warren, 1979).

Henna and its active colouring ingredient, 2-hydroxy-1,4-naphthoquinone, were tested for mutagenicity in *S. typhimurium* TA98, TA100, TA1535, TA1537 and TA1538. Henna was not mutagenic to any strain, but 2-hydroxy-1,4-naphthoquinone was mutagenic to TA98, only in the absence of S9 (Stamberg *et al.*, 1979).

2-Amino-5-methoxy-2'(or 3')-methylindamine and 2-amino-5-methoxy-2'(or 3')-methylindoaniline were isolated from an oxidative reaction mixture of 2,5-diaminotoluene and 2,4-diaminotoluene. They were highly mutagenic to *S. typhimurium* TA98 in the presence of an exogenous metabolic system (Matsuki *et al.*, 1981).

In a study of heritable translocation, groups of 25 male Sprague-Dawley CD rats were painted twice weekly for 10 weeks on the shaved dorsal skin with 0.5 ml of a semi-permanent dye formulation (comprising base ingredients plus 0.12% CI Disperse Blue 1, 0.04% CI Disperse Black 9, 0.01% HC Red No. 3, 0.21% HC Yellow No. 3, 0.50% HC Blue No. 1, 0.06% Acid Orange No. 3, 0.07% CI Disperse Violet No. 11 and 0.01% HC Yellow No. 2) or to 0.5 ml of an oxidative dye formulation (comprising base ingredients plus 2.2% *para*-phenylenediamine, 3.1% *N,N*-bis(2-hydroxyethyl)-*para*-phenylenediamine sulfate, 1.0% resorcinol and *meta*-aminophenol, mixed 1:1 with 6% hydrogen peroxide just prior to use). Animals were then mated with untreated female rats. Male F_1 progeny were subsequently mated with other untreated females, and the resulting pregnancies were arrested at day 16 of gestation. No difference in average litter size or frequency of successful matings at the F_1 mating was observed between controls and the two exposed groups. Furthermore, there was no effect on the number of live fetuses, implantations or resorptions at the F_2 mating (total litters analysed: 275 controls, 261 oxidation dye group and 271 semi-permanent dye group) (Burnett *et al.*, 1981).

5. Summary of Data Reported and Evaluation

5.1 Exposure data

Since the early twentieth century, hairdressers have made use of a wide range of products, including hair colourants and bleaches, shampoos and conditioners, hair styling preparations and nail and skin care products. Several thousand chemicals are found in formulations of these products. Barbers generally cut only men's hair and make limited use of some of the above products, such as hair dyes, in their work.

Hair colourants are classified as permanent (primarily aromatic amines and amino-phenols with hydrogen peroxide), semi-permanent (nitro-substituted aromatic amines, aminophenols, aminoanthraquinones and azo dyes) and temporary (high-molecular-weight or insoluble complexes and metal salts, such as lead acetate). The numerous individual chemicals used in hair colourants have varied over time. Only permanent and semi-permanent hair colourants are used to a significant extent by hairdressers, while consumers at home use any of the three types.

Hairdressers may also be exposed to volatile solvents, propellants and aerosols (from hair sprays), formaldehyde (an antibacterial agent), methacrylates (in nail care products) and trace quantities of nitrosamines, which have been reported in many hair care products.

It is estimated that there are several million hairdressers and barbers worldwide. Few exposure measurements are available. Approximately 35% of women and 10% of men in Europe, Japan and the USA use hair colourants.

5.2 Human carcinogenicity data

There is consistent evidence from five (all from Europe) of the six large cohort studies of an excess risk for cancer of the urinary bladder in male hairdressers and barbers. The increase was significant in three studies, and the overall risk relative to that in the general population amounted to about 1.6. In 12 case–control studies, male hairdressers and barbers had an overall relative risk of about 1.2; smoking was adjusted for in three of these case–control studies, conducted in North America, and these did not show an overall excess risk. The risk for cancer of the urinary bladder was less consistently increased in corresponding studies in women: positive results were obtained in five cohort studies and negative results in three; none was significant. An overall relative risk for lung cancer of about 1.3 was seen among male and female hairdressers in cohort studies. One case–control study from Australia found a significant excess risk for non-Hodgkin's lymphoma among female hairdressers; a nonsignificant excess of this malignancy was noted in one cohort study from Denmark in men and women and in one case–control study from the USA in men.

One cohort study, from Finland, found a significant excess risk for ovarian cancer; two other studies, in the USA and Japan, found nonsignificant risks, and a fourth, in Switzerland, showed no effect. Excess risks were seen among male hairdressers for cancers of the buccal cavity and pharynx and prostate in one study from Switzerland; increased risks for cancers at these sites were not reported in another cohort study, from the United Kingdom.

Personal use of hair colourants has been studied in seven case–control studies of cancer of the urinary bladder. Overall, these do not indicate an excess risk; however, one study from Denmark found an association with personal use of briliantine, although it had methodological limitations. Following a report in 1976 of an excess of breast cancers among hair dye users in New York, USA, six case–control studies and one cohort study examined this subject. None found evidence of a significant excess among hair dye users overall. One case–control study of non-Hodgkin's lymphoma from Iowa and Minnesota showed a significantly increased risk among male users of hair colouring products. A second case–control study, from Nebraska, showed an excess risk for this malignancy among female users of hair colourants but showed no excess among a smaller number of male users. The case–control study from Nebraska also found a significant excess of multiple myeloma among female users of permanent hair dyes, and another study from Iowa reported a nonsignificant excess of this malignancy in male users of hair colourants. One cohort study in the USA showed no excess risk among hair dye users for all lymphomas combined. One case–control study of neuroblastoma and one of Wilms' tumour showed significantly increased risks for the offspring of mothers who had used hair dyes during pregnancy. Single studies have reported significant excess risks for Hutchinson's melanotic freckle, Hodgkin's disease, leukaemia, malignant tumours of the brain and cancers of the salivary gland, cervix and lower female genital tract. Other studies showed no such excesses.

The higher prevalence of smokers reported among male hairdressers and barbers in some studies is consistent with the overall excess of lung cancer but cannot readily explain the magnitude of the increase in risk for cancer of the urinary bladder in the European cohort studies. In particular, studies in Switzerland and Denmark have shown significant excesses of cancer of the urinary bladder unaccompanied by appreciable excesses of lung cancer, which further weigh against smoking as the sole explanation for the overall excess. Specific exposures of hairdressers and barbers have not been evaluated in epidemiological studies.

5.3 Animal carcinogenicity data

Various commercially available hair dye formulations and various laboratory preparations of hair dyes were tested for carcinogenicity in mice or rats by skin application in many studies and by subcutaneous injection in a single study in rats. In one study by skin application in rats, a particular formulation was associated with an increased incidence of pituitary adenomas in females. The other studies either showed no increased incidence of tumours at any site or were inadequate for evaluation.

5.4 Other relevant data

Contact dermatitis is a common clinical dermatological problem in hairdressers. Because hairdressers use a wide variety of multicomponent chemical products, it is difficult to determine the specific etiology of their dermatitis, although cutaneous nickel allergy and atopic status have been suggested to play a role. Moreover, many of the products used contain both irritants and sensitizers. Pulmonary toxicity has been associated with the use of hair lacquer by consumers and hairdressers.

No study has reported a significant excess of congenital malformations, early or late fetal death or low birth weight among the offspring of male or female barbers or hairdressers.

No increase was observed in chromosomal aberration frequencies in the lymphocytes of humans exposed to commercial hair colourants which included hydrogen peroxide application. In this and another study, no increase in sister chromatid exchange frequency was found.

A number of different commercial permanent and semi-permanent hair colourants were tested for their mutagenic activity *in vitro*. Many were mutagenic to bacteria. Less than half of the preparations applied to rats resulted in the excretion of bacterial mutagens in urine. Application of a semi-permanent and an oxidation dye colourant topically to male rats had no effect on the reproductive performance of the treated rats and did not induce heritable translocations, as judged by a mating protocol.

5.5 Evaluation[1]

There is *limited evidence* that occupation as a hairdresser or barber entails exposures that are carcinogenic.

---

[1]For definition of the italicized terms, see Preamble, pp. 26–30.

There is *inadequate evidence* that personal use of hair colourants entails exposures that are carcinogenic.

Overall evaluations

Occupation as a hairdresser or barber entails exposures that *are probably carcinogenic (Group 2A)*.

Personal use of hair colourants *cannot be evaluated as to its carcinogenicity (Group 3)*.

6. References

Ahlbom, A., Navier, I.L., Norell, S., Olin, R. & Spännare, B. (1986) Nonoccupational risk indicators for astrocytomas in adults. *Am. J. Epidemiol.*, **124**, 334–337

Albano, G., Carere, A., Crebelli, R. & Zito, R. (1982) Mutagenicity of commercial hair dyes in *Salmonella typhimurium* TA98. *Food Chem. Toxicol.*, **20**, 171–175

Alderson, M. (1980) Cancer mortality in male hairdressers. *J. Epidemiol. Community Health*, **34**, 182–185

Almaguer, D.A. & Blade, L.M. (1990) *Health Hazard Evaluation Report. Buckeye Hills Career Center, Rio Grande, Ohio* (HETA Report 88-153-2072), Cincinnati, OH, National Institute for Occupational Safety and Health

Almaguer, D. & Klein, M. (1991) *Health Hazard Evaluation Report. Northwest Vocational School, Cincinnati, Ohio* (HETA Report 89-170-2100), Cincinnati, OH, National Institute for Occupational Safety and Health

Ameille, J., Guillon, F., Pagès, M.G., Proteau, J. & Boudène, C. (1984) Inhalation of capillary laquers and pulmonary thesaurosis. Real or false problem? An experimental study in rats (Fr.). *Arch. Mal. prof.*, **45**, 208–210

Ameille, J., Pagès, M.G., Capron, F., Proteau, J. & Rochemaure, J. (1985) Respiratory pathology induced by inhalation of hair lacquer (Fr.). *Rev. Pneumol. clin.*, **41**, 325–330

Ammenheuser, M. & Warren, M.E. (1979) Detection of mutagens in the urine of rats following topical application of hair dyes. *Mutat. Res.*, **66**, 241–245

Anon. (1966) *Encyclopaedia Britannica*, Vol. 7, London, William Benton, p. 816

Anthony, H.M. & Thomas, G.M. (1970) Tumors of the urinary bladder: an analysis of the occupations of 1,030 patients in Leeds, England. *J. natl Cancer Inst.*, **45**, 879–895

Armstrong, B.K. & Holman, C.D'A.J. (1985) Hutchinson's melanotic freckle melanoma and the use of non-permanent hair dyes (Letter to the Editor). *Br. J. Cancer*, **52**, 135

Babish, J.G., Scarlett, J.M., Voekler, S.E., Gutenmann, W.H. & Lisk, D.J. (1991) Urinary mutagens in cosmetologists and dental personnel. *J. Toxicol. environ. Health*, **34**, 197–206

Barker, G. (1985) Surfactants in shampoos. In: Rieger, M.M., ed., *Surfactants in Cosmetics*, New York, Marcel Dekker, pp. 251–292

Bartek, M.J., LaBudde, J.A. & Maibach, H.I. (1972) Skin permeability *in vivo*: comparison in rat, rabbit, pig and man. *J. invest. Dermatol.*, **58**, 114–123

Baxter, P.J. & McDowall, M.E. (1986) Occupation and cancer in London: an investigation into nasal and bladder cancer using the Cancer Atlas. *Br. J. ind. Med.*, **43**, 44–49

Beernaert, H., Herpol-Borremans, M. & De Cock, F. (1987) Determination of 1,4-dioxane in cosmetic products by headspace gas chromatography. *Belg. J. Food Chem. Biotechnol.*, **42**, 131–135

Bergmann, M., Flance, I.J. & Blumenthal, H.T. (1958) Thesaurosis following inhalation of hair spray. A clinical and experimental study. *New Engl. J. Med.*, **258**, 471–476

Blainey, A.D., Ollier, S., Cundell, D., Smith, R.E. & Davies, R.J. (1986) Occupational asthma in a hairdressing salon. *Thorax*, **41**, 42–50

Blair, A., Linos, A., Stewart, P.A., Burmeister, L.F., Gibson, R., Everett, G., Schuman, L. & Cantor, K.P. (1993) Evaluation of risks for non-Hodgkin's lymphoma by occupation and industry exposures from a case–control study. *Am. J. ind. Med.*, **23**, 301–312

Boffetta, P., Stellman, S.D. & Garfinkel, L. (1989) A case–control study of multiple myeloma nested in the American Cancer Society prospective study. *Int. J. Cancer*, **43**, 554–559

Brown, L.M., Everett, G.D., Burmeister, L.F. & Blair, A. (1992) Hair dye use and multiple myeloma in white men. *Am. J. public Health*, **82**, 1673–1674

Brunner, M.J., Giovacchini, R.P., Wyatt, J.P., Dunlap, F.E. & Calendra, J.C. (1963) Pulmonary disease and hair-spray polymers: a disputed relationship. *J. Am. med. Assoc.*, **184**, 851–857

Bunin, G.R., Kramer, S., Marrero, O. & Meadows, A.T. (1987) Gestational risk factors for Wilms' tumor: results of a case–control study. *Cancer Res.*, **47**, 2972–2977

Burch, J.D., Craib, K.J.P., Choi, B.C.K., Miller, A.B., Risch, H.A. & Howe, G.R. (1987) An exploratory case–control study of brain tumors in adults. *J. natl Cancer Inst.*, **78**, 601–609

Burnett, C.M. & Goldenthal, E.I. (1988) Multigeneration reproduction and carcinogenicity studies in Sprague-Dawley rats exposed topically to oxidative hair-colouring formulations containing *p*-phenylenediamine and other aromatic amines. *Food Chem. Toxicol.*, **26**, 467–474

Burnett, C.M., Lanman, B.M., Giovacchini, R., Wolcott, R., Scala, R. & Keplinger, M. (1975) Long-term toxicity studies on oxidation hair dyes. *Food Cosmet. Toxicol.*, **13**, 353–357

Burnett, C.M., Goldenthal, E.I., Harris, S.B., Wazeter, F.X., Strausburg, J., Kapp, R. & Voelker, R. (1976) Teratology and percutaneous toxicity studies on hair dyes. *J. Toxicol. environ. Health*, **1**, 1027–1040

Burnett, C.M., Corbett, J.F. & Lanman, B.M. (1977) Hair dyes and aplastic anemia. *Drug Chem. Toxicol.*, **1**, 45–61

Burnett, C.M., Fuchs, C.M. & Corbett, J.F. (1979) Mutagenicity studies on urine concentrates from female users of dark hair color products. *Drug Chem. Toxicol.*, **2**, 283–293

Burnett, C., Jacobs, M.M., Seppala, A. & Shubik, P. (1980) Evaluation of the toxicity and carcinogenicity of hair dyes. *J. Toxicol. environ. Health*, **6**, 247–257

Burnett, C., Loehr, R. & Corbett, J. (1981) Heritable translocation study on two hair dye formulations. *Fundam. appl. Toxicol.*, **1**, 325–328

Calendra, J. & Kay, J.A. (1958) The effects of aerosol hair sprays on experimental animals. *Proc. Sci. Sect. Toilet Goods Assoc.*, **30**, 41–44

Cantor, K.P., Blair, A., Everett, G., VanLier, S., Burmeister, L., Dick, F.R., Gibson, R.W. & Schuman, L. (1988) Hair dye use and risk of leukaemia and lymphoma. *Am. J. public Health*, **78**, 570–571

Cavignaux, L. (1962) Confirmed intoxications (Fr.). *Cahiers Med. interprof.*, **2**, 28

Claude, J., Kunze, E., Frentzel-Beyme, R., Paczkowski, K., Schneider, J. & Schubert, H. (1986) Life-style and occupational risk factors in cancer of the lower urinary tract. *Am. J. Epidemiol.*, **124**, 578–589

Clausen, T. (1989) Hair coloring preparations. In: Elvers, B., Hawkins, S. Ravenscroft, M., Rounsaville, J.F. & Schulz, G., eds, *Ullmann's Encyclopedia of Industrial Chemistry*, 5th ed., Vol. A12, New York, VCH Publishers, pp. 583–588

Clemmesen, J. (1977) Statistical studies in the aetiology of malignant neoplasms. V. Trends and risks, Denmark 1943–72. *Acta pathol. microbiol. scand.*, **Suppl. 261**

Clemmesen, J. (1981) Epidemiological studies into the possible carcinogenicity of hair dyes. *Mutat. Res.*, **87**, 65–79

Cole, P., Monson, R.R., Haning, H. & Friedell, G.H. (1971) Smoking and cancer of the lower urinary tract. *New Engl. J. Med.*, **284**, 129–134

Cole, P., Hoover, R. & Friedell, G.H. (1972) Occupation and cancer of the lower urinary tract. *Cancer*, **29**, 1250–1261

Commission of the European Communities (1976) Council Directive 76/768/EEC of 27 July 1976 on the approximation of the laws of the Member States relating to cosmetic products. *Off. J. Eur. Commun.*, **L262**, 169–200

Commission of the European Communities (1990) Proposal for a Council Directive on the approximation of the laws of the Member States relating to cosmetic products. *Off. J. Eur. Comm.*, **C322**, 29–77

Commission of the European Communities (1991) Thirteenth Commission Directive of 12 March 1991 (91/814/EEC) on the approximation of the laws of the Member States relating to cosmetic products. *Off. J. Eur. Commun.*, **L91**, 59–62

Commission of the European Communities (1992) Fifteenth Commission Directive of 21 October 1992 (92/86/EEC) on the approximation of the laws of the Member States relating to cosmetic products. *Off. J. Eur. Commun.*, **L325**, 18–22

Conway, W.D. & Lethco, E.J. (1960) Aromatic amine impurities in Yellow AB and Yellow OB food dyes. *Anal. Chem.*, **32**, 838–841

Corbett, J.F. (1976) Hair dyes—their chemistry and toxicology. *Cosmet. Toiletries*, **91**, 21–28

Corbett, J.F. (1988) Hair coloring. *Clin. Dermatol.*, **6**, 93–101

Cordle, F. & Thompson, G.E. (1981) An epidemiologic assessment of hair dye use. *Regul. Toxicol. Pharmacol.*, **31**, 388–400

Cosmetic, Toiletry, and Fragrance Association (1991) *International Cosmetic Ingredient Dictionary*, Washington DC

Cosmetic, Toiletry, and Fragrance Association (1992) *Theory and Practice of Hair Waving*, Washington DC

Cosmetic, Toiletry, and Fragrance Association (undated) *Hairdressers*, Washington DC

Court Brown, W.M., Buckton, K.E., Jacobs, P.A., Tough, I.M., Kuenssberg, E.V. & Knox, J.D.E. (1966) *Chromosome Studies on Adults* (Eugenics Laboratory Memoirs 42), London, Cambridge University Press

Cronin, E. & Kullavanijaya, P. (1979) Hand dermatitis in hairdressers. *Acta dermatovenereol.*, **59**, 47–50

DiNardo, J.C., Picciano, J.C., Schnetzinger, R.W., Morris, W.E. & Wolf, B.A. (1985) Teratological assessment of five oxidative hair dyes in the rat. *Toxicol. appl. Pharmacol.*, **78**, 163–166

Draize, J.H., Nelson, A.A., Newburger, S.H. & Kelley, E.A. (1959) Inhalation toxicity studies of six types of aerosol hair sprays. *Proc. sci. Sect. Toilet Goods Assoc.*, **31**, 28–32

Dubrow, R. & Wegman, D.H. (1982) *Occupational Characteristics of White Male Cancer Victims in Massachusetts, 1971–1973*, Cincinnati, OH, National Institute for Occupational Safety and Health

Dubrow, R. & Wegman, D.H. (1983) Setting priorities for occupational cancer research and control: synthesis of the results of occupational disease surveillance studies. *J. natl Cancer Inst.*, **71**, 1123–1142

Dubrow, R. & Wegman, D.H. (1984) Cancer and occupation in Massachusetts: a death certificate study. *Am. J. ind. Med.*, **6**, 207–230

Dunham, L.J., Rabson, A.S., Stewart, H.L., Frank, A.S. & Young, J.L. (1968) Rates, interview, and pathology study of cancer of the urinary bladder in New Orleans, Louisiana. *J. natl Cancer Inst.*, **41**, 683–709

Eisenbrand, G., Blankart, M., Sommer, H. & Weber, B. (1991) *N*-Nitrosoalkanolamines in cosmetics. In: O'Neill, I.K., Chen, J. & Bartsch, H., eds, *Relevance to Human Cancer of N-Nitroso Compounds, Tobacco Smoke and Mycotoxins* (IARC Scientific Publications No. 105), Lyon, IARC, pp. 238–241

Eriksson, M. & Karlsson, M. (1992) Occupational and other environmental factors and multiple myeloma: a population based case–control study. *Br. J. ind. Med.*, **49**, 95–103

Fan, T.Y., Goff, U., Song, L., Fine, D.H., Arsenault, G.P. & Biemann, K. (1977) *N*-Nitrosodiethanolamine in cosmetics, lotions and shampoos. *Food Cosmet. Toxicol.*, **15**, 423–430

Feinland, R., Platko, F.E., White, L., DeMarco, R., Varco, J.J. & Wolfram, L.J. (1980) Hair preparations. In: Mark, H.F., Othmer, D.F., Overberger, C.G., Seaborg, G.T. & Grayson, N., eds, *Kirk-Othmer Encyclopedia of Chemical Technology*, 3rd ed., Vol. 12, New York, John Wiley & Sons, pp. 80–117

Ferguson, L.R. & Baguley, B.C. (1988) Verapamil as a co-mutagen in the *Salmonella*/mammalian microsome mutagenicity test. *Mutat. Res.*, **209**, 57–62

Ferguson, L.R., Roberton, A.M. & Berriman, J. (1990) Direct-acting mutagenic properties of some hair dyes used in New Zealand. *Mutat. Res.*, **245**, 41–46

Fisher, A.A. & Dooms-Goossens, A. (1976) Persulfate hair bleach reactions. Cutaneous and respiratory manifestations. *Arch. Dermatol.*, **112**, 1407–1410

Flodin, U., Redriksson, M. & Persson, B. (1987) Multiple myeloma and engine exhausts, fresh wood, and creosote: a case–referent study. *Am. J. ind. Med.*, **12**, 519–529

Fregert, S. (1986) Contact allergens and prevention of contact dermatitis. *J. Allergy clin. Immunol.*, **78**, 1071–1072

Freni-Titulaer, L.W.J., Kelley, D.B., Grow, A.G., McKinley, T.W., Arnett, F.C. & Hochberg, M.C. (1989) Connective tissue disease in southeastern Georgia: a case–control study of etiologic factors. *Am. J. Epidemiol.*, **130**, 404–409

Froines, J.R. & Garabrant, D.H. (1986) Quantitative evaluation of manicurists exposure to methyl, ethyl and isobutyl methacrylate during production of synthetic fingernails. *Appl. ind. Hyg.*, **1**, 70–74

Gagliardi, L., Ambroso, M., Mavro, J., Furno, F. & Discalzi, G. (1992) Exposure to paraphenylenediamine in hairdressing parlours. *Int. J. cosmet. Sci.*, **14**, 19–31

Gallagher, R.P., Threlfall, W.J., Band, P.R. & Spinelli, J.J. (1989) *Occupational Mortality in British Columbia 1950–1984*, Vancouver, BC, Workers' Compensation Board of British Columbia

Garfinkel, J., Selvin, S. & Brown, S.M. (1977) Possible increased risk of lung cancer among beauticians. *J. natl Cancer Inst.*, **58**, 141–143

Gerkens, R., Zucchini, G. & Ambroso, M. (1989) Exposure to methylene chloride in hairdressing salons (Ger.). *Aerosol Rep.*, **28**, 121–129

Gershon, S.D., Goldberg, M.A. & Rieger, M.M. (1972) Permanent waving. In: Balsam, M.S. & Sagarin, E., eds, *Cosmetics—Science and Technology*, 2nd ed., New York, Wiley-Interscience, pp. 167–250

Giles, G.G., Lickiss, J.N., Baikie, M.J., Lowenthal, R.M. & Panton, J. (1984) Myeloproliferative and lymphoproliferative disorders in Tasmania, 1972–80: occupational and familial aspects. *J. natl Cancer Inst.*, **72**, 1233–1240

Giovacchini, R.P., Becker, G.H., Brunner, M.J. & Dunlap, F.E. (1965) Pulmonary disease and hair-spray polymers. Effect of long-term exposure of dogs. *J. Am. med. Assoc.*, **193**, 298–299

Goulet, L. & Thériault, G. (1991) Stillbirth and chemical exposure of pregnant workers. *Scand. J. Work Environ. Health*, **17**, 25–31

Green, A., Willett, W.C., Colditz, G.A., Stampfer, M.J., Bain, C., Rosner, B., Hennekens, C.H. & Speizer, F.E. (1987) Use of permanent hair dyes and risk of breast cancer. *J. natl Cancer Inst.*, **79**, 253–257

Gubéran, E., Raymond, L. & Sweetnam, P.M. (1985) Increased risk for male bladder cancer among a cohort of male and female hairdressers from Geneva. *Int. J. Epidemiol.*, **14**, 549–554

Guerra, L., Bardazzi, F. & Tosti, A. (1992) Contact dermatitis in hairdressers' clients. *Contact Derm.*, **26**, 108–111

Guidotti, S., Wright, W.E. & Peters, J.M. (1982) Multiple myeloma in cosmetologists. *Am. J. ind. Med.*, **3**, 169–171

Gunter, B.J., Rostand, R.A. & Philbin, E. (1976) *Health Hazard Evaluation Determination. Radiant Lady Beauty Salon, Inc.* (HHE Report 75-128-262), Cincinnati, OH, National Institute for Occupational Safety and Health

Hartge, P., Hoover, R., Altman, R., Austin, D.F., Cantor, K.P., Child, M.A., Key, C.R., Mason, T.J., Marrett, L.D., Myers, M.H., Narayana, A.S., Silverman, D.T., Sullivan, J.W., Swanson, G.M., Thomas, D.B. & West, D.W. (1982) Use of hair dyes and risk of bladder cancer. *Cancer Res.*, **42**, 4784–4787

Hedner, K., Högstedt, B., Kolnig, A.-M., Mark-Vendel, E., Strömbeck, B. & Mitelman, F. (1982) Sister chromatid exchanges and structural chromosome aberrations in relation to age and sex. *Hum. Genet.*, **62**, 305–309

Hennekens, C.H., Rosner, B., Belanger, C., Speizer, F.E., Bain, C.J. & Peto, R. (1979) Use of permanent hair dyes and cancer among registered nurses. *Lancet*, **i**, 1390–1393

Hofer, H., Bornatowicz, N. & Reindl, E. (1983) Analysis of human chromosomes after repeated hair dyeing. *Food chem. Toxicol.*, **21**, 785–789

Hoffman, C.S., Jr (1973) Beauty salon air quality measurements. *Cosmet. Toiletries Fragrance Assoc. Cosmet. J.*, **5**, 16–21

Holman, C.D'A.J. & Armstrong, B.K. (1983) Hutchinson's melanotic freckle melanoma associated with non-permanent hair dyes. *Br. J. Cancer*, **48**, 599–601

Holness, D.L. & Nethercott, J.R. (1990) Dermatitis in hairdressers. *Dermatol. Clin.*, **8**, 119–126

Hopkins, J.E. & Manoharan, A. (1985) Severe aplastic anaemia following the use of hair dye: report of two cases and review of literature. *Postgrad. med. J.*, **61**, 1003–1005

Howe, G.R., Burch, J.D., Miller, A.B., Cook, G.M., Esteve, J., Morrison, B., Gordon, P., Chambers, L.W., Fodor, G. & Winsor, G.M. (1980) Tobacco use, occupation, coffee, various nutrients, and bladder cancer. *J. natl Cancer Inst.*, **64**, 701–713

Hrubec, Z., Blair, A.E., Rogot, E. & Vaught, J. (1992) *Mortality Risks by Occupation Among US Veterans of Known Smoking Status 1954–1980*, Vol. 1 (NIH Publ. No. 92-3407), Bethesda, MD, National Institutes of Health

IARC (1979) *IARC Monographs on the Evaluation of the Carcinogenic Risk of Chemicals to Humans*, Vol. 19, *Some Monomers, Plastics and Synthetic Elastomers, and Acrolein*, Lyon, pp. 379–380

Ippen, H., Seubert, S., Seubert, A., Bertram, H.P. & Kemper, F.H. (1981) Investigations on the dermatologic assessment of lead acetate as a hair-dyeing agent (Ger.). *Ärztlich. Kosmet.*, **11**, 93–98

Isacoff, H. (1979) Cosmetics. In: Mark, H.F., Othmer, D.F., Overberger, C.G., Seaborg, G.T. & Grayson, N., eds, *Kirk-Othmer Encyclopedia of Chemical Technology*, 3rd ed., Vol. 7, New York, John Wiley & Sons, pp. 143–176

Ivanov, B., Praskova, L., Mileva, M., Bulanova, M. & Georgieva, I. (1978) Spontaneous chromosomal aberration levels in human peripheral lymphocytes. *Mutat. Res.*, **52**, 421–426

Iyer, G., Kannan, K. & Khan, R.R. (1985) Toxicology of hairdyes: an overview. *J. Sci. ind. Res.*, **44**, 392–402

Jacobs, M.M., Burnett, C.M., Penicnak, A.J., Herrera, J.A., Morris, W.E., Shubik, P., Apaja, M. & Grenroth, G. (1984) Evaluation of the toxicity and carcinogenicity of hair dyes in Swiss mice. *Drug. chem. Toxicol.*, **7**, 573–586

Jain, M., Morgan, R.W. & Elinson, L. (1977) Hair dyes and bladder cancer (Letter to the Editor). *Can. med. Assoc. J.*, **117**, 1131, 1133

Jensen, O.M., Knudsen, J.B., McLaughlin, J.K. & Sørensen, B.L. (1988) The Copenhagen case–control study of renal pelvis and ureter cancer: role of smoking and occupational exposures. *Int. J. Cancer*, **41**, 557-561

Kiese, M. & Rauscher, E. (1968) The absorption of *p*-toluenediamine through human skin in hair dyeing. *Toxicol. appl. Pharmacol.*, **13**, 325–331

Kinkel, H.J. & Holzmann, S. (1973) Study of long-term percutaneous toxicity and carcinogenicity of hair dyes (oxidizing dyes) in rats. *Food Cosmet. Toxicol.*, **11**, 641–648

Kinlen, L.J., Harris, R., Garrod, A. & Rodriguez, K. (1977) Use of hair dyes by patients with breast cancer: a case–control study. *Br. med. J.*, **ii**, 366–368

Kirkland, D.J., Lawler, S.D. & Venitt, S. (1978a) Chromosomal damage and hair dyes. *Lancet*, **ii**, 124–128

Kirkland, D.J., Lawler, S.D. & Venitt, S. (1978b) Chromosomal damage and hair dyes (Letter to the Editor). *Lancet*, **ii**, 272

Kirkland, D.J., Honeycombe, J.R., Lawler, S.D., Venitt, S. & Crofton-Sleigh, C. (1981) Sister-chromatid exchanges before and after hair dyeing. *Mutat. Res.*, **90**, 279–286

Kleinhans, D. & Ranneberg, K.M. (1988) Immediate reactions after ammonium persulfate in bleaching powders (Ger.). *Allergologie*, **11**, 194–195

Koenig, K.L., Pasternack, B.S., Shore, R.E. & Strax, P. (1991) Hair dye use and breast cancer: a case–control study among screening participants. *Am. J. Epidemiol.*, **133**, 985-995

Kohler, J. (1989a) Waving. In: Elvers, B., Hawkins, S. Ravenscroft, M., Rounsaville, J.F. & Schulz, G., eds, *Ullmann's Encyclopedia of Industrial Chemistry*, 5th ed., Vol. A12, New York, VCH Publishers, pp. 588–591

Kohler, J. (1989b) Hair straightening preparations. In: Elvers, B., Hawkins, S. Ravenscroft, M., Rounsaville, J.F. & Schulz, G., eds, *Ullmann's Encyclopedia of Industrial Chemistry*, 5th ed., Vol. A12, New York, VCH Publishers, p. 591

Kono, S., Tokudome, S., Ikeda, M., Yoshimura, T. & Kuratsune, M. (1983) Cancer and other causes of death among female beauticians. *J. natl Cancer Inst.*, **70**, 443–446

Kramer, S., Ward, E., Meadows, A.T. & Malone, K.E. (1987) Medical and drug risk factors associated with neuroblastoma: a case–control study. *J. natl Cancer Inst.*, **78**, 797–804

Kritchevsky, W. (1937) *Hydrotropic Fatty Material and Method of Making Same* (US Patent 2,089,212)

Kronoveter, K. (1977) *Health Hazard Evaluation Determination. Hair Zoo, Penfield, New York* (RHE Report 76-82-361), Cincinnati, OH, National Institute for Occupational Safety and Health

Kuijten, R.R., Bunin, G.R., Nass, C.C. & Meadows A.T. (1990) Gestational and familial risk factors for childhood astrocytoma: results and a case–control study. *Cancer Res.*, **50**, 2608–2612

Kuijten, R.R., Bunin, G.R., Nass, C.C. & Meadows, A.T. (1992) Parental occupation and childhood astrocytoma: results of a case–control study. *Cancer Res.*, **52**, 782–786

Landthaler, M., Burg, G. & Zirbs, S. (1981) Colourant and nickel allergy in hairdressers (Ger.). *Hautarzt*, **32**, 281–284

Lang, G. (1989a) Hair cleansing and care preparations. In: Elvers, B., Hawkins, S. Ravenscroft, M., Rounsaville, J.F. & Schulz, G., eds, *Ullmann's Encyclopedia of Industrial Chemistry*, 5th ed., Vol. A12, New York, VCH Publishers, pp. 576–580

Lang, G. (1989b) Hairstyling preparations. In: Elvers, B., Hawkins, S. Ravenscroft, M., Rounsaville, J.F. & Schulz, G., eds, *Ullmann's Encyclopedia of Industrial Chemistry*, 5th ed., Vol. A12, New York, VCH Publishers, pp. 580–583

Liebscher, K.D. & Spengler, J. (1989) Toxicology and legal aspects. In: Elvers, B., Hawkins, S. Ravenscroft, M., Rounsaville, J.F. & Schulz, G., eds, *Ullmann's Encyclopedia of Industrial Chemistry*, 5th ed., Vol. A12, New York, VCH Publishers, pp. 593–597

Liem, D.H. (1977) Analysis of antimicrobial compounds in cosmetics. *Cosmet. Toiletries*, **92**, 59–72

Lindemayr, H. (1984) Eczema in hairdressers (Ger.). *Dermatosen*, **32**, 5–13

Lockwood, K. (1961) On the etiology of bladder tumors in København–Frederiksberg. An enquiry of 369 patients and 369 controls. *Acta pathol. microbiol. scand.*, **51** (Suppl. 145)

Lodén, M. (1986a) The *in vitro* permeability of human skin to benzene, ethylene glycol, formaldehyde and n-hexane. *Acta pharmacol. toxicol.*, **58**, 382–389

Lodén, M. (1986b) The effect of 4 barrier creams on the absorption of water, benzene, and formaldehyde into excised human skin. *Contact Derm.*, **14**, 292–296

Lowsma, H.B., Jones, R. & Pendergast, J.A. (1966) Effects of respired polyvinylpyrrolidone aerosol in rats. *Toxicol. appl. Pharmacol.*, **9**, 571–582

Lynde, C.W. & Mitchell, J.C. (1982) Patch test results in 66 hairdressers 1973–81. *Contact Derm.*, **8**, 302–307

Lynge, E. & Thygesen, L. (1988) Use of surveillance systems for occupational cancer: data from the Danish national system. *Int. J. Epidemiol.*, **17**, 493–500

Maibach, H.I. & Wolfram, L.J. (1981) Percutaneous penetration of hair dyes. *J. Soc. cosmet. Chem.*, **32**, 223–229

Malker, H.S.R., McLaughlin, J.K., Silverman, D.T., Ericsson, J.L.E., Stone, B.J., Weiner, J.A., Malker, B.K. & Blot, W.J. (1987) Occupational risks for bladder cancer among men in Sweden. *Cancer Res.*, **47**, 6763–6766

Malkinson, F.D. & Gehlmann, L. (1977) Factors affecting percutaneous absorption. In: Drill, V.A. & Lazar, P., eds, *Cutaneous Toxicity*, New York, Academic Press, pp. 63–81

Mareš, P. & Baran, P. (1989) Occupation of pregnant women in relation to the course and outcome of pregnancy (Czech.). *Cs. Gynekol.*, **54**, 1–6

Markowitz, J.A., Szklo, M., Sensenbrenner, L.L. & Warm, S. (1985) Hair dyes and acute nonlymphocytic leukaemia (Abstract). *Am. J. Epidemiol.*, **122**, 523

Marks, J.G., Jr (1986) Occupational skin disease in hairdressers. *State Art Rev. occup. Med.*, **1**, 273–284

Marks, T.A., Gupta, B.N., Ledoux, T.A. & Staples, R.E. (1981) Teratogenic evaluation of 2-nitro-*p*-phenylenediamine, 4-nitro-*o*-phenylenediamine, and 2,5-toluenediamine sulfate in the mouse. *Teratology*, **24**, 253–265

Marzulli, F.N., Watlington, P.M. & Maibach, H.I. (1978) Exploratory skin penetration findings relating to the use of lead acetate hair dyes. *Curr. Probl. Dermatol.*, **7**, 196–204

Marzulli, F.N., Anjo, D.M. & Maibach, H.I. (1981) In vivo skin penetration studies of 2,4-toluene-diamine, 2,4-diaminoanisole, 2-nitro-*p*-phenylenediamine, *p*-dioxane and *N*-nitrosodiethanol-amine in cosmetics. *Food Cosmet. Toxicol.*, **19**, 743–747

Matsuki, Y., Fukuhara, K., Inoue, Y., Yui, T. & Nambara, T. (1981) Characterization of amino-indamines and aminoindoanilines formed by oxidative hair dyeing and their mutagenicity. *J. pharmacol. Dyn.*, **4**, 269–274

Matsunaga, K., Hosokawa, K., Suzuki, M., Arima, Y. & Hayakawa, R. (1988) Occupational allergic contact dermatitis in beauticians. *Contact Derm.*, **18**, 94–96

McDonald, A.D., Armstrong, B., Cherry, N.M., Delorme, C., Diodati-Nolin, A., McDonald, J.C. & Robert, D. (1986) Spontaneous abortion and occupation. *J. occup. Med.*, **28**, 1232–1238

McDonald, A.D., McDonald, J.C., Armstrong, B., Cherry, N.M., Delorme, C., Nolin, A.D. & Robert, D. (1987) Occupation and pregnancy outcome. *Br. J. ind. Med*, **44**, 521–526

McDonald, A.D., McDonald, J.C., Armstrong, B., Cherry, N.M., Côté, R., Lavoie, J., Nolin, A.D. & Robert, D. (1988a) Fetal death and work in pregnancy. *Br. J. ind. Med.*, **45**, 148–157

McDonald, A.D., McDonald, J.C., Armstrong, B., Cherry, N.M., Côté, R., Lavoie, J., Nolin, A.D. & Robert D. (1988b) Congenital defects and work in pregnancy. *Br. J. ind. Med.*, **45**, 581–588

McDonough, E.G. (1937) *Truth About Cosmetics*, New York, The Drug and Cosmetic Industry

McDowall, M.E. (1985) *Occupational Reproductive Epidemiology. The Use of Routinely Collected Statistics in England and Wales 1980–82, Office of Population Censuses and Survey* (Studies on Medical and Population Subjects No. 50), London, Her Majesty's Stationery Office

McLaughlin, A.I.G., Bidstrup, P.L. & Konstam, M. (1963) The effect of hair lacquer sprays on the lung. *Food Cosmet. Toxicol.*, **1**, 171–188

McLaughlin, J.K., Linet, M.S., Stone, B.J., Blot, W.J., Fraumeni, J.F., Jr, Malker, H.S.R., Weiner, J.A. & Ericsson, J.L.E. (1988) Multiple myeloma and occupation in Sweden. *Arch. environ. Health*, **43**, 7–10

Menck, H.R., Pike, M.C., Henderson, B.E. & Jing, J.S. (1977) Lung cancer risk among beauticians and other female workers: brief communication. *J. natl Cancer Inst.*, **59**, 1423–1425

Milham, S. (1983) *Occupational Mortality in Washington State, 1950–1979* (NIOSH Research Report), Washington DC, US Department of Health, Education, and Welfare

Moore, M.R., Meredith, P.A., Watson, W.S., Sumner, D.J., Taylor, M.K. & Goldberg, A. (1980) The percutaneous absorption of lead-203 in humans from cosmetic preparations containing lead acetate, as assessed by whole-body counting and other techniques. *Food Cosmet. Toxicol.*, **18**, 399–405

Morrison, A.S., Ahlbom, A., Verhoek, W.G., Aoki, K., Leck, I., Ohno, Y. & Obata, K. (1985) Occupation and bladder cancer in Boston, USA, Manchester, UK, and Nagoya, Japan. *J. Epidemiol. Community Health*, **39**, 294–300

Nasca, P.C., Lawrence, C.E., Greenwald, P., Chorost, S., Arbuckle, J.T. & Paulson, A. (1980) Relationship of hair dye use, benign breast disease, and breast cancer. *J. natl Cancer Inst.*, **64**, 23–28

Nasca, P.C., Baptiste, M.S., Field, N.A., Metzger, B.B. & DeMartino, R. (1990) An epidemiologic case–control study of breast cancer (Abstract). *Am. J. Epidemiol.*, **132**, 790–791

Nethercott, J.R., MacPherson, M., Choi, B.C.K. & Nixon, P. (1986) Contact dermatitis in hairdressers. *Contact Derm.*, **14**, 73–79

Neuberger, J.S., Brownson, R.C., Morantz, R.A. & Chin, T.D.Y. (1991) Association of brain cancer with dental x-rays and occupation in Missouri. *Cancer Detect. Prev.*, **15**, 31–34

Neutel, C.I., Nair, R.C. & Last, J.M. (1978) Are hair dyes associated with bladder cancer? (Letter to the Editor). *Can. med. Assoc. J.*, **119**, 307–308

Nomura, A., Kolonel, L.N. & Yoshizawa, C.N. (1989) Smoking, alcohol, occupation, and hair dye use in cancer of the lower urinary tract. *Am. J. Epidemiol.*, **130**, 1159–1163

Office of Population Censuses and Surveys (1978) *Occupational Mortality Decennial Supplement, 1970–1972, England and Wales*, London, Her Majesty's Stationery Office

Office of Population Censuses and Surveys (1986) *Occupational Mortality Decennial Supplement, 1979–80, 1982–83, Great Britain*, London, Her Majesty's Stationery Office

Ohno, Y., Aoki, K., Obata, K. & Morrison, A.S. (1985) Case–control study of urinary bladder cancer in metropolitan Nagoya. *Natl Cancer Inst. Monogr.*, **69**, 229–234

Osorio, A.M., Bernstein, L., Garabrant, D.H. & Peters, J.M. (1986) Investigation of lung cancer among female cosmetologists. *J. occup. Med.*, **28**, 291–295

Østerlind, A., Tucker, M.A., Stone, B.J. & Jensen, O.M. (1988a) The Danish case–control study of cutaneous malignant melanoma. IV. No association with nutritional factors, alcohol, smoking or hair dyes. *Int. J. Cancer*, **42**, 825–828

Østerlind, A., Tucker, M.A., Hou-Jensen, K., Stone, B.J., Engholm, G. & Jensen, O.M. (1988b) The Danish case–control study of cutaneous malignant melanoma. I. Importance of host factors. *Int. J. Cancer*, **42**, 200–206

Palmer, A., Renzetti, A.D., Jr & Gillam, D. (1979) Respiratory disease prevalence in cosmetologists and its relationship to aerosol sprays. *Environ. Res.*, **19**, 136–153

Pearce, N.E. & Howard, J.K. (1986) Occupation, social class and male cancer mortality in New Zealand, 1974–78. *Int. J. Epidemiol.*, **15**, 456–462

Pepys, J., Hutchcroft, B.J. & Breslin, A.B.X. (1976) Asthma due to inhaled chemical agents— persulphate salts and henna in hairdressers. *Clin. Allergy*, **6**, 399–404

Persson, B., Dahlander, A.-M., Fredriksson, M., Brage, H.N., Ohlson, C.-G. & Axelson, O. (1989) Malignant lymphomas and occupational exposures. *Br. J. ind. Med.*, **46**, 516–520

Petri, M. & Allbritton, J. (1992) Hair product use in systemic lupus erythematosus. A case–control study. *Arthritis Rheum.*, **38**, 625–629

Pottern, L.M., Heineman, E.F., Olsen, J.H., Raffn, E. & Blair, A. (1992) Multiple myeloma among Danish women: employment history and workplace exposures. *Cancer Causes Control*, **3**, 427–432

Powers, D.H. (1972) Shampoos. In: Balsam, M.S. & Sagarin, E., eds, *Cosmetics—Science and Technology*, 2nd ed., New York, Interscience Publishers, pp. 73–116

Pukkala, E., Nokso-Koivisto, P. & Roponen, P. (1992) Changing cancer risk patterns among Finnish hairdressers. *Int. Arch. occup. environ. Health*, **64**, 39–42

Rajan, B. (1992) *Hairdressing Preparations. A Review Paper for CEC*, Bootle, Health and Safety Executive

Rastogi, S.C. (1990) Headspace analysis of 1,4-dioxane in products containing polyethoxylated surfactants by gas chromatography–mass spectrometry. *Chromatographia*, **29**, 441–445

Registrar General (1958) *The Registrar General's Decennial Supplement, England and Wales, 1951, Occupational Mortality*, Part II, Vol. 2, *Tables*, London, Her Majesty's Stationery Office

Registrar General (1971) *The Registrar General's Decennial Supplement, England and Wales, 1961, Occupational Mortality Tables*, London, Her Majesty's Stationery Office

Renzetti, A.D., Jr, Conrad, J., Watanabe, S., Palmer, A. & Armstrong, J. (1980) Thesaurosis from hair-spray exposure. A non-disease. Validation studies of an epidemiologic survey of cosmetologists. *Environ. Res.*, **22**, 130–138

Risch, H.A., Burch, J.D., Miller, A.B., Hill, G.B., Steele, R. & Howe, G.R. (1988) Occupational factors and the incidence of cancer of the bladder in Canada. *Br. J. ind. Med.*, **45**, 361–367

Rojanapo, W., Kupradinun, P., Tepsuwan, A., Chutimataewin, S. & Tanyakaset, M. (1986) Carcino-genicity of an oxidation product of *p*-phenylenediamine. *Carcinogenesis*, **7**, 1997–2002

Şardaş, S., Karakaya, A.E. & Şener, B. (1986) Determination of 2,4-diaminotoluene in human urine. *J. Fac. Pharm. Gazi*, **3**, 89–94

Sayad, R.S., Stevenson, M.P., Skory, L.K. & Jordan, J.W. (1976) Methylene chloride in hair sprays. *Soap Cosmet. chem. Spec.*, **52**, 87–90, 134–136

Scalia, S. & Menegatti, E. (1991) Assay of 1,4-dioxane in commercial cosmetic products by HPLC. *Farmaco*, **46**, 1365–1370

Schwaiblmair, M., Baur, X. & Fruhmann, G. (1990) Bronchial asthma caused by hair bleach in a hair-dresser (Ger.). *Dtsch. med. Wschr.*, **115**, 695–697

Searle, C.E. & Jones, E.L. (1977) Effects of repeated applications of two semi-permanent hair dyes to the skin of A and DBAf mice. *Br. J. Cancer*, **36**, 467–478

Shafer, N. & Shafer, R.W. (1976) Potential of carcinogenic effects of hair dyes. *N.Y. State J. Med.*, **76**, 394–396

Shibata, A., Sasaki, R., Hamajima, N. & Aoki, K. (1989) Mortality of hematopoietic disorders and hair dye use among barbers. *Acta haematol. jpn.*, **52**, 116–118

Shilling, S. & Lalich, N.R. (1984) Maternal occupation and industry and the pregnancy outcome of US married women, 1980. *Public Health Rep.*, **99**, 152–161

Shore, R.E., Pasternack, B.S., Thiessen, E.U., Sadow, M., Forbes, R. & Albert, R.E. (1979) A case–control study of hair dye use and breast cancer. *J. natl Cancer Inst.*, **62**, 277–283

Silverman, D.T., Levin, L.I., Hoover, R.N. & Hartge, P. (1989) Occupational risks of bladder cancer in the United States: I. White men. *J. natl Cancer Inst.*, **81**, 1472–1480

Silverman, D.T., Levin, L.I. & Hoover, R.N. (1990) Occupational risks of bladder cancer among white women in the United States. *Am. J. Epidemiol.*, **132**, 453–461

Skov, T. & Lynge, E. (1991) Non-Hodgkin's lymphoma and occupation in Denmark. *Scand. J. Soc. Med.*, **19**, 162–169

Skov, T., Andersen, A., Malker, H., Pukkala, E., Weiner, J. & Lynge, E. (1990) Risk for cancer of the urinary bladder among hairdressers in the Nordic countries. *Am. J. ind. Med.*, **17**, 217–223

Spinelli, J.J., Gallagher, R.P., Band, P.R. & Threlfall, W.J. (1984) Multiple myeloma, leukaemia, and cancer of the ovary in cosmetologists and hairdressers. *Am. J. ind. Med.*, **6**, 97–102

Spitz, M.R., Fueger, J.J., Goepfert, H. & Newell, G.R. (1990) Salivary gland cancer. A case–control investigation of risk factors. *Arch. Otolaryngol. Head Neck Surg.*, **116**, 1163–1166

Stamberg, J., Werczberger, R. & Koltin, Y. (1979) Non-mutagenicity of the hair dye, henna, in the Ames test. *Mutat. Res.*, **62**, 383–387

Starr, J.C., Yunginger, J. & Brahser, G.W. (1982) Immediate type I asthmatic response to henna following occupational exposure in hairdressers. *Ann. Allergy*, **48**, 98–99

Stavraky, K.M., Clarke, E.A. & Donner, A. (1979) Case–control study of hair dye use by patients with breast cancer and endometrial cancer. *J. natl Cancer Inst.*, **63**, 941–945

Stavraky, K.M., Clarke, E.A. & Donner, A. (1981) A case–control study of hair-dye use and cancers of various sites. *Br. J. Cancer*, **43**, 236–239

Stovall, G.K., Levin, L. & Oler, J. (1983) Occupational dermatitis among hairdressers. A multifactor analysis. *J. occup. Med.*, **25**, 871–878

Teta, M.J., Walrath, J., Wister Meigs, J. & Flannery, J.T. (1984) Cancer incidence among cosmetologists. *J. natl Cancer Inst.*, **72**, 1051–1057

Thomssen, E.G. (1947) *Modern Cosmetics*, New York, Drug and Cosmetic Industry, pp. 337–348, 365–376

Tikkanen, J. (1986) *Synnynnäisten Sydänvikojen Riskitekijät* [Risk factors for congenital heart disease], Thesis, Helsinki, Health Services Research, National Board of Health

Tikkanen, J., Kurppa, K., Timonen, H., Holmberg, P.C., Kuosma, E. & Rantala, K. (1988) Cardio-vascular malformations, work attendance and occupational exposures during pregnancy in Finland. *Am. J. ind. Med.*, **14**, 197–204

Turanitz, K., Kovac, R., Tuschl, H. & Pavlicek, E. (1983) Investigations on the effect of repeated hair dyeing on sister chromatid exchanges. *Food Chem. Toxicol.*, **21**, 791–793

US Consumer Product Safety Commission (1974) Vinyl chloride as an ingredient of drug and cosmetic aerosol products. *Fed. Regist.*, **39**, 30830

US Environmental Protection Agency (1993) Protection of stratospheric ozone. *Fed. Regist.*, **58**, 15014–15049

US Food and Drug Administration (1979) Nitrosamine-contaminated cosmetics; call for industry action; request for data. *Fed. Regist.*, **44**, 21365–21367

US Food and Drug Administration (1980) Lead acetate; listing as a color additive in cosmetics that color the hair on the scalp. *Fed. Regist.*, **45**, 72112–72116

US Food and Drug Administration (1991) *Cosmetic Handbook*, Washington DC, Department of Health and Human Services

Valeyre, D., Perret, G., Amouroux, J., Saumon, G., Georges, R., Pre, J. & Battesti, J.-P. (1983) Diffuse interstitial pulmonary disease due to prolonged inhalation of hair spray. *Lung*, **161**, 19–26

Vaughan, T.L., Daling, J.R. & Starzyk, P.M. (1984) Fetal death and maternal occupation. An analysis of birth records in the State of Washington. *J. occup. Med.*, **26**, 676–678

Viadana, E., Bross, I.D.J. & Houten, L. (1976) Cancer experience of men exposed to inhalation of chemicals or to combustion products. *J. occup. Med.*, **18**, 787–792

Vineis, P. & Magnani, C. (1985) Occupation and bladder cancer in males: a case–control study. *Int. J. Cancer*, **35**, 599–606

Vivoli, G. (1966) Experimental investigations of pulmonary lesions caused by prolonged inhalations of hair varnishes (Ital.). *Ig. Mod.*, **19**, 67–88

Walker, J.F. (1975) *Formaldehyde*, 3rd ed., New York, Robert E. Krieger

Wall, F.E. (1954) Shampoos and other hair preparations. In: Kirk, R.E. & Othmer, D.F., eds, *Encyclopedia of Chemical Technology*, Vol. 12, New York, Interscience, pp. 221–243

Wall, F.E. (1972) Bleaches, hair colorings and dye removers. In: Balsam, M.S. & Sagarin, E., eds, *Cosmetics Science and Technology*, 2nd ed., Vol. 2, New York, Wiley-Interscience, pp. 279–343

Watanabe, T., Hirayama, T. & Fukui, S. (1990) Mutagenicity of commercial hair dyes and detection of 2,7-diaminophenazine. *Mutat. Res.*, **244**, 303–308

Weinberg, F. (1980) Highlights on hair dyes. *Consum. Res. Mag.*, **63**, 19–21

Wernick, T., Lanman, B.M. & Fraux, J.L. (1975) Chronic toxicity, teratologic and reproduction studies with hair dyes. *Toxicol. appl. Pharmacol.*, **32**, 450–460

Willat, A.F. (1939) *Permanent Waving of Hair* (US Patent 2,180,380)

Wilson, C.H. (1974) Fluorometric determination of formaldehyde in cosmetic products. *J. Soc. Cosmet. Chem.*, **25**, 67–71

Winkel, F.M. (1936) *Hair Waving Unit* (US Patent 2,051,063)

Wolfram, L.J. & Maibach, H.I. (1985) Percutaneous penetration of hair dyes. *Arch. dermatol. Res.*, **277**, 235–241

Wynder, E.L. & Goodman, M. (1983) Epidemiology of breast cancer and hair dyes. *J. natl Cancer Inst.*, **71**, 481–488

Wynder, E.L., Onderdonk, J. & Mantel, N. (1963) An epidemiological investigation of cancer of the bladder. *Cancer*, **16**, 1388–1407

Zahm, S.H., Weisenburger, D.D., Babbitt, P.A., Saal, R.C., Vaught, J.B. & Blair, A. (1992) Use of hair coloring products and the risk of lymphoma, multiple myeloma, and chronic lymphocytic leukemia. *Am. J. public Health*, **82**, 990–997

Zviak, C. (1986a) Hair bleaching. In: Zviak, C., ed., *The Science of Hair Care*, New York, Marcel Dekker, pp. 213–233

Zviak, C. (1986b) Hair coloring—nonoxidation coloring. In: Zviak, C., ed., *The Science of Hair Care*, New York, Marcel Dekker, pp. 235–261

Zviak, C. (1986c) Oxidation coloring. In: Zviak, C., ed., *The Science of Hair Care*, New York, Marcel Dekker, pp. 263–286

Zviak, C. (1986d) Permanent waving and hair straightening. In: Zviak, C., ed., *The Science of Hair Care*, New York, Marcel Dekker, pp. 183–212

Zviak, C. & Camp, M. (1986) Laws and regulations. In: Zviak, C., ed., *The Science of Hair Care*, New York, Marcel Dekker, pp. 345–385

HAIR DYES

CI ACID ORANGE 3

1. Exposure Data

1.1 Chemical and physical data

1.1.1 *Synonyms, structural and molecular data*

Chem. Abstr. Serv. Reg. No.: 6373-74-6; replaces 74968-36-8

Chem. Abstr. Name: 5-[(2,4-Dinitrophenyl)amino]-2-(phenylamino)benzene-sulfonic acid, monosodium salt

Colour Index No.: 10385

Synonyms: 2-Anilino-5-(2,4-dinitroanilino)benzenesulfonic acid, monosodium salt; sodium 4-(2,4-dinitroanilino)diphenylamine-2-sulfonate

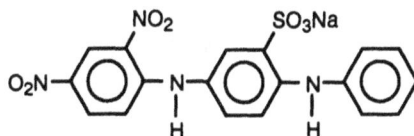

$C_{18}H_{13}N_4O_7S.Na$ Mol. wt: 452.39

1.1.2 *Chemical and physical properties*

(a) *Description*: Dark orange-brown microcrystals (US National Toxicology Program, 1988)

(b) *Spectroscopy data*: Infrared and nuclear magnetic resonance spectral data have been reported (US National Toxicology Program, 1988).

(c) *Solubility*: Very soluble in water (> 2% w/w) and ethanol (Society of Dyers and Colourists, 1971).

1.1.3 *Trade names, technical products and impurities*

Some trade names are: Acid Fast Yellow AG; Acid Fast Yellow E 5R; Acid Leather Light Brown G; Acid Orange 3; Acid Yellow E; Airedale Yellow E; Amido Yellow E; Amido Yellow EA; Amido Yellow EA-CF; Anthralan Yellow RRT; Coranil Brown H EPS; Derma Fur Yellow RT; Derma Yellow P; Dimacide Yellow N-5RL; Duasyn Acid Yellow RRT; Elbenyl Orange A-3RD; Erio Fast Yellow AE; Erio Fast Yellow AEN; Erio Yellow AEN; Erionyl Yellow E-AEN; Fast Light Yellow E; Fenalan Yellow E; Heliacid Light Yellow 4R; Intranyl Orange T-4R; Kiton Fast Yellow A; Lanaperl Yellow Brown GT; Light Fast Yellow

ES; Lissamine Fast Yellow AE; Lissamine Fast Yellow AES; Lissamine Yellow AE; Multacid Yellow 3R; Multicuer Brown MPH; Nailamide Yellow Brown E-L; Nylocrom Yellow 3R; Nylomine Acid Yellow B-RD; Nylosan Yellow E-3R; Polan Yellow E-3R; Sellacid Yellow AEN; Solanile Yellow E; Sulfacid Light Yellow 5RL; Superian Yellow R; Tectilon Orange 3GT; Tertracid Light Yellow 2R; Unitertracid Light Yellow RR; Vondacid Fast Yellow AE; Vondacid Light Yellow AE; Xylene Fast Yellow ES.

A technical product was reported to contain approximately 65–67% CI Acid Orange 3 (US National Toxicology Program, 1988), together with approximately 16% sodium chloride and 19% sodium sulfate.

1.1.4 *Analysis*

No data were available to the Working Group.

1.2 Production and use

1.2.1 *Production*

CI Acid Orange 3 was first synthesized by Schmidlin in 1911 and has been produced commercially since the 1920s. It is prepared by the condensation of 1-chloro-2,4-dinitro-benzene with 5-amino-2-anilinobenzenesulfonic acid (Society of Dyers and Colourists, 1971).

At present, approximately 900 kg of CI Acid Orange 3 are used annually in the USA, according to industry estimates.

1.2.2 *Use*

CI Acid Orange 3 has been used as a dye in semi-permanent hair colouring products since the late 1950s. These products are generally shampooed into the hair, lathered and then allowed to remain in contact with the hair and scalp for 30–45 min. At the concentrations (up to 0.2%) used in these preparations, CI Acid Orange 3 is in solution (Frenkel & Brody, 1973; US National Toxicology Program, 1988). It is also used to dye textiles (US Environmental Protection Agency, 1990).

1.3 Occurrence

1.3.1 *Natural occurrence*

CI Acid Orange 3 is not known to occur as a natural product.

1.3.2 *Occupational exposure*

At one site where upholstery fabric was printed and powder acid dyes were used for dyeing nylon fibres, an industrial hygiene study was conducted to estimate dust exposures during weighing of the powder dyes. The principal dyes handled were CI Acid Black 107, CI Acid Brown 298 and CI Acid Orange 3. Spectrophotometric estimates of the average airborne concentration of active colourant were 10 μg/m^3 using personal filters and < 0.01 μg/m^3 using area filters (US Environmental Protection Agency, 1990).

On the basis of a survey conducted in the USA between 1981 and 1983, the US National Institute for Occupational Safety and Health estimated that a total of 22 238 workers, including 14 728 women, may have been exposed to CI Acid Orange 3 in beauty salons (US National Library of Medicine, 1992).

1.4 Regulations and guidelines

No data were available to the Working Group.

2. Studies of Cancer in Humans

No data were available to the Working Group.

3. Studies of Cancer in Experimental Animals

3.1 Oral administration

3.1.1 *Mouse*

Groups of 50 male and 50 female B6C3F$_1$ mice, eight to nine weeks of age, were given 0, 125 or 250 (males) or 0, 250 or 500 (females) mg/kg bw CI Acid Orange 3 (90% pure, ≤ 1% impurities other than water and acetone) by gavage in corn oil on five days per week for 103 weeks and were sacrified at 112–113 weeks of age. Mean body weights of high-dose mice were 5–11% lower than those of vehicle controls after week 74. Survival at the end of the study was: males—control, 38/50; low-dose, 25/50; and high-dose, 26/50; females—control, 23/50; low-dose, 23/50; and high-dose, 24/50. Treatment-related nephrotoxicity occurred in animals of each sex. Survival of males was reduced after week 100; this was attributed to the nephrotoxicity. There was no significant increase in the incidence of any tumour. Epithelial hyperplasia of the urinary bladder was observed in one low-dose and three high-dose females. One low-dose female had a squamous-cell carcinoma of the urinary bladder (US National Toxicology Program, 1988).

3.1.2 *Rat*

Groups of 50 male and 50 female Fischer 344/N rats, six to seven weeks of age, were given 0, 375 or 750 mg/kg bw CI Acid Orange 3 (90% pure, ≤ 1% impurities other than water and acetone) by gavage in corn oil on five days per week for 103 weeks and were sacrificed at 110–112 weeks of age. Survival of high-dose male rats (after week 33) and high-dose female rats (after week 14) was significantly lower than that of vehicle controls and was attributed to nephrotoxicity. Final survival rates were: males—control, 36/50; low-dose, 30/50; and high-dose 0/50 ($p < 0.001$); females—control, 43/50; low-dose, 34/50; and high-dose, 7/50

($p < 0.001$). The primary cause of death in treated animals was a spectrum of non-neoplastic renal lesions. Renal pelvic epithelial hyperplasia was seen in 0/50 control, 6/50 low-dose and 13/50 high-dose males and 0/50 control, 2/50 low-dose and 13/50 high-dose females. Transitional-cell carcinomas of the renal pelvis were observed only in high-dose female rats (6/50; $p < 0.001$, life table test) at 87–104 weeks; 18 animals were still alive at 87 weeks. No significant increase in the incidence of tumours at any site was reported in male rats, but, because of a marked reduction in survival, the high-dose group was considered to be inadequate for an assessment of carcinogenic activity (US National Toxicology Program, 1988).

4. Other Relevant Data

4.1 Absorption, distribution, metabolism and excretion

No data were available to the Working Group.

4.2 Toxic effects

4.2.1 *Humans*

No data were available to the Working Group.

4.2.2 *Experimental systems*

In 14-day studies, groups of five Fischer 344/N rats of each sex received 0, 94, 187, 375, 750 or 1500 mg/kg bw CI Acid Orange 3 (purity, 90%) and groups of five B6C3F$_1$ mice of each sex received 0, 62, 125, 250, 500 or 1000 mg/kg bw CI Acid Orange 3 in corn oil by gavage for 14 consecutive days. No compound-related toxic effect was observed (US National Toxicology Program, 1988).

In 13-week studies, groups of 10 Fischer 344/N rats of each sex received 0, 94, 187, 375, 750 or 1500 mg/kg bw CI Acid Orange 3 and groups of 10 B6C3F$_1$ mice of each sex received 0, 250, 500, 1000 or 2000 mg/kg bw in corn oil by gavage on five days per week. Dose-related kidney lesions were observed in rats and mice of each sex, including variable degrees of degeneration and necrosis of epithelial cells in the proximal convoluted tubules, increased basophilia of tubular epithelium and granular casts in the tubules. A marked reduction in survival was observed in female rats that received the highest dose (US National Toxicology Program, 1988).

In the two-year studies in Fischer 344/N rats and B6C3F$_1$ mice described above, the primary cause of death was dose-related kidney lesions (US National Toxicology Program, 1988).

Acid Orange 3 was present at a low concentration (0.2%) in semi-permanent hair colouring formulations evaluated in a 13-week study of dermal toxicity in rabbits (Burnett et al., 1976) and in a two-year feeding study in dogs (Wernick et al., 1975), described in detail on p. 97. No treatment-related toxicity was detected in either study. [The Working Group noted that the dose of each component of the formulation was very low and unlikely to have been toxic.]

4.3 Reproductive and developmental effects

4.3.1 *Humans*

No data were available to the Working Group.

4.3.2 *Experimental systems*

No data were available to the Working Group on the reproductive and developmental effects of CI Acid Orange 3 alone. This compound was present at low concentrations in semi-permanent hair colouring formulations evaluated in a study of fertility and reproductive performance in rats (0.2%) (Wernick *et al.*, 1975; see p. 99), in a study of heritable translocation in rats (0.06%) (Burnett *et al.*, 1981; see p. 104) and in studies of teratogenesis in rats (0.2%) (Wernick *et al.*, 1975; Burnett *et al.*, 1976) and rabbits (0.2%) (Wernick *et al.*, 1975) (see p. 100). No treatment-related adverse effect was detected. [The Working Group noted that the dose of each component of the formulation was very low and unlikely to be toxic.]

4.4 Genetic and related effects

4.4.1 *Humans*

No data were available to the Working Group.

4.4.2 *Experimental systems* (see also Table 1 and Appendices 1 and 2)

CI Acid Orange 3 was mutagenic to *Salmonella typhimurium* in the presence and absence of metabolic activation.

Table 1. Genetic and related effects of CI Acid Orange 3

Test system	Result		Dose (LED/HID) (μg/ml)	Reference
	Without exogenous metabolic system	With exogenous metabolic system		
SA0, *Salmonella typhimurium* TA100, reverse mutation	+	+	167.0000	Zeiger *et al.* (1988)
SA5, *Salmonella typhimurium* TA1535, reverse mutation	–	–	500.0000	Zeiger *et al.* (1988)
SA9, *Salmonella typhimurium* TA98, reverse mutation	+	+	50.0000	Zeiger *et al.* (1988)
SAS, *Salmonella typhimurium* TA97, reverse mutation	(+)	(+)	167.0000	Zeiger *et al.* (1988)

+, positive; (+), weakly positive; –, negative

5. Summary of Data Reported and Evaluation

5.1 Exposure data

CI Acid Orange 3 is used to a limited extent as a dye in semi-permanent hair colouring products and in the dyeing of textiles.

5.2 Human carcinogenicity data

No data were available to the Working Group.

5.3 Animal carcinogenicity data

CI Acid Orange 3 was tested for carcinogenicity by gavage in one study in mice and in one study in rats. In mice, there was no significant increase in the incidence of tumours. A significant increase in the incidence of transitional-cell carcinomas of the renal pelvis was observed in female rats given the high dose. The data on high-dose male rats could not be evaluated owing to their poor survival.

5.4 Other relevant data

CI Acid Orange 3 caused renal toxicity in rats and mice. It was mutagenic to bacteria.

5.5 Evaluation[1]

There is *inadequate evidence* in humans for the carcinogenicity of CI Acid Orange 3.

There is *limited evidence* in experimental animals for the carcinogenicity of CI Acid Orange 3.

Overall evaluation

CI Acid Orange 3 *is not classifiable as to its carcinogenicity to humans (Group 3).*

6. References

Burnett, C., Goldenthal, E.I., Harris, S.B., Wazeter, F.X., Strausburg, J., Kapp, R. & Voelker, R. (1976) Teratology and percutaneous toxicity studies on hair dyes. *J. Toxicol. environ. Health*, **1**, 1027–1040

Burnett, C., Loehr, R. & Corbett, J. (1981) Heritable translocation study on two hair dye formulations. *Fundam. appl. Toxicol.*, **1**, 325–328

---

[1]For definition of the italicized terms, see Preamble, pp. 26–30.

Frenkel, E.P. & Brody, F. (1973) Percutaneous absorption and elimination of an aromatic hair dye. *Arch. environ. Health*, **27**, 401–404

Society of Dyers and Colourists (1971) *Colour Index*, 3rd ed., Vol. 4, Bradford, Yorkshire, p. 4007

US Environmental Protection Agency (1990) *Textile Dye Weighing Monitoring Study* (EPA Report No. EPA-560/5-90-009), Washington DC, Office of Toxic Substances

US National Library of Medicine (1992) *Registry of Toxic Effects of Chemical Substances* (RTECS No. DB5042500), Bethesda, MD

US National Toxicology Program (1988) *Toxicology and Carcinogenesis Studies of CI Acid Orange 3 (CAS No. 6373-74-6) in F344/N Rats and B6C3F$_1$ Mice (Gavage Studies)* (NTP Technical Report 335; NIH Publ. No. 89-2591), Research Triangle Park, NC

Wernick, T., Lanman, B.M. & Fraux, J.L. (1975) Chronic toxicity, teratology and reproduction studies with hair dyes. *Toxicol. appl. Pharmacol.*, **32**, 450–460

Zeiger, E., Anderson, B., Haworth, S., Lawlor, T. & Mortelmans, K. (1988) *Salmonella* mutagenicity tests: IV. Results from the testing of 300 chemicals. *Environ. Mol. Mutag.*, **11** (Suppl. 12), 1–158

HC BLUE NO. 1

1. Exposure Data

1.1 Chemical and physical data

1.1.1 *Synonyms, structural and molecular data*

Chem. Abstr. Serv. Reg. No.: 2784-94-3

Chem. Abstr. Name: 2,2'-([4-(Methylamino)-3-nitrophenyl]imino)bis(ethanol)

Synonyms: N^4,N^4-Bis(2-hydroxyethyl)-N^1-methyl-2-nitro-*para*-phenylenediamine; HC Blue 1; HC Blue Number 1; 2,2'-([4-(methylamino)-3-nitrophenyl]imino)di(ethanol)

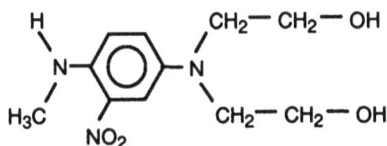

$C_{11}H_{17}N_3O_4$ Mol. wt: 255.27

1.1.2 *Chemical and physical properties of the substance*

From US National Toxicology Program (1985), unless otherwise specified

(a) *Description*: Dark-blue microcrystals or blue–black amorphous powder

(b) *Melting-point*: 101.5–104 °C

(c) *Spectroscopy data*: Infrared, ultraviolet and nuclear magnetic resonance spectral data have been reported.

(d) *Solubility*: Slightly soluble in water (0.38% w/w) (Frenkel & Brody, 1973); soluble in ethanol, methanol and acetone

(e) *Octanol/water partition coefficient (P)*: 17.2

1.1.3 *Trade names, technical products and impurities*

HC Blue No. 1 has been available commercially with a purity ≥ 95%, with 2-([4-(methyl-amino)-3-nitrophenyl]imino)ethanol (< 5 %) as a possible impurity.

1.1.4 *Analysis*

A thin-layer chromatographic method with spectrophotometric analysis has been reported for determination of HC Blue No. 1 in biological fluids (Frenkel & Brody, 1973).

1.2 Production and use

1.2.1 *Production*

HC Blue No. 1 was produced commercially by the reaction of 4-fluoro-3-nitrobenzen-amine with ethylene oxide (see IARC, 1985, 1987) to form 2,2-[(4-fluoro-3-nitrophenyl)-imino]bis(ethanol); this intermediate was reacted with methylamine to form HC Blue No. 1.

HC Blue No. 1 is not known to be produced or used currently anywhere in the world. Production and use of HC Blue No. 1 began in the late 1960s and was discontinued in the mid-1980s. In the early 1980s, approximately 6-8 tonnes of HC Blue No. 1 were used annually in the USA, according to industry estimates.

1.2.2 *Use*

HC Blue No. 1 was used exclusively as a dye in semi-permanent hair colouring products. These products were generally shampooed into the hair, lathered and then allowed to remain in contact with the hair and scalp for 30-45 min. The concentration of HC Blue No. 1 used in these preparations ranged from 1 to 2% (Frenkel & Brody, 1973; US National Toxicology Program, 1985).

1.3 Occurrence

1.3.1 *Natural occurrence*

HC Blue No. 1 is not known to occur as a natural product.

1.3.2 *Occupational exposure*

No data were available to the Working Group.

1.4 Regulations and guidelines

The production and use of HC Blue No. 1 were discontinued in the mid-1980s.

2. Studies of Cancer in Humans

No data were available to the Working Group.

3. Studies of Cancer in Experimental Animals

3.1 Oral administration

3.1.1 *Mouse*

Groups of 50 male and 50 female B6C3F$_1$ mice, 53 days of age, were fed 0, 1500 or 3000 mg/kg (ppm) (males) or 0, 3000 or 6000 ppm (females) HC Blue No. 1 ($\sim$ 97% pure) in the diet for 103 weeks and were killed at 112–115 weeks of age. Final mean body weights were reduced by 10–12% in treated males and 21–29% in treated females compared with controls. Survival at the end of the study was: males—control, 33/50; low-dose, 37/50; and high-dose, 30/50; females—control, 36/50; low-dose, 28/50; and high-dose, 24/50 (p = 0.026, life table test). Survival of female mice was reduced after 91 weeks, and many high-dose females that died early had hepatocellular carcinomas. In male and female mice, both doses of HC Blue No. 1 increased the incidence of hepatocellular carcinomas (males: control, 11/50; low-dose, 20/50; and high-dose, 30/50 (p < 0.001, incidental tumour trend test); females: control, 1/50; low-dose, 24/48; and high-dose, 47/49 (p < 0.001, incidental tumour trend test)). The incidence of hepatocellular adenomas was increased in both low-dose groups (males: control, 4/50; low-dose, 17/50 (p = 0.003, incidental tumour test); and high-dose, 10/50; females: control, 2/50; low-dose, 11/48 (p = 0.004, incidental tumour test); and high-dose, 4/49). In male mice, the incidences of thyroid follicular hyperplasia (control, 3/47; low-dose, 7/49; high-dose, 14/50) and thyroid follicular adenomas (control, 0/47; low-dose, 0/49; high-dose, 5/50 (p = 0.027, incidental tumour test)) were increased. The historical incidence of thyroid follicular adenomas at the study laboratory was 0–6% (US National Toxicology Program, 1985; Kari *et al.*, 1989a).

In a subsequent study, in which only the liver was examined, two groups of 48 female B6C3F$_1$ mice, six weeks of age, were fed 0.3% [3000 mg/kg of diet] (ppm) highly purified HC Blue No. 1 or recrystallized, charcoal-filtered commercial HC Blue No. 1 in the diet for 24 months. One group of 48 female mice served as controls. Highly purified HC Blue No. 1 increased the incidences of hepatocellular adenomas (10/46 *versus* 1/48 controls) and of hepatocellular carcinoms (41/46 *versus* 2/48 controls), as did commercial HC Blue No. 1 (hepatocellular adenomas: 10/46 *versus* 1/48 controls; hepatocellular carcinomas: 44/46 *versus* 2/48 controls). Three additional groups of 24 or 48 females received 0.3% recrystallized, charcoal-filtered commercial HC Blue No. 1 in the diet for nine months followed by 15 months without treatment, for 15 months in the diet followed by nine months without treatment or every other week for 24 months. All three treatment regimens resulted in an increase in the number of mice with benign and malignant hepatocellular tumours. Data from the five experiments are summarized in Table 1 (Burnett & Corbett, 1987).

3.1.2 *Rat*

Groups of 50 male and 50 female Fischer 344/N rats, 53 days of age, were fed 0, 1500 or 3000 mg/kg (ppm) of diet HC Blue No. 1 (∼ 97% pure) for 103 weeks and were killed at 112–115 weeks of age. From about week 50, the body weights of high-dose females were depressed by > 10% compared with controls. Survival at the end of the study was not affected by treatment (males—control, 39/50; low-dose, 34/50; and high-dose, 41/50; females—control, 40/50; low-dose, 38/50; and high-dose, 41/50). HC Blue No. 1 increased the incidences of pulmonary adenomatous hyperplasia (control, 2/50; low-dose, 5/49; high-dose, 8/50) and pulmonary adenomas/carcinomas (control, 1/50; low-dose, 3/49; high-dose, 7/50; p = 0.034, incidental tumour test) in females. The mean historical incidence of pulmonary adenomas and carcinomas in the laboratory was 2% (range, 0–3%). Male rats also had an increased incidence of pulmonary adenomatous hyperplasia (control, 3/50; low-dose, 5/50; high-dose, 7/50). A significant positive trend was seen in the incidence of

Table 1. Hepatocellular tumour incidences in female B6C3F$_1$ mice fed various preparations of HC Blue No. 1 in the diet

Treatment regimen	Incidence of hepatocellular tumours		
	Adenomas	Carcinomas	Combined
HC Blue No. 1 (highly purified) continuously for 24 months	10/46	41/46	45/46
HC Blue No. 1 (recrystallized, charcoal filtered) continuously for 24 months	10/46	44/46	46/46
HC Blue No. 1 (recrystallized, charcoal filtered) for 9 months followed by control diet for 15 months	10/22	13/22	20/22
HC Blue No. 1 (recrystallized, charcoal filtered) for 15 months followed by control diet for 9 months	4/23	19/23	20/23
HC Blue No. 1 (recrystallized, charcoal filtered) every other week for 24 months	21/46	25/46	40/46
Controls	1/48	2/48	3/48

From Burnett & Corbett (1987)

uterine stromal polyps (control, 5/50; low-dose, 9/50; and high-dose, 14/50; $p = 0.022$, incidental tumour trend test) and of neoplastic nodules or neoplastic nodules and carcinomas (combined) in the livers of male rats, although the incidences in the treated groups were not significantly greater than those in controls (US National Toxicology Program, 1985; Kari *et al.*, 1989a).

4. Other Relevant Data

4.1 Absorption, distribution, metabolism and excretion

4.1.1 *Humans*

About 85 g of a commercial semi-permanent hair dye formulation containing 1.48% HC Blue No. 1 enriched with 113.6 μCi/mg [ring-^{14}C]-labelled HC Blue No. 1 was applied on two occasions to the hair of human volunteers, worked in gently for 5–8 min and allowed to remain in contact with the hair and scalp for an additional 30 min. On the first occasion, the hair was shaven, and radiolabel accounting for 0.09–0.15% of that applied was detected in the urine over a seven-day period; half was excreted in the urine after 18 h. On the second occasion, the hair was shaven only after 30 days: cumulative absorption was 0.15% on the first day and 0.5% on the 30th day; half of the radiolabel was excreted after 138 h (Maibach & Wolfram, 1981; Wolfram & Maibach, 1985). [The Working Group noted that in neither study were urinary metabolites identified, so that the metabolic fate of HC Blue No. 1 in humans remains unknown.]

4.1.2 *Experimental systems*

The same commercial hair dye formulation as used above was applied to the scalp hair of rhesus monkeys and allowed to remain in contact for 30 min. Radiolabel accounting for

0.12–0.13% of that applied was detected in urine over a seven-day period; half was excreted in the urine after 40 h (Maibach & Wolfram, 1981; Wolfram & Maibach, 1985).

Following intraperitoneal or subcutaneous injection of 2.5, 3.5, 4.0, 5.0 or 100 mg/kg bw HC Blue No. 1 (98% pure, containing four minor components) to adult Fischer rats or rabbits, over 90% was recovered in bile or urine within 6 h of administration. Following application of about 1 mg/cm^2 (250 μg/ml in saline) HC Blue No. 1 to the skin, about 1% of the dose was recovered in the bile and slightly more in the urine of rats and an average of 4.5% of the dose in the urine of rabbits after 48 h (Frenkel & Brody, 1973).

[The Working Group noted that urinary metabolites were not identified in these three studies].

Up to 40% of radiolabel was recovered in the urine of B6C3F$_1$ mice and Fischer 344/N rats after oral administration by gavage of 100 mg/kg bw [ring-^{14}C]HC Blue No. 1 (29 mCi/mmol [113.6 μCi/mg]; 97% pure). HC Blue No. 1 administered orally to B6C3F$_1$ mice yielded three metabolites in equal proportions, which were more water soluble than the parent compound; one was a glucuronide of the parent compound. Metabolism of [ring-^{14}C]HC Blue No. 1 (200 μM [51 mg]) by hepatocytes isolated from mice and rats yielded profiles similar to those seen *in vivo*. High-performance liquid chromatography separation showed that HC Blue No. 1 is metabolized extensively in mice to five major metabolites. Thermospray liquid chromatography–mass spectrometry of these metabolites provided tentative evidence for nitroreduction, *N*-demethylation and conjugation (glucuronidation of a demethylated product and acetylation). In rats, HC Blue No. 1 produced three metabolites similar to those found in mice (Kari *et al.*, 1988, 1989b, 1990a,b).

4.2 Toxic effects

4.2.1 *Humans*

No data were available to the Working Group.

4.2.2 *Experimental systems*

Concentrations of 0, 1500 or 3000 ppm (mg/kg of diet) HC Blue No. 1 (~ 97% pure) were administered in the diet to Fischer 344/N rats of each sex and to male B6C3F$_1$ mice, and concentrations of 0, 3000 or 6000 ppm (mg/kg of diet) were given to female B6C3F$_1$ mice, for 103 weeks. The calculated average daily doses were 66 and 38 mg/kg bw for male rats, 74 and 153 mg/kg bw for female rats, 309 and 582 mg/kg bw for male mice, and 778 and 1634 mg/kg bw for female mice. No toxicologically significant non-neoplastic lesion was found in rats or mice of either sex (US National Toxicology Program, 1985; Kari *et al.*, 1989a).

HC Blue No. 1 was present at 1.6% in semi-permanent hair colouring formulations evaluated in a 13-week study of dermal toxicity in rabbits (Burnett *et al.*, 1976), at 0.3% in a 20-month study of dermal toxicity in mice (Jacobs *et al.*, 1984) and at 1.54% in a two-year feeding study in dogs (Wernick *et al.*, 1975), described in detail on p. 97. No treatment-related toxicity was detected. [The Working Group noted that the dose of each component of the formulation was very low and unlikely to have been toxic.]

4.3 Reproductive and developmental effects

4.3.1 *Humans*

No data were available to the Working Group.

4.3.2 *Experimental systems*

No data were available to the Working Group on the reproductive and developmental effects of HC Blue No. 1 alone. The compound was present at low concentrations in semi-permanent hair colouring formulations evaluated in a study of fertility and reproductive performance in rats (1.54%) (Wernick *et al.*, 1975; see p. 99), in a study of heritable trans-location in rats (0.5%) (Burnett *et al.*, 1981; see p. 104) and in studies of teratogenesis in rats (Wernick *et al.*, 1975, 1.54%; Burnett *et al.*, 1976, 1.6%) and rabbits (1.54%) (Wernick *et al.*, 1975) (see p. 100). No treatment-related adverse effect was detected. [The Working Group noted that the dose of each component of the formulation was very low and unlikely to have been toxic.]

4.4 Genetic and related effects

4.4.1 *Humans*

No data were available to the Working Group.

4.4.2 *Experimental systems* (see also Tables 2 and 3 and Appendices 1 and 2)

Both commercial preparations and purified samples of HC Blue No. 1 have been tested for genetic and related effects. The results of some tests indicate that the bacterial mutagenicity and DNA adducts seen after exposure to commercial HC Blue No. 1 are due to impurities and not to the main component (Abu-Shakra *et al.*, 1991). Commercial samples of HC Blue No. 1 induced mutations in *Salmonella typhimurium* and mutations at both the *hprt* locus of cultured Chinese hamster ovary cells and the *tk* locus of mouse lymphoma L5178Y cells. In contrast, purified samples did not induce mutation in *S. typhimurium*, *Escherichia coli*, *Saccharomyces cerevisiae*, *Schizosaccharomyces pombe* or *Drosophila melanogaster* or at the *hprt* locus of Chinese hamster V79 cells; a weak response was, however, obtained at the *tk* locus of mouse lymphoma L5178Y cells. The negative results in *S. typhimurium* were obtained at doses of the purified material up to 50-fold higher than the effective doses needed when commercial HC Blue No. 1 samples were tested.

Purified and commercial HC Blue No. 1 preparations induced unscheduled DNA synthesis in primary cultures of rat hepatocytes. Purified samples were found to induce unscheduled DNA synthesis in primary cultures of mouse, Syrian hamster, rabbit and rhesus monkey hepatocytes.

Sister chromatid exchange frequency was increased in cultured Chinese hamster ovary cells exposed to purified and commercial HC Blue No. 1 and in primary cultures of mouse hepatocytes exposed to a commercial preparation. Chromosomal aberrations were induced in primary mouse but not rat hepatocyte cultures by commercial HC Blue No. 1. A commercial HC Blue No. 1 preparation increased the frequency of chromosomal aberrations in Chinese hamster ovary cells *in vitro* in the presence of a metabolic activation system, whereas one study with purified HC Blue No. 1 showed no increase in chromosomal aberrations; however, in the latter study, it was tested at a lower concentration and only in the absence of an exogenous metabolic activation system. A commercial HC Blue No. 1 was reported not to induce morphological transformation of Syrian hamster embryo cells.

Purified HC Blue No. 1 induced micronuclei in the bone marrow of female ICR mice exposed *in vivo* intraperitoneally but did not increase the frequency in the bone marrow of male CBA, male or female CD-1 or male ICR mice. A commercial sample of HC Blue No. 1 (97%) did not induce micronuclei in male or female B6C3F$_1$ mice exposed by oral administration.

Commercial HC Blue No. 1 inhibited gap-junctional intercellular communication in Chinese hamster lung V79 cells at non-cytotoxic doses.

It was reported in an abstract that presumably commercial samples (concentration unspecified) of HC Blue No. 1 induced S-phase synthesis in the livers of male but not female mice exposed *in vivo*. The samples did not induce unscheduled DNA synthesis in the livers of mice or rats exposed *in vivo* but induced unscheduled DNA synthesis in primary cultures of mouse, Syrian hamster and cynomolgus monkey hepatocytes. The samples induced hepatocyte proliferation in mice but not in rats treated *in vivo* (Mirsalis *et al.*, 1986).

5. Summary of Data Reported and Evaluation

5.1 Exposure data

HC Blue No. 1 was used as a semi-permanent hair dye until the mid-1980s, when its production and use were discontinued.

5.2 Human carcinogenicity data

No data were available to the Working Group.

5.3 Animal carcinogenicity data

HC Blue No. 1 was tested for carcinogenicity by administration in the diet in two studies in mice, one of which was restricted to females, and in one study in male and female rats. In one study in male and female mice and in several experiments in the study of females, it significantly increased the incidence of hepatocellular adenomas and/or carcinomas in mice of each sex and increased the incidence of thyroid follicular-cell adenomas in males. An increase in the combined incidence of pulmonary adenomas and carcinomas was seen in female but not in male rats.

5.4 Other relevant data

Commercial samples of HC Blue No. 1 bound to DNA and induced mutation in bacteria. They induced DNA damage, gene mutation and chromosomal anomalies and inhibited intercellular communication in cultured mammalian cells.

Table 2. Genetic and related effects of purified HC Blue No. 1

Test system	Result		Dose[a] (LED/HID)	Reference
	Without exogenous metabolic system	With exogenous metabolic system		
SA0, *Salmonella typhimurium* TA100, reverse mutation	–	–	2500.0000	Shahin & Bugaut (1983)[b]
SA0, *Salmonella typhimurium* TA100, reverse mutation	–	–	2500.0000	Oberly et al. (1990)[c]
SA5, *Salmonella typhimurium* TA1535, reverse mutation	–	–	2500.0000	Shahin & Bugaut (1983)
SA5, *Salmonella typhimurium* TA1535, reverse mutation	–	–	2500.0000	Oberly et al. (1990)
SA7, *Salmonella typhimurium* TA1537, reverse mutation	–	–	2500.0000	Shahin & Bugaut (1983)
SA7, *Salmonella typhimurium* TA1537, reverse mutation	–	–	2500.0000	Oberly et al. (1990)
SA8, *Salmonella typhimurium* TA1538, reverse mutation	–	–	2500.0000	Shahin & Bugaut (1983)
SA9, *Salmonella typhimurium* TA98, reverse mutation	–	–	2500.0000	Shahin & Bugaut (1983)
SA9, *Salmonella typhimurium* TA98, reverse mutation	–	–	2500.0000	Oberly et al. (1990)
SA9, *Salmonella typhimurium* TA98, reverse mutation	–	0	1000.0000	Abu-Shakra et al. (1991)[d]
ECW, *Escherichia coli* WP2, *uvrA*⁻, *trp*⁻, reverse mutation	–	–	2500.0000	Oberly et al. (1990)
SCG, *Saccharomyces cerevisiae*, *ade* and *trp* conversions	–	–	12700.0000	Loprieno et al. (1983)[e]
SZF, *Schizosaccharomyces pombe*, forward mutation, *ade* and *rad*	–	–	12700.0000	Loprieno et al. (1983)
DMX, *Drosophila melanogaster*, sex-linked recessive lethal mutation	–		5100.00 injection	Darroudi et al. (1983)[f]
URP, Unscheduled DNA synthesis, rat primary hepatocytes	+	0	0.1000	Williams et al. (1989)[g]
URP, Unscheduled DNA synthesis, rat primary hepatocytes	+	0	5.0000	Hill et al. (1990)
UIA, Unscheduled DNA synthesis, mouse primary hepatocytes	+	0	5.0000	Hill et al. (1990)
UIA, Unscheduled DNA synthesis, Syrian hamster primary hepatocytes	+	0	5.0000	Hill et al. (1990)
UIA, Unscheduled DNA synthesis, rabbit primary hepatocytes	+	0	50.0000	Hill et al. (1990)
UIA, Unscheduled DNA synthesis, rhesus monkey primary hepatocytes	+	0	50.0000	Hill et al. (1990)
G9H, Gene mutation, Chinese hamster lung V79 cells, *hprt* locus	–	–	25500.0000	Loprieno et al. (1983)
G5T, Gene mutation, mouse lymphoma L5178Y cells, *tk* locus	–	(+)	25.0000	Oberly et al. (1990)
SIC, Sister chromatid exchange, Chinese hamster ovary cells *in vitro*	–	0	1600.0000 × 1 h	Darroudi et al. (1983)

Table 2 (contd)

Test system	Result		Dose[a] (LED/HID)	Reference
	Without exogenous metabolic system	With exogenous metabolic system		
SIC, Sister chromatid exchange, Chinese hamster ovary cells *in vitro*	+	0	100.0000 × 24 h	Darroudi *et al.* (1983)
CIC, Chromosomal aberrations, Chinese hamster ovary cells *in vitro*	–	0	400.0000	Darroudi *et al.* (1983)
UHT, Unscheduled DNA synthesis, human HeLa cells	–	–	7600.0000	Loprieno *et al.* (1983)
MVM, Micronucleus test, male CBA mouse bone marrow	–		100.0000 ip × 3	Darroudi *et al.* (1983)
MVM, Micronucleus test, female ICR mouse bone marrow	+		1000.0000 ip × 1	Parton *et al.* (1990)[h]
MVM, Micronucleus test, male ICR mouse bone marrow	–		1000.0000 ip × 1	Parton *et al.* (1990)[h]
MVM, Micronucleus test, male and female CD-1 mouse bone marrow	–		1000.0000 ip × 1	Parton *et al.* (1990)[h]
BID, Binding (covalent) to TA98 DNA *in vitro* (^{32}P-postlabelling)	–	0	12000.0000[i]	Abu–Shakra *et al.* (1991)[d]

+ , positive; (+), weakly positive; –, negative; 0, not tested

[a]In-vitro tests, μg/ml; in-vivo tests, mg/kg bw

[b]Synthesized and purified industrial sample with one recrystallization in ethanol

[c]Industrial sample with one ethanol recrystallization, purity > 98%

[d]High-performance liquid chromatography (HPLC)-purified

[e]Provided by l'Oréal (ref. MPIp37) as a pure product

[f]Pure form supplied by l'Oréal

[g]Purified preparation

[h]> 98% pure

[i]12 000 μg/ml equivalent; HPLC-purified sample derived from HPLC fractionation of 240 mg HC Blue 1 added to 20 ml incubation mixture

Table 3. Genetic and related effects of commercial HC Blue No. 1

Test system	Result — Without exogenous metabolic system	Result — With exogenous metabolic system	Dose[a] (LED/HID)	Reference
SA0, *Salmonella typhimurium* TA100, reverse mutation	+	+	50.0000	Zeiger et al. (1988)[b]
SA5, *Salmonella typhimurium* TA1535, reverse mutation	−	−	500.0000	Zeiger et al. (1988)
SA9, *Salmonella typhimurium* TA98, reverse mutation	+	+	50.0000	Zeiger et al. (1988)
SA9, *Salmonella typhimurium* TA98, reverse mutation	+	0	1000.0000	Abu–Shakra et al. (1991)[c]
SA9, *Salmonella typhimurium* TA98, reverse mutation	+	0	0.0000	Casciano et al. (1985)[d]; abstr.
SAS, *Salmonella typhimurium* TA98NR, reverse mutation	+	0	0.0000	Casciano et al. (1985)[d]; abstr.
SAS, *Salmonella typhimurium* TA97, reverse mutation	+	+	50.0000	Zeiger et al. (1988)
URP, Unscheduled DNA synthesis, rat primary hepatocytes	+	0	50.0000	US National Toxicology Program (1985)[b]
URP, Unscheduled DNA synthesis, rat primary hepatocytes	+	0	1.0000	Williams et al. (1989)[e]
UIA, Unscheduled DNA synthesis, mouse primary hepatocytes	+	0	0.0000	Mirsalis et al. (1986)[d]; abstr.
UIA, Unscheduled DNA synthesis, Syrian hamster primary hepatocytes	+	0	0.0000	Mirsalis et al. (1986)[d]; abstr.
UIA, Unscheduled DNA synthesis, cynomologus monkey primary hepatocytes	+	0	0.0000	Mirsalis et al. (1986)[d]; abstr.
UIH, Unscheduled DNA synthesis, human primary hepatocytes	+	0	0.0000	Mirsalis et al. (1986)[d]; abstr.
G5T, Gene mutation, mouse lymphoma L5178Y cells, *tk* locus	+	0	20.0000	Myhr & Caspary (1991)[b]
GCO, Gene mutation, Chinese hamster ovary cells, *hprt* locus	+	0	0.0000	Casciano et al. (1985); abstr.
SIM, Sister chromatid exchange, mouse hepatocytes *in vitro*	(+)	0	10.0000	Kari et al. (1990a)[b]
SIC, Sister chromatid exchange, Chinese hamster ovary cells *in vitro*	+	(+)	119.0000	Loveday et al. (1990)[b]
CIC, Chromosomal aberrations, Chinese hamster ovary cells *in vitro*	−	+	960.0000	Loveday et al. (1990)[b]
CIM, Chromosomal aberrations, mouse hepatocytes *in vitro*	+	0	10.0000	Kari et al. (1990a,b)[b]
CIR, Chromosomal aberrations, rat hepatocytes *in vitro*	−	0	100.0000	Kari et al. (1990b)

Table 3 (contd)

Test system	Result — Without exogenous metabolic system	Result — With exogenous metabolic system	Dose[a] (LED/HID)	Reference
TCS, Cell transformation, Syrian hamster embryo cells, clonal assay	−	0	50.0000	Pienta & Kawalek (1981)[d]
UPR, Unscheduled DNA synthesis, rat hepatocytes in vivo	−		0.0000	Mirsalis et al. (1986)[d]; abstr.
UVM, Unscheduled DNA synthesis, male B6C3F$_1$ mouse hepatocytes in vivo	−		360.0000, 7 days	Mirsalis et al. (1988); abstr.
UVM, Unscheduled DNA synthesis, female B6C3F$_1$ mouse hepatocytes in vivo	−		720.0000, 7 days	Mirsalis et al. (1988); abstr.
MVM, Micronucleus test, male B6C3F$_1$ mouse bone marrow	−		360.0000, 7 days	Mirsalis et al. (1988); abstr.
MVM, Micronucleus test, female B6C3F$_1$ mouse bone marrow	−		720.0000, 7 days	Mirsalis et al. (1988); abstr.
*, S-Phase synthesis, male B6C3F$_1$ mouse hepatocytes in vivo	+		360.0000, 7 days	Mirsalis et al. (1988)[d]; abstr.
*, S-Phase synthesis, female B6C3F$_1$ mouse hepatocytes in vivo	−		720.0000, 7 days	Mirsalis et al. (1988)[d]; abstr.
BID, Binding (covalent) to TA98 DNA in vitro (P^{32}-postlabelling)	+	0	12000.0000	Abu–Shakra et al. (1991)
ICR, Inhibition of cell-cell communication, Chinese hamster lung V79 cells	+	0	50.0000	Kari et al. (1990a)

+, positive; (+), weakly positive; −, negative; 0, not tested; ?, inconclusive (variable response in several experiments within an adequate study); 0.0000, dose not given

[a] In-vitro tests, µg/ml; in-vivo tests, mg/kg bw

[b] Commercial HC Blue 1, Lot No. 3670379, approximately 97% pure

[c] Commercial HC Blue 1, Lot No. 68379913

[d] Purity unspecified

[e] Commercial sample

* Not displayed on profile

Purified samples of HC Blue No. 1 did not bind to DNA or induce mutation in bacteria. They did not induce mitotic recombination in yeasts and did not induce mutation in insects. They induced DNA damage, sister chromatid exchange and, weakly, gene mutation but not chromosomal aberrations in cultured mammalian cells. DNA damage was not induced in cultured human cells (HeLa). Micronuclei were induced in the bone marrow of female mice of one strain exposed *in vivo*.

5.5 Evaluation[1]

There is *inadequate evidence* in humans for the carcinogenicity of HC Blue No. 1.

There is *sufficient evidence* in experimental animals for the carcinogenicity of HC Blue No. 1.

Overall evaluation

HC Blue No. 1 is *possibly carcinogenic to humans (Group 2B)*.

6. References

Abu-Shakra, A., Johnson, L., Earley, K., Jameson, C.W., Kari, F.W., Gupta, R. & Langenbach, R. (1991) Isolation of the mutagenic and DNA adduct-inducing components from a commercial preparation of HC Blue 1 using *Salmonella* (TA98) bioassay-directed HPLC fractionation. *Mutat. Res.*, **260**, 377–385

Burnett, C.M. & Corbett, J.F. (1987) Failure of short-term in vitro mutagenicity tests to predict animal carcinogenicity of hair dyes. *Food Chem. Toxicol.*, **25**, 703–707

Burnett, C., Goldenthal, E.I., Harris, S.B., Wazeter, F.X., Strausburg, J., Kapp, R. & Voelker, R. (1976) Teratology and percutaneous toxicity studies on hair dyes. *J. Toxicol. environ. Health*, **1**, 1027-1040

Burnett, C., Loehr, R. & Corbett, J. (1981) Heritable translocation study on two hair dye formulations. *Fundam. appl. Toxicol.*, **1**, 325–328

Casciano, D.A., Shaddock, J.G., Hass, B.S. & Spalding, J.W. (1985) *N*-Methylamino-2-nitro-4-*N'*,*N'*-bis(2-hydroxyethyl)aminobenzene (HC-Blue No. 1) is genotoxic as judged by the hepatocyte/-DNA repair, Chinese hamster ovary hypoxanthine-guanine phosphoribosyl transferase and *Salmonella* assays (Abstract). *Environ. Mutag.*, **7** (Suppl. 3), 19

Darroudi, F., Sobels, F.H. & Natarajan, A.T. (1983) Evaluation of the mutagenic potential of the hair dye *N*-methylamino-2-nitro-4-*N'*,*N'*-bis(2-hydroxyethyl)aminobenzene in a battery consisting of *Drosophila* and mammalian cytogenetic assays. *Mutat. Res.*, **116**, 169–178

Frenkel, E.P. & Brody, F. (1973) Percutaneous absorption and elimination of an aromatic hair dye. *Arch. environ. Health*, **27**, 401–404

Hill, L.E., Parton, J.W., Probst, G.S. & Garriott, M.L. (1990) Mutagenicity evaluation of HC Blue No. 1 and HC Blue No. 2. II. Effect on the in vitro induction of unscheduled DNA synthesis in rat, mouse, rabbit, hamster and monkey primary hepatocytes. *Mutat. Res.*, **241**, 145–150

---

[1]For definition of the italicized terms, see Preamble, pp. 26–30.

IARC (1985) *IARC Monographs on the Evaluation of the Carcinogenic Risk of Chemicals to Humans*, Vol. 36, *Allyl Compounds, Aldehydes, Epoxides and Peroxides*, Lyon, pp. 189–226

IARC (1987) *IARC Monographs on the Evaluation of Carcinogenic Risks to Humans*, Suppl. 7, *Overall Evaluations of Carcinogenicity: An Updating of* IARC Monographs *Volumes 1–42*, Lyon, pp. 205–207

Jacobs, M.M., Burnett, C.M., Penicnak, A.J., Herrera, J.A., Morris, W.E., Shubik, P., Apaja, M. & Granroth, G. (1984) Evaluation of the toxicity and carcinogenicity of hair dyes in Swiss mice. *Drug Chem. Toxicol.*, 7, 573–586

Kari, F.W., Rudo, K., Volosin, J., Jenkins, W., Driscoll, S. & Langenbach, R. (1988) Comparative metabolism of two structurally similar nitrophenylene-diamine dyes (HC Blue 1 and HC Blue 2) by mouse hepatocytes (Abstract No. 505). *Proc. Am. Assoc. Cancer Res.*, 29, 127

Kari, F.W., Mennear, J.H., Farnell, D., Thompson, R.B. & Huff, J.E. (1989a) Comparative carcinogenicity of two structurally similar phenylenediamine dyes (HC Blue No. 1 and HC Blue No. 2) in F344/N rats and B6C3F$_1$ mice. *Toxicology*, 56, 155–165

Kari, F.W., Driscoll, S., Parker, C., Rudo, K., Tomer, K. & Langenbach, R. (1989b) Species comparisons regarding comparative metabolism of two structurally similar nitrophenylene-diamines (HC Blue 1 and HC Blue 2) (Abstract No. 651). *Proc. Am. Assoc. Cancer Res.*, 30, 164

Kari, F.W., Driscoll, S.M., Abu-Shakra, A., Strom, S.C., Jenkins, W.L., Volosin, J.S., Rudo, K.M. & Langenbach, R. (1990a) Comparative metabolism and genotoxicity of the structurally similar nitrophenylenediamine dyes, HC Blue 1 and HC Blue 2, in mouse hepatocytes. *Cell. Biol. Toxicol.*, 6, 139–155

Kari, F.W., Driscoll, S., Parker, C., Rudo, K., Tomer, K. & Langenbach, R. (1990b) Species comparisons regarding comparative metabolism of two structurally similar phenylenediamines (HC Blue 1 and HC Blue 2). *Prog. clin. biol. Res.*, 340D, 305–314

Loprieno, N., Mariani, L. & Rusciano, D. (1983) Lack of genotoxic properties of the hair-dye component *N*-methylamino-2-nitro-4-*N'*,*N'*-bis(2-hydroxyethyl)aminobenzene, in mammalian cells *in vitro*, and in yeasts. *Mutat. Res.*, 116, 161–168

Loveday, K.S., Anderson, B.E., Resnick, M.A. & Zeiger, E. (1990) Chromosome aberration and sister chromatid exchange tests in Chinese hamster ovary cells *in vitro*. V: Results with 46 chemicals. *Environ. mol. Mutag.*, 16, 272–303

Maibach, H.I. & Wolfram, L.J. (1981) Percutaneous penetration of hair dyes. *J. Soc. Cosmet. Chem.*, 32, 223–229

Mirsalis, J.C., Steinmetz, K.L., Bakke, J.P., Tyson, C.K., Soh, E.K.W., Hamilton, C.M., Ramsay, M.J. & Spalding, J.W. (1986) Genotoxicity and tumor promoting capabilities of blue hair dyes in rodent and primate liver (Abstract No. 147). *Environ. Mutag.*, 8 (Suppl. 6), 55–56

Mirsalis, J.C., Steinmetz, K.L., Blazak, W.F., Bakke, J.P., Hamilton, C.M., Stewart, B.E., Deahl, J.T. & Cunningham, G.D. (1988) Evaluation of genotoxicity and hepatic hyperplasia in mice following exposure to HC Blue # 1 and HC Blue # 2 *via* dosed feed (Abstract No. 171). *Environ. mol. Mutag.*, 11 (Suppl. 11), 71

Myhr, B.C. & Caspary, W.J. (1991) Chemical mutagenesis at the thymidine kinase locus in L5178Y mouse lymphoma cells: results for 31 coded compounds in the National Toxicology Program. *Environ. mol. Mutag.*, 18, 51–83

Oberly, T.J., Kokkino, A.J., Bewsey, B.J. & Richardson, K.K. (1990) Mutagenic evaluation of HC Blue No. 1 and HC Blue No. 2. III. Effects in the *Salmonella typhimurium/Escherichia coli* reversion assay and the mouse lymphoma L5178Y TK$^{+/-}$ forward mutation assay. *Mutat. Res.*, 241, 151–159

Parton, J.W., Beyers, J.E. & Garriott, M.L. (1990) Mutagenicity evaluation of HC Blue No. 1 and HC Blue No. 2. I. Effect of the induction of micronuclei in mouse bone marrow cells. *Mutat Res.*, **241**, 139–144

Pienta, R.J. & Kawalek, J.C. (1981) Transformation of hamster embryo cells by aromatic amines. *Natl Cancer Inst. Monogr.*, **58**, 243–251

Shahin, M.M. & Bugaut, A. (1983) Mutagenic evaluation of the monocyclic aromatic amine *N*-methyl-amino-2-nitro-4-*N'*,*N'*-bis(2-hydroxyethyl)-aminobenzene in the *Salmonella typhimurium*/mammalian microsome test. *Mutat. Res.*, **116**, 155–159

US National Toxicology Program (1985) *Toxicology and Carcinogenesis Studies of HC Blue No. 1 (CAS No. 2784-94-3) in F344/N Rats and B6C3F$_1$ Mice (Feed Studies)* (NTP Technical Report 271; NIH Publ. No. 85-2527), Research Triangle Park, NC

Wernick, T., Lanman, B.M. & Fraux, J.L. (1975) Chronic toxicity, teratologic and reproduction studies with hair dyes. *Toxicol. appl. Pharmacol.*, **32**, 450–460

Williams, G.M., Mori, H. & McQueen, C.A. (1989) Structure–activity relationships in the rat hepatocyte DNA-repair test for 300 chemicals. *Mutat. Res.*, **221**, 263–286

Wolfram, L.J. & Maibach, H.I. (1985) Percutaneous penetration of hair dyes. *Arch. dermatol. Res.*, **277**, 235–241

Zeiger, E., Anderson, B., Haworth, S., Lawlor, T. & Mortelmans, K. (1988) *Salmonella* mutagenicity tests: IV. Results from the testing of 300 chemicals. *Environ. mol. Mutag.*, **11** (Suppl. 12), 1–158

HC BLUE NO. 2

1. Exposure Data

1.1 Chemical and physical data

1.1.1 Synonyms, structural and molecular data

Chem. Abstr. Serv. Reg. No.: 33229-34-4

Chem. Abstr. Name: 2,2'-([4-([2-Hydroxyethyl]amino)-3-nitrophenyl]imino)bis(ethanol)

Synonyms: HC Blue 2; HC Blue Number 2; 2,2'-([4-([2-hydroxyethyl]amino)-3-nitrophenyl]imino)di(ethanol); N^1,N^4,N^4-tris(2-hydroxyethyl)-2-nitro-para-phenylenediamine

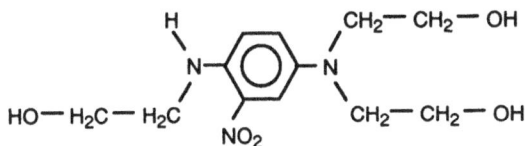

$C_{12}H_{19}N_3O_5$ Mol. wt: 285.30

1.1.2 Chemical and physical properties of the substance

From US National Toxicology Program (1985)

(a) Description: Dark-blue microcrystalline (75% pure) or blackish-blue amorphous powder (98% pure), with a copper cast

(b) Melting-point: 93–98 °C (98% pure)

(c) Spectroscopy data: Infrared, ultraviolet and nuclear magnetic resonance spectral data have been reported.

(d) Solubility: Soluble in water, ethanol, methanol and acetone

(e) Octanol/water partition coefficient (P): 1.7

1.1.3 Trade names, technical products and impurities

HC Blue No. 2 is available commercially with a purity ≥ 95% with possible impurities, including methylamine (≤ 1%), 1,2-dihydroxyethane (≤ 1%) and water (≤ 1%). It is also available in a technical grade containing 55–90% dye, 10–30% inorganic salts and 2,2-[(4-amino-3-nitrophenyl)imino]bis(ethanol) (≤ 7%) as a possible impurity.

1.1.4 *Analysis*

No data were available to the Working Group.

1.2 Production and use

1.2.1 *Production*

The form of HC Blue No. 2 that is ≥ 95% pure is produced commercially by the reaction of 4-fluoro-3-nitrobenzenamine with ethylene oxide (see IARC, 1985, 1987) to form 2,2-[(4-fluoro-3-nitrophenyl)imino]bis(ethanol); this intermediate is reacted with mono-ethanolamine to form HC Blue No. 2. The technical grade is produced by reaction of 2-nitro-*para*-phenylenediamine (see IARC, 1978) with ethylene oxide or 2-chloroethanol.

Production and use of HC Blue No. 2 began in the late 1950s. Approximately 9–11 tonnes are used annually in the USA, according to industry estimates.

1.2.2 *Use*

HC Blue No. 2 is used exclusively as a dye in semi-permanent hair colouring products. These products are generally shampooed into the hair, lathered and then allowed to remain in contact with the hair and scalp for 30–45 min. The concentration of HC Blue No. 2 used in these preparations ranges from 1.6 to 2% (Frenkel & Brody, 1973; US National Toxicology Program, 1985).

1.3 Occurrence

1.3.1 *Natural occurrence*

HC Blue No. 2 is not known to occur as a natural product.

1.3.2 *Occupational exposure*

No data were available to the Working Group.

1.4 Regulations and guidelines

No data were available to the Working Group.

2. Studies of Cancer in Humans

No data were available to the Working Group.

3. Studies of Cancer in Experimental Animals

3.1 Oral administration

3.1.1 *Mouse*

Groups of 50 male and 50 female B6C3F$_1$ mice, seven weeks of age, were fed 0, 5000 or 10 000 mg/kg (ppm) (males) or 0, 10 000 or 20 000 ppm (females) HC Blue No. 2 (about 98%

pure) in the diet for 104 weeks and were killed at 112–113 weeks of age. Final mean body weights of treated males were similar to those of controls; however, those of treated females were 15% (low-dose) and 22% (high-dose) lower than those of controls. Survival at the end of the study was: males—control, 24/50; low-dose, 24/50; and high-dose, 34/50; females—control, 35/50; low-dose, 28/50; and high-dose, 20/50 ($p < 0.005$, life table test). The reduced survival of female mice was attributed to infection of the ovaries and uteri with *Klebsiella* sp. No significant increase in the incidence in any tumour was observed (US National Toxicology Program, 1985; Kari *et al.*, 1989a). [The Working Group noted that the reduced survival of females precluded adequate evaluation of the study.]

3.1.2 *Rat*

Groups of 50 male and 50 female Fischer 344/N rats, six to seven weeks of age, were fed 0, 5000 or 10 000 mg/kg of diet (ppm) (males) or 0, 10 000 or 20 000 mg/kg ppm (females) HC Blue No. 2 ($\sim$ 98% pure) in the diet for 103 weeks and were killed at 110–112 weeks of age. Final mean body weights were depressed by less than 10% in treated males but by 13% (low-dose) and 22% (high-dose) in females. No adverse effect on survival was observed in males (control, 32/50; low-dose, 38/50; high-dose, 42/50) or females (control, 41/50; low-dose, 40/50; high-dose, 39/50). The incidence of C-cell adenomas of the thyroid in males was 7/50 control, 2/50 low-dose and 5/49 high-dose; the incidence of C-cell carcinomas was 0/50 control, 3/50 low-dose and 5/49 high-dose ($p = 0.029$, incidental tumour trend test). The trend in combined incidence (7/50, 5/50 and 10/49) was not significant. There was no excess of thyroid tumours in females. No other significant increase in the incidence of tumours was reported; however, malignant mixed mesenchymal tumours of the kidney were detected in 2/50 high-dose female rats and none of 1863 historical controls. A negative trend in the incidence of fibroadenomas of the mammary gland was seen in female rats (control, 20/50; low-dose, 10/50; high-dose, 4/50 [$p < 0.001$, Cochran Armitage test for trend]) (US National Toxicology Program, 1985; Kari *et al.*, 1989a).

4. Other Relevant Data

4.1 Absorption, distribution, metabolism and excretion

4.1.1 *Humans*

About 85 g of a commercial semi-permanent hair dye formulation containing 1.77% HC Blue No. 2 enriched with 378.6 μCi/mg [ring-^{14}C]-labelled HC Blue No. 2 was applied to the hair of human volunteers, worked in gently for 5–8 min and allowed to remain in contact with the hair and scalp for an additional 30 min. After 30 days, radiolabel accounting for less than 0.1% of that applied was detected in the urine; half was excreted in urine after 52 h (Wolfram & Maibach, 1985). [The Working Group noted that urinary metabolites were not identified, so that the metabolic fate of HC Blue No. 2 in humans remains unknown.]

4.1.2 *Experimental systems*

Up to 40% of radiolabel was recovered in the urine of B6C3F$_1$ mice and Fischer 344/N rats after oral administration by gavage of 100 mg/kg bw [ring-^{14}C]-labelled HC Blue No. 2

(0.1 mCi/mmol [35 µCi/mg]; 98% pure). Metabolism of HC Blue No. 2 (200 µM [57 mg]) by hepatocytes isolated from mice and rats yielded profiles similar to those seen *in vivo*. High-performance liquid chromatography separation showed that HC Blue No. 2 is metabolized extensively in mice to one major metabolite, which has not been characterized (Kari *et al.*, 1988, 1989b, 1990a,b).

4.2 Toxic effects

4.2.1 *Humans*

No data were available to the Working Group.

4.2.2 *Experimental systems*

Concentrations of 0, 5000 or 10 000 ppm (mg/kg) HC Blue No. 2 (98% pure) were administered in the diet to male Fischer 344/N rats for 103 weeks and to male B6C3F$_1$ mice for 104 weeks and concentrations of 0, 10 000 or 20 000 ppm (mg/kg) to female rats for 103 weeks and to female mice for 104 weeks. The calculated average daily doses were 194 and 391 mg/kg bw for male rats, 465 and 1001 mg/kg bw for female rats, 1321 and 2243 mg/kg bw for male mice, and 2362 and 5609 mg/kg for female mice. A dose-related increase in the incidence of hyperostosis of the skull was observed in male and female rats (US National Toxicology Program, 1985; Kari *et al.*, 1989a).

HC Blue No. 2 was present at low concentrations in semi-permanent hair colouring formulations evaluated in a 13-week study of dermal toxicity in rabbits (1.7%) (Burnett *et al.*, 1976) and in a two-year feeding study in dogs (1.63%) (Wernick *et al.*, 1975), described in detail on p. 97. No treatment-related adverse effect was detected. [The Working Group noted that the dose of each component of the formulation was very low and unlikely to have been toxic.]

4.3 Reproductive and developmental effects

4.3.1 *Humans*

No data were available to the Working Group.

4.3.2 *Experimental systems*

No data were available to the Working Group on the reproductive and developmental effects of HC Blue No. 2 alone. The compound was present at low concentrations in semi-permanent hair colouring formulations evaluated in a study of fertility and reproductive performance in rats (Wernick *et al.*, 1975, 1.63%; see p. 99) and in studies of teratogenesis in rats (Wernick *et al.*, 1975, 1.63%; Burnett *et al.*, 1976, 1.70%) and rabbits (Wernick *et al.*, 1975, 1.63%) (see p. 100). No treatment-related adverse effect was detected. [The Working Group noted that the dose of each component of the formulations was very low and unlikely to have been toxic.]

4.4 Genetic and related effects

4.4.1 *Humans*

No data were available to the Working Group.

4.4.2 *Experimental systems* (see also Table 1 and Appendices 1 and 2)

Although two different lots of HC Blue No. 2 have been used in most of the short-term tests (98.5% and 99.8% purity), they appear to induce similar responses when tested in the same assay system.

HC Blue No. 2 induced mutation in *Salmonella typhimurium* but did not induce reverse mutation in *Escherichia coli*. It induced mutations at the *tk* locus of mouse lymphoma L5178Y cells and induced unscheduled DNA synthesis in cultures of primary hepatocytes from mice, rats, Syrian hamsters and rabbits, but not in those from monkeys. HC Blue No. 2 induced sister chromatid exchange in cultured Chinese hamster ovary cells and, weakly, in female B6C3F$_1$ mouse primary hepatocytes. Chromosomal aberrations were not induced in Chinese hamster ovary cells or in primary cultures of rat or mouse hepatocytes.

HC Blue No. 2 did not inhibit gap-junctional communication in Chinese hamster lung V79 cells, but it elicited a slight, dose-dependent increase in communication at non-cytotoxic concentrations.

HC Blue No. 2 did not induce micronuclei in mouse bone-marrow in three assays (one of which was with the lower purity sample).

As reported in two abstracts, HC Blue No. 2 did not increase proliferation of hepatocytes from rats and mice treated *in vivo* (Mirsalis *et al.*, 1986, 1988), but it enhanced S-phase DNA synthesis in male (but not female) mouse hepatocytes. It did not induce unscheduled DNA synthesis in the livers of mice or rats in feeding studies.

5. Summary of Data Reported and Evaluation

5.1 Exposure data

HC Blue No. 2 is used as a semi-permanent hair dye.

5.2 Human carcinogenicity data

No data were available to the Working Group.

5.3 Animal carcinogenicity data

HC Blue No. 2 was tested for carcinogenicity by administration in the diet in one study in mice and in one study in rats. No significant increase in tumour incidence was observed in either species, but the data on female mice could not be adequately evaluated.

5.4 Other relevant data

HC Blue No. 2 induced gene mutation in bacteria. It induced DNA damage, gene mutation and sister chromatid exchange but not chromosomal aberrations or inhibition of intercellular communication in cultured mammalian cells. Micronuclei were not induced in the bone marrow of mice exposed *in vivo*.

Table 1. Genetic and related effects of HC Blue No. 2

Test system	Result		Dose[a] (LED/HID)	Reference
	Without exogenous metabolic system	With exogenous metabolic system		
98–98.5% Purity sample[b]				
SA0, *Salmonella typhimurium* TA100, reverse mutation	–	–	5000.0000	Zeiger et al. (1988)
SA5, *Salmonella typhimurium* TA1535, reverse mutation	–	–	5000.0000	Zeiger et al. (1988)
SA7, *Salmonella typhimurium* TA1537, reverse mutation	(+)	(+)	1667.0000	Zeiger et al. (1988)
SA9, *Salmonella typhimurium* TA98, reverse mutation	+	+	500.0000	Zeiger et al. (1988)
SAS, *Salmonella typhimurium* TA97, reverse mutation	(+)	(+)	3333.0000	Zeiger et al. (1988)
GST, Gene mutation, mouse lymphoma L5178Y cells, *tk* locus	+	0	30.0000	Myhr & Caspary (1991)
SIC, Sister chromatid exchange, Chinese hamster ovary cells *in vitro*	+	+	240.0000	Loveday et al. (1990)
SIM, Sister chromatid exchange, mouse hepatocytes *in vitro*	(+)	0	50.0000	Kari et al. (1990a)
CIC, Chromosomal aberrations, Chinese hamster ovary cells *in vitro*	–	–	2500.0000	Loveday et al. (1990)
CIM, Chromosomal aberrations, mouse hepatocytes *in vitro*	–	0	100.0000	Kari et al. (1990a,b)
CIR, Chromosomal aberrations, rat hepatocytes *in vitro*	–	0	100.0000	Kari et al. (1990b)
ICR, Inhibition of cell–cell communication, Chinese hamster lung V79 cells	–	0	40.0000	Kari et al. (1990b)
99.8% Purity sample[c]				
SA0, *Salmonella typhimurium* TA100, reverse mutation	–	–	2500.0000	Oberly et al. (1990)
SA5, *Salmonella typhimurium* TA1535, reverse mutation	–	–	2500.0000	Oberly et al. (1990)
SA7, *Salmonella typhimurium* TA1537, reverse mutation	–	(+)	2500.0000	Oberly et al. (1990)
SA9, *Salmonella typhimurium* TA98, reverse mutation	+	+	160.0000	Oberly et al. (1990)
ECW, *Escherichia coli* WP2, $uvrA^-$, trp^-, reverse mutation	–	–	2500.0000	Oberly et al. (1990)
URP, Unscheduled DNA synthesis, male rat primary hepatocytes	+	0	50.0000	Hill et al. (1990)
UIA, Unscheduled DNA synthesis, male mouse primary hepatocytes	+	0	10.0000	Hill et al. (1990)
UIA, Unscheduled DNA synthesis, male hamster primary hepatocytes	+	0	50.0000	Hill et al. (1990)
UIA, Unscheduled DNA synthesis, male rabbit primary hepatocytes	+	0	50.0000	Hill et al. (1990)

Table 1 (contd)

Test system	Result		Dose[a] (LED/HID)	Reference
	Without exogenous metabolic system	With exogenous metabolic system		
UIA, Unscheduled DNA synthesis, male rhesus monkey primary hepatocytes	–	0	500.0000	Hill et al. (1990)
G5T, Gene mutation, mouse lymphoma L5178Y cells, tk locus	+	+	200.0000	Oberly et al. (1990)
MVM, Micronucleus test, CD-1 mouse bone marrow	–		1000.0000 ip × 1	Parton et al. (1990)
MVM, Micronucleus test, ICR mouse bone marrow	–		1000.0000 ip × 1	Parton et al. (1990)
Purity unspecified				
URP, Unscheduled DNA synthesis, rat primary hepatocytes	+	0	0.0000	Mirsalis et al. (1986); abstr.
UPR, Unscheduled DNA synthesis, rat hepatocytes in vivo	–		0.0000	Mirsalis et al. (1986); abstr.
UVM, Unscheduled DNA synthesis, male mouse hepatocytes in vivo	–		1200.0000 diet 7 days	Mirsalis et al. (1986); abstr.
UVM, Unscheduled DNA synthesis, female mouse hepatocytes in vivo	–		2400.0000 diet 7 days	Mirsalis et al. (1988); abstr.
MVM, Micronucleus test, male B6C3F1 mouse bone marrow in vivo	–		1200.0000 diet 7 days	Mirsalis et al. (1988); abstr.
MVM, Micronucleus test, female B6C3F1 mouse bone marrow in vivo	–		2400.0000 diet 7 days	Mirsalis et al. (1988); abstr.
*, S-Phase synthesis, male B6C3F1 mouse hepatocytes in vivo	+		1200.0000 diet	Mirsalis et al. (1988); abstr.
*, S-Phase synthesis, female B6C3F1 mouse hepatocytes in vivo	–		2400.0000 diet	Mirsalis et al. (1988); abstr.

+, positive; (+), weakly positive; –, negative; 0, not tested
[a] In-vitro tests, μg/ml; in-vivo tests, mg/kg bw
[b] Approximately 98.5% pure
[c] Lot No. 1-329, Clairol, 99.8% pure
* Not displayed on profile

5.5 Evaluation[1]

There is *inadequate evidence* in humans for the carcinogenicity of HC Blue No. 2.

There is *inadequate evidence* in experimental animals for the carcinogenicity of HC Blue No. 2.

Overall evaluation

HC Blue No. 2 is *not classifiable as to its carcinogenicity to humans (Group 3).*

6. References

Burnett, C., Goldenthal, E.I., Harris, S.B., Wazeter, F.X., Strausburg, J., Kapp, R. & Voelker, R. (1976) Teratology and percutaneous toxicity studies on hair dyes. *J. Toxicol. environ. Health*, **1**, 1027–1040

Frenkel, E.P. & Brody, F. (1973) Percutaneous absorption and elimination of an aromatic hair dye. *Arch. environ. Health*, **27**, 401–404

Hill, L.E., Parton, J.W., Probst, G.S. & Garriott, M.L. (1990) Mutagenicity evaluation of HC Blue No. 1 and HC Blue No. 2. II. Effect on the in vitro induction of unscheduled DNA synthesis in rat, mouse, rabbit, hamster and monkey primary hepatocytes. *Mutat. Res.*, **241**, 145–150

IARC (1978) *IARC Monographs on the Evaluation of the Carcinogenic Risk of Chemicals to Man*, Vol. 16, *Some Aromatic Amines and Related Nitro Compounds—Hair Dyes, Colouring Agents and Miscellaneous Industrial Chemicals*, Lyon, pp. 73–82

IARC (1985) *IARC Monographs on the Evaluation of the Carcinogenic Risk of Chemicals to Humans*, Vol. 36, *Allyl Compounds, Aldehydes, Epoxides and Peroxides*, Lyon, pp. 189–226

IARC (1987) *IARC Monographs on the Evaluation of Carcinogenic Risks to Humans*, Suppl. 7, *Overall Evaluations of Carcinogenicity: An Updating of* IARC Monographs *Volumes 1 to 42*, Lyon, pp. 205–207

Kari, F.W., Rudo, K., Volosin, J., Jenkins, W., Driscoll, S. & Langenbach, R. (1988) Comparative metabolism of two structurally similar nitrophenylene-diamine dyes (HC Blue 1 and HC Blue 2) by mouse hepatocytes (Abstract No. 505). *Proc. Am. Assoc. Cancer Res.*, **29**, 127

Kari, F.W., Mennear, J.H., Farnell, D., Thompson, R.B. & Huff, J.E. (1989a) Comparative carcinogenicity of two structurally similar phenylenediamine dyes (HC Blue No. 1 and HC Blue No. 2) in F344/N rats and B6C3F$_1$ mice. *Toxicology*, **56**, 155–165

Kari, F.W., Driscoll, S., Parker, C., Rudo, K., Tomer, K. & Langenbach, R. (1989b) Species comparisons regarding comparative metabolism of two structurally similar nitrophenylenediamines (HC Blue 1 and HC Blue 2) (Abstract No. 651). *Proc. Am. Assoc. Cancer Res.*, **30**, 164

Kari, F.W., Driscoll, S.M., Abu-Shakra, A., Strom, S.C., Jenkins, W.L., Volosin, J.S., Rudo, K.M. & Langenbach, R. (1990a) Comparative metabolism and genotoxicity of the structurally similar nitrophenylenediamine dyes, HC Blue 1 and HC Blue 2, in mouse hepatocytes. *Cell. Biol. Toxicol.*, **6**, 139–155

Kari, F.W., Driscoll, S., Parker, C., Rudo, K., Tomer, K. & Langenbach, R. (1990b) Species comparisons regarding comparative metabolism of two structurally similar phenylenediamines (HC Blue 1 and HC Blue 2). *Prog. clin. biol. Res.*, **340D**, 305–314

---

[1]For definition of the italicized terms, see Preamble, pp. 26–30.

Kari, F.W., Driscoll, S., Parker, C., Rudo, K., Tomer, K. & Langenbach, R. (1990b) Species comparisons regarding comparative metabolism of two structurally similar phenylenediamines (HC Blue 1 and HC Blue 2). *Prog. clin. biol. Res.*, **340D**, 305–314

Loveday, K.S., Anderson, B.E., Resnick, M.A. & Zeiger, E. (1990) Chromosome aberration and sister chromatid exchange tests in Chinese hamster ovary cells *in vitro*. V: Results with 46 chemicals. *Environ. mol. Mutag.*, **16**, 272–303

Mirsalis, J.C., Steinmetz, K.L., Bakke, J.P., Tyson, C.K., Loh, E.K.N., Hamilton, C.M., Ramsey, M.J. & Spalding, J.W. (1986) Genotoxicity and tumor promoting capability of blue hair dyes in rodent and primate liver (Abstract No. 147). *Environ. Mutag.*, **8** (Suppl. 6), 55–56

Mirsalis, J.C., Steinmetz, K.L., Blazak, W.F., Bakke, J.P., Hamilton, C.M., Stewart, B.E., Deahl, J.T. & Cunningham, G.D. (1988) Evaluation of genotoxicity and hepatic hyperplasia in mice following exposure to HC Blue # 1 and HC Blue # 2 via dosed feed (Abstract No. 171). *Environ. mol. Mutag.*, **11** (Suppl. 11), 71

Myhr, B.C. & Caspary, W.J. (1991) Chemical mutagenesis at the thymidine kinase locus in L5178Y mouse lymphoma cells: results for 31 coded compounds in the National Toxicology Program. *Environ. mol. Mutag.*, **18**, 51–83

Oberly, T.J., Kokkino, A.J., Bewsey, B.J. & Richardson, K.K. (1990) Mutagenic evaluation of HC Blue No. 1 and HC Blue No. 2. III. Effects in the *Salmonella typhimurium/Escherichia coli* reversion assay and the mouse lymphoma L5178Y TK$^{+/-}$ forward mutation assay. *Mutat. Res.*, **241**, 151–159

Parton, J.W., Beyers, J.E. & Garriott, M.L. (1990) Mutagenicity evaluation of HC Blue No. 1 and HC Blue No. 2. I. Effect of the induction of micronuclei in mouse bone marrow cells. *Mutat. Res.*, **241**, 139–144

US National Toxicology Program (1985) *Toxicology and Carcinogenesis Studies of HC Blue No. 2 (CAS No. 33229-34-4) in F344/N Rats and B6C3F₁ Mice (Feed Studies)* (NTP Technical Report 293; NIH Publ. No. 85-2549), Research Triangle Park, NC

Wernick, T., Lanman, B.M. & Fraux, J.L. (1975) Chronic toxicity, teratologic and reproduction studies with hair dyes. *Toxicol. appl. Pharmacol.*, **32**, 450–460

Wolfram, L.J. & Maibach, H.I. (1985) Percutaneous penetration of hair dyes. *Arch. dermatol. Res.*, **277**, 235–241

Zeiger, E., Anderson, B., Haworth, S., Lawlor, T. & Mortelmans, K. (1988) *Salmonella* mutagenicity tests: IV. Results from the testing of 300 chemicals. *Environ. mol. Mutag.*, **11** (Suppl. 12), 1–158

HC RED NO. 3

1. Exposure Data

1.1 Chemical and physical data

1.1.1 Synonyms, structural and molecular data

Chem. Abstr. Serv. Reg. No.: 2871-01-4

Chem. Abstr. Name: 2-[(4-Amino-2-nitrophenyl)amino]ethanol

Synonyms: 2-(4-Amino-2-nitroanilino)ethanol; HC Red 3; HC Red Number 3; 4-(2-hydroxyethyl)amino-3-nitroaniline; N^1-(2-hydroxyethyl)-2-nitro-para-phenylenediamine

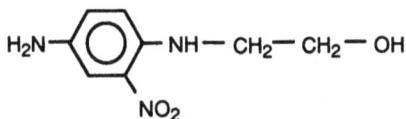

$C_8H_{11}N_3O_3$ Mol. wt: 197.19

1.1.2 Chemical and physical properties

From US National Toxicology Program (1986)

(a) Description: Fine, dark-maroon crystals, with a greenish cast

(b) Melting-point: 124–128 °C

(c) Spectroscopy data: Infrared, ultraviolet and nuclear magnetic resonance spectral data have been reported.

(d) Solubility: Soluble in water (0.28% w/w), ethanol and acetone

(e) Octanol/water partition coefficient (P): 1.9

1.1.3 Trade names, technical products and impurities

HC Red No. 3 is available commercially at a purity ≥ 95%, with aminoquinoxaline, aminonaphthyridine (US National Toxicology Program, 1986) and 2-[(4-[4-amino-2-nitrophenyl]amino-2-nitrophenyl)amino] ethanol (< 1%) as possible impurities.

1.1.4 Analysis

No data were available to the Working Group.

1.2 Production and use

1.2.1 *Production*

HC Red No. 3 is produced by the reaction of 4-fluoro-3-nitrobenzenamine with mono-ethanolamine. Production and use of this dye began in the late 1950s. Approximately 2300 kg are used annually in the USA, according to industry estimates.

1.2.2 *Use*

HC Red No. 3 is used exclusively as a dye in semi-permanent hair colour products. These products are generally shampooed into the hair, lathered and then allowed to remain in contact with the hair and scalp for 30–45 min. The concentration of HC Red No. 3 used in these preparations ranges from 0.1 to 5% (Frenkel & Brody, 1973; US National Toxicology Program, 1986).

1.3 Occurrence

1.3.1 *Natural occurrence*

HC Red No. 3 is not known to occur as a natural product.

1.3.2 *Occupational exposure*

No data were available to the Working Group.

On the basis of a survey conducted in the USA between 1981 and 1983, the US National Institute for Occupational Safety and Health estimated that a total of 42 485 workers, including 32 059 women, were potentially exposed as beauticians and cosmetologists to HC Red No. 3 (US National Library of Medicine, 1992).

1.4 Regulations and guidelines

No data were available to the Working Group.

2. Studies of Cancer in Humans

No data were available to the Working Group.

3. Studies of Cancer in Experimental Animals

3.1 Oral administration

3.1.1 *Mouse*

Groups of 50 male and 50 female B6C3F$_1$ mice, eight weeks of age, were administered 0, 125 or 250 mg/kg bw HC Red No. 3 (97% pure) by gavage in corn oil on five days a week for

104 weeks and were sacrificed at 113 weeks of age. Body weight gain and survival were reduced in all groups of females because of a reproductive tract infection. Survival at the end of the study was: males—control, 30/50; low-dose, 41/50; and high-dose, 29/50; females—control, 12/50; low-dose, 8/50; and high-dose, 9/50. The incidence of hepatocellular adenomas in males was control, 11/50; low-dose, 6/50; high-dose, 16/50; the incidence of hepatocellular carcinomas was, control, 17/50; low-dose, 9/50; high-dose, 21/50. There was an increased incidence of hepatocellular adenomas and carcinomas combined in high-dose male mice (control, 25/50; low-dose, 15/50; high-dose, 35/50), which was significant ($p = 0.017$, incidental tumour test), but not after pair-wise comparison. The incidence in historical controls in the testing laboratory was 109/298 ($37 \pm 12\%$) (US National Toxicology Program, 1986). [The Working Group noted the poor survival of females and the unusually . high incidence of hepatocellular carcinomas in male controls.]

3.1.2 *Rat*

Groups of 50 male and 50 female Fischer 344/N rats, seven to eight weeks of age, were administered 0, 250 or 500 mg/kg bw HC Red No. 3 (97% pure) by gavage in corn oil on five days a week for 105 weeks and were sacrificed at 113–114 weeks of age. The treatment had no effect on body weight gain throughout the study and did not reduce survival in males or females. Survival at the end of the experiment was: males—control, 34/50; low-dose, 34/50; high-dose, 32/50; females—control, 39/50; low-dose, 38/50; high-dose, 34/50. The incidence of mammary gland fibroadenomas was significantly ($p = 0.019$, incidental tumour test) increased in low-dose females (control, 14/50 *versus* low-dose, 24/50) but not in high-dose females (11/50) (US National Toxicology Program, 1986). [The Working Group noted the absence of a dose–response relationship.]

4. Other Relevant Data

4.1 Absorption, distribution, metabolism and excretion

No data were available to the Working Group.

4.2 Toxic effects

4.2.1 *Humans*

No data were available to the Working Group.

4.2.2 *Experimental systems*

In the studies reported above, no compound-related toxic effect was reported (US National Toxicology Program, 1986).

HC Red No. 3 was present at low concentrations (0.02%) in semi-permanent hair colouring formulations evaluated in a two-year feeding study in dogs (Wernick *et al.*, 1975) and in a 20-month study of dermal toxicity in mice (Jacobs *et al.*, 1984, 0.3%), described in detail on p. 97. No treatment-related adverse effect was detected. [The Working Group noted that the dose of each component of the formulations was very low and unlikely to have been toxic.]

4.3 Reproductive and developmental effects

4.3.1 *Humans*

No data were available to the Working Group.

4.3.2 *Experimental systems*

No data were available to the Working Group on the reproductive and developmental effects of HC Red No. 3 alone. The compound was present at low concentrations in semi-permanent hair colouring formulations evaluated in a study of fertility and reproductive performance in rats (Wernick *et al.*, 1975, 0.02%; see p. 99), in a study of heritable translocation in rats (Burnett *et al.*, 1981, 0.01%; see p. 104), and in studies of teratogenesis in rats and rabbits (Wernick *et al.*, 1975) (see p. 100). No treatment-related adverse effect was detected. [The Working Group noted that the dose of each component of the formulations was very low and unlikely to have been toxic.]

4.4 Genetic and related effects

4.4.1 *Humans*

No data were available to the Working Group.

4.4.2 *Experimental systems* (see also Table 1 and Appendices 1 and 2)

HC Red No. 3 was mutagenic to *Salmonella typhimurium*.

Table 1. Genetic and related effects of HC Red No. 3

Test system	Result		Dose (LED/HID) (µg/ml)	Reference
	Without exogenous metabolic system	With exogenous metabolic system		
SA0, *Salmonella typhimurium* TA100, reverse mutation	+	+	50.0000	Zeiger *et al.* (1988)
SA5, *Salmonella typhimurium* TA1535, reverse mutation	–	–	1667.0000	Zeiger *et al.* (1988)
SA9, *Salmonella typhimurium* TA98, reverse mutation	+	+	1.7000	Zeiger *et al.* (1988)
SAS, *Salmonella typhimurium* TA97, reverse mutation	+	+	1.7000	Zeiger *et al.* (1988)

+, positive; –, negative

5. Summary of Data Reported and Evaluation

5.1 Exposure data

HC Red No. 3 is used as a semi-permanent hair dye.

5.2 Human carcinogenicity data

No data were available to the Working Group.

5.3 Animal carcinogenicity data

HC Red No. 3 was tested for carcinogenicity by gavage in one study in mice and in one study in rats. There was a significant increase in the incidence of hepatocellular adenomas and carcinomas combined in male mice administered the high dose; poor survival precluded evaluation of the females. No increase in the incidence of treatment-related tumours was seen in rats of either sex.

5.4 Other relevant data

HC Red No. 3 was mutagenic to bacteria.

5.5 Evaluation[1]

There is *inadequate evidence* in humans for the carcinogenicity of HC Red No. 3.

There is *inadequate evidence* in experimental animals for the carcinogenicity of HC Red No. 3.

Overall evaluation

HC Red No. 3 is *not classifiable as to its carcinogenicity to humans (Group 3)*.

6. References

Burnett, C., Loehr, R. & Corbett, J. (1981) Heritable translocation study on two hair dye formulations. *Fundam. appl. Toxicol.*, **1**, 325–328

Frenkel, E.P. & Brody, F. (1973) Percutaneous absorption and elimination of an aromatic hair dye. *Arch. environ. Health*, **27**, 401–404

---

[1]For definition of the italicized terms, see Preamble, pp. 26–30.

US National Library of Medicine (1992) *Registry of Toxic Effects of Chemical Substances* (RTECS No. KJ6500000), Bethesda, MD

US National Toxicology Program (1986) *Toxicology and Carcinogenesis Studies of HC Red No. 3 (CAS No. 2871-01-4) in F344/N Rats and B6C3F$_1$ Mice (Gavage Studies)* (NTP Technical Report 281; NIH Publ. No. 86-2537), Research Triangle Park, NC

Wernick, T., Lanman, B.M. & Fraux, J.L. (1975) Chronic toxicity, teratologic and reproduction studies with hair dyes. *Toxicol. appl. Pharmacol.*, **32**, 450–460

Zeiger, E., Anderson, B., Haworth, S., Lawlor, T. & Mortelmans, K. (1988) *Salmonella* mutagenicity tests: IV. Results from the testing of 300 chemicals. *Environ. mol. Mutag.*, **11** (Suppl. 12), 1–158

HC YELLOW NO. 4

1. Exposure Data

1.1 Chemical and physical data

1.1.1 Synonyms, structural and molecular data

Confusion has existed over the structure of HC Yellow No. 4. In the second edition of the *Directory of Cosmetic and Toiletry Ingredients* (Cosmetic, Toiletry, and Fragrance Association, 1982), the structure shown for HC Yellow No. 4 had both hydroxyethyl groups on the amine and an assigned CAS No. of 52551-67-4 (2-[bis(2-hydroxyethyl)amino]-5-nitrophenol; *N,N*-bis(2-hydroxyethyl)-2-amino-5-nitrophenol). In the third edition of the *Directory of Cosmetic and Toiletry Ingredients* (Cosmetic, Toiletry, and Fragrance Association, 1991), the structure was corrected on the basis of additional structural analysis, to show one hydroxyethyl group on the amine and the other at the *ortho* position on the ring. This structure and its CAS No. (US National Toxicology Program, 1992) are given below.

Chem. Abstr. Serv. Reg. No.: 59820-43-8

Chem. Abstr. Name: 2-[(2-[2-Hydroxyethoxy]-4-nitrophenyl)amino]ethanol

Synonyms: *N,O*-Di(2-hydroxyethyl)-2-amino-5-nitrophenol; HC Yellow 4; 2-[3-nitro-6-(*beta*-hydroxyethylamino)phenoxy] ethanol

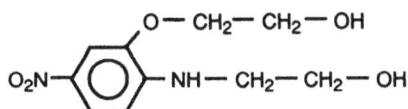

$C_{10}H_{14}N_2O_5$ Mol. wt: 242.23

1.1.2 Chemical and physical properties of the substance

From US National Toxicology Program (1992)

(a) *Description*: Fluffy, bright-yellow powder

(b) *Melting-point*: 145–147 °C

(c) *Spectroscopy data*: Infrared, ultraviolet and nuclear magnetic resonance spectral data have been reported.

(d) *Solubility*: Soluble in water (0.14% w/w), ethanol and acetone

1.1.3 Trade names, technical products and impurities

HC Yellow No. 4 is commercially available at a purity ≥ 93%, with *N*-(2-hydroxyethyl)-2-hydroxy-4-nitroaniline (0.3–7%) (US National Toxicology Program, 1992), 2-

(2-amino-5-nitrophenoxy)ethanol ($< 5\%$) and 2,2'-[(2-hydroxy-4-nitrophenyl)imino]bis-(ethanol) ($< 1\%$) as possible impurities.

1.1.4 *Analysis*

No data were available to the Working Group.

1.2 Production and use

1.2.1 *Production*

HC Yellow No. 4 is produced by the reaction of 2-hydroxy-4-nitrobenzenamine with 2-chloroethanol and sodium hydroxide. Production of this dye began in the late 1950s and was estimated to be 2300 kg in the USA in 1976 (US National Toxicology Program, 1992). Currently, approximately 900 kg are used annually in the USA, according to industry estimates.

1.2.2 *Use*

HC Yellow No. 4 is used exclusively as a dye in semi-permanent hair colour products. These products are generally shampooed into the hair, lathered and then allowed to remain in contact with the hair and scalp for 30–45 min. The concentration of HC Yellow No. 4 used in these preparations ranges from 0.1 to 1.0% (Frenkel & Brody, 1973; US National Toxicology Program, 1992).

1.3 Occurrence

1.3.1 *Natural occurrence*

HC Yellow No. 4 is not known to occur as a natural product.

1.3.2 *Occupational exposure*

No data were available to the Working Group.

An estimated 4000 workers in department stores and beauty shops in the USA were exposed to HC Yellow No. 4 in 1974 (US National Toxicology Program, 1992).

1.4 Regulations and guidelines

No data were available to the Working Group.

2. Studies of Cancer in Humans

No data were available to the Working Group.

3. Studies of Cancer in Experimental Animals

3.1 Oral administration

3.1.1 *Mouse*

Groups of 50 male and 50 female B6C3F$_1$ mice, six weeks of age, were fed diets containing 0, 5000 or 10 000 mg/kg of diet (ppm) HC Yellow No. 4 ($> 93\%$ pure; major impurity tentatively identified as N-(2-hydroxyethyl)-2-hydroxy-4-nitroaniline, $\sim$ 7%) for up to 104 weeks and were killed at 110–111 weeks of age. The mean body weights of high-dose mice were 20–30% lower than those of controls during the second year of the study. Survival at the end of the study was: males—control, 28/50; low-dose, 29/50; and high-dose, 35/50; females—control, 43/50; low-dose, 38/50; and high-dose, 43/50. No significant increase in the incidence of tumours was found in treated animals as compared with controls (US National Toxicology Program, 1992).

3.1.2 *Rat*

Groups of 50 male and 50 female Fischer 344/N rats, six weeks of age, were fed diets containing 0, 2500 or 5000 mg/kg of diet (ppm) (males) and 0, 5000 or 10 000 ppm (females) HC Yellow No. 4 (> 93% pure; major impurity tentatively identified as N-(2-hydroxyethyl)-2-hydroxy-4-nitroaniline, $\sim$ 7%) for up to 104 weeks and were killed at 110–111 weeks of age. The mean body weights of high-dose female rats were significantly lower than those of controls. Survival at the end of the experiment was: males—control, 21/50; low-dose, 29/50; and high-dose, 28/50; females—control, 27/50; low-dose, 31/50; and high-dose, 34/50. The incidence of adenomas of the pituitary gland was increased in male rats (control, 17/45; low-dose, 20/49; high-dose, 28/49; p = 0.034, logistic regression trend test), but the increase was barely significant in a pair-wise comparison (p = 0.047, logistic regression trend test). The incidence in historical controls in all National Toxicology Program feed studies was 29.7 $\pm$ 11.5% (range, 12–60%). Similarly, the incidence of pituitary gland hyperplasia in males was dose-dependently increased (control, 8/45; low-dose, 13/49; high-dose, 18/49; p = 0.026, logistic regression trend test). The incidence of pituitary gland tumours was not increased in female rats (US National Toxicology Program, 1992).

4. Other Relevant Data

4.1 Absorption, distribution, metabolism and excretion

No data were available to the Working Group.

4.2 Toxic effects

4.2.1 *Humans*

No data were available to the Working Group.

4.2.2 *Experimental systems*

During 14-day studies, groups of five Fischer 344/N rats of each sex received 0, 5000, 10 000, 20 000, 40 000 or 80 000 ppm (mg/kg) and B6C3F$_1$ mice of each sex received 0, 1250, 2500, 5000, 10 000 or 20 000 ppm HC Yellow No. 4 (purity, > 93%) in the feed. All animals survived to the end of the studies. No dose-related toxic effect was observed (US National Toxicology Program, 1992).

In 13-week studies, groups of 10 Fischer 344/N rats of each sex were fed diets containing 0, 2500, 5000, 10 000, 20 000 or 40 000 ppm (mg/kg) and 10 B6C3F$_1$ mice of each sex were fed diets containing 0, 5000, 10 000, 20 000, 40 000 or 80 000 ppm HC Yellow No. 4. All rats survived to the end of the studies. Compound-related deaths occurred in male and female mice at the two highest dose levels. Mineralization of the renal papilla occurred in all male rats fed 40 000 ppm. Thyroid pigmentation occurred in rats receiving 40 000 ppm and in 40/46 male mice; a dose-related increase in the incidence of pigmentation was observed in female mice, except for those at the highest dose, most of which died within the first two weeks of the study. The nature of the pigment was not determined. Uterine atrophy occurred in female rats fed 20 000 and 40 000 ppm and in female mice fed 40 000 and 80 000 ppm. Lymphoid depletion and atrophy of the spleen occurred in male mice that received 40 000 or 80 000 ppm and in female mice that received 80 000 ppm. Atrophy of the thymus occurred in male and female mice that received 40 000 or 80 000 ppm (US National Toxicology Program, 1992).

In the two-year studies described above, no compound-related lesion was seen in exposed rats. Male and female mice had a dose-related increase in the incidence of thyroid gland pigmentation and follicular-cell hyperplasia. The predominant impurity, tentatively identified as N-(2-hydroxyethyl)-2-hydroxy-4-nitroaniline, was suggested to have contributed to the increased incidence of thyroid follicular-cell hyperplasia (US National Toxicology Program, 1992).

HC Yellow No. 4 was present at a low concentration in semi-permanent hair colouring formulations evaluated in a 13-week study of dermal toxicity in rabbits (Burnett et al., 1976; 0.4%) and in a two-year feeding study in dogs (Wernick et al., 1975; 0.3%), described in detail on p. 97. No treatment-related adverse effect was detected. [The Working Group noted that the dose of each component of the formulations was very low and unlikely to have been toxic.]

4.3 Reproductive and developmental effects

4.3.1 Humans

No data were available to the Working Group.

4.3.2 Experimental systems

No data were available to the Working Group on the reproductive and developmental effects of HC Yellow No. 4 alone. The compound was present at low concentrations in semi-permanent hair colouring formulations evaluated in a study of fertility and reproductive performance in rats (Wernick et al., 1975, 0.3%; see p. 99) and in studies of teratogenesis in rats (Wernick et al., 1975, 0.3%; Burnett et al., 1976, 0.4%) and rabbits (Wernick et al., 1975, 0.3%) (see p. 100). No treatment-related adverse effect was detected. [The Working Group noted that the dose of each component of the formulations was very low and unlikely to have been toxic.]

4.4 Genetic and related effects

4.4.1 *Humans*

No data were available to the Working Group.

4.4.2 *Experimental systems* (see also Table 1 and Appendices 1 and 2)

HC Yellow No. 4 (purity > 93%) induced mutation in *Salmonella typhimurium*. In one of the two experiments, in spite of the presence of a precipitate at all doses that induced a significant response, increasing numbers of mutants were observed as increasing amounts of test material were added to the plates. HC Yellow No. 4 induced sex-linked recessive lethal mutation in *Drosophila melanogaster* after injection but not in a feeding experiment in adults. It did not induce reciprocal translocations when injected into the flies.

HC Yellow No. 4 induced sister chromatid exchange in Chinese hamster ovary cells in culture, but equivocal results were obtained for chromosomal aberration in the same cells.

5. Summary of Data Reported and Evaluation

5.1 Exposure data

HC Yellow No. 4 is used as a semi-permanent hair dye.

5.2 Human carcinogenicity data

No data were available to the Working Group.

5.3 Animal carcinogenicity data

HC Yellow No. 4 was tested for carcinogenicity by administration in the diet in one study in mice and in one study in rats. No significant increase in tumour incidence was found in mice. The incidence of adenomas of the pituitary gland was increased in male rats but not in females.

5.4 Other relevant data

HC Yellow No. 4 induced gene mutation in bacteria and in insects. Chromosomal aberrations were not induced in insects, and equivocal results for this end-point were obtained in cultured mammalian cells. Sister chromatid exchange was induced in mammalian cells.

5.5 Evaluation[1]

There is *inadequate evidence* in humans for the carcinogenicity of HC Yellow No. 4.

---

[1]For definition of the italicized terms, see Preamble, pp. 26–30.

Table 1. Genetic and related effects of HC Yellow No. 4

Test system	Result		Dose[a] (LED/HID)	Reference
	Without exogenous metabolic system	With exogenous metabolic system		
SA0, *Salmonella typhimurium* TA100, reverse mutation	+	+	5.0000[b]	Mortelmans et al. (1986)
SA5, *Salmonella typhimurium* TA1535, reverse mutation	(+)	(+)	5000.0000[b]	Mortelmans et al. (1986)
SA7, *Salmonella typhimurium* TA1537, reverse mutation	+	+	50.0000[b]	Mortelmans et al. (1986)
SA9, *Salmonella typhimurium* TA98, reverse mutation	+	+	50.0000[b]	Mortelmans et al. (1986)
DMX, *Drosophila melanogaster*, sex-linked recessive lethal mutation	−		10000.0000 feeding	Woodruff et al. (1985)
DMX, *Drosophila melanogaster*, sex-linked recessive lethal mutation	+		10000.0000 injection	Woodruff et al. (1985)
DMH, *Drosophila melanogaster*, reciprocal translocation	−		10000.0000 injection	Woodruff et al. (1985)
SIC, Sister chromatid exchange, Chinese hamster ovary cells *in vitro*	+	−	167.0000	US National Toxicology Program (1992)
CIC, Chromosomal aberrations, Chinese hamster ovary cells *in vitro*	−	?	3000.0000	US National Toxicology Program (1992)

+, positive; (+), weakly positive; −, negative; 0, not tested; ?, inconclusive (variable response in several experiments within an adequate study)
[a]In-vitro tests, μg/ml; in-vivo tests, mg/kg bw
[b]Precipitate present in plates

There is *inadequate evidence* in experimental animals for the carcinogenicity of HC Yellow No. 4.

Overall evaluation

HC Yellow No. 4 is *not classifiable as to its carcinogenicity to humans (Group 3).*

6. References

Burnett, C., Goldenthal, E.I., Harris, S.B., Wazeter, F.X., Strausburg, J., Kapp, R. & Voelker, R. (1976) Teratology and percutaneous toxicity studies on hair dyes. *J. Toxicol. environ. Health*, **1**, 1027–1040

Cosmetic, Toiletry, and Fragrance Association (1982) *Directory of Cosmetic and Toiletry Ingredients*, 2nd ed., Washington DC

Cosmetic, Toiletry, and Fragrance Association (1991) *Directory of Cosmetic and Toiletry Ingredients*, 3rd ed., Washington DC

Frenkel, E.P. & Brody, F. (1973) Percutaneous absorption and elimination of an aromatic hair dye. *Arch. environ. Health*, **27**, 401–404

Mortelmans, K., Haworth, S., Lawlor, T., Speck, W., Tainer, B. & Zeiger, E. (1986) *Salmonella* mutagenicity tests: II. Results from the testing of 270 chemicals. *Environ. Mutag.*, **8** (Suppl. 7), 1–119

US National Toxicology Program (1992) *Toxicology and Carcinogenesis Studies of HC Yellow No. 4 (CAS No. 59820-43-8) in F344/N Rats and B6C3F$_1$ Mice (Feed Studies)* (NTP Tech. Rep. No. 419; NIH Publ. No. 92-3150), Research Triangle Park, NC

Wernick, T., Lanman, B.M. & Fraux, J.L. (1975) Chronic toxicity, teratologic and reproduction studies with hair dyes. *Toxicol. appl. Pharmacol.*, **32**, 450–460

Woodruff, R.C., Mason, J.M., Valencia, R. & Zimmering, S. (1985) Chemical mutagenesis testing in *Drosophila*. V. Results of 53 coded compounds tested for the National Toxicology Program. *Environ. Mutag.*, **7**, 677–702

2-AMINO-4-NITROPHENOL

1. Exposure Data

1.1 Chemical and physical data

1.1.1 *Synonyms, structural and molecular data*

Chem. Abstr. Serv. Reg. No.: 99-57-0
Chem. Abstr. Name: 2-Amino-4-nitrophenol
Colour Index No.: 76530
Synonyms: 1-Amino-2-hydroxy-5-nitrobenzene; 1-hydroxy-2-amino-4-nitrobenzene; 2-hydroxy-5-nitroaniline; 4-nitro-2-aminophenol; *para*-nitro-*ortho*-aminophenol

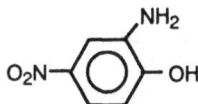

$C_6H_6N_2O_3$ Mol. wt: 154.12

1.1.2 *Chemical and physical properties*

(a) *Description*: Yellow-brown to orange prisms (Lide, 1991)
(b) *Melting-point*: 143–145 °C (anhydrous) (Aldrich Chemical Co., 1992); 80–90 °C (hydrated) (Lide, 1991)
(c) *Spectroscopy data*: Infrared, ultraviolet and nuclear magnetic resonance spectral data have been reported (Pouchert, 1981, 1983; US National Toxicology Program, 1988; Sadtler Research Laboratories, 1980, 1991).
(d) *Solubility*: Soluble in ethanol, acetone, acetic acid and diethyl ether; sparingly soluble in water (US National Toxicology Program, 1988; Lide, 1991)
(e) *Octanol/water partition coefficient (P)*: 13.5 (Bronaugh & Congdon, 1984)

1.1.3 *Trade names, technical products and impurities*

Trade name: Rodol 42 (Jos. H. Lowenstein & Sons, 1991)
2-Amino-4-nitrophenol is available commercially with the following specifications: purity, 96% (min.); ash, 0.1% (max.); iron, 100 ppm (mg/kg) (max.); lead (see IARC, 1980a, 1987a), 5 ppm (mg/kg) (max.); and arsenic (see IARC, 1980b, 1987b), 2 ppm (mg/kg) (max.). It is also available in research quantities at purities ranging from 90 to > 99%

(Riedel-de-Haen, 1990; Heraeus, 1991; Jos. H. Lowenstein & Sons, 1991; Lancaster Synthesis, 1991; TCI America, 1991; Aldrich Chemical Co., 1992; Fluka Chemie AG, 1993).

1.1.4 *Analysis*

No data were available to the Working Group.

1.2 Production and use

1.2.1 *Production*

2-Amino-4-nitrophenol is produced by the reaction of 2,4-dinitrophenol with sodium sulfide (Farris, 1978). It was first synthesized by Agfa in 1898 (Society of Dyers and Colourists, 1971).

At present, approximately 150 kg of 2-amino-4-nitrophenol are used in hair colouring products in the USA annually, according to industry estimates. It is produced by one company each in Brazil, China, Czechoslovakia, France, Germany, India and the United Kingdom and by three companies in Japan (Chemical Information Services, 1991).

1.2.2 *Use*

2-Amino-4-nitrophenol is used as an intermediate in the manufacture of CI Mordant Brown 33 and CI Mordant Brown 1, which are used for dyeing leather, nylon, silk, wool and fur (US National Toxicology Program, 1988). It is also used in some countries as a dye in semi-permanent hair colour products to produce gold-blond shades. These products are generally shampooed into the hair, lathered and then allowed to remain in contact with the hair and scalp for 30–45 min. For this application, 2-amino-4-nitrophenol is mixed at levels up to 0.5% with a blend of several other dyes in a shampoo base to produce the final colour or tint (Frenkel & Brody, 1973; US National Toxicology Program, 1988). It has also been used in permanent hair colouring products.

1.3 Occurrence

1.3.1 *Natural occurrence*

2-Amino-4-nitrophenol is not known to occur as a natural product.

1.3.2 *Occupational exposure*

No data were available to the Working Group.

On the basis of a survey conducted in the USA between 1981 and 1983, the US National Institute for Occupational Safety and Health estimated that a total of 20 256 workers, including 17 049 women, were potentially exposed to 2-amino-4-nitrophenol in an estimated 2232 beauty shops (US National Library of Medicine, 1992).

1.3.3 *Other*

2-Amino-4-nitrophenol and 4-amino-2-nitrophenol are reportedly formed by environmental degradation (reduction) of 2,4-dinitrophenol, which is used as a fungicide on wood (Mitra & Vaidyanathan, 1982).

1.4 Regulations and guidelines

The use of 2-amino-4-nitrophenol in cosmetic products is prohibited in the European Economic Community (Commission of the European Communities, 1976, 1990, 1991).

2. Studies of Cancer in Humans

No data were available to the Working Group.

3. Studies of Cancer in Experimental Animals

3.1 Oral administration

3.1.1 *Mouse*

Groups of 50 male and 50 female B6C3F$_1$ mice, seven to eight weeks of age, were administered 0, 125 or 250 mg/kg bw 2-amino-4-nitrophenol (98% pure) [impurities unspecified] by gavage in corn oil (10 ml/kg bw) on five days a week for up to 103 weeks. The mean body weight of low-dose females was up to 17% greater than that of the controls; the body weights of the other treated groups were comparable with those of vehicle controls. No significant difference in survival was observed at termination of the study in treated and control groups of either sex (males: control, 28/50; low-dose, 29/50 and high-dose, 23/50; females: control, 28/50; low-dose, 31/50; and high-dose, 30/50). The incidence of combined haemangiomas and haemangiosarcomas at all sites in high-dose male mice was significantly higher (5/50) than that in controls (0/50; $p < 0.05$, Fisher exact test); however, these tumours were not considered to be related to the treatment since their incidence in historical controls at the study laboratory was 16/149 (11 $\pm$ 10%) and that in all studies of the National Toxicology Program was 101/1743 (6 $\pm$ 5%) (US National Toxicology Program, 1988).

3.1.2 *Rat*

Groups of 50 male and 50 female Fischer 344/N rats, six weeks of age, were administered 0, 125 or 250 mg/kg bw 2-amino-4-nitrophenol (98% pure) [impurities unspecified] by gavage in corn oil (5 ml/kg bw) on five days a week for up to 103 weeks. Mean body weights of low-dose and high-dose males were 6 and 10% lower than those of controls, respectively; values for female rats were comparable to those of controls. Survival of high-dose males was significantly lower than that of controls ($p < 0.001$, Cox and Tarone's method); no significant difference was found for females. Survival at the end of the study was, in males, control, 32/50; low-dose, 24/50; high-dose, 10/50, and, in females, control, 25/50; low-dose, 27/50; high-dose, 31/50. Hyperplasia of the renal tubular epithelium was observed only in male rats (control, 1/50; low-dose, 4/48; high-dose, 5/50); the difference was not significant. Renal tubular-cell adenomas were also observed in treated males (control, 0/50; low-dose, 1/48; high-dose, 3/50); among male rats that lived beyond week 100, when the first renal tubular-cell tumour was observed, the incidence in high-dose animals (3/20) was significantly higher than that in controls ($0/39; p = 0.035$, Fisher exact test). Two liver-cell neoplastic nodules and one hepatocellular carcinoma were observed in high-dose male rats. The historical incidence of neoplastic nodules or hepatocellular carcinomas at the study laboratory was $3/149$ ($2 \pm 3\%$) and that of renal-cell adenomas, $0/149$. In all studies of the National Toxicology Program, renal-cell adenomas occurred in $9/1695$ ($0.5 \pm 0.9\%$) (US National Toxicology Program, 1988).

4. Other Relevant Data

4.1 Absorption, distribution, metabolism and exctretion

4.1.1 Humans

No data were available to the Working Group.

4.1.2 Experimental systems

Percutaneous absorption of ^{14}C-2-amino-4-nitrophenol (specific radioactivity, 10 mCi/mmol [65 μCi/mg]; purity, 98%) was studied *in vitro* by partitioning between excised human abdominal skin preparations and water. 2-Amino-4-nitrophenol appeared to bind to skin components (Bronaugh & Congdon, 1984).

Percutaneous absorption through the skin of Sprague-Dawley rats of each sex was examined following application of two hair dye formulations: formulation 1 contained 1.54% ^{14}C-2-amino-4-nitrophenol; formulation 2 contained 0.77% ^{14}C-2-amino-4-nitrophenol, 1,4-diaminobenzene (1,4-phenylenediamine), 2,4-diaminoanisole, oleic acid and isopropanol and was mixed with equal amounts of a 6% hydrogen peroxide solution. After one and five days, 0.21 and 0.36% of the radiolabel administered in formulation 1 and 1.12 and 1.67% of that administered in formulation 2 had been absorbed (calculated as combined radiolabel in urine, faeces, expired air and carcass, without treated skin area). Absorbed material was excreted predominantly in the urine within 24 h after the initial application (Hofer *et al.*, 1982).

Five days after oral administration by gavage of 2 ml ^{14}C-2-amino-4-nitrophenol (0.2% in saline), $68.3\% \pm 9.4$ (SD) of the radiolabel had been excreted in the urine and $25.4\% \pm 6.9$ in the faeces. Within 3 h, about 4% of the radiolabel was eliminated in the bile. Following subcutaneous injection of the same dose, 89% of the dose was eliminated after one day, predominantly in the urine (Hofer *et al.*, 1982). [The Working Group noted that metabolites were not identified in the urine, bile or faeces in either study.]

2-Amino-4-nitrophenol was the predominant metabolite formed enzymatically by nitroreduction following oral administration of 2,4-dinitrophenol (22.5 mg/kg bw) to ICR mice. It had an elimination half-time from the plasma of 46 h, while that of the isomer 4-amino-2-nitrophenol was 26 h (Robert & Hagardorn, 1985).

4.2 Toxic effects

4.2.1 Humans

No data were available to the Working Group.

4.2.2 *Experimental systems*

The LD_{50} of 2-amino-4-nitrophenol in rats has been reported as 246 mg/kg bw after intraperitoneal injection (US National Toxicology Program, 1988) and 2400 mg/kg bw after oral administration (Lloyd *et al.*, 1977). The LD_{50} in mice after intraperitoneal injection was reported to be 143 mg/kg bw (Mikstacki, 1985).

During 15-day studies, groups of five Fischer 344/N rats and $B6C3F_1$ mice of each sex received 0, 313, 625, 1250, 2500 or 5000 mg/kg bw 2-amino-4-nitrophenol (purity, 98%) in corn oil by gavage. Reduced survival was observed in all animals that received 2500 or 5000 mg/kg; diarrhoea was observed in all treated rats except those receiving the lowest dose (US National Toxicology Program, 1988).

In 13-week studies, groups of 10 Fischer 344/N rats and $B6C3F_1$ mice of each sex received 2-amino-4-nitrophenol at doses of 0, 62.5, 125, 250, 500 or 1000 mg/kg bw by gavage in corn oil. Survival was reduced by the highest dose in both species. Diarrhoea was observed in rats that received 500 or 1000 mg/kg. Mild to severe mineralization of the renal cortex and mild to severe degeneration of the renal tubular epithelium were observed in male rats that received 500 or 1000 mg/kg and in females that received 1000 mg/kg. Degeneration and necrosis of the renal tubular epithelium, with some indication of regeneration, were observed in mice that received 1000 mg/kg (US National Toxicology Program, 1988).

In the two-year studies described above, nephropathy was present in nearly all exposed male rats and was presumed to have contributed to the reduced survival of those given 250 mg/kg. The more severe nephropathy was associated with a spectrum of non-neoplastic lesions characteristic of reduced renal function and renal secondary hyperparathyroidism, i.e., parathyroid hyperplasia, fibrous osteodystrophy, calcification of the heart and other organs (US National Toxicology Program, 1988).

2-Amino-4-nitrophenol was present at a low concentration in an oxidative hair colouring formulation evaluated in a 13-week study of dermal toxicity in rabbits (Burnett *et al.*, 1976, 0.4%) and in a semi-permanent formulation evaluated in a two-year feeding study in dogs (Wernick *et al.*, 1975; 0.05%), described in detail on p. 97. No treatment-related adverse effect was detected. [The Working Group noted that the dose of each component of the formulations was very low and unlikely to have been toxic.]

4.3 Reproductive and developmental effects

4.3.1 *Humans*

No data were available to the Working Group.

4.3.2 *Experimental systems*

No data were available to the Working Group on the reproductive and developmental effects of 2-amino-4-nitrophenol alone. The compound was present at low concentrations in semi-permanent hair colouring formulations evaluated in a study of fertility and reproductive performance in rats and in studies of teratogenesis in rats and rabbits (Wernick *et al.*, 1975, 0.05%; see p. 99). It was also present (at 0.4%) in oxidative and semi-permanent formulations evaluated in a study of teratogenesis (Burnett *et al.*, 1976) and in a two-generation study of reproduction in rats (Burnett & Goldenthal, 1988) (see p. 100). No treatment-related adverse effect was detected. [The Working Group noted that the dose of each component of the formulations was very low and unlikely to have been toxic.]

4.4 Genetic and related effects

4.4.1 *Humans*

No data were available to the Working Group.

4.4.2 *Experimental systems* (see also Table 1 and Appendices 1 and 2)

2-Amino-4-nitrophenol did not induce mutation in bacteriophage but was mutagenic to *Salmonella typhimurium*, to the fungus *Sordaria brevicollis* and at the *tk* locus in mouse lymphoma L5178Y cells. It induced sister chromatid exchange and chromosomal aberrations in cultured Chinese hamster ovary cells.

Neither micronuclei, chromosomal aberrations nor dominant lethal effects were induced in rodents exposed *in vivo*.

5. Summary of Data Reported and Evaluation

5.1 Exposure data

2-Amino-4-nitrophenol is used as an intermediate in the manufacture of certain azo dyes. It is also used in semi-permanent hair colouring products and has been used in permanent hair colours.

5.2 Human carcinogenicity data

No data were available to the Working Group.

5.3 Animal carcinogenicity data

2-Amino-4-nitrophenol was tested for carcinogenicity by gavage in one study in mice and one study in rats. No significant increase in the incidence of tumours was observed in mice or in female rats. The incidence of renal-cell adenomas was increased in male rats.

5.4 Other relevant data

2-Amino-4-nitrophenol caused renal toxicity in rats and mice. The effect occurred at a lower dose in male than in female rats.

Table 1. Genetic and related effects of 2-amino-4-nitrophenol

Test system	Result Without exogenous metabolic system	With exogenous metabolic system	Dose[a] (LED/HID)	Reference
BPF, Bacteriophage T4D, forward mutation	−	0	305.1000	Kvelland (1985)
SA0, *Salmonella typhimurium* TA100, reverse mutation	−	−	500.0000	Shahin et al. (1982)
SA0, *Salmonella typhimurium* TA100, reverse mutation	−	−	1667.0000	Zeiger et al. (1987)[b]
SA5, *Salmonella typhimurium* TA1535, reverse mutation	−	−	500.0000	Shahin et al. (1982)
SA5, *Salmonella typhimurium* TA1535, reverse mutation	−	−	1667.0000	Zeiger et al. (1987)[b]
SA7, *Salmonella typhimurium* TA1537, reverse mutation	−	−	500.0000	Shahin et al. (1982)
SA7, *Salmonella typhimurium* TA1537, reverse mutation	−	−	1667.0000	Zeiger et al. (1987)[b]
SA8, *Salmonella typhimurium* TA1538, reverse mutation	0	+	10.0000	Ames et al. (1975)
SA8, *Salmonella typhimurium* TA1538, reverse mutation	+	+	25.0000	Garner & Nutman (1977)
SA8, *Salmonella typhimurium* TA1538, reverse mutation	+	(+)	25.0000	Shahin et al. (1982)
SA9, *Salmonella typhimurium* TA98, reverse mutation	+	(+)	5.0000	Shahin et al. (1982)
SA9, *Salmonella typhimurium* TA98, reverse mutation	(+)	+[c]	50.0000	Zeiger et al. (1987)[b]
PLM, *Sordaria brevicollis*, ascospore mutation	+	0	246.0000	Yu-Sun (1981)
G5T, Gene mutation, mouse lymphoma L5178Y cells, *tk* locus	+	0	50.0000	US National Toxicology Program (1988)[b]
SIC, Sister chromatid exchange, Chinese hamster ovary cells *in vitro*	+	+	16.7000	US National Toxicology Program (1988)[b]
CIC, Chromosomal aberrations, Chinese hamster ovary cells *in vitro*	+	+	199.0000	US National Toxicology Program (1988)[b]
MVR, Micronucleus test, CFY rats bone-marrow cells *in vivo*	−		2500.0000 po × 2	Hossack & Richardson (1977)
CBA, Chromosomal aberrations, mouse bone-marrow cells *in vivo*	−		71.3500 ip	Mikstacki (1985)
CVA, Chromosomal aberrations, mouse Ehrlich ascites tumour cells *in vivo*	−		71.3500 ip	Mikstacki (1985)
DLR, Dominant lethal mutation, CD rats	−		20.0000 ip × 24	Burnett et al. (1977)

+, positive; (+), weakly positive; −, negative; 0, not tested

[a] In-vitro tests, μg/ml; in-vivo tests, mg/kg bw

[b] Results from two laboratories

[c] Hamster liver S9; negative result with rat liver S9

2-Amino-4-nitrophenol induced mutation in bacteria, fungi and cultured mammalian cells and sister chromatid exchange and chromosomal aberrations in cultured mammalian cells. It did not induce micronuclei, chromosomal aberrations or dominant lethal mutation in rodents exposed *in vivo*.

5.5 Evaluation[1]

There is *inadequate evidence* in humans for the carcinogenicity of 2-amino-4-nitrophenol.

There is *limited evidence* in experimental animals for the carcinogenicity of 2-amino-4-nitrophenol.

Overall evaluation

2-Amino-4-nitrophenol *is not classifiable as to its carcinogenicity to humans (Group 3).*

6. References

Aldrich Chemical Co. (1992) *Aldrich Catalog/Handbook of Fine Chemicals 1992- 1993*, Milwaukee, WI, p. 75

Ames, B.N., Kammen, H.O. & Yamasaki, E. (1975) Hair dyes are mutagenic: identification of a variety of mutagenic ingredients. *Proc. natl Acad Sci. USA*, **72**, 2423–2427

Bronaugh, R.L. & Congdon, E.R. (1984) Percutaneous absorption of hair dyes: correlation with partition coefficients. *J. invest. Dermatol.*, **83**, 124–127

Burnett, C.M. & Goldenthal, E.I. (1988) Multigeneration reproduction and carcinogenicity studies in Sprague-Dawley rats exposed topically to oxidative hair-coloring formulations containing *p*-phenylenediamine and other aromatic amines. *Food Chem. Toxicol.*, **26**, 467–474

Burnett, C., Goldenthal, E.I., Harris, S.B., Wazeter, F.X., Strausburg, J., Kapp, R. & Voelker, R. (1976) Teratology and percutaneous toxicity studies on hair dyes. *J. Toxicol. environ. Health*, **1**, 1027–1040

Burnett, C., Loehr, R. & Corbett, J. (1977) Dominant lethal mutagenicity study on hair dyes. *J. Toxicol. environ. Health*, **2**, 657–662

Chemical Information Services (1991) *Directory of World Chemical Producers*, Dallas, TX, p. 39

Commission of the European Communities (1976) Council Directive 76/768/EEC of 27 July 1976. *Off. J. Eur. Commun.*, **L262**, 169–200

Commission of the European Communities (1990) Proposal for a Council Directive on the approximation of the laws of the Member States relating to cosmetic products of 15 November 1990. *Off. J. Eur. Commun.*, **C322**, 29–77

Commission of the European Communitites (1991) Commission Directive 91/184/EEC of 12 March 1991. *Off. J. Eur. Commun.*, **L91**, 59–62

Farris, R.E. (1978) Aminophenols. In: Mark, H.F., Othmer, D.F., Overberger, C.G., Seaborg, G.T. & Grayson, M., eds, *Kirk-Othmer Encyclopedia of Chemical Technology*, 3rd ed., Vol. 2, New York, John Wiley & Sons, pp. 422–440

---

[1]For definition of the italicized terms, see Preamble, pp. 26–30.

Fluka Chemie AG (1993) *Fluka Chemika-BioChemika*, Buchs, p. 93

Frenkel, E.P. & Brody, F. (1973) Percutaneous absorption and elimination of an aromatic hair dye. *Arch. environ. Health*, **27**, 401–404

Garner, R.C. & Nutman, C.A. (1977) Testing of some azo dyes and their reduction products for mutagenicity using *Salmonella typhimurium* TA1538. *Mutat. Res.*, **44**, 9–19

Heraeus (1991) *Feinchemikalien Forschungsbedarf* (Refined chemicals and research supply), Karlsruhe, p. 70

Hofer, H., Schwach, G.W. & Fenzl, C. (1982) Percutaneous absorption of 2-amino-4-nitrophenol in the rat. *Food Chem. Toxicol.*, **20**, 921–923

Hossack, D.J.N. & Richardson, J.C. (1977) Examination of the potential mutagenicity of hair dye constituents using the micronucleus test. *Experientia*, **33**, 377–378

IARC (1980a) *IARC Monographs on the Evaluation of the Carcinogenic Risk of Chemicals to Humans*, Vol. 23, *Some Metals and Metallic Compounds*, Lyon, pp. 325–415

IARC (1980b) *IARC Monographs on the Evaluation of the Carcinogenic Risk of Chemicals to Humans*, Vol. 23, *Some Metals and Metallic Compounds*, Lyon, pp. 39–141

IARC (1987a) *IARC Monographs on the Evaluation of Carcinogenic Risks to Humans*, Suppl. 7, *Overall Evaluations of Carcinogenicity: An Updating of* IARC Monographs *Volumes 1 to 42*, Lyon, pp. 230–232

IARC (1987b) *IARC Monographs on the Evaluation of Carcinogenic Risks to Humans*, Suppl. 7, *Overall Evaluations of Carcinogenicity: An Updating of* IARC Monographs *Volumes 1 to 42*, Lyon, pp. 100–106

Jos. H. Lowenstein & Sons (1991) *Specifications: Rodol 42 (4-Nitro-2-aminophenol Pure)*, New York

Kvelland, I. (1985) Mutagenicity of five hair dyes in bacteriophage T4D. *Hereditas*, **102**, 151–154

Lancaster Synthesis (1991) *MTM Research Chemicals/Lancaster Catalogue 1991/92*, Windham, NH, MTM Plc, p. 69

Lide, D.R., ed. (1991) *CRC Handbook of Chemistry and Physics*, 72nd ed., Boca Raton, FL, CRC Press, p. 3–377

Lloyd, G.K., Liggett, M.P., Kynoch, S.R. & Davies, R.E. (1977) Assessment of the acute toxicity and potential irritancy of hair dye constituents. *Food Cosmet. Toxicol.*, **15**, 607–610

Mikstacki, A. (1985) Evaluation of mutagenicity of some aromatic amines, used as hair dyes, by chromosomal aberration tests *in vivo*. *Genet. pol.*, **26**, 109–116

Mitra, D. & Vaidyanathan, C.S. (1982) Comparative phytotoxicity of nitrophenolic soil pollutants and their microbial metabolites to the growth of cucumber (*Cucumis sativus* L.) seedlings. *Plant Soil*, **69**, 467–471

Pouchert, C.J. (1981) *The Aldrich Library of Infrared Spectra*, 3rd ed., Milwaukee, WI, Aldrich Chemical Co., p. 823

Pouchert, C.J. (1983) *The Aldrich Library of NMR Spectra*, 2nd ed., Vol. 1, Milwaukee, WI, Aldrich Chemical Co., p. 1166

Riedel-de Haen (1990) *Laboratory Chemicals 1990*, Seelze, p. 61

Robert, T.A. & Hagardorn, A.N. (1985) Plasma levels and kinetic disposition of 2,4-dinitrophenol and its metabolites 2-amino-4-nitrophenol and 4-amino-2-nitrophenol in the mouse. *J. Chromatogr.*, **344**, 177–186

Sadtler Research Laboratories (1980) *Sadtler Standard Spectra 1980*, Philadelphia, PA

Sadtler Research Laboratories (1991) *Sadtler Standard Spectra 1981–1991, Supplementary Index*, Philadelphia, PA

Shahin, M.M., Bugaut, A. & Kalopissis, G. (1982) Mutagenicity of aminonitrophenol compounds in *Salmonella typhimurium*: a study of structural–activity relationships. *Int. J. cosmet. Sci.*, **4**, 25–35

Society of Dyers and Colourists (1971) *Colour Index*, 3rd ed., Vol. 4, Bradford, Yorkshire, p. 4647

TCI America (1991) *Organic Chemicals 91/92 Catalog*, Portland, OR, p. 78

US National Library of Medicine (1992) *Registry of Toxic Effects of Chemical Substances* (RTECS No. SJ6300000), Bethesda, MD

US National Toxicology Program (1988) *Toxicology and Carcinogenesis Studies of 2-Amino-4-nitrophenol (CAS No. 99-57-0) in F344/N Rats and B6C3F₁ Mice (Gavage Studies)* (NTP Tech. Rep. No. 339; NIH Publ. No. 88-2595), Research Triangle Park, NC

Wernick, T., Lanman, B.M. & Fraux, J.L. (1975) Chronic toxicity, teratologic, and reproduction studies with hair dyes. *Toxicol. appl. Pharmacol.*, **32**, 450–460

Yu-Sun, C.C., Carter L.A., Sandoval, L. & Thompson, A. (1981) Mutagenicity of 4-nitroquinoline 1-oxide and three hair dye compounds in *Sordaria brevicollis*. *Neurospora Newslett.*, **28**, 22

Zeiger, E., Anderson, B., Haworth, S., Lawlor, T., Mortelmans, K. & Speck, W. (1987) *Salmonella* mutagenicity tests: III. Results from the testing of 255 chemicals. *Environ. Mutag.*, **9** (Suppl. 9), 1–110

2-AMINO-5-NITROPHENOL

1. Exposure Data

1.1 Chemical and physical data

1.1.1 *Synonyms, structural and molecular data*

Chem. Abstr. Serv. Reg. No.: 121-88-0
Chem. Abstr. Name: 2-Amino-5-nitrophenol
Colour Index No.: 76535
Synonyms: 3-Hydroxy-4-aminonitrobenzene; 2-hydroxy-4-nitroaniline; 3-nitro-6-aminophenol; 5-nitro-2-aminophenol

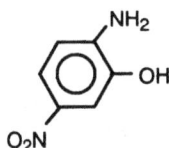

$C_6H_6N_2O_3$ Mol. wt: 154.12

1.1.2 *Chemical and physical properties*

(a) *Description*: Olive-brown, brown to orange crystalline solid (US National Toxicology Program, 1988; Jos. H. Lowenstein & Sons, 1991)

(b) *Melting-point*: 200 °C (decomposes) (Aldrich Chemical Co., 1992); 207–208 °C (Lide, 1991); 198–202 °C (98% pure) (Jos. H. Lowenstein & Sons, 1991)

(c) *Spectroscopy data*: Infrared, ultraviolet and nuclear magnetic resonance spectral data have been reported (Sadtler Research Laboratories, 1980; Pouchert, 1981; US National Toxicology Program, 1988; Sadtler Research Laboratories, 1991).

(d) *Solubility*: Slightly soluble in water (US National Toxicology Program, 1988); soluble in ethanol, acetone and benzene (Lide, 1991)

1.1.3 *Trade names, technical products and impurities*

Trade names: Ursol Yellow Brown A; Rodol YBA

2-Amino-5-nitrophenol is available commercially with the following specifications: purity, 98% (min.); ash, 0.05% (max.); iron, 40 ppm (mg/kg) (max.); lead (see IARC, 1980a, 1987a), 5 ppm (mg/kg) (max.); and arsenic (see IARC, 1980b, 1987b), 2 ppm (mg/kg) (max.).

It is also available in research quantities, at purities ranging from 90 to 99% (Jos. H. Lowenstein & Sons, 1991; TCI America, 1991; Aldrich Chemical Co., 1992; Fluka Chemie AG, 1993).

1.1.4 *Analysis*

No data were available to the Working Group.

1.2 Production and use

1.2.1 *Production*

2-Amino-5-nitrophenol is produced from 2-aminophenol by reaction with acetic anhydride to form 2-methylbenzoxazole, which is nitrated and hydrolysed to form 2-amino-5-nitrophenol (Farris, 1978). It was first synthesized by Kaltwasser and Oehrn in 1920 (Society of Dyers and Colourists, 1971).

2-Amino-5-nitrophenol is produced by one company each in France and Germany and by three companies in Japan (Chemical Information Services, 1991). It is not produced in commercial quantities in the USA. Between 1973 and 1979, US imports averaged 13.4 tonnes per year (US National Toxicology Program, 1988).

1.2.2 *Use*

2-Amino-5-nitrophenol is used as an intermediate in the manufacture of several azo dyes, including CI Solvent Red 8, which is used for colouring synthetic resins, lacquers, inks and wood stains (US National Toxicology Program, 1988).

2-Amino-5-nitrophenol is also used in many countries as a dye in semi-permanent hair colouring products to produce red and gold-blond shades. These products are generally shampooed into the hair, lathered and then allowed to remain in contact with the hair and scalp for 30–45 min. For this application, 2-amino-5-nitrophenol is mixed (at levels up to 0.5%) with a blend of several other dyes in a shampoo base to produce the final colour or tint desired (Frenkel & Brody, 1973; US National Toxicology Program, 1988). It has been used (and still is to a limited extent) in permanent hair colouring products.

1.3 Occurrence

1.3.1 *Natural occurrence*

2-Amino-5-nitrophenol is not known to occur as a natural product.

1.3.2 *Occupational exposure*

No data were available to the Working Group.

On the basis of a survey conducted in the USA between 1981 and 1983, the US National Institute for Occupational Safety and Health estimated that a total of 14 512 workers, including 11 827 women, were potentially exposed to 2-amino-5-nitrophenol in 1339 beauty salons (US National Library of Medicine, 1992).

1.4 Regulations and guidelines

The use of 2-amino-5-nitrophenol in cosmetic products is prohibited in the European Economic Community (Commission of the European Communities, 1976, 1990, 1991).

2. Studies of Cancer in Humans

No data were available to the Working Group.

3. Studies of Cancer in Experimental Animals

3.1 Oral administration

3.1.1 *Mouse*

Groups of 50 male and 50 female B6C3F$_1$ mice, seven to eight weeks of age, were administered 0, 400 or 800 mg/kg bw 2-amino-5-nitrophenol (98% pure) by gavage in corn oil (10 ml/kg) on five days a week for up to 103 weeks and were killed at 112 weeks of age. The mean body weights of high-dose males were 8–11% lower than those of vehicle controls from week 29 to week 74, whereas those of low-dose males were greater than those of vehicle controls throughout most of the study. The mean body weights of low-dose and high-dose female mice were 5–9 and 8–13% lower than those of vehicle controls from week 69 to the end of the study, respectively. Survival of high-dose males after week 20 and of females after week 22 was reduced compared with that of controls ($p < 0.001$, Cox and Tarone's test). Survival at termination of the study was: males—control, 31/50; low-dose, 36/50; and high-dose, 12/50; females—control, 37/50; low-dose, 36/50; and high-dose, 10/50. No significant increase in the incidence of tumours was observed in treated groups when compared with controls (US National Toxicology Program, 1988). [The Working Group noted the high mortality in the high-dose groups.]

3.1.2 *Rat*

Groups of 50 male and 50 female Fischer 344/N rats, six to seven weeks of age, were administered 0, 100 or 200 mg/kg bw 2-amino-5-nitrophenol (98% pure) by gavage in corn oil (5 ml/kg) on five days a week for up to 103 weeks and were killed at 111 weeks of age. Mean body weights of male and female high-dose rats were 5–10 and 4–5% lower than those of controls after weeks 33 and 93, respectively. Survival of high-dose males and females after week 75 and that of low-dose males and females after week 99 was significantly lower than that of vehicle controls ($p < 0.001$, Cox and Tarone's test). Survival at termination was: males—control, 33/50; low-dose, 16/50; and high-dose, 4/50; females—control, 30/50; low-dose, 32/50; and high-dose, 29/50. The incidence of pancreatic acinar-cell adenomas was significantly increased in low-dose (10/50; $p = 0.002$, incidental tumour test) but not in high-dose (3/49) males in comparison with controls (1/50). One acinar-cell carcinoma was also seen in a low-dose male (US National Toxicology Program, 1988). [The Working Group noted the poor survival of treated males.]

4. Other Relevant Data

4.1 Absorption, distribution, metabolism and excretion

No data were available to the Working Group.

4.2 Toxic effects

4.2.1 *Humans*

No data were available to the Working Group.

4.2.2 *Experimental systems*

The LD_{50} of 2-amino-5-nitrophenol in rats has been reported to be greater than 4000 mg/kg bw by oral administration and greater than 800 mg/kg bw by intraperitoneal injection (Burnett *et al.*, 1977).

During 16-day studies, groups of five Fischer 344/N rats of each sex received 0, 156, 313, 625, 1250 or 2500 mg/kg bw 2-amino-5-nitrophenol (purity, 98%), and groups of five B6C3F$_1$ mice of each sex received 0, 313, 625, 1250, 2500 or 5000 mg/kg bw, by gavage in corn oil. A reduction in survival in relation to dose was observed in female mice (US National Toxicology Program, 1988).

In 13-week studies, groups of 10 Fischer 344/N rats and B6C3F$_1$ mice of each sex received 0, 100, 200, 400, 800 or 1600 mg/kg bw 2-amino-5-nitrophenol by gavage in corn oil. A dose-related reduction in survival was observed in rats. Rats receiving 400–1600 mg/kg and mice receiving 1600 mg/kg had acute or chronic perivasculitis of the vessels of the caecum and colon (US National Toxicology Program, 1988).

In the two-year studies described above, acute and chronic inflammation of the caecum and colon were observed in low- and high-dose male rats, high-dose female rats and high-dose male mice; the conditions were associated with the accumulation of an orange, granular pigment in the submucosa of the intestine. Focal ulceration of the intestinal mucosa was often present (US National Toxicology Program, 1988).

2-Amino-5-nitrophenol was present at low concentrations in an oxidative hair colouring formulation evaluated in a 13-week study of dermal toxicity in rabbits (Burnett *et al.*, 1976, 0.5%) and in a semi-permanent formulation evaluated in a 20-month study of dermal toxicity in mice (Jacobs *et al.*, 1984, 0.15%), described in detail on p. 97. No treatment-related adverse effect was detected. [The Working Group noted that the dose of each component of the formulations was very low and unlikely to have been toxic.]

4.3 Reproductive and developmental effects

4.3.1 *Humans*

No data were available to the Working Group.

4.3.2 *Experimental systems*

No data were available to the Working Group on the reproductive and developmental effects of 2-amino-5-nitrophenol alone. The compound was present at low concentrations in oxidative hair colouring formulations evaluated in a two-generation study of reproduction in rats (Burnett & Goldenthal, 1988, 2%) and in a study of teratogenesis in rats (Burnett *et al.*, 1976, 0.5%), described in detail on p. 100. No treatment-related adverse effect was detected. [The Working Group noted that the dose of each component of the formulations was very low and unlikely to have been toxic.]

4.4 Genetic and related effects

4.4.1 *Humans*

No data were available to the Working Group.

4.4.2 *Experimental systems* (see also Table 1 and Appendices 1 and 2)

2-Amino-5-nitrophenol induced mutation in bacteriophage, *Salmonella typhimurium* and at the *tk* locus in mouse lymphoma L5178Y cells. It also induced sister chromatid exchange and chromosomal aberrations in cultured Chinese hamster ovary cells.

2-Amino-5-nitrophenol did not induce dominant lethal mutation in rats exposed *in vivo*.

5. Summary of Data Reported and Evaluation

5.1 Exposure data

2-Amino-5-nitrophenol is used as an intermediate in the manufacture of certain azo dyes. It is also used in semi-permanent and permanent hair colouring products.

5.2 Human carcinogenicity data

No data were available to the Working Group.

5.3 Animal carcinogenicity data

2-Amino-5-nitrophenol was tested for carcinogenicity by gavage in one study in mice and one study in rats. In mice, no significant increase in tumour incidence was observed in the low-dose groups; data on the high-dose groups could not be evaluated owing to high mortality rates. An increased incidence of pancreatic acinar-cell tumours was observed in male rats.

5.4 Other relevant data

Oral treatment with 2-amino-5-nitrophenol was associated with inflammation of the lower intestinal tract in mice and rats.

2-Amino-5-nitrophenol induced gene mutation in bacteria and gene mutation, sister chromatid exchange and chromosomal aberrations in cultured mammalian cells. It did not induce dominant lethal mutation in rats.

Table 1. Genetic and related effects of 2-amino-5-nitrophenol

Test system	Result Without exogenous metabolic system	With exogenous metabolic system	Dose[a] (LED/HID)	Reference
BPF, Bacteriophage T4D, forward mutation	+	0	256.4000	Kvelland (1985)
SA0, *Salmonella typhimurium* TA100, reverse mutation	–	0	770.0000	Chiu et al. (1978)
SA0, *Salmonella typhimurium* TA100, reverse mutation	(+)	–	500.0000	Shahin et al. (1982)
SA0, *Salmonella typhimurium* TA100, reverse mutation	(+)	(+)	1667.0000	Zeiger et al. (1987)
SA5, *Salmonella typhimurium* TA1535, reverse mutation	(+)	–	500.0000	Shahin et al. (1982)
SA5, *Salmonella typhimurium* TA1535, reverse mutation	–	–	5000.0000	Zeiger et al. (1987)
SA7, *Salmonella typhimurium* TA1537, reverse mutation	(+)	(+)	500.0000	Shahin et al. (1982)
SA7, *Salmonella typhimurium* TA1537, reverse mutation	(+)	(+)	500.0000	Zeiger et al. (1987)
SA8, *Salmonella typhimurium* TA1538, reverse mutation	+	0	5.0000	Ames et al. (1975)
SA8, *Salmonella typhimurium* TA1538, reverse mutation	+	+	50.0000	Shahin et al. (1982)
SA9, *Salmonella typhimurium* TA98, reverse mutation	+	0	7.7000	Chiu et al. (1978)
SA9, *Salmonella typhimurium* TA98, reverse mutation	+	+	25.0000	Shahin et al. (1982)
SA9, *Salmonella typhimurium* TA98, reverse mutation	+	+	167.0000	Zeiger et al. (1987)
GST, Gene mutation, mouse lymphoma L5178Y cells, *tk* locus	+	0	25.0000	US National Toxicology Program (1988)
SIC, Sister chromatid exchange, Chinese hamster ovary cells *in vitro*	+	+	13.3000	US National Toxicology Program (1988)
CIC, Chromosomal aberrations, Chinese hamster ovary cells *in vitro*	+	+	49.5000	US National Toxicology Program (1988)
DLR, Dominant lethal mutation, CD rats	–		20.0000 ip × 24	Burnett et al. (1977)

+, positive; (+), weakly positive; –, negative; 0, not tested
[a]In-vitro tests, μg/ml; in-vivo tests, mg/kg bw

5.5 Evaluation[1]

There is *inadequate evidence* in humans for the carcinogenicity of 2-amino-5-nitro-phenol.

There is *limited evidence* in experimental animals for the carcinogenicity of 2-amino-5-nitrophenol.

Overall evaluation

2-Amino-5-nitrophenol *is not classifiable as to its carcinogenicity to humans (Group 3)*.

6. References

Aldrich Chemical Co. (1992) *Aldrich Catalog/Handbook of Fine Chemicals 1992–1993*, Milwaukee, WI, p. 75

Ames, B.N., Kammen, H.O. & Yamasaki, E. (1975) Hair dyes are mutagenic: identification of a variety of mutagenic ingredients. *Proc. natl Acad Sci. USA*, **72**, 2423–2427

Burnett, C.M. & Goldenthal, E.I. (1988) Multigeneration reproduction and carcinogenicity studies in Sprague-Dawley rats exposed topically to oxidative hair-coloring formulations containing p-phenylenediamine and other aromatic amines. *Food Chem. Toxicol.*, **26**, 467–474

Burnett, C., Goldenthal, E.I., Harris, S.B., Wazeter, F.X., Strausburg, J., Kapp, R. & Voelker, R. (1976) Teratology and percutaneous toxicity studies on hair dyes. *J. Toxicol. environ. Health*, **1**, 1027–1040

Burnett, C., Loehr, R. & Corbett, J. (1977) Dominant lethal mutagenicity study on hair dyes. *J. Toxicol. environ. Health*, **2**, 657–662

Chemical Information Services (1991) *Directory of World Chemical Producers*, Dallas, TX, p. 39

Chiu, C.W., Lee, L.H., Wang, C.Y. & Bryan, G.T. (1978) Mutagenicity of some commercially available nitro compounds for *Salmonella typhimurium*. *Mutat. Res.*, **58**, 11–22

Commission of the European Communities (1976) Council Directive 76/768/EEC of 27 July 1976. *Off. J. Eur. Commun.*, **L262**(27.9), 169–200

Commission of the European Communities (1990) Proposal for a Council Directive on the approximation of the laws of the Member States relating to cosmetic products of 15 November 1990. *Off. J. Eur. Commun.*, **C322**, 29–77

Commission of the European Communities (1991) Commission Directive 91/184/EEC of 12 March 1991. *Off. J. Eur. Commun.*, **L91**, 59–62

Farris, R.E. (1978) Aminophenols. In: Mark, H.F., Othmer, D.F., Overberger, C.G., Seaborg, G.T. & Grayson, M., eds, *Kirk-Othmer Encyclopedia of Chemical Technology*, 3rd ed., Vol. 2, New York, John Wiley & Sons, pp. 422–440

Fluka Chemie AG (1993) *Fluka Chemika-Biochemika*, Buchs, p. 93

Frenkel, E.P. & Brody, F. (1973) Percutaneous absorption and elimination of an aromatic hair dye. *Arch. environ. Health*, **27**, 401–404

---

[1]For definition of the italicized terms, see Preamble, pp. 26–30.

IARC (1980a) *IARC Monographs on the Evaluation of the Carcinogenic Risk of Chemicals to Humans*, Vol. 23, *Some Metals and Metallic Compounds*, Lyon, pp. 325–415

IARC (1980b) *IARC Monographs on the Evaluation of the Carcinogenic Risk of Chemicals to Humans*, Vol. 23, *Some Metals and Metallic Compounds*, Lyon, pp. 39–141

IARC (1987a) *IARC Monographs on the Evaluation of Carcinogenic Risks to Humans*, Suppl. 7, *Overall Evaluations of Carcinogenicity: An Updating of* IARC Monographs *Volumes 1 to 42*, Lyon, pp. 230–232

IARC (1987b) *IARC Monographs on the Evaluation of Carcinogenic Risks to Humans*, Suppl. 7, *Overall Evaluations of Carcinogenicity: An Updating of* IARC Monographs *Volumes 1 to 42*, Lyon, pp. 100–106

Jacobs, M.M., Burnett, C.M., Penicnak, A.J., Herrera, J.A., Morris, W.E., Shubik, P., Apaja, M. & Granroth, G. (1984) Evaluation of the toxicity and carcinogenicity of hair dyes in Swiss mice. *Drug chem. Toxicol.*, **7**, 573–586

Jos. H. Lowenstein & Sons (1991) *Specifications: Rodol YBA (5-Nitro-2-aminophenol Pure)*, New York

Kvelland, I. (1985) Mutagenicity of five hair dyes in bacteriophage T4D. *Hereditas*, **102**, 151–154

Lide, D.R., ed. (1991) *CRC Handbook of Chemistry and Physics*, 72nd ed., Boca Raton, FL, CRC Press, p. 3–377

Pouchert, C.J. (1981) *The Aldrich Library of Infrared Spectra*, 3rd ed., Milwaukee, WI, Aldrich Chemical Co., p. 823

Sadtler Research Laboratories (1980) *Sadtler Standard Spectra. 1980 Cumulative Index*, Philadelphia, PA

Sadtler Research Laboratories (1991) *Sadtler Standard Spectra, 1981–1991 Supplementary Index*, Philadelphia, PA

Shahin, M.M., Bugaut, A. & Kalopissis, G. (1982) Mutagenicity of aminonitrophenol compounds in *Salmonella typhimurium*: a study of structural activity relationships. *Int. J. cosmet. Sci.*, **4**, 25–35

Society of Dyers and Colourists (1971) *Colour Index*, 3rd ed., Vol. 4, Bradford, Yorkshire, p. 4647

TCI America (1991) *Organic Chemicals 91/92 Catalog*, Portland, OR, p. 78

US National Library of Medicine (1992) *Registry of Toxic Effects of Chemical Substances* (RTECS No. SJ6302500), Bethesda, MD

US National Toxicology Program (1988) *Toxicology and Carcinogenesis Studies of 2-Amino-5-nitrophenol (CAS No. 121-88-0) in F344/N Rats and B6C3F1 Mice (Gavage Studies)* (NTP Tech. Rep. No. 344; NIH Publ. No. 88-2590), Research Triangle Park, NC

Zeiger, E., Anderson, B., Haworth, S., Lawlor, T., Mortelmans, K. & Speck, W. (1987) *Salmonella* mutagenicity tests: III. Results from the testing of 255 chemicals. *Environ. Mutag.*, **9** (Suppl.9), 1–110

1,4-DIAMINO-2-NITROBENZENE
(2-Nitro-*para*-phenylenediamine)

This substance was considered by a previous Working Group, in 1977 (IARC, 1978a). Since that time, new data have become available, and these have been incorporated into the monograph and taken into consideration in the evaluation.

1. Exposure Data

1.1 Chemical and physical data

1.1.1 *Synonyms, structural and molecular data*

Chem. Abstr. Serv. Reg. No.: 5307-14-2
Chem. Abstr. Name: 2-Nitro-1,4-benzenediamine
IUPAC Systematic Name: 2-Nitro-*para*-phenylenediamine
Colour Index No.: 76070
Synonyms: 4-Amino-2-nitroaniline; CI Oxidation Base 22; 2,5-diaminonitrobenzene; 2-nitro-4-aminoaniline; 2-nitro-1,4-benzenediamine; 2-nitro-1,4-diaminobenzene; 2-nitro-1,4-phenylenediamine; nitro-*para*-phenylenediamine; *ortho*-nitro-*para*-phenylenediamine; NPD

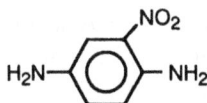

$C_6H_7N_3O_2$ Mol. wt: 153.14

1.1.2 *Chemical and physical properties of the substance*

(a) *Description*: Reddish-brown crystalline powder, with a greenish cast (Cosmetic Ingredient Review Expert Panel, 1985)

(b) *Melting-point*: 137–140 °C (95–99% pure) (Janssen Chimica, 1990; Aldrich Chemical Co., 1992); 142–144 °C (97.5–100% pure) (Jos. H. Lowenstein & Sons, 1991)

(c) *Spectroscopy data*: Infrared, ultraviolet and nuclear magnetic resonance spectral data have been reported (Sadtler Research Laboratories, 1980; Pouchert, 1981, 1983; Sadtler Research Laboratories, 1991).

(*d*) *Solubility*: Slightly soluble in water (0.18% w/w), ethanol, polar organic compounds and benzene; soluble in acetone and diethyl ether (Marzulli *et al.*, 1981)

(*e*) *Octanol/water partition coefficient (P)*: log P, 3.7 (Cosmetic Ingredient Review Expert Panel, 1985)

1.1.3 *Trade names, technical products and impurities*

Some trade names are Durafur Brown 2R; Fouramine 2R; Fourrine 36; Fourrine Brown 2R; Ursol Brown RR; Zoba Brown RR.

1,4-Diamino-2-nitrobenzene is available commercially in purities ranging from 95 to 100%, with 4-amino-3-nitroacetanilide as a possible impurity (from incomplete hydrolysis of the acetylated intermediate; Cosmetic Ingredient Review Expert Panel, 1985). It has the following specifications: ash, 0.1% (max.); iron, 40 ppm (mg/kg) (max.); lead (see IARC, 1980a, 1987a), 5 ppm (mg/kg) (max.); and arsenic (see IARC, 1980b, 1987b), 2 ppm (mg/kg) (max.). It is also available in research quantities at purities ranging from 90 to 99% (Janssen Chimica, 1990; Jos. H. Lowenstein & Sons, 1991; Aldrich Chemical Co., 1992; Fluka Chemie AG, 1993).

1.1.4 *Analysis*

Qualitative and quantitative determinations of 1,4-diamino-2-nitrobenzene and its derivatives are made using paper chromatography, high-performance liquid chromatography, reverse-phase liquid chromatography and thin-layer chromatography and by spectrophotometric methods and electrophoresis (Cosmetic Ingredient Review Expert Panel, 1985).

1.2 Production and use

1.2.1 *Production*

1,4-Diamino-2-nitrobenzene was first synthesized in 1907 (Society of Dyers and Colourists, 1971a). It is prepared by the reaction of 1,4-diaminobenzene (*para*-phenylenediamine; see IARC, 1978b) with acetic anhydride to form 1,4-bis(acetylamino)benzene, which is nitrated and hydrolysed (Cosmetic Ingredient Review Expert Panel, 1985).

Approximately 150 kg of 1,4-diamino-2-nitrobenzene are used in hair colouring products in the USA annually, according to industry estimates. It is produced by one company each in France and Germany (Chemical Information Services, 1991).

1.2.2 *Use*

1,4-Diamino-2-nitrobenzene is used as a dye in semi-permanent hair colouring products. These products are generally shampooed into the hair, lathered and then allowed to remain in contact with the hair and scalp for 30–45 min. (US National Cancer Institute, 1979; Cosmetic Ingredient Review Expert Panel, 1985).

1,4-Diamino-2-nitrobenzene is also used as an ingredient in permanent hair dye formulations, at levels of up to about 1% (Cosmetic Ingredient Review Expert Panel, 1985).

The active ingredient in these dyes reacts in an oxidative coupling reaction with hydrogen peroxide within the hair shafts to produce the permanent colours. 1,4-Diamino-2-nitrobenzene is used to produce light-brown and reddish shades (US National Cancer Institute, 1979). In a similar process, it is used in fur dyeing to produce a red-brown colour, or to add red shading when used in combination with other oxidation bases (Society of Dyers and Colourists, 1971b; US National Cancer Institute, 1979).

1.3 Occurrence

1.3.1 *Natural occurrence*

1,4-Diamino-2-nitrobenzene is not known to occur as a natural product.

1.3.2 *Occupational exposure*

No data were available to the Working Group.

On the basis of a survey conducted in the USA between 1981 and 1983, the US National Institute for Occupational Safety and Health estimated that a total of 29 422 workers, including 23 531 women, may have been exposed to 1,4-diamino-2-nitrobenzene in 3160 facilities (US National Library of Medicine, 1992).

1.4 Regulations and guidelines

The use of 1,4-diamino-2-nitrobenzene as a hair dye is not permitted in Italy or Denmark (Liebscher & Spengler, 1989).

2. Studies of Cancer in Humans

No data were available to the Working Group.

3. Studies of Cancer in Experimental Animals

3.1 Oral administration

3.1.1 *Mouse*

Groups of 50 male and 50 female B6C3F$_1$ mice, six weeks of age, were fed diets containing 2200 or 4400 mg/kg of diet (ppm) 1,4-diamino-2-nitrobenzene (commercial grade; melting-point, 138–139 °C [purity unspecified]) for 78 weeks, followed by a 12-week (males and low-dose females) or 13-week (high-dose females) observation period before sacrifice. Control groups of 20 males and 20 females were maintained on basal diet for up to 90 weeks. Dose-related mean body weight depression (15–20%) was observed in both males and females throughout the experiment. Survival rates, analysed by Tarone's test, did not differ significantly among males or females. Survival at the end of the study was: males, 18/20 (controls), 46/50 (low-dose), 49/50 (high-dose); females, 20/20 (controls), 45/50 (low-dose),

43/50 (high-dose). In females, the incidences of hepatocellular adenomas were: control, 1/20; low-dose, 10/49; and high-dose, 14/48 [$p = 0.01$, Cochran Armitage test for trend]; three hepatocarcinomas occurred in high-dose females. No difference in the incidence of hepatocellular tumours was observed in males, and there was no increase in the incidence of other tumours in either sex (US National Cancer Institute, 1979). The histopathological findings in the livers of female mice in this study were confirmed by Reznik and Ward (1979).

3.1.2 Rat

Groups of 50 male and 50 female Fischer 344/N rats, six weeks of age, were fed diets containing 550 or 1100 mg/kg of diet (ppm) (males) and 1100 or 2200 ppm (females) 1,4-diamino-2-nitrobenzene (commercial grade [purity unspecified]) for 78 weeks, followed by a 27-week observation period before all surviving animals were killed. Control groups of 20 males and 20 females were maintained on basal diet for up to 105 weeks. A dose-related mean body weight depression of approximately 10% was apparent in male rats from week 12 until week 87. Female rats had a dose-related mean body weight depression (> 10%) throughout the study. Survival rates, analysed by Tarone's test, were not significantly different between treated and control animals of either sex. Survivors at the end of the study were: males, 16/20 (controls), 46/50 (low-dose), 47/50 (high-dose); females, 18/20 (controls), 45/50 (low-dose), 38/50 (high-dose). No significant increase in the incidence of tumours was observed (US National Cancer Institute, 1979).

4. Other Relevant Data

4.1 Absorption, distribution, metabolism and excretion

4.1.1 Humans

About 85 g of a commercial semi-permanent hair dye formulation containing 1.36% 1,4-diamino-2-nitrobenzene enriched with ^{14}C-labelled compound at 0.576 μCi/mg was applied on two occasions to the hair of human volunteers, worked in gently for 5–8 min and allowed to remain in contact with the hair and scalp for an additional 30 min. On the first occasion, the hair was clipped, and radiolabel accounting for 0.14% of that applied was detected in the urine over a seven-day period; half was excreted in the urine after 24 h. On the second occasion, the hair was clipped only after 30 days: cumulative absorption was 0.19% on the first day and 0.75% on the 30th day; half of the radiolabel was excreted after 150 h. Urinary metabolites were not identified (Wolfram & Maibach, 1985).

4.1.2 Experimental systems

The same commercial hair dye formulation as used above was applied to the scalp hair of rhesus monkeys and allowed to remain in contact for 30 min. Radiolabel accounting for 0.55% of that applied was detected in urine over a seven-day period; half was excreted in the urine after 24 h. Urinary metabolites were not identified (Wolfram & Maibach, 1985).

[14]C-1,4-Diamino-2-nitrobenzene (1.32 mci/mmol [8.6 μCi/mg]) in acetone was applied to the forearms of adult rhesus monkeys of each sex and to the backs of immature

Pitman-Moore white swine (4 $\mu g/cm^2$). The skin contact area ranged from 3 to 15 cm^2. Skin penetration over the 24-h exposure period was 29.9% of the applied dose in monkeys and 17.7% in swine. The peak rate of excretion of radiolabel in urine occurred between 4 and 8 h in monkeys and between 8 and 12 h in swine. Urinary metabolites were not identified (Marzulli et al., 1981).

Male Sprague-Dawley rats were injected intraperitoneally or intravenously with ^{14}C-1,4-diamino-2-nitrobenzene (6.2 mCi/mmol [6.5 μCi/mg]; radiochemical purity, > 99%) in isotonic buffer solution (pH 7.4) at a dose of 2.6 mg/kg bw. After intraperitoneal injection, 37.4% of the radiolabel was excreted in the urine and 54.3% in the faeces within 24 h; total excretion over four days amounted to 96% of the dose. Within 24 h after intravenous injection to cannulated rats, 42.2% of the radiolabel was excreted in the bile, 34.5% in urine, 8.1% in faeces and 0.65% in the digestive tract. The highest concentration of radiolabel was found at 1 h, except in the small and large intestines where it was found after 3 h, followed by a rapid decrease in concentration. Only small amounts of radiolabel were present in tissues after 48 h. After intraperitoneal injection, the urinary metabolites identified were N^1,N^4-diacetyl-1,2,4-triaminobenzene (N^1,N^4-diacetyl-2-amine-p-phenylenediamine), representing 13.4% of the urinary radiolabel, and N^4-acetyl-1,4-diamino-2-nitrobenzene (N^4-acetyl-2-nitro-p-phenylenediamine), representing 5.8%. Evidence was obtained for the presence of conjugates of unstable metabolites (Nakao & Takeda, 1983).

In an extension of the previous study, the N-acetylation reaction following intraperitoneal administration of 1,4-diamino-2-nitrobenzene, 1,2,4-triaminobenzene or various N-acetylated metabolites was examined in male Sprague-Dawley rats given injections of 30 or 100 mg/kg bw in a 2% carboxymethyl cellulose sodium salt solution. 1,4-Diamino-2-nitrobenzene was metabolized to N^4-acetyl-1,4-diamino-2-nitrobenzene, N^4-acetyl-1,2,4-triaminobenzene and N^1,N^4-diacetyl-1,2,4-triaminobenzene by regioselective N^4-acetylation and subsequent nitroreduction, followed by regioselective N^1-acetylation (Nakao et al., 1987).

1,2,4-Triaminobenzene and its N^4-acetyl derivative were shown to be intermediates in the anaerobic metabolism of 1,4-diamino-2-nitrobenzene and N^4-acetyl-1,2-diamino-2-nitrobenzene in liver microsomes and cytosol from male Sprague-Dawley rats. The cytosolic nitro-reducing activity was attributed to xanthine oxidase, aldehyde oxidase and, possibly, other unknown enzymes (Nakao et al., 1991).

4.2 Toxic effects

4.2.1 Humans

A case of psoriasis-like contact dermatitis was reported following use of a semi-permanent hair dye containing 1,4-diamino-2-nitrobenzene; a patch test carried out with 1% of the compound was positive (Perno & Lisi, 1990).

4.2.2 Experimental systems

In a study of the transformation of lymphocytes into blastocytes, reduced uptake of ^3H-thymidine was observed following incubation of human peripheral blood cultures with

1,4-diamino-2-nitrobenzene (purity, 97%) for 48 or 72 h at concentrations of 25, 50 or 100 µg/ml water (Smith *et al.*, 1976).

The oral LD_{50} of the compound in oil-in-water suspension was 3080 mg/kg bw in Charles River CD rats; the intraperitoneal LD_{50} in dimethyl sulfoxide was 348 mg/kg bw in rats (Burnett *et al.*, 1977). The oral LD_{50} of the compound in water was 2100 mg/kg bw in male Wistar rats (Gloxhuber *et al.*, 1972). The intraperitoneal LD_{50} of the compound in CFW mice was reported to be 214 mg/kg bw (Mikstacki, 1985).

During a 13-week study, groups of 10 Wistar rats of each sex were fed diets containing 500 mg/kg 1,4-diamino-2-nitrobenzene [purity unspecified] to give a calculated daily intake of 30–50 mg/kg bw. No change was found in body weight, blood or urine parameters or in the histological appearance of a range of tissues in comparison with controls (Gloxhuber *et al.*, 1972).

In the chronic feeding study described on pp. 187–188, no significant compound-related non-neoplastic lesion or toxic effect was observed in rats or mice when compared with controls (US National Cancer Institute, 1979).

1,4-Diamino-2-nitrobenzene was present at low concentrations in an oxidative hair colouring formulation evaluated in a 13-week study of dermal toxicity in rabbits (Burnett *et al.*, 1976; 1.1%), in a semi-permanent formulation tested in a two-year feeding study in dogs (Wernick *et al.*, 1975, 0.24%) and in a 20-month study of dermal toxicity in mice (Jacobs *et al.*, 1984, 0.85%), described in detail on p. 97. No treatment-related adverse effect was detected. [The Working Group noted that the dose of each component of the formulations was very low and unlikely to have been toxic.]

4.3 Reproductive and developmental effects

4.3.1 *Humans*

No data were available to the Working Group.

4.3.2 *Experimental systems*

1,4-Diamino-2-nitrobenzene was present at low concentrations in semi-permanent hair colouring formulations evaluated in a study of fertility and reproductive performance in rats and in studies of teratogenesis in rats and rabbits (Wernick *et al.*, 1975, 0.24%; see p. 99) and in an oxidative formulation evaluated in a two-generation study of reproduction (Burnett & Goldenthal, 1988, 1.1%) and in a study of teratogenesis in rats (Burnett *et al.*, 1976, 1.1%) (see p. 100). No treatment-related adverse effect was detected. [The Working Group noted that the dose of each component of the formulations was very low and unlikely to have been toxic.]

1,4-Diamino-2-nitrobenzene [purity unspecified] in sterile distilled water was injected subcutaneously into groups of 25–69 pregnant CD-1 mice on gestation days 6–15 at doses of 0, 32, 64, 128, 160, 192, 224 or 256 mg/kg per day (Marks *et al.*, 1981). Maternal body weight gain during gestation days 1–10 was significantly reduced in all treated groups, and doses of 128 mg/kg per day and above significantly reduced maternal weight gain throughout pregnancy. Maternal mortality occurred at doses of 224 and 256 mg/kg per day. The average number of implants per litter was significantly reduced with 32, 128 and 160 mg/kg per day, but not at higher doses. The frequency of resorptions was significantly increased at 224 and 256 mg/kg per day, but the average number of live fetuses per litter was significantly reduced only with 32, 128 and 256 mg/kg per day. Average fetal body weights were significantly reduced with 128 mg/kg per day and above, and the number of stunted fetuses was significantly increased with 224 and 256 mg/kg per day. The percentage of malformed fetuses (cleft palate, fused ribs, bilateral open eye) was significantly increased at doses of 160 mg/kg per day and above. Under the conditions of this study, 1,4-diamino-2-nitrobenzene was developmentally toxic to CD-1 mice at doses that were also toxic to pregnant dams.

4.4 Genetic and related effects

4.4.1 *Humans*

No data were available to the Working Group.

4.4.2 *Experimental systems* (see also Tables 1 and 2 and Appendices 1 and 2)

1,4-Diamino-2-nitrobenzene was mutagenic to *Salmonella typhimurium*, to *Escherichia coli* and at the *tk* locus in mouse lymphoma L5178Y cells. It was neither mutagenic to *Neurospora crassa* nor recombinogenic in *Saccharomyces cerevisiae*. 1,4-Diamino-2-nitro-benzene induced dominant lethal mutation and chromosomal aberrations in germ cells of *Drosophila melanogaster* (abstract).

Unscheduled DNA synthesis was not induced in primary cultures of rat hepatocytes, whereas an extremely low dose was reported to do so in HeLa cells. Sister chromatid exchange was induced by 1,4-diamino-2-nitrobenzene in cultured Chinese hamster ovary cells, and it induced structural chromosomal aberrations *in vitro* in Chinese hamster cells and in human lymphocytes. It enhanced morphological transformation of primary Syrian hamster embryo cells, BALB/c 3T3 and C3H/10T½ mouse cells and enhanced Moloney mouse sarcoma–leukaemia virus complex induction of transformation of mouse C3H2K cells.

1,4-Diamino-2-nitrobenzene did not induce sister chromatid exchange in bone-marrow cells of Chinese hamsters treated *in vivo* orally or intraperitoneally. In mice dosed intraperitoneally, it did not induce chromosomal aberrations in bone-marrow cells or in previously injected Ehrlich ascites tumour cells. The dye was also inactive in inducing micronuclei in polychromatic erythrocytes of rat bone marrow after treatment by gavage. No dominant lethal mutation was observed in rats following intraperitoneal treatment.

The addition of hydrogen peroxide to 1,4-diamino-2-nitrobenzene had inconsistent effects upon mutagenic responses in *S. typhimurium* TA98 (Yoshikawa *et al.*, 1976, 1977).

1,2,4-Triaminobenzene, a metabolite of 1,4-diamino-2-nitrobenzene, was mutagenic to bacteria but did not induce sperm-head abnormality in mice after intraperitoneal injection.

5. Summary of Data Reported and Evaluation

5.1 Exposure data

1,4-Diamino-2-nitrobenzene is used in permanent and semi-permanent hair dye formulations and for dyeing fur.

Table 1. Genetic and related effects of 1,4-diamino-2-nitrobenzene

Test system	Result Without exogenous metabolic system	Result With exogenous metabolic system	Dose[a] (LED/HID)	Reference
SA0, *Salmonella typhimurium* TA100, reverse mutation	–	–	25.0000	Byeon et al. (1975)
SAO, *Salmonella typhimurium* TA100, reverse mutation	+	0	0.0000	McMahon et al. (1979)
SA0, *Salmonella typhimurium* TA100, reverse mutation	–	–	50.0000	de Giovanni-Donnelly (1981)
SA0, *Salmonella typhimurium* TA100, reverse mutation	+	0	5.0100	Probst et al. (1981)
SA0, *Salmonella typhimurium* TA100, reverse mutation	+	+	50.0000	Gentile et al. (1987)
SA0, *Salmonella typhimurium* TA100, reverse mutation	+	+	50.0000	Zeiger et al. (1988)
SA0, *Salmonella typhimurium* TA100, reverse mutation	(+)	–	25.0000	Byeon et al. (1975)
SA5, *Salmonella typhimurium* TA1535, reverse mutation	–	(+)	50.0000	Zeiger et al. (1988)
SA5, *Salmonella typhimurium* TA1535, reverse mutation	0	+	50.0000	Shahin et al. (1985)
SA7, *Salmonella typhimurium* TA1537, reverse mutation	0	+	10.0000	Ames et al. (1975)
SA8, *Salmonella typhimurium* TA1538, reverse mutation	+	+	2.5000	Searle et al. (1975)
SA8, *Salmonella typhimurium* TA1538, reverse mutation	+	+	6.2500	Byeon et al. (1975)
SA8, *Salmonella typhimurium* TA1538, reverse mutation	0	+	250.0000	Venitt & Searle (1976)
SA8, *Salmonella typhimurium* TA1538, reverse mutation	+	+	25.0000	Garner & Nutman (1977)
SA8, *Salmonella typhimurium* TA1538, reverse mutation	+	0	25.0000	Ammenheuser & Warren (1979)
SA8, *Salmonella typhimurium* TA1538, reverse mutation	+	+	10.0000	de Giovanni-Donnelly (1981)
SA8, *Salmonella typhimurium* TA1538, reverse mutation	+	0	5.0100	Probst et al. (1981)
SA8, *Salmonella typhimurium* TA1538, reverse mutation	0	+	50.0000	Shahin et al. (1985)
SA9, *Salmonella typhimurium* TA98, reverse mutation	+	+	25.0000	Byeon et al. (1975)
SA9, *Salmonella typhimurium* TA98, reverse mutation	+	+	25.0000	Yoshikawa et al. (1976)
SA9, *Salmonella typhimurium* TA98, reverse mutation	+	+	5.0000	Dunkel & Simmon (1980)
SA9, *Salmonella typhimurium* TA98, reverse mutation	+	+	20.0000	de Giovanni-Donnelly (1981)
SA9, *Salmonella typhimurium* TA98, reverse mutation	+	0	0.0000	Ishidate et al. (1981)
SA9, *Salmonella typhimurium* TA98, reverse mutation	+	0	5.0100	Probst et al. (1981)
SA9, *Salmonella typhimurium* TA98, reverse mutation	+	+	5.0000	Gentile et al. (1987)

Table 1 (contd)

Test system	Result — Without exogenous metabolic system	Result — With exogenous metabolic system	Dose[a] (LED/HID)	Reference
SA9, *Salmonella typhimurium* TA98, reverse mutation	+	+	5.0000	Zeiger et al. (1988)
SAS, *Salmonella typhimurium* TA97, reverse mutation	0	+	50.0000	Shahin et al. (1985)
SAS, *Salmonella typhimurium* TA97, reverse mutation	+	+	17.0000	Zeiger et al. (1988)
SCG, *Saccharomyces cerevisiae* D4, *trp5* conversion	−	0	0.0000	Mayer & Goin (1980)
SCH, *Saccharomyces cerevisiae* D3, *ade2* mitotic recombination	−	−	500.0000	Mayer & Goin (1980)
NCR, *Neurospora crassa*, reverse mutation	−	0	400.0000	Ong (1978)
DMC, *Drosophila melanogaster*, chromosomal aberrations in germ cells	+		1000.0000, 24 h	Laethem & Wu (1985); abstr.
DML, *Drosophila melanogaster*, dominant lethal mutation	+		1000.0000	Laethem & Wu (1985); abstr.
URP, Unscheduled DNA synthesis, rat primary hepatocytes	(+)	0	100.0000	Williams et al. (1982)
URP, Unscheduled DNA synthesis, rat primary hepatocytes	−	0	153.0000	Probst et al. (1981)
G5T, Gene mutation, mouse lymphoma L5178Y cells, *tk* locus	+	0	25.0000	Palmer et al. (1977)
G5T, Gene mutation, mouse lymphoma L5178Y cells, *tk* locus	+	0	50.0000	Oberty et al. (1984)
SIC, Sister chromatid exchange, Chinese hamster ovary cells in vitro	+	0	15.0000	Perry & Searle (1977)
CIC, Chromosomal aberrations, Chinese hamster prostate cells in vitro	+	0	25.0000	Kirkland & Venitt (1976)
CIC, Chromosomal aberrations, Chinese hamster lung fibroblasts in vitro	+ +	0 0	0.0000 20.0000	Ishidate & Odashima (1977); Ishidate et al. (1981)
CIT, Chromosomal aberrations, mouse C3H/10T½ fibroblasts in vitro	+	0	1.5300	Benedict (1976)
TBM, Cell transformation, BALB/c 3T3 mouse cells	+	0	0.0000	Sivak & Tu (1985)
TCM, Cell transformation, C3H/10T½ mouse cells	+	0	1.5300	Benedict (1976)
TCS, Cell transformation, Syrian hamster embryo cells, clonal assay	+	0	0.5000	Pienta & Kawalek (1981)
TEV, Cell transformation, Moloney sarcoma virus in mouse C3H2K cells	−		0.0000	Yoshikura et al. (1979)
UHT, Unscheduled DNA synthesis, HeLa cells	+	0	0.0150	Martin et al. (1978)

Table 1 (contd)

Test system	Result		Dose[a] (LED/HID)	Reference
	Without exogenous metabolic system	With exogenous metabolic system		
CHL, Chromosomal aberrations, human lymphocytes in vitro	+	0	50.0000	Searle et al. (1975)
SVA, Sister chromatid exchange, Chinese hamster bone-marrow cells in vivo	-		300.0000 ip	Neal & Probst (1983)
SVA, Sister chromatid exchange, Chinese hamster bone-marrow cells in vivo	-		500.0000 po	Neal & Probst (1983)
MVR, Micronucleus test, CFY rats in vivo	-		1000.0000 po × 2	Hossack & Richardson (1977)
CBA, Chromosomal aberrations, CFW mouse bone-marrow cells in vivo	-		107.0000 ip	Mikstacki (1985)
CBA, Chromosomal aberrations, mouse Ehrlich ascites tumour cells in vivo	-		0.0000	Bogajewski & Bogajewska (1982); abstr.
CVA, Chromosomal aberrations, mouse Ehrlich ascites tumour cells in vivo	-		107.0000 ip	Mikstacki (1985)
DLR, Dominant lethal mutation, CD rats	-		20.0000 ip × 24	Burnett et al. (1977)
DLR, Dominant lethal mutation, Holtzman rats	-		40.0000 ip × 30	Sheu & Green (1979)

+, positive; (+), weakly positive; −, negative; 0, not tested
[a]In-vitro tests, μg/ml; in-vivo tests, mg/kg bw; 0.0000, not given

Table 2. Genetic and related effects of 1,2,4-triaminobenzene

Test system	Result		Dose[a] (LED/HID)	Reference
	Without exogenous metabolic system	With exogenous metabolic system		
SAO, *Salmonella typhimurium* TA100, reverse mutation	+	0	19.0000	Mitchell (1978)
SA9, *Salmonella typhimurium* TA98, reverse mutation	+	+	19.0000[b]	Mitchell (1978)
SA8, *Salmonella typhimurium* TA1538, reverse mutation	−	+	25.0000	Garner & Nutman (1977)
SPM, sperm morphology, (CBA × BALB/c)F₁ mouse *in vivo*	−		25 × 5 ip	Topham (1980)

+, positive; (+), weakly positive; −, negative; 0, not tested

[a]In-vitro tests, μg/ml; in-vivo tests, mg/kg bw

[b]S9 was detoxifying

5.2 Human carcinogenicity data

No data were available to the Working Group.

5.3 Animal carcinogenicity data

1,4-Diamino-2-nitrobenzene was tested for carcinogenicity by oral administration in the diet in one study in mice and in one study in rats. An increased incidence of liver-cell tumours was observed in female mice. No increase in the incidence of tumours was observed in male mice or in rats.

5.4 Other relevant data

1,4-Diamino-2-nitrobenzene induced gene mutation in bacteria and in cultured mammalian cells. It did not induce gene mutation, mitotic crossing over or gene conversion in yeasts. It induced chromosomal aberrations, sister chromatid exchange and cell transformation in cultured mammalian cells and chromosomal aberrations in human lymphocytes *in vitro*. Equivocal responses were obtained for DNA damage induction in cultured rodent cells.

There was no evidence for induction of sister chromatid exchange, micronuclei, chromosomal aberrations or dominant lethal mutation in rodents dosed *in vivo*.

1,2,4-Triaminobenzene, a metabolite of 1,4-diamino-2-nitrobenzene, was mutagenic to bacteria.

5.5 Evaluation[1]

There is *inadequate evidence* in humans for the carcinogenicity of 1,4-diamino-2-nitrobenzene.

There is *limited evidence* in experimental animals for the carcinogenicity of 1,4-diamino-2-nitrobenzene.

Overall evaluation

1,4-Diamino-2-nitrobenzene *is not classifiable as to its carcinogenicity to humans (Group 3)*.

6. References

Aldrich Chemical Co. (1992) *Aldrich Catalog/Handbook of Fine Chemicals 1992–1993*, Milwaukee, WI, p. 931

Ames, B.N., Kammen, H.O. & Yamasaki, E. (1975) Hair dyes are mutagenic: identification of a variety of mutagenic ingredients. *Proc. natl Acad Sci. USA*, 72, 2423–2427

---

[1]For definition of the italicized terms, see Preamble, pp. 26–30.

Ammenheuser, M.M. & Warren, M.E. (1979) Detection of mutagens in the urine of rats following topical application of hair dyes. *Mutat. Res.*, **66**, 241–245

Benedict, W.F. (1976) Morphological transformation and chromosome aberrations produced by two hair dye components. *Nature*, **260**, 368–369

Bogajewski, J. & Bogajewska, G. (1982) Comparison of determinations of chromosomal aberrations in anaphases and metaphases (Abstract No. 20). *Mutat. Res.*, **97**, 173–174

Burnett, C.M. & Goldenthal, E.I. (1988) Multigeneration reproduction and carcinogenicity studies in Sprague-Dawley rats exposed topically to oxidative hair-coloring formulations containing *p*-phenylenediamine and other aromatic amines. *Food Chem. Toxicol.*, **26**, 467–474

Burnett, C., Goldenthal, E.I., Harris, S.B., Wazeter, F.X., Strausburg, J., Kapp, R. & Voelker, R. (1976) Teratology and percutaneous toxicity studies on hair dyes. *J. Toxicol. environ. Health*, **1**, 1027–1040

Burnett, C., Loehr, R. & Corbett, J. (1977) Dominant lethal mutagenicity study on hair dyes. *J. Toxicol. environ. Health*, **2**, 657–622

Byeon, W.H., Paik, S.G. & Lee, S.Y. (1975) Mutagenicity of phenylenediamines and their derivatives (I) (Kor.). *Kor. J. Microbiol.*, **13**, 51–58

Chemical Information Services (1991) *Directory of World Chemical Producers*, Dallas, TX, p. 436

Cosmetic Ingredient Review Expert Panel (1985) Final report on the safety assessment of 2-nitro-*p*-phenylenediamine and 4-nitro-*o*-phenylenediamine. *J. Am. Coll. Toxicol.*, **4**, 161–202

Dunkel, V.C. & Simmon, V.F. (1980) Mutagenic activity of chemicals previously tested for carcinogenicity in the National Cancer Institute Bioassay Program. In: Montesano R., Bartsch, H. & Tomatis, L., eds, *Molecular and Cellular Aspects of Carcinogen Screening Tests* (IARC Scientific Publications No. 27), Lyon, IARC, pp. 283–302

Fluka Chemie AG (1993) *Fluka Chemika-BioChemika*, Buchs, p. 967

Garner, R.C. & Nutman, C.A. (1977) Testing of some azo dyes and their reduction products for mutagenicity using *Salmonella typhimurium* TA1538. *Mutat. Res.*, **44**, 9–19

Gentile, J.M., Gentile, G.J. & Plewa, M.J. (1987) Mutagenicity of selected aniline derivatives to *Salmonella* following plant activation and mammalian hepatic activation. *Mutat. Res.*, **188**, 185–196

de Giovanni-Donnelly, R. (1981) The comparative response of *Salmonella typhimurium* strains TA1538, TA98 and TA100 to various hair dye components. *Mutat. Res.*, **91**, 21–25

Gloxhuber, C., Potokar, M., Reese, G. & Flemming, P. (1972) Toxicologic examination of direct hair dyes (Ger.). *J. Soc. Cosmet. Chem.*, **23**, 259–269

Hossack, D.J.N. & Richardson, J.C. (1977) Examination of the potential mutagenicity of hair dye constituents using the micronucleus test. *Experientia*, **33**, 377–378

IARC (1978a) *IARC Monographs on the Evaluation of the Carcinogenic Risk of Chemicals to Man*, Vol. 16, *Some Aromatic Amines and Related Nitro Compounds—Hair Dyes, Colouring Agents and Miscellaneous Industrial Chemicals*, Lyon, pp. 73–82

IARC (1978b) *IARC Monographs on the Evaluation of the Carcinogenic Risk of Chemicals to Man*, Vol. 16, *Some Aromatic Amines and Related Nitro Compounds—Hair Dyes, Colouring Agents and Miscellaneous Industrial Chemicals*, Lyon, pp. 125–142

IARC (1980a) *IARC Monographs on the Evaluation of the Carcinogenic Risk of Chemicals to Humans*, Vol. 23, *Some Metals and Metallic Compounds*, Lyon, pp. 325–415

IARC (1980b) *IARC Monographs on the Evaluation of the Carcinogenic Risk of Chemicals to Humans*, Vol. 23, *Some Metals and Metallic Compounds*, Lyon, pp. 39–41

IARC (1987a) *IARC Monographs on the Evaluation of Carcinogenic Risks to Humans*, Suppl. 7, *Overall Evaluations of Carcinogenicity: An Updating of* IARC Monographs *Volumes 1 to 42*, Lyon, pp. 230–232

IARC (1987b) *IARC Monographs on the Evaluation of Carcinogenic Risks to Humans*, Suppl. 7, *Overall Evaluations of Carcinogenicity: An Updating of* IARC Monographs *Volumes 1 to 42*, Lyon, pp. 100–106

Ishidate, M., Jr & Odashima, S. (1977) Chromosome tests with 134 compounds on Chinese hamster cells *in vitro*—a screening for chemical carcinogens. *Mutat. Res.*, **48**, 337–354

Ishidate, M., Jr, Sofuni, T. & Yoshikawa, K. (1981) Chromosomal aberration tests *in vitro* as a primary screening tool for environmental mutagens and/or carcinogens. *Gann Monogr. Cancer Res.*, **27**, 95–108

Jacobs, M.M., Burnett, C.M., Penicnak, A.J., Herrera, J.A., Morris, W.E., Shubik, P., Apaja, M. & Granroth, G. (1984) Evaluation of the toxicity and carcinogenicity of hair dyes in Swiss mice. *Drug Chem. Toxicol.*, **7**, 573–586

Janssen Chimica (1990) *1991 Catalog Handbook of Fine Chemicals*, Beerse, p. 888

Jos H. Lowenstein & Sons (1991) *Specifications: Rodol Brown 2R (2-Nitro-1,4-diaminobenzene)*, New York

Kirkland, D.J. & Venitt, S. (1976) Cytotoxicity of hair colourant constituents: chromosome damage induced by two nitrophenylenediamines in cultured Chinese hamster cells. *Mutat. Res.*, **40**, 47–56

Laethem, R.M. & Wu, C.K. (1985) Induced lethality and chromosome damage by 2-nitro-*p*-phenylenediamine in *Drosophila melanogaster* (Abstract No. 4.4). *Genetics*, **110**, S17

Liebscher, K.D. & Spengler, J. (1989) Toxicology and legal aspects. In: Elvers, B., Hawkins, S., Ravenscroft, M., Rounsaville, J.F. & Schulz, G., eds, *Ullmann's Encyclopedia of Industrial Chemistry*, 5th ed., Vol. A12, New York, VCH Publishers, pp. 593–597

Marks, T.A., Gupta, B.N., Ledoux, T.A. & Staples, R.E. (1981) Teratogenic evaluation of 2-nitro-*p*-phenylenediamine, 4-nitro-*o*-phenylenediamine, and 2,5-toluenediamine sulfate in the mouse. *Teratology*, **24**, 253–265

Martin, C.N., McDermid, A.C. & Garner, R.C. (1978) Testing of known carcinogens and noncarcinogens for their ability to induce unscheduled DNA synthesis in HeLa cells. *Cancer Res.*, **38**, 2621–2627

Marzulli, F.N., Anjo, D.M. & Maibach, H.I. (1981) In vivo skin penetration studies of 2,4-toluenediamine, 2,4-diaminoanisole, 2-nitro-*p*-phenylene-diamine, *p*-dioxane and *N*-nitrosodiethanolamine in cosmetics. *Food Cosmet. Toxicol.*, **19**, 743–747

Mayer, V.W. & Goin, C.J. (1980) Induction of mitotic recombination by certain hair-dye chemicals in *Saccharomyces cerevisiae*. *Mutat. Res.*, **78**, 243–252

McMahon, R.E., Cline, J.C. & Thompson, C.Z. (1979) Assay of 855 test chemicals in ten tester strains using a new modification of the Ames test for bacterial mutagens. *Cancer Res.*, **38**, 682–693

Mikstacki, A. (1985) Evaluation of mutagenicity of some aromatic amines, used as hair dyes, by chromosomal aberration tests *in vivo*. *Genet. pol.*, **26**, 109–116

Mitchell, I.diG. (1978) Microbial assays for mutagenicity: a modified liquid culture method compared with the agar plate system for precision and sensitivity. *Mutat. Res.*, **54**, 1–16

Nakao, M. & Takeda, Y. (1983) Distribution, excretion and metabolism of nitro-*p*-phenylenediamine in rats. *J. Toxicol. environ. Health*, **11**, 93–100

Nakao, M., Gotoh, Y., Matsuki, Y., Hiratsuka, A. & Watabe, T. (1987) Metabolism of the hair dye component, nitro-*p*-phenylenediamine, in the rat. *Chem. pharm. Bull.*, **35**, 785–791

Nakao, M., Goto, Y., Hiratsuka, A. & Watabe, T. (1991) Reductive metabolism of nitro-*p*-phenylene-diamine by rat liver. *Chem. pharm. Bull.*, **39**, 177–180

Neal, S.B. & Probst, G.S. (1983) Chemically-induced sister-chromatid exchange *in vivo* in bone marrow of Chinese hamsters. *Mutat. Res.*, **113**, 33–43

Oberly, T.J., Bewsey B.J. & Probst, G.S. (1984) An evluation of the L5178Y TK$^{+/-}$ mouse lymphoma forward mutation assay using 42 chemicals. *Mutat. Res.*, **125**, 291–306

Ong, T. (1978) Use of the spot, plate and suspension test systems for the detection of the mutagenicity of environmental agents and chemicals carcinogens in *Neurospora crassa*. *Mutat. Res.*, **53**, 297–308

Palmer, K.A., Denunzio, A. & Green, S. (1977) The mutagenic assay of some hair dye components using the thymidine kinase locus of L5178Y mouse lymphoma cells. *J. environ. Pathol. Toxicol.*, **1**, 87–91

Perno, P. & Lisi, P. (1990) Psoriasis-like contact dermatitis from a hair nitro dye. *Contact Derm.*, **23**, 123–124

Perry, P.E. & Searle, C.E. (1977) Induction of sister chromatid exchanges in Chinese hamster cells by the hair dye constituents 2-nitro-*p*-phenylenediamine and 4-nitro-*o*-phenylenediamine. *Mutat. Res.*, **56**, 207–210

Pienta, R.J. & Kawalek, J.C. (1981) Transformation of hamster embryo cells by aromatic amines. *Natl Cancer Inst. Monogr.*, **58**, 243–251

Pouchert, C.J. (1981) *The Aldrich Library of Infrared Spectra*, 3rd ed., Milwaukee, WI, Aldrich Chemical Co., p. 827

Pouchert, C.J. (1983) *The Aldrich Library of NMR Spectra*, 2nd ed., Vol. 1, Milwaukee, WI, Aldrich Chemical Co., p. 1172

Probst, G.S., McMahon, R.E., Hill, L.E., Thompson, C.Z., Epp, J.K. & Neal, S.B. (1981) Chemically-induced unscheduled DNA synthesis in primary rat hepatocyte cultures: a comparison with bacterial mutagenicity using 218 compounds. *Environ. Mutag.*, **3**, 11–32

Reznik, G. & Ward, J.M. (1979) Carcinogenicity of the hair-dye component 2-nitro-*p*-phenylene-diamine: induction of eosinophilic hepatocellular neoplasms in female B6B3F$_1$ mice. *Food Cosmet. Toxicol.*, **17**, 493–500

Sadtler Research Laboratories (1980) *Sadtler Standard Spectra 1980, Cumulative Index*, Philadelphia, PA

Sadtler Research Laboratories (1991) *Sadtler Standard Spectra 1981–1991, Supplementary Index*, Philadelphia, PA

Searle, C.E., Harnden D.G., Venitt, S. & Gyde, O.H.B. (1975) Carcinogenicity and mutagenicity tests of some hair colourants and constituents. *Nature*, **255**, 506–507

Shahin, M.M., Chopy, C. & Lequesne, N. (1985) Comparison of mutation induction by six monocyclic aromatic amines in *Salmonella typhimurium* tester strains TA97, TA1537 and TA1538. *Environ. Mutag.*, **7**, 535–546

Sheu, C.-J.W. & Green, S. (1979) Dominant lethal assay of some hair-dye components in random-bred male rats. *Mutat. Res.*, **68**, 85–98

Sivak, A. & Tu, A.S. (1985) Use of rodent hepatocytes for metabolic activation in transformation assays. In: Kakunaga, T. & Yamasaki, H., eds, *Transformation Assay of Established Cell Lines: Mechanisms and Application* (IARC Scientific Publications No. 67), Lyon, IARC, pp. 121–135

Smith, N.S., Bishun, N.P. & Williams, D. (1976) Depression of lymphocyte transformation by two hair dye constituents. *Microbios Lett.*, **1**, 205–208

Society of Dyers and Colourists (1971a) *Colour Index*, 3rd ed., Vol. 4, Bradford, Yorkshire, p. 4644

Society of Dyers and Colourists (1971b) *Colour Index*, 3rd ed., Vol. 3, Bradford, Yorkshire, p. 3264

Topham, J.C. (1980) The detection of carcinogen-induced sperm head abnormalities in mice. *Mutat. Res.*, **69**, 149–155

US National Cancer Institute (1979) *Bioassay of 2-Nitro-p-phenylenediamine for Possible Carcinogenicity (CAS No. 5307-14-2)* (NCI-CG-TR-169; NIH Publ. No. 79-1725), Bethesda, MD

US National Library of Medicine (1992) *Registry of Toxic Effects of Chemical Substances* (RTECS No. ST3000000), Bethesda, MD

Venitt, S. & Searle, C.E. (1976) Mutagenicity and possible carcinogenicity of hair colourants and constituents. In: Rosenfeld, C. & Davis, W., eds, *Environmental Pollution and Carcinogenic Risks* (IARC Scientific Publications No. 13), Lyon, IARC, pp. 263–271

Wernick, T., Lanman, B.M. & Fraux, J.L. (1975) Chronic toxicity, teratologic and reproduction studies with hair dyes. *Toxicol. appl. Pharmacol.*, **32**, 450–460

Williams, G.M., Laspia, M.F. & Dunkel, V.C. (1982) Reliability of the hepatocyte primary culture/DNA repair test in testing of coded carcinogens and noncarcinogens. *Mutat. Res.*, **97**, 359–370

Wolfram, L.J. & Maibach, H.I. (1985) Percutaneous penetration of hair dyes. *Arch. dermatol. Res.*, **277**, 235–241

Yoshikawa, K., Uchino, H. & Kurata, H. (1976) Studies on the mutagenicity of hair dye (Jpn.). *Bull. natl Inst Hyg. Sci.*, **94**, 28–32

Yoshikawa, K., Uchino, H., Tateno, N. & Kurata, H. (1977) Mutagenic activities of the samples prepared with raw material of hair dye (Jpn.). *Bull. natl. Inst Hyg. Sci.*, **95**, 15–24

Yoshikura, H., Kuchino, T. & Matsushima, T. (1979) Carcinogenic chemicals enhance mouse leukemia virus infection in contact-inhibited culture: a new simple method of screening carcinogens. *Cancer Lett.*, **7**, 203–208

Zeiger, E., Anderson, B., Haworth, S., Lawlor, T. & Mortelmans, K. (1988) *Salmonella* mutagenicity tests: IV. Results from the testing of 300 chemicals. *Environ. mol. Mutag.*, **11** (Suppl. 12), 1–158

COSMETIC COLOURANT

D&C RED NO. 9 (CI Pigment Red 53:1)

This substance was considered by a previous Working Group, in 1974 (IARC, 1975). Since that time, new data have become available, and these have been incorporated into the monograph and taken into consideration in the evaluation.

D&C Red No. 9 is a grade of CI Pigment Red 53:1 (Colour Index No. 15585:1), which is certified for use in drugs and cosmetics (US Food & Drug Administration, 1974).

1. Exposure Data

1.1 Chemical and physical data

1.1.1 Synonyms, structural and molecular data

Chem. Abstr. Serv. Reg. No.: 5160-02-1; replaces 12237-52-4; 12238-39-0; 12238-41-4; 12238-43-6; 24777-23-9; 52627-68-6; 68894-03-1

Chem. Abstr. Name: 5-Chloro-2-[(2-hydroxy-1-naphthalenyl)azo]-4-methyl benzene-sulfonic acid, barium salt (2:1)

Colour Index No.: 15585:1

Synonyms: CI Pigment Red 53, Ba salt; CI Pigment Red 53, barium salt (2:1); D and C Red No. 9; Pigment Red 53:1; Lake Red C; Red Lake C

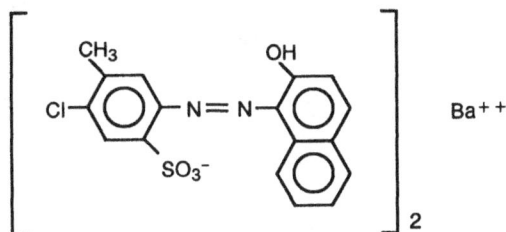

$[C_{17}H_{12}ClN_2O_4S]_2.Ba$ Mol. wt: 888.6

1.1.2 Chemical and physical properties

(a) *Description*: Red powder (Benemelis, 1973)

(b) *Melting-point*: 343–345 °C (decomposes) (US National Toxicology Program, 1982)

(c) *Density*: 1.66 g/cm^3 (Benemelis, 1973)

(d) *Spectroscopy data*: Infrared and ultraviolet spectral data have been reported (US National Toxicology Program, 1982).

(e) *Solubility*: Slightly soluble in water and ethanol; insoluble in acetone and benzene (Society of Dyers and Colourists, 1982)

1.1.3 *Trade names, technical products and impurities*

D&C Red No. 9 is required to contain a minimum of 87% pure colour for sale as a drug and cosmetic colourant (US Food and Drug Administration, 1974).

Analysis of commercial samples of D&C Red No. 9 revealed the presence of 11 aromatic azo compounds (subsidiary colours), at levels of up to 27 ppm (mg/kg), derived from aromatic amine impurities in the Red Lake C Amine (2-amino-4-methyl-5-chlorobenzene-sulfonic acid) precursor (Naganuma *et al.*, 1983).

1.1.4 *Analysis*

The amount of pure colourant in colour additives can be determined by a titrimetric method using titanous chloride as an indicator (Williams, 1984).

1.2 Production and use

1.2.1 *Production*

The first commercial production of CI Pigment Red 53:1 was in 1903. The method of manufacture involves three steps: diazotization, preparation of the coupling intermediate and coupling. The diazotization step involves reacting 2-amino-4-methyl-5-chlorobenzene-sulfonic acid with hydrochloric acid and sodium nitrite to form the diazonium chloride moiety. The coupling step involves mixing the diazonium chloride solution with the coupling component (β-naphthol), then adding barium chloride to form CI Pigment Red 53:1 (Benemelis, 1973). To meet specifications for use in drugs and cosmetics, purified starting materials may be required (US Food and Drug Administration, 1979).

Production of US Food and Drug Administration-certified D&C Red No. 9 was 13 tonnes in 1970, 28 tonnes in 1975, 38 tonnes in 1980 and 0.5 tonnes in 1987; the last year in which it was approved as a D&C colour was 1988 (Marmion, 1991). Approximate US production of CI Pigment Red 53:1 was 430 tonnes in 1950, 990 tonnes in 1970, 1240 tonnes in 1975, 1770 tonnes in 1980, 2020 tonnes in 1985 and 1960 tonnes in 1990 (Benemelis, 1973; US International Trade Commission, 1977, 1981, 1986, 1991). CI Pigment Red 53:1 is produced by one company each in Belgium, Canada, Denmark, India and Japan and by four companies in the USA (Chemical Information Services, 1991).

1.2.2 *Use*

D&C Red No. 9 is used in some countries in the cosmetic and drug industry in such applications as a lipstick colourant, mouthwashes, dentifrices and drugs (Dry Color Manufacturers Association, 1987).

CI Pigment Red 53:1 (as Red Lake C) is widely used in printing inks. It has been used extensively in letter press and offset inks and also in gravure inks, in which its transparency is important. The non-resinated form is used in water- and solvent-based flexographic inks. It also finds substantial use in coated papers and crayons. Because of its good heat resistance, it is used in polystyrene and rubber, in tin printing and in baking enamels (Society of Dyers and Colourists, 1971; Benemelis, 1973; Dry Color Manufacturers Association, 1987). Resinated CI Pigment Red 53:1 (as Red Lake C) is also used extensively in flexographic inks, in which it provides a stronger, cleaner, yellower colour than the non-resinated grade (Benemelis, 1973).

1.3 Occurrence

1.3.1 *Natural occurrence*

D&C Red No. 9 is not known to occur as a natural product.

1.3.2 *Occupational exposure*

No data were available to the Working Group.

On the basis of a survey conducted in the USA between 1981 and 1983, the US National Institute for Occupational Safety and Health estimated that a total of 122 313 workers, including 23 095 women, were potentially exposed occupationally to CI Pigment Red 53:1. The compound was observed in 43 industries, but the greatest number of potentially exposed workers were employed in the printing trades (US National Library of Medicine, 1992).

1.4 Regulations and guidelines

D&C Red No. 9 was provisionally allowed in the European Economic Community for use in cosmetic products (with a maximum of 3% in products intended to come into contact with mucous membranes) except those intended to be applied in the vicinity of the eyes, in particular eye make-up and eye make-up remover (Commission of the European Communities, 1976, 1990, 1991). This application was prohibited in 1992 (Commission of the European Community, 1992).

D&C Red No. 9 was provisionally listed by the US Food and Drug Administration for use in internally and externally applied drugs and cosmetics (US Food and Drug Administration, 1974; Dry Color Manufacturers Association, 1987), including (i) use in lipsticks and other cosmetics intended to be applied to the lips at not more than 3.0% pure pigment by weight of each lipstick or other lip cosmetic; (ii) use in a dentifrice at not more than 0.002% of the pure pigment by weight of the dentifrice or in a mouthwash at not more than 0.005% of the pure dye by weight of the mouthwash; and (iii) use in drugs subject to ingestion, other than mouthwashes and dentifrices at not more than 0.1 mg per day. In 1988, these applications were prohibited (US Food and Drug Administration, 1979, 1987, 1988).

2. Studies of Cancer in Humans

No data were available to the Working Group.

3. Studies of Cancer in Experimental Animals

3.1 Oral administration

3.1.1 *Mouse*

Groups of 50 male and 50 female B6C3F$_1$ mice, six weeks of age, were fed diets containing 1000 or 2000 mg/kg (ppm) D&C Red No. 9 (89.8% pure; major impurities, sodium and barium sulfates) for 103 weeks, followed by an observation period of two weeks before all survivors were killed. A control group of 50 males and 50 females was fed basal diet for 104 (males) and 105 (females) weeks. Mean body weights of treated males and control mice were comparable, although, after week 50, the mean body weights of high-dose females were slightly lower than those of controls. No significant difference was observed in survival in any group: males (control, 42/50; low-dose, 40/50; high-dose, 39/50) and females (control, 40/50; low-dose, 40/50; high-dose, 41/50). The incidence of hepatocellular carcinomas was significantly increased in treated males (control, 4/50; low-dose, 9/50; high-dose, 11/50; $p < 0.038$, Cochran-Armitage trend test). The historical incidence of hepatocellular carcinomas in male mice at the study laboratory was 65/297 (22%). The incidence of hepatocellular adenomas in males was 4/50 controls, 4/50 low-dose and 4/50 high-dose. The combined incidences of hepatocellular adenomas and carcinomas were not significantly different. No significant difference was found in the incidence of tumours of other sites. In female mice, no significant increase in tumours was observed at any site (US National Toxicology Program, 1982). [The Working Group considered that the marginally significant increase in trend of hepatocellular carcinomas in male mice is neither biologically significant nor related to treatment.]

3.1.2 *Rat*

Groups of 25 male and 25 female Osborne-Mendel rats, three weeks of age, were fed 0, 100, 500, 2500 or 10 000 mg/kg of diet (ppm) D&C Red No. 9 (purity, $\geq 86\%$ [impurities unspecified]) for up to 103–108 weeks, when all surviving animals were killed. About 80% of rats in all groups survived 18 months or longer. There was no significant increase in the incidence of tumours at any site (Davis & Fitzhugh, 1962).

Groups of 50 male and 50 female Fischer 344/N rats, six weeks of age, were fed 0, 1000 or 3000 mg/kg of diet (ppm) D&C Red No. 9 (89.8% pure; major impurities, sodium and barium sulfates) for 103 weeks, followed by an observation period of one week before surviving animals were killed. Mean body weights were comparable in treated and control rats. Survival at the end of the study was males: 35/50 controls, 44/50 low dose, 30/50 high dose; females: 38/50 controls, 40/50 low dose and 41/50 high dose. The incidence of splenic sarcomas was significantly increased in high-dose males (26/48 *versus* 0/50 in low-dose and 0/50 in controls; $p < 0.001$, Fisher exact test). 'Neoplastic nodules of the liver' occurred in males: in 0/50 controls, 6/50 at the low dose and 7/49 at the high dose ($p = 0.02$, Cochran-Armitage trend test), and in females: in 1/50 controls, 1/50 at the low dose and 5/50 at the high dose (p for trend < 0.05, Cochran-Armitage trend test). The incidence in historical controls at the study laboratory was 5/140 (3.6%) (US National Toxicology Program, 1982; Weinberger *et al.*, 1985).

3.2 Skin application

Mouse

Groups of 50 male and 50 female ICR (Swiss Webster-derived) mice [age unspecified] received topical applications of 1 mg D&C Red No. 9 (90.0% pure [impurities unspecified]) in 0.1 ml water to an area of approximately 6 cm2 of clipped back skin, twice a week for 18 months. Three groups of 50 male and 50 female controls received applications of water alone. No difference in survival was observed at 18 months. No skin tumour was found. Although various tumours developed in the mammary glands and internal organs, no treatment-related difference in incidence was found (Carson, 1984).

4. Other Relevant Data

4.1 Absorption, distribution, metabolism and excretion

No data were available to the Working Group.

4.2 Toxic effects

4.2.1 *Humans*

D&C Red No. 9 has been associated with contact dermatitis following cosmetic use (Sugai *et al.*, 1977).

4.2.2 *Experimental systems*

D&C Red No. 9 was tested for toxicity in Fischer 344 rats and B6C3F$_1$ mice in a range-finding study for carcinogenicity testing (US National Toxicology Program, 1982). Groups of five males and five females of each species received feed containing 6000, 12 500, 25 000, 50 000 or 100 000 ppm (mg/kg) of the pigment for 14 days. None of the rats, but 1/5 male mice receiving 12 500 ppm, 4/5 males and 3/5 females receiving 25 000 ppm and all mice treated with higher doses died. The spleens of all dosed rats and mice were dark red and enlarged, and the livers and kidneys were dark red to reddish tan.

In a subchronic study, groups of 10 rats of each sex received feed containing 0, 3000, 6000, 12 500 or 50 000 ppm (mg/kg) D&C Red No. 9 for 91 days (US National Toxicology Program, 1982). The respective doses in mice were 0, 600, 1250, 2500, 5000 and 10 000 ppm. Mean body weight gains were not altered in any of the groups, but spleens were affected in all of them. Typically, in rats, congestion and lymphoreticular hyperplasia were seen; in addition, haemosiderosis of the liver was found in the high-dose male and female rats. All except one male and one female rat survived the treatment. Mice that received 1250 ppm or more had congestion of the spleen and haemosiderin deposits.

In Osborne Mendel rats, splenomegaly was a common finding after two years' feeding of up to 20 000 ppm (mg/kg) D&C Red No. 9 (Davis & Fitzhugh, 1962).

4.3 Reproductive and prenatal effects

No data were available to the Working Group.

4.4 Genetic and related effects

4.4.1 *Humans*

No data were available to the Working Group.

4.4.2 *Experimental systems* (see also Table 1 and Appendices 1 and 2)

D&C Red No. 9 was not mutagenic to *Salmonella typhimurium* in most studies; the two weakly positive responses that were recorded were obtained at doses well above those at which precipitation was first observed (100 μg per plate). [The Working Group considered that the effect was due to a substance other than that which precipitated.] D&C Red No. 9 did not induce mutation at the *tk* locus in mouse lymphoma L5178Y cells, sister chromatid exchange or chromosomal damage in Chinese hamster ovary cells or unscheduled DNA synthesis in rat hepatocytes *in vitro*.

After oral administration to rats, D&C Red No. 9 did not induce unscheduled DNA synthesis in the liver or micronucleus formation in bone marrow.

5. Summary of Data Reported and Evaluation

5.1 Exposure data

D&C Red No. 9 (a certified grade of CI Pigment Red 53:1) is used in lipsticks, mouthwashes, dentifrices and drugs in some countries. CI Pigment Red 53:1 has been used extensively since the 1940s as a pigment in printing inks, coated papers, crayons, rubber and baking enamels.

5.2 Human carcinogenicity data

No data were available to the Working Group.

5.3 Animal carcinogenicity data

D&C Red No. 9 was tested for carcinogenicity by administration in the diet in one study in mice and in two studies in rats and by skin painting in one study in mice. In one study, it produced splenic sarcomas in male rats and increased the incidence of neoplastic liver nodules in animals of each sex. No treatment-related increase in the incidence of tumours was observed in mice.

Table 1. Genetic and related effects of D&C Red No. 9

Test system	Result Without exogenous metabolic system	Result With exogenous metabolic system	Dose[a] (LED/HID)	Reference
SA0, *Salmonella typhimurium* TA100, reverse mutation	-	-	167.0000	Brown *et al.* (1979)
SA0, *Salmonella typhimurium* TA100, reverse mutation	-	-	0.0000	Muzzall & Cook (1979)
SA0, *Salmonella typhimurium* TA100, reverse mutation	-	-	5000.0000[b]	Zeiger *et al.* (1988)
SA5, *Salmonella typhimurium* TA1535, reverse mutation	-	-	167.0000	Brown *et al.* (1979)
SA5, *Salmonella typhimurium* TA1535, reverse mutation	-	-	0.0000	Muzzall & Cook (1979)
SA5, *Salmonella typhimurium* TA1535, reverse mutation	-	-	5000.0000[b]	Zeiger *et al.* (1988)
SA7, *Salmonella typhimurium* TA1537, reverse mutation	-	-	167.0000	Brown *et al.* (1979)
SA7, *Salmonella typhimurium* TA1537, reverse mutation	-	-	0.0000	Muzzall & Cook (1979)
SA7, *Salmonella typhimurium* TA1537, reverse mutation	-	0	5000.0000[b]	Zeiger *et al.* (1988)
SA8, *Salmonella typhimurium* TA1538, reverse mutation	-	-	167.0000	Brown *et al.* (1979)
SA9, *Salmonella typhimurium* TA98, reverse mutation	-	-	167.0000	Brown *et al.* (1979)
SA9, *Salmonella typhimurium* TA98, reverse mutation	-	-	0.0000	Muzzall & Cook (1979)
SA9, *Salmonella typhimurium* TA98, reverse mutation	(+)	-	5000.0000[b]	Zeiger *et al.* (1988)
SAS, *Salmonella typhimurium* TA97, reverse mutation	(+)	-	5000.0000[b]	Zeiger *et al.* (1988)
URP, Unscheduled DNA synthesis, rat primary hepatocytes *in vitro*	-	0	50.0000	Kornbrust & Barfknecht (1985)
URP, Unscheduled DNA synthesis, rat primary hepatocytes *in vitro*	-	0	1.0000	Williams *et al.* (1989)
GST, Gene mutation, mouse lymphoma L5178Y cells, *tk* locus	-	-	15.0000	Myhr & Caspary (1991)
SIC, Sister chromatid exchange, Chinese hamster ovary cells *in vitro*	-	-	500.0000	Ivett *et al.* (1989)
CIC, Chromosomal aberrations, Chinese hamster ovary cells *in vitro*	-	-	250.0000	Ivett *et al.* (1989)
UPR, Unscheduled DNA synthesis, rat hepatocytes *in vivo*	-		500.0000 × 1 po	Kornbrust & Barfknecht (1985)
UPR, Unscheduled DNA synthesis, rat hepatocytes *in vivo*	-		2000.0000 × 1 po	Westmoreland & Gatehouse (1992)
MVR, Micronucleus test, rat bone-marrow *in vivo*	-		2000.0000 × 1 po	Westmoreland & Gatehouse (1992)

(+), weakly positive; −, negative; 0, not tested
[a]In-vitro tests, μg/ml; in-vivo tests, mg/kg bw; 0.0000, not given
[b]Precipitate present at all doses

5.4 Other relevant data

D&C Red No. 9 caused splenic toxicity in rats and mice.

D&C Red No. 9 was inactive in all studies in which it was tested, including assays for gene mutation in bacteria and in cultured mammalian cells, DNA damage in cultured mammalian cells and in rodents *in vivo*, sister chromatid exchange and chromosomal aberrations in cultured mammalian cells and micronucleus formation in the bone marrow of rats treated orally.

5.5 Evaluation[1]

There is *inadequate evidence* in humans for the carcinogenicity of D&C Red No. 9.

There is *limited evidence* in experimental animals for the carcinogenicity of D&C Red No. 9.

Overall evaluation

D&C Red No. 9 *is not classifiable as to its carcinogenicity to humans (Group 3).*

6. References

Benemelis, R. (1973) Red Lake C. In: Patton, T.C., ed., *Pigment Handbook*, Vol. 1, *Properties and Economics*, New York, John Wiley & Sons, pp. 493–496

Brown, J.P., Dietrich, P.S. & Bakner, C.M. (1979) Mutagenicity testing of some drug and cosmetic dye lakes with the *Salmonella*/mammalian microsome assay. *Mutat. Res.*, **66**, 181–185

Carson, S. (1984) Skin painting studies in mice with 14 FD&C and D&C colors: FD&C Blue No. 1, Red No. 3, and Yellow No. 5, D&C Red No. 7, Red No. 9, Red No. 10, Red No. 19, Red No. 21, Red No. 27, Red No. 31, Red No. 36, Orange No. 5, Orange No. 10 and Orange No. 17. *J. Toxicol. cutaneous ocular Toxicol.*, **3**, 357–370

Chemical Information Services (1991) *Directory of World Chemical Producers*, Dallas, TX, p. 508

Commission of the European Communities (1976) Council Directive of 27 July 1976 on the approximation of the laws of the Member States relating to cosmetic products. *Off. J. Eur. Commun.*, **L262**, 169–200

Commission of the European Communities (1990) Proposal for a Council Directive on the approximation of the laws of the Member States relating to cosmetic products. *Off. J. Eur. Commun.*, **C322**, 29–77

Commission of the European Communities (1991) 13th Commission Directive of 12 March 1991 adapting to technical progress Annexes II, III, IV, V, VI and VII of Council Directive 76/768/EEC on the approximation of the laws of the Member States relating to cosmetic products. *Off. J. Eur. Commun.*, **L91**, 59–62

Commission of the European Communities (1992) Fifteenth Commission Directive 92/86/EEC of 21 October 1992 adapting to technical progress Annexes II, III, IV, V, VI and VII of Council Directive 76/768/EEC on the approximation of the laws of the Member States relating to cosmetic products. *Off. J. Eur. Commun.*, **L325**, 18–22

---

[1]For definition of the italicized terms, see Preamble, pp. 26–30.

Davis, K.J. & Fitzhugh, O.G. (1962) Pathological changes noted in rats fed D&C Red No. 9 for two years. *Toxicol. appl. Pharmacol.*, **4**, 200–205

Dry Color Manufacturers Association (1987) The future of Red Lake C. *Am. Ink Maker*, **65**, 17–18

IARC (1975) *IARC Monographs on the Evaluation of Carcinogenic Risk of Chemicals to Man*, Vol. 8, *Some Aromatic Azo Compounds*, Lyon, pp. 107–111

Ivett, J.L., Brown, B.M., Rodgers, C., Anderson, B.E., Resnick, M.A. & Zeiger, E. (1989) Chromosomal aberrations and sister chromatid exchange tests in Chinese hamster ovary cells *in vitro*. IV. Results with 15 chemicals. *Environ. Mutag.*, **14**, 165–187

Kornbrust, D. & Barfknecht, T. (1985) Testing of 24 food, drug, cosmetic and fabric dyes in the in vitro and the in vivo/in vitro rat hepatocyte primary culture/DNA repair assays. *Environ. Mutag.*, **7**, 101–120

Marmion, D.M. (1991) *Handbook of US Colorants. Foods, Drugs, Cosmetics and Medical Devices*, 3rd ed., New York, John Wiley & Sons, pp. 86–89

Miyagoshi, M., Hayakawa, Y. & Nagayama, T. (1983) Studies on the mutagenicity of cosmetic azo dyes (Jpn.). *Eisei Kagaku (J. hyg. Chem.)*, **29**, 212–220

Muzzall, J.M. & Cook, W.L. (1979) Mutagenicity test of dyes used in cosmetics with the *Salmonella*/-mammalian microsome test. *Mutat. Res.*, **67**, 1–8

Myhr, B.C. & Caspary, W.J. (1991) Chemical mutagenesis at the thymidine kinase locus in L5178Y mouse lymphoma cells: results for 31 coded compounds in the National Toxicology Program. *Environ. mol. Mutag.*, **18**, 51–83

Naganuma, M., Ohtsu, Y., Katsumura, Y., Matsuoka, M., Morikawa, Y., Tanaka, M. & Mitsui, T. (1983) Analysis of subsidiary colors in D&C Red No. 9 and its purification: development of non-allergenic D&C Red No. 9. *J. Soc. cosmet. Chem.*, **34**, 273–284

Society of Dyers and Colourists (1971) *Colour Index*, 3rd ed., Vol. 3, Bradford, Yorkshire, pp. 3308–3309

Society of Dyers and Colourists (1982) *Colour Index*, 3rd ed., *Pigments and Solvent Dyes*, Bradford, Yorkshire, p. 300

Sugai, T., Takahashi, Y. & Takagi, T. (1977) Pigmented cosmetic dermatitis and coal tar dyes. *Contact Derm.*, **3**, 249–256

US Food & Drug Administration (1974) Foods and drugs. *US Code Fed. Regul.*, **Title 21**, pp. 179, 198

US Food and Drug Administration (1979) General specifications and general restrictions for provisional color additives for use in foods, drugs, and cosmetics; temporary tolerances. *Fed. Regist.*, **44**, 48964–48967

US Food and Drug Administration (1987) D&C Red No. 8 and D&C Red No. 9; permanent listing for use in ingested drug and cosmetic lip products and externally applied drugs and cosmetics; confirmation of effective date and further treatment. *Fed. Regist.*, **52**, 21302–21306

US Food and Drug Administration (1988) Revocation of regulations; D&C Red No. 8 and D&C Red No. 9. *Fed. Regist.*, **53**, 26766–26768

US International Trade Commission (1977) *Synthetic Organic Chemicals, US Production and Sales, 1975* (USITC Publication 804), Washington DC, US Government Printing Office, pp. 52, 79

US International Trade Commission (1981) *Synthetic Organic Chemicals, US Production and Sales, 1980* (USITC Publication 1183), Washington DC, US Government Printing Office, p. 103

US International Trade Commission (1986) *Synthetic Organic Chemicals, US Production and Sales, 1985* (USITC Publication 1892), Washington DC, US Government Printing Office, p. 87

US International Trade Commission (1991) *Synthetic Organic Chemicals, US Production and Sales, 1990* (USITC Publication 2470), Washington DC, US Government Printing Office, pp. 5-3

US National Library of Medicine (1992) *Registry of Toxic Effects of Chemical Substances* (RTECS No. DB5500000), Bethesda, MD

US National Toxicology Program (1982) *Carcinogenesis Bioassay of D&C Red No. 9 (CAS No. 5160-02-1) in F344/N Rats and B6C3F$_1$ Mice (Feed Study)* (NTP Tech. Rep. No. 225; NIH Publ. No. 82-1781), Research Triangle Park, NC

Weinberger, M.A., Albert, R.H. & Montgomery, S.B. (1985) Splenotoxicity associated with splenic sarcomas in rats fed high doses of D&C Red No. 9 or aniline hydrochloride. *J. natl Cancer Inst.*, **75**, 681–690

Westmoreland, C. & Gatehouse, D. (1992) D and C Red No. 9: genotoxic or non-genotoxic carcinogen? *Mutat. Res.*, **281**, 163–167

Williams, S., ed. (1984) *Official Methods of Analysis of the Association of Official Analytical Chemists*, 14th ed., Arlington, VA, Association of Official Analytical Chemists, pp. 641–647

Williams, G.M., Mori, H. & McQueen, C.A. (1989) Structure–activity relationships in the rat hepatocyte DNA-repair test for 300 chemicals. *Mutat. Res.*, **221**, 263–286

Zeiger, E., Anderson, B., Haworth, S., Lawlor, T. & Mortelmans, K. (1988) *Salmonella* mutagenicity tests: IV. Results from the testing of 300 chemicals. *Environ. mol. Mutag.*, **11** (Suppl. 12), 1–158

INDUSTRIAL DYESTUFFS

MAGENTA AND CI BASIC RED 9

These substances were considered by a previous Working Group, in 1973 (IARC, 1974a). Since that time, new data have become available, and these have been incorporated into the monograph and taken into consideration in the evaluation.

Magenta is a mixture of several closely related homologues in varying proportions, with zero (CI Basic Red 9), one (magenta I) and two (magenta II) methyl functions on a 4,4′,4″-triaminotriarylmethane structure in the form of their hydrochloride salts. Small amounts of magenta III (with three methyl functions) may be present in magenta. The term 'basic fuchsin' has been used as a synonym for magenta, but also for CI Basic Red 9 and magenta I.

1. Exposure Data

1.1 Chemical and physical data

1.1.1 *Synonyms, structural and molecular data*

Magenta I

Chem. Abstr. Serv. Reg. No.: 632-99-5; replaces 8053-09-6
Chem. Abstr. Name: 4-[(4-Aminophenyl)(4-imino-2,5-cyclohexadien-1-ylidene)methyl]-2-methylbenzenamine, monohydrochloride
Colour Index No.: 42510
Synonyms: Basic fuchsin; basic fuchsine; basic magenta; Basic Violet 14; CI Basic Violet 14; CI Basic Violet 14, monohydrochloride; fuchsin; fuchsine; rosaniline; rosaniline chloride; rosaniline hydrochloride; rosanilinium chloride

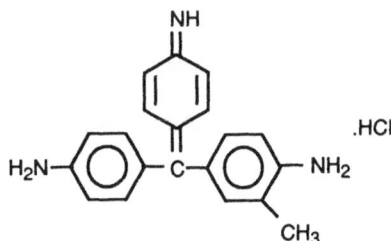

$C_{20}H_{19}N_3.HCl$ Mol. wt: 337.85

Magenta II

Chem. Abstr. Serv. Reg. No.: 26261-57-4

Chem. Abstr. Name: 4-[(4-Aminophenyl)(4-imino-3-methyl-2,5-cyclohexadien-1-ylidene)methyl]-2-methylbenzenamine, monohydrochloride

Synonym: Dimethyl fuchsin

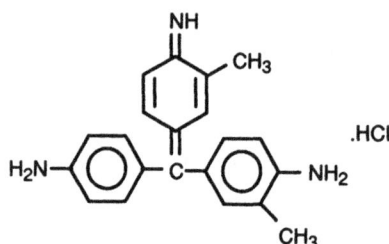

$C_{21}H_{21}N_3 \cdot HCl$ Mol. wt: 351.9

Magenta III

Chem. Abstr. Serv. Reg. No.: 3248-91-7; replaces 100359-07-7

Chem. Abstr. Name: 4-[(4-Amino-3-methylphenyl)(4-imino-3-methyl-2,5-cyclohexa-dien-1-ylidene)methyl]-2-methylbenzenamine, monohydrochloride

Colour Index No.: 42520

Synonyms: Basic Violet 2; CI Basic Violet 2; neofuchsine; new fuchsine; new magenta; trimethyl fuchsin; isorubine

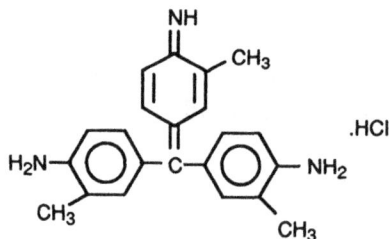

$C_{22}H_{23}N_3 \cdot HCl$ Mol. wt: 365.9

CI Basic Red 9

Chem. Abstr. Serv. Reg. No.: 569-61-9; replaces 70426-60-7; 131883-55-1

Chem. Abstr. Name: 4-[(4-Aminophenyl)(4-imino-2,5-cyclohexadien-1-ylidene)methyl]-benzenamine, monohydrochloride

Colour Index No.: 42500

Synonyms: Basic fuchsin; basic parafuchsine; Basic Red 9; basic rubine; CI Basic Red 9, monohydrochloride; *para*-fuchsin; *para*-fuchsine; parafuchsin; parafuchsine; para-magenta; pararosaniline; pararosaniline chloride; pararosaniline hydrochloride; *para*-rosaniline hydrochloride

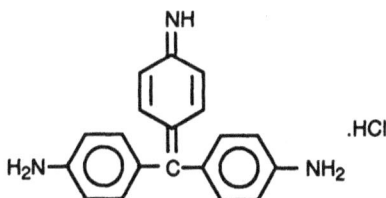

C$_{19}$H$_{17}$N$_3$.HCl   Mol. wt: 323.82

1.1.2 *Chemical and physical properties of the substances*

Magenta I (CI 42510)

(a) *Description*: Dark-green crystalline powder (Green, 1990)

(b) *Melting-point*: 250 °C (decomposes) (Green, 1990)

(c) *Spectroscopy data*: Infrared and ultraviolet spectral data have been reported (Sadtler Research Laboratories, 1980; Pouchert, 1981, Green, 1990; Sadtler Research Laboratories, 1991).

(d) *Solubility*: Soluble in water (4 mg/ml), ethanol (30 mg/ml), ethylene glycol methyl ether (30 mg/ml) (Green, 1990) and methanol (Sadtler Research Laboratories, 1980)

(e) *Reactivity*: Destroyed by strong oxidizing agents; readily reduced to leuco-bases with a variety of reducing reagents; sensitive to photochemical oxidation (Bannister & Elliott, 1983)

CI Basic Red 9 (CI 42500)

(a) *Description*: Dark-green crystalline powder (Green, 1990)

(b) *Melting-point*: 268–270 °C (decomposes) (Green, 1990)

(c) *Spectroscopy data*: Infrared, ultraviolet and nuclear magnetic resonance spectral data have been reported (Sadtler Research Laboratories, 1980; Pouchert, 1981; US National Toxicology Program, 1986; Green, 1990; Sadtler Research Laboratories, 1991).

(d) *Solubility*: Soluble in water (2–3 mg/ml), ethanol (2–25 mg/ml), ethylene glycol methyl ether (50–70 mg/ml) (Green, 1990) and methanol (Sadtler Research Laboratories, 1980)

(e) *Reactivity*: Destroyed by strong oxidizing agents; readily reduced to leuco-bases with a variety of reducing reagents sensitive to photochemical oxidation (Bannister & Elliott, 1983)

1.1.3 *Trade names, technical products and impurities*

Magenta I

Some trade names are: Aizen Magenta; Astra Fuchsine B; Basic Magenta E 200; C-WR Violet 8; Calcozine Fuchsine HO; Calcozine Magenta RTN; Calcozine Magenta XX; Cerise

B; Diabasic Magenta; Diamond Fuchsine; Fuchsine A; Fuchsine CS; Fuchsine G; Fuchsine HO; Fuchsine N; Fuchsine RTN; Fuchsine SBP; Fuchsine Y; Magenta DP; Magenta E; Magenta G; Magenta PN; Magenta S; Magenta Superfine; Orient Basic Magenta; 12418 Red

Magenta, a cationic triarylmethane dye, is commonly, but not always, a homologous mixture of dyes; in a given lot, any homologue may be dominant. The Biological Stain Commission has determined, however, that for a lot to perform satisfactorily in all the usual applications embraced by the protocol of the Commission, CI Basic Red 9 (CI 42500) must comprise not less than 50% of the total dye present; other components that may be found are magenta I (CI 42510), magenta II and magenta III (CI 42520). Both CI Basic Red 9 and magenta III can be produced directly as pure products; however, to obtain pure magenta I and magenta II, free of the other homologue, chromatographic separation must be used (Green, 1990).

Magenta I is commercially available as a biological stain-grade product (Aldrich Chemical Co., 1992).

CI Basic Red 9

Some trade names are: Calcozine Magenta N; Fuchsine DR 001; Fuchsine SP; Fuchsine SPC; Orient Para Magenta Base

CI Basic Red 9 is available commercially as a certified biological stain at a purity of approximately 95%; it is also available at a purity of at least 88% (Aldrich Chemical Co., 1992).

1.1.4 *Analysis*

A rapid method for the assay of triarylmethane dyes (Knecht method) is titration with titanium trichloride to a colourless end-point (Bannister & Elliott, 1983).

1.2 Production and use

1.2.1 *Production*

The first triarylmethane dyes were synthesized in the late 1850s. Their structure was established by Otto Fischer and Emil Fischer in 1878 after the identification of pararosaniline (CI Basic Red 9) (Bannister & Elliott, 1983). Magenta was being produced for sale in England before 1874 (Bannister & Olin, 1965). It has been produced commercially in the USA since at least 1921 (US Tariff Commission, 1922).

In the United Kingdom, the process for manufacturing magenta has involved condensation of *ortho*-toluidine (see IARC, 1982a, 1987a) and formaldehyde (see IARC, 1982b, 1987b) in the presence of nitrotoluene, resulting mainly in the production of magenta III (Howe, 1977).

Magenta I is prepared by the reaction of a mixture of aniline (see IARC 1982c, 1987c), *ortho*- and *para*-toluidine and their hydrochlorides with nitrobenzene or a mixture of nitrobenzene and *ortho*-nitrotoluene in the presence of ferrous chloride, ferrous oxide and zinc chloride (US National Library of Medicine, 1992a). CI Basic Red 9 is prepared by the reaction of aniline with formaldehyde in the presence of hydrogen chloride, forming 4,4'-methylenedianiline (see IARC, 1986), which is then heated with aniline and aniline hydrochloride in the presence of nitrobenzene and ferric chloride (US National Library of Medicine, 1992a).

CI Basic Red 9 (CI 42500) is produced by one company in Brazil and by two companies in the USA, and magenta I (CI 42510) is produced by one company each in India and the United Kingdom (Chemical Information Services, 1991).

No recent data were available on the production of magenta or CI Basic Red 9. US production data for magenta I were last reported for 1964, when the combined production of five US producers was reported as 53 tonnes (US Tariff Commission, 1965). US production of CI Basic Red 9 was estimated as greater than 0.9 tonnes in 1972 and 0.5 tonnes in 1975 (US National Library of Medicine, 1992a).

1.2.2 *Use*

The triarylmethane dyes have been used extensively as textile dyes. Magenta and CI Basic Red 9 are of brilliant hue, exhibit high tinctorial strength, are relatively inexpensive and may be applied to a wide range of substrates. They are not, however, very stable to light and washing, and the use of triarylmethane dyes on textiles has decreased as dyes of other chemical classes with superior properties have become available. Interest in this class of dyes was revived with the introduction of polyacrylonitrile fibres (see IARC, 1979). Triaryl-methane dyes are readily adsorbed on these fibres and are surprisingly more light- and wash-fast than when they are used on natural fibres. The most important commercial black dye for acid-modified fibres is a mixture of the classical triarylmethane dyes, malachite green and magenta I (Bannister & Elliott, 1983).

Current use of triarylmethane dyes is mainly for nontextile purposes. Substantial quantities are used in the preparation of organic pigments for printing inks and in printing, in which cost and brilliance are more important than light fastness. Triarylmethane dyes and their colourless precursors (carbinols and lactones) are used extensively in high-speed photo-duplicating and photoimaging systems. They are also used for specialty applications such as tinting automobile antifreeze solutions and toilet sanitary preparations, in the manufacture of carbon paper, in ink for typewriter ribbons and in jet printing for high-speed computer printers. Triarylmethane dyes may be used to colour other substrates, such as leather, fur, anodized aluminium, glass, waxes, polishes, soaps, plastics, drugs and cosmetics. They are also used extensively as microbiological stains (Bannister & Elliott, 1983).

CI Basic Red 9 can be *N*-phenylated with excess aniline and benzoic acid to form *N,N',N''*-triphenylaminotriphenylmethane hydrochloride (Spirit Blue; CI Solvent Blue 23) (Bannister & Elliott, 1983).

1.3 Occurrence

1.3.1 *Natural occurrence*

Magenta and CI Basic Red 9 are not known to occur as natural products.

1.3.2 *Occupational exposure*

At one textile plant where socks were dyed, several classes of compounds were used for dyeing acrylic/modacrylic, wool, nylon, polyester and cotton fibres. Over 200 dyes were handled during the survey at this facility, comprising acid, disperse, basic (including magenta I), reactive and direct dyes. Spectrophotometric estimates of the average airborne concentration of active colourant were 90 $\mu g/m^3$ using personal filters and 60 $\mu g/m^3$ using area filters (US Environmental Protection Agency, 1990).

On the basis of a survey conducted in the USA between 1981 and 1983, the US National Institute for Occupational Safety and Health estimated that a total of 12 691 workers, including 8288 women, were potentially exposed to magenta I in six industries and that a total of 907 workers, including 733 women, may have been exposed to CI Basic Red 9 in four industries (US National Library of Medicine, 1992b).

1.4 Regulations and guidelines

Magenta I is allowed for use exclusively in cosmetic products not intended to come into contact with the mucous membranes (Commission of the European Communities, 1976, 1990, 1991).

2. Studies of Cancer in Humans

2.1 Case report

Rehn (1895) described three cases of bladder cancer among 45 workers employed in the manufacture of magenta (fuchsin) at a dye factory in Frankfurt, Germany. The cases had worked in the process for 15–29 years. The author mentioned that the process involved exposure to aniline, toluidine and nitrobenzene.

2.2 Cohort studies

Case and Pearson (1954) studied men who had been employed for at least six months between 1910 and 1952 in the manufacture of magenta in the British chemical industry. Detailed job histories were derived from nominal rolls of employees in factories. Workers who had been exposed to benzidine or 1- or 2-naphthylamine were excluded. Bladder cancer occurrence was determined from factory and hospital records. Deaths were identified from alphabetical lists of death certificates, and the numbers were compared with mortality rates for England and Wales for the same period (1921[Case *et al.*, 1954]–52). Results were analysed for subjects who had worked in magenta manufacture, with and without concomitant exposure to auramine. Among 85 subjects who had been engaged in the manufacture of magenta and not in the manufacture of auramine, five cases of bladder cancer were observed, with exposures ranging from one to 19 years, and three deaths from bladder cancer, with 0.13 expected (standardized mortality ratio [SMR], 23.08; $p < 0.005$). One case of bladder cancer was observed among nine subjects who had been exposed to both magenta and auramine, but no death was seen from this cause (0.02 expected). [The Working Group noted that the process for the manufacture of magenta involved exposure to other aromatic amines used as intermediates.]

Rubino *et al.* (1982) studied 53 male workers who had been employed for at least one month in the manufacture of 'new fuchsin' (magenta III) and safranine T between 1922 and 1970 at a factory in the Province of Torino, Italy. Manufacture and use of magenta III had been discontinued in 1970–72. These workers were a subset of a cohort of 906 workers. Subjects engaged in the manufacture and use of 1- or 2-naphthylamine or benzidine were excluded from the study. Subjects and their work histories were identified from factory personnel records, and the workers were followed for mortality from 1946 to 1976, as identified from factory records and from municipal registries of current residence. Working conditions were reported to have resulted in severe exposure to magenta. Five deaths from bladder cancer were observed, while 0.08 were expected (SMR, 62.50; $p < 0.001$) on the basis of mortality rates for Italy in 1951–76. The cases had had exposure to magenta III (CI No. 42520) and safranine T (Basic Red 2, CI No. 50240) for 12–40 years. The authors noted that the processes for the manufacture of magenta and safranine T involved exposure to *ortho*-toluidine, *ortho*-aminoazotoluene (see IARC, 1975), 2,5-diaminotoluene (see IARC, 1978), 4,4'-methylenebis(2-methylaniline) (see IARC, 1974b, 1987d) and *ortho*-nitro-toluene.

Follow-up to 1981 (Decarli *et al.*, 1985) and 1989 (Piolatto *et al.*, 1991) of the 906 workers included 54 workers employed in the manufacture of magenta III and safranine T. No additional death from bladder cancer was reported after 1976.

2.3 Case–control study

Vineis and Magnani (1985) studied 512 prevalent and incident male cases of bladder cancer and 596 hospital-based controls between 1978 and 1983 in the Province of Torino, Italy—the same area considered in the cohort study described above. Complete occupational histories and related information were obtained by hospital interviews. Exposures to specific chemicals, including magenta, were estimated from ILO occupation and industry titles, using information on the industrial uses of these chemicals as described in published sources. On the basis of industrial branches in which magenta exposure could have occurred, 41 cases were classified as having been exposed prior to the age of 60, to give a relative risk of 1.8 (95% confidence interval, 1.1–2.9). On the basis of job titles in which exposure to magenta could have occurred, two cases were classified as having been exposed prior to the age of 60, with an associated relative risk of 3.0 (95% confidence interval, 0.4–20.0). [The Working Group noted that exposure to other aromatic amines could not be excluded].

3. Studies of Cancer in Experimental Animals

3.1 Oral administration

3.1.1 *Mouse*

Magenta I

Groups of 30 male and 30 female stock mice [strain and age unspecified] were treated intragastrically with 0 or 6 mg magenta I [purity unspecified] in arachis oil twice weekly for 52 weeks [about 600 mg/kg bw per week], to give a total dose of 624 mg per mouse. Controls were given subcutaneous injections of arachis oil. The mice were held as long as possible, and at 90 weeks 21/30 control and 23/30 treated males and 21/30 control and 17/30 treated females were still alive. Only gross lesions were examined microscopically. No treatment-related increase in the incidence of tumours was observed in mice of either sex; one liver-cell tumour was observed in a treated female (Bonser *et al.*, 1956). [The Working Group noted the inadequate study design.]

CI Basic Red 9

Groups of 50 male and 50 female B6C3F$_1$ mice, 6–10 weeks of age, were administered 0, 500 or 1000 mg/kg of diet (ppm) CI Basic Red 9 in the diet for 103 weeks and were killed at 110–115 weeks of age. Two lots of the test chemical were used, with purities of 93 and 99% (water was the major impurity). Mean body weights of treated mice were lower than those of controls throughout the study. At the end of the experiment, 42/50 control, 32/50 low-dose and 36/50 high-dose males and 31/50 control, 12/50 low-dose and 6/50 high-dose females were alive ($p < 0.001$). In male mice, CI Basic Red 9 caused a dose-related increase in the incidence of hepatocellular carcinomas (control, 10/50; low-dose, 20/50; high-dose, 27/50; $p < 0.001$, incidental tumour trend test). The incidence of hepatocellular adenomas was 22/50 (control), 21/50 (low-dose) and 17/50 (high-dose). The combined incidence of liver tumours was 29/50 (control), 37/50 (low-dose) and 41/50 (high-dose) ($p = 0.005$, incidental tumour trend test). In female mice, the compound caused a dose-related increase in the incidence of hepatocellular carcinomas (control, 3/49; low-dose, 19/50; high-dose, 37/49; $p < 0.001$, Cochran-Armitage trend test). The incidence of hepatocellular adenomas was 2/49 control, 18/50 low-dose ($p < 0.001$, Fischer exact test) and 4/49 high-dose. The combined incidence of liver tumours in females was 5/49 control, 35/50 low-dose and 41/49 high-dose ($p < 0.001$, Cochran-Armitage trend test). An increase in the incidence of benign and malignant adrenal phaeochromocytomas (combined) was found in females (control, 1/48; low-dose, 8/47; high-dose, 8/45; $p = 0.015$, Cochran-Armitage trend test) (US National Toxicology Program, 1986).

3.1.2 *Rat*

Magenta I

Groups of 40 male and 40 female Sprague-Dawley rats, 12 weeks old, were treated intragastrically with 0 or 400 mg/kg bw magenta I (CI 42510) [purity unspecified] in 0.9%

saline solution twice a week. Controls were given saline only. After two weeks, the dose of 400 mg/kg was found to be toxic, and treatment was discontinued for one week; after a further six weeks, half of the original dose (200 mg/kg bw) was used for the remaining treatment, for life. Average survival times were 104 weeks for control males, 59 weeks for treated males, 92 weeks for control females and 49 weeks for treated females. No treatment-related increase in the incidence of tumours was observed in rats of either sex (Ketkar & Mohr, 1982). [The Working Group noted the poor survival in the treated groups and the inadequate reporting of the study.]

CI Basic Red 9

In the same study, groups of 40 male and 40 female Sprague-Dawley rats, 12 weeks old, were treated intragastrically twice a week with 0 or 600 mg/kg bw CI Basic Red 9 [purity unspecified] in 0.9% saline. The dose of 600 mg/kg was found to be toxic and, after 12 weeks, treatment was discontinued for one week; after a further six weeks, half of the original dose (300 mg/kg bw) was used for the remaining treatment, for life. Average survival times were 104 weeks for control males, 70 weeks for treated males, 92 weeks for control female and 69 weeks for treated females. No treatment-related increase in the incidence of tumours was observed in rats of either sex (Ketkar & Mohr, 1982). [The Working Group noted the poor survival in the treated groups and the inadequate reporting of the study.]

Groups of 50 male and 50 female Fischer 344/N rats, six to seven weeks of age, were administered 0, 1000 or 2000 mg/kg of diet (ppm) (males) and 0, 500 or 1000 ppm (females) CI Basic Red 9 in the diet for 103 weeks and were killed at 110–113 weeks of age. Two lots of the test chemical were used, with purities of 93 and 99% (water was the major impurity). Increased mortality was seen in high-dose males and females, and, at the end of the experiment, 36/50 control, 29/50 low-dose and 0/50 high-dose males and 37/50 control, 35/50 low-dose and 14/50 high-dose females were still alive. CI Basic Red 9 caused significant increases in the incidences of benign and malignant tumours at various sites in both males and females (Table 1) (US National Toxicology Program, 1986).

3.1.3 *Hamster*

Magenta I

Groups of 40 male and 40 female outbred Syrian golden hamsters, 12 weeks old, were treated intragastrically with 0, 400 or 600 mg/kg bw magenta I (CI 42510) [purity unspecified] in 0.9% saline solution twice a week for life. In the high-dose group, the majority of animals died within the first 10 weeks of treatment; the lower dose was well tolerated, and body weight development and average survival times were similar to those of controls. After 72 weeks of treatment, 17/40 control and 17/40 low-dose males and 3/40 control and 0/40 low-dose females were still alive; by 88 weeks of treatment, all treated and control animals had died. No treatment-related increase in the incidence of tumours was observed in hamsters of either sex (Green *et al*., 1979). [The Working Group noted the high mortality in the control and treated groups, especially in females.]

Table 1. Trends in tumour incidences at specific sites in Fischer 344/N rats fed diets containing CI Basic Red 9

Tumour site and type	Control	Low-dose	High-dose	p (trend)[a]
Males				
Dose (mg/kg diet)	0	1000	2000	
Skin				
Squamous–cell carcinoma	0/50	1/50	10/50	< 0.001
Trichoepithelioma	0/50	0/50	7/50	= 0.001
Sebaceous adenoma	0/50	0/50	5/50	= 0.006
Subcutis				
Fibroma	2/50	20/50	16/50	< 0.001
Zymbal gland				
Carcinoma	1/50	1/50	13/50	< 0.001
Thyroid gland				
Follicular adenoma	0/49	0/46	9/44	< 0.001
Follicular carcinoma	0/49	5/46	18/44	< 0.001
Combined	0/49	5/46	25/44	< 0.001
Liver				
Hepatocellular neoplastic nodule	5/50	14/50	6/50	= 0.447
Hepatocellular carcinoma	0/50	2/50	8/50	= 0.001
Combined	5/50	15/50	14/50	= 0.021
Females				
Dose (mg/kg diet)	0	500	1000	
Subcutis				
Fibroma	0/50	15/50	10/50	= 0.005
Zymbal gland				
Carcinoma	0/50	2/50	7/50	= 0.003
Thyroid				
Follicular adenoma	0/47	0/48	4/50	= 0.017
Follicular carcinoma	0/47	2/48	2/50	> 0.05
Combined	0/47	2/48	6/50	= 0.009

From US National Toxicology Program (1986)
[a]Cochran-Armitage trend test

CI Basic Red 9

In the same study, similar groups of hamsters were treated intragastrically with 0, 300 or 600 mg/kg bw CI Basic Red 9 [purity unspecified] in 0.9% saline solution twice a week for life. In the high-dose group, the majority of animals died within the first 10 weeks of treatment; the lower dose was well tolerated, and body weight development and average survival times were similar to those of controls. After 72 weeks of treatment, 17/40 control and 15/40 low-dose males and 3/40 control and 3/40 low-dose females were still alive; by 88 weeks of treatment, all treated and control animals had died. No treatment-related increase in the incidence of tumours was observed in hamsters of either sex (Green et al., 1979). [The

Working Group noted the high mortality in control and treated animals, especially in females.]

3.2 Subcutaneous administration

Rat

In a study reported in a short communication, a group of 20 BD III rats [sex unspecified] was treated once a week with 10 mg of an aqueous solution of 1% CI Basic Red 9 [purity unspecified] for a maximum of 515 days (total dose, 650 mg). The mean life span was 545 days in treated rats and 780 days in controls. The first local sarcoma appeared at 300 days, after a total dose of 370 mg of the dye. Spindle-cell sarcomas were found in 7/12 rats surviving after the appearance of the first tumour, compared to a spontaneous incidence of sarcomas in these rats of less than 0.5% (Druckrey *et al.*, 1956).

4. Other Relevant Data

4.1 Absorption, distribution, metabolism and excretion

No data were available to the Working Group.

4.2 Toxic effects

4.2.1 *Humans*

No data were available to the Working Group.

4.2.2 *Experimental systems*

CI Basic Red 9 (93% pure) was tested for subchronic toxicity in groups of 10 male and 10 female Fischer 344/N rats and B6C3F$_1$ mice fed diets containing 0, 250, 500, 1000, 2000 or 4000 ppm (mg/kg) CI Basic Red 9 for 13 weeks (US National Toxicology Program, 1986). Body weight gain was reduced in female rats at the two highest doses, by 14 and 37%, and in male rats at the high dose, by 40%. Two females and one male rat in the high-dose group died before the end of the study. Adenomatous goitre was seen in 9/9 females and 9/10 males in the high-dose group; diffuse hyperplasia of the thyroid gland occurred in 7/10 females given 2000 ppm and in 1/10 males given 4000 ppm. Pituitary basophilic hypertrophy was found in 8/9 female and 5/7 male rats that received 4000 ppm and in 1/10 female and 1/9 male rats that received 2000 ppm. None of these lesions was found in controls. Fatty changes in the liver were observed in 1/10 male and 4/10 female rats in the high-dose groups. In mice, body weight gain was at least 10% lower than that in controls in males in the high-dose group and in females that received 1000 ppm or more. Clinical signs of toxicity were not observed.

A longer study was performed in rats to observe effects on the thyroid gland (US National Toxicology Program, 1986). Groups of 10 male Fischer 344/N rats were fed diets containing 0 or 2000 ppm (mg/kg) and groups of 10 females, 0 or 1000 ppm CI Basic Red 9

(93 and 99% pure) for 52 weeks. Thyroid glands were palpated regularly; serum thyroxin levels were determined during the first and second week of quarantine and at weeks 13, 26, 39 and 52. The final mean body weights of treated males were 13% lower than that of controls and those of females were 9% lower. Of the male rats, 1/10 had hyperplasia, 1/10 an adenoma and 1/10 a carcinoma of the follicular epithelium of the thyroid gland at the end of treatment. Follicular cysts of the thyroid gland were observed in 2/10 females and 1/10 males. The relative weight of thyroid glands was 1.69 times that of the controls in males and 1.13 times that of controls in females. The concentration of thyroxin was significantly lower than that of controls by week 13 in males and by week 52 in females. The ratio of thyroxin level in dosed groups to that in controls was 0.52 in males and 0.64 in females at 52 weeks. Four of 10 males had fatty changes of the liver, two had focal necrosis of the liver and one, a neoplastic nodule.

4.3 Reproductive and prenatal effects

No data were available to the Working Group.

4.4 Genetic and related effects

4.4.1 *Humans*

No data were available to the Working Group.

4.4.2 *Experimental systems* (see also Table 2 and Appendices 1 and 2)

No data were available on the genetic and related effects of magenta.

CI Basic Red 9 induced repairable DNA damage in bacterial differential toxicity assays, in the absence of activation. It was generally not mutagenic to *Salmonella typhimurium*; some activity was observed in the presence of exogenous activating systems, especially those derived from Syrian hamster liver. It induced forward mutation in *Escherichia coli* in the absence of exogenous metabolism. It did not induce mitotic recombination in *Saccharomyces cerevisiae*.

Conflicting reports were obtained for induction of unscheduled DNA synthesis in rat hepatocytes *in vitro*: in a single study, it induced unscheduled DNA synthesis in primary hepatocytes from Syrian hamsters but not from rats. The compound gave inconclusive responses in two tests for mutation at the *tk* locus in mouse lymphoma L5178Y cells and positive responses in another. CI Basic Red 9 did not induce chromosomal rearrangement or sister chromatid exchange in Chinese hamster ovary cells. It induced morphological transformation of Syrian hamster embryo cells in the presence, but not in the absence, of an exogenous activating system from hamster liver. It also induced transformation of BALBc/3T3 mouse cells and enhanced Rauscher leukaemia virus-induced transformation of Fischer rat embryo cells.

Oral administration of CI Basic Red 9 to mice or rats resulted in urine that was mutagenic to *S. typhimurium*. The dye did not induce mitotic recombination in *S. cerevisiae* or mutation in *S. typhimurium* recovered from the peritoneal cavity of mice, and it did not induce mutation in *S. typhimurium* after intramuscular administration.

Table 2. Genetic and related effects of CI Basic Red 9 (*para*-rosaniline)

Test system	Result		Dose[a] (LED/HID)	Reference
	Without exogenous metabolic system	With exogenous metabolic system		
PRB, Prophage induction, SOS repair test, DNA strand breaks, cross-links or related damage	–	0	500.0000	Speck et al. (1978)
ECL, *Escherichia coli pol* A+/pol A–W3110-P3478 differential toxicity (liquid suspension)	+	0	20.0000	Rosenkranz & Poirier (1979)
BRD, *Escherichia coli* WP2/WP67/CM871, differential toxicity	+	–	155.0000	De Flora et al. (1984a)
SA0, *Salmonella typhimurium* TA100, reverse mutation	–	–	250.0000	Simmon (1979a)
SA0, *Salmonella typhimurium* TA100, reverse mutation	–	–	1070.0000	De Flora (1981)
SA0, *Salmonella typhimurium* TA100, reverse mutation	–	+[b]	167.0000	Dunkel et al. (1984)
SA0, *Salmonella typhimurium* TA100, reverse mutation	–	+	17.0000	Mortelmans et al. (1986)
SA2, *Salmonella typhimurium* TA102, reverse mutation	–	0	0.0000	De Flora et al. (1984b)
SA5, *Salmonella typhimurium* TA1535, reverse mutation	–	–	125.0000	Rosenkranz & Poirier (1979)
SA5, *Salmonella typhimurium* TA1535, reverse mutation	–	–	250.0000	Simmon (1979a)
SA5, *Salmonella typhimurium* TA1535, reverse mutation	–	–	1070.0000	De Flora (1981)
SA5, *Salmonella typhimurium* TA1535, reverse mutation	–	–	167.0000	Dunkel et al. (1984)
SA5, *Salmonella typhimurium* TA1535, reverse mutation	–	(+)	500.0000	Mortelmans et al. (1986)
SA7, *Salmonella typhimurium* TA1537, reverse mutation	–	–	250.0000	Simmon (1979a)
SA7, *Salmonella typhimurium* TA1537, reverse mutation	–	–	1070.0000	De Flora (1981)
SA7, *Salmonella typhimurium* TA1537, reverse mutation	–	–	167.0000	Dunkel et al. (1984)
SA7, *Salmonella typhimurium* TA1537, reverse mutation	–	–	167.0000	Mortelmans et al. (1986)
SA8, *Salmonella typhimurium* TA1538, reverse mutation	–	–	125.0000	Rosenkranz & Poirier (1979)
SA8, *Salmonella typhimurium* TA1538, reverse mutation	–	–	250.0000	Simmon (1979a)
SA8, *Salmonella typhimurium* TA1538, reverse mutation	–	–	1070.0000	De Flora (1981)
SA8, *Salmonella typhimurium* TA1538, reverse mutation	–	–	167.0000	Dunkel et al. (1984)
SA9, *Salmonella typhimurium* TA98, reverse mutation	–	–	250.0000	Simmon (1979a)
SA9, *Salmonella typhimurium* TA98, reverse mutation	–	–	1070.0000	De Flora (1981)
SA9, *Salmonella typhimurium* TA98, reverse mutation	–	(+)[c]	167.0000	Dunkel et al. (1984)
SA9, *Salmonella typhimurium* TA98, reverse mutation[d]	0	+	0.0000	Arni et al. (1985)
SA9, *Salmonella typhimurium* TA98, reverse mutation	–	+	50.0000	Mortelmans et al. (1986)
SAS, *Salmonella typhimurium* TA1586, reverse mutation	–	–	250.0000	Simmon (1979a)

Table 2 (contd)

Test system	Result		Dose[a] (LED/HID)	Reference
	Without exogenous metabolic system	With exogenous metabolic system		
SAS, *Salmonella typhimurium* TA97, reverse mutation	–	(+)	1600.0000	De Flora et al. (1984b)
ECF, *Escherichia coli* exclusive of strain K12, forward mutation	+	(+)	5000.0000	Hayes et al. (1984)
ECW, *Escherichia coli* WP2 *uvrA*, reverse mutation	–	–	167.0000	Dunkel et al. (1984)
SCH, *Saccharomyces cerevisiae*, homozygosis by mitotic recombination	–		300.0000	Simmon (1979b)
URP, Unscheduled DNA synthesis, rat primary hepatocytes *in vitro*	–	0	1.0000	Williams et al. (1982)
URP, Unscheduled DNA synthesis, rat primary hepatocytes *in vitro*	+	0	2.2000	US National Toxicology Program (1986)
URP, Unscheduled DNA synthesis, rat primary hepatocytes *in vitro*	–	0	3.2400	Kornbrust & Barfknecht (1984)
UIA, Unscheduled DNA synthesis, Syrian hamster primary hepatocytes *in vitro*	+	0	3.2400	Kornbrust & Barfknecht (1984)
GST, Gene mutation, mouse lymphoma L5178Y cells *tk* locus	+	+	1.0000	Mitchell et al. (1988)
GST, Gene mutation, mouse lymphoma L5178Y cells, *tk* locus	?	–	7.5000	Myhr & Caspary (1988)
SIC, Sister chromatid exchange, Chinese hamster cells *in vitro*	–	–	15.0000	Anderson et al. (1990)
CIC, Chromosomal aberrations, Chinese hamster cells *in vitro*	–	–	50.0000	Anderson et al. (1990)
TBM, Cell transformation, BALB/c 3T3 mouse cells	+	0	0.0400	Dunkel et al. (1981)
TCS, Cell transformation, Syrian hamster embryo cells, clonal assay	–	0	1.0000	Pienta et al. (1977)
TCS, Cell transformation, Syrian hamster embryo cells, clonal assay	–	+	2.0000	Pienta & Kawalek (1981)
TRR, Cell transformation, RLV/Fischer rat embryo cells	+	0	1.4000	Dunkel et al. (1981)
BFA, Urine from mouse, microbial mutagenicity	+	+	0.0000 × 1 po	Haworth et al. (1981); abstr.
BFA, Urine from mouse and rat, microbial mutagenicity	+	+	120.0000 × 2 po	Lawlor et al. (1987)
HMM, Host-mediated assay, *Salmonella typhimurium* in mice	–		1600.0000 × 1 po	Simmon et al. (1979)
HMM, Host-mediated assay, *Salmonella typhimurium* in mice	–		1600.0000 × 1 im	Simmon et al. (1979)
HMM, Host-mediated assay, *Saccharomyces cerevisiae* in mice	–		1600.0000 × 1 po	Simmon et al. (1979)

+, positive; (+), weakly positive; –, negative; 0, not tested; ?, inconclusive (variable response in several experiments within an adequate study)

[a] In-vitro tests, µg/ml; in-vivo tests, mg/kg bw; 0.0000, not given

[b] Positive in 2/4 laboratories

[c] Positive in 1/4 laboratories

[d] Automated COBAS Bact apparatus also positive

5. Summary of Data Reported and Evaluation

5.1 Exposure data

Magenta and CI Basic Red 9, a common constituent of magenta, were first produced commercially in the late nineteenth century in Germany. As the industry developed in the early twentieth century, it converted in some countries, such as Italy and the United Kingdom, from production of magenta (prepared from a mixture of aniline and *ortho*-toluidine) to production of magenta III (prepared from *ortho*-toluidine without aniline).

Magenta and CI Basic Red 9 have been used to dye textile fibres, in the preparation of pigments for printing inks and in other specialty applications, such as biological stains.

5.2 Human carcinogenicity data

Two small cohorts of workers engaged in the manufacture of magenta were studied in the United Kingdom and Italy. Marked excesses of cancer of the urinary bladder were identified. Although efforts were made to exclude workers exposed to 2-naphthylamine and benzidine, both cohorts may also have been exposed to aromatic amines present as intermediates and suspected to be urinary bladder carcinogens, such as *ortho*-toluidine.

5.3 Animal carcinogenicity data

No adequate study was available to evaluate the carcinogenicity in experimental animals of magenta or of magenta I, magenta II or magenta III.

CI Basic Red 9 was tested for carcinogenicity in one study in mice and in one study in rats by oral administration in the diet and in one study in rats by subcutaneous administration. After oral administration, the compound induced hepatocellular carcinomas in male and female mice and in male rats; adrenal gland phaeochromocytomas in female mice; benign and malignant skin tumours in male rats; and subcutaneous fibromas, thyroid gland follicular-cell tumours and Zymbal gland carcinomas in male and female rats. Subcutaneous administration to rats resulted in a high incidence of local sarcomas.

5.4 Other relevant data

CI Basic Red 9 lowers thyroxin levels and caused hypertrophy of the thyroid in rats and mice.

CI Basic Red 9 induced DNA damage in bacteria, but conflicting results were obtained in assays for gene mutation. Mitotic recombination was not induced in yeast. In cultured mammalian cells, there was no induction of sister chromatid exchange or chromosomal aberrations, but DNA damage and cell transformation were induced; assays for gene mutation gave inconsistent results.

5.5 Evaluations[1]

There is *inadequate evidence* in humans for the carcinogenicity of magenta.

There is *inadequate evidence* in humans for the carcinogenicity of CI Basic Red 9.

There is *sufficient evidence* that the manufacture of magenta entails exposures that are carcinogenic.

There is *sufficient evidence* in experimental animals for the carcinogenicity of CI Basic Red 9.

There is *inadequate evidence* in experimental animals for the carcinogenicity of magenta.

Overall evaluation

The manufacture of magenta *entails exposures that are carcinogenic (Group 1).*

CI Basic Red 9 *is possibly carcinogenic to humans (Group 2B).*

Magenta containing CI Basic Red 9 is *possibly carcinogenic to humans (Group 2B).*

6. References

Aldrich Chemical Co. (1992) *Aldrich Catalog/Handbook of Fine Chemicals 1992–1993*, Milwaukee, WI, p. 115

Anderson, B.E., Zeiger, E., Shelby, M.D., Resnick, M.A., Gulati, D.K., Ivett, J.L. & Loveday, K.S. (1990) Chromosome aberration and sister chromatid exchange test results with 42 chemicals. *Environ. Mutag.*, **16** (Suppl. 18), 55–137

Arni, P., Dollenmeier, P. & Müller, D. (1985) Automated modification of the Ames test with COBAS Bact. *Mutat. Res.*, **144**, 137–140

Bannister, D.W. & Elliott, J. (1983) Triphenylmethane and related dyes. In: Mark, H.F., Othmer, D.F., Overberger, C.G., Seaborg, G.T. & Grayson, N., eds, *Kirk-Othmer Encyclopedia of Chemical Technology*, 3rd ed., Vol. 23, New York, John Wiley & Sons, pp. 399–412

Bannister, D.W. & Olin, A.D. (1965) Dyes and dye intermediates. In: Kirk, R.E. & Othmer, D.F., eds, *Encyclopedia of Chemical Technology*, 2nd ed., Vol. 7, New York, John Wiley & Sons, p. 464

Bonser, G.M., Clayson, D.B. & Jull, J.W. (1956) The induction of tumours of the subcutaneous tissues, liver and intestine in the mouse by certain dye-stuffs and their intermediates. *Br. J. Cancer*, **10**, 653–667

Case, R.A.M. & Pearson, J.T. (1954) Tumours of the urinary bladder in workmen engaged in the manufacture and use of certain dyestuff intermediates in the British chemical industry. II. Further consideration of the role of aniline and of the manufacture of auramine and magenta (fuchsine) as possible causative agents. *Br. J. ind. Med.*, **11**, 213–216

Case, R.A.M., Hosker, M.E., McDonald, D.B. & Pearson, J.T. (1954) Tumours of the urinary bladder in workmen engaged in the manufacture and use of certain dyestuff intermediates in the British chemical industry. I. The role of aniline, benzidine, alpha-naphthylamine, and beta-naphthyl-amine. *Br. J. ind. Med.*, **11**, 75–104

---

[1]For definition of the italicized terms, see Preamble, pp. 26–30.

Chemical Information Services (1991) *Directory of World Chemical Producers*, Dallas, TX, pp. 64, 512

Commission of the European Communities (1976) Council Directive 76/768/EEC of 27 July 1976 on the approximation of the laws of the Member States relating to cosmetic products. *Off. J. Eur. Commun.*, **L262**, 169–200

Commission of the European Communities (1990) Proposal for a Council Directive on the approximation of the laws of the Member States relating to cosmetic products. *Off. J. Eur. Commun.*, **C322**, 29–77

Commission of the European Communities (1991) Thirteen Commission Directive of 12 March 1991 (91/184/EEC). *Off. J. Eur. Commun.*, **L91**, 59–62

Decarli, A., Peto, J., Piolatto, G. & La Vecchia, C. (1985) Bladder cancer mortality of workers exposed to aromatic amines: analysis of models of carcinogenesis. *Br. J. Cancer*, **51**, 707–712

De Flora, S. (1981) Study of 106 organic and inorganic compounds in the *Salmonella*/microsome test. *Carcinogenesis*, **2**, 283–298

De Flora, S., Zanacchi, P., Camoirano, A., Bennicelli, C. & Badolati, G.S. (1984a) Genotoxic activity and potency of 135 compounds in the Ames reversion test and in a bacterial DNA-repair test. *Mutat. Res.*, **133**, 161–198

De Flora, S., Camoirano, A., Zanacchi, P. & Bennicelli, C. (1984b) Mutagenicity testing with TA97 and TA102 of 30 DNA-damaging compounds, negative with other *Salmonella* strains. *Mutat. Res.*, **134**, 159–165

Druckrey, H., Nieper, H.A. & Lo, H.W. (1956) Carcinogenic action of parafuchsin in an injection study in rats. (Short communication) (Ger.). *Naturwissenschaften*, **43**, 543–544

Dunkel, V.C., Pienta, R.J., Sivak, A. & Traul, K.A. (1981) Comparative neoplastic transformation responses of Balb/3T3 cells, Syrian hamster embryo cells, and Rauscher murine leukemia virus-infected Fischer 344 rat embryo cells to chemical carcinogens. *J. natl Cancer Inst.*, **67**, 1303–1315

Dunkel, V.C., Zeiger, E., Brusick, D., McCoy, E., McGregor, D., Mortelmans, K., Rosenkranz, H.S. & Simmon, V.F. (1984) Reproducibility of microbial mutagenicity assays: I. Tests with *Salmonella typhimurium* and *Escherichia coli* using a standardized protocol. *Environ. Mutag.*, **6** (Suppl. 2), 1–254

Green, F.J. (1990) *The Sigma-Aldrich Handbook of Stains, Dyes and Indicators*, Milwaukee, WI, Aldrich Chemical Co., pp. 126–129

Green, U., Holste, J. & Spikermann, A.R. (1979) A comparative study of the chronic effects of magenta, paramagenta, and phenyl-β-naphthylamine in Syrian golden hamsters. *J. Cancer Res. clin Oncol.*, **95**, 51–55

Haworth, S.R., Lawlor, T.E., Lilja, H.S., Douglas, J.F., Cameron, T. & Dunkel, V.C. (1981) Mutagenicity evaluation of urine collected from rodents treated with either 2-acetylaminofluorene (2AAF), *p*-rosaniline, 8-hydroxyquinoline or aniline HCl (Abstract Ea-5). *Environ. Mutag.*, **3**, 379

Hayes, S., Gordon, A., Sadowski, I. & Hayes, C. (1984) RK bacterial test for independently measuring chemical toxicity and mutagenicity: short-term forward selection assay. *Mutat. Res.*, **130**, 97–106

Howe, J.R. (1977) Is there a cancer risk in the laboratory use of magenta and related dyes? *Lab. Pract.*, **26**, 87–91

IARC (1974a) *IARC Monographs on the Evaluation of Carcinogenic Risk of Chemicals to Man*, Vol. 4, *Some Aromatic Amines, Hydrazine and Related Substances, N-Nitroso Compounds and Miscellaneous Alkylating Agents*, Lyon, pp. 57–64

IARC (1974b) *IARC Monographs on the Evaluation of Carcinogenic Risk of Chemicals to Man*, Vol. 4, *Some Aromatic Amines, Hydrazine and Related Substances, N-Nitroso Compounds and Miscellaneous Alkylating Agents*, Lyon, pp. 73–77

IARC (1975) *IARC Monographs on the Evaluation of Carcinogenic Risk of Chemicals to Man*, Vol. 8, *Some Aromatic Azo Compounds*, Lyon, pp. 61–74

IARC (1978) *IARC Monographs on the Evaluation of Carcinogenic Risk of Chemicals to Man*, Vol. 16, *Some Aromatic Amines and Related Nitro Compounds—Hair Dyes, Colouring Agents and Miscellaneous Industrial Chemicals*, Lyon, pp. 97–109

IARC (1979) *IARC Monographs on the Evaluation of the Carcinogenic Risk of Chemicals to Humans*, Vol. 19, *Some Monomers, Plastics and Synthetic Elastomers, and Acrolein*, Lyon, pp. 73–113

IARC (1982a) *IARC Monographs on the Evaluation of the Carcinogenic Risk of Chemicals to Humans*, Vol. 27, *Some Aromatic Amines, Anthraquinones and Nitroso Compounds, and Inorganic Fluorides Used in Drinking-water and Dental Preparations*, Lyon, pp. 155–175

IARC (1982b) *IARC Monographs on the Evaluation of the Carcinogenic Risk of Chemicals to Humans*, Vol. 29, *Some Industrial Chemicals and Dyestuffs*, Lyon, pp. 345–389

IARC (1982c) *IARC Monographs on the Evaluation of the Carcinogenic Risk of Chemicals to Humans*, Vol. 27, *Some Aromatic Amines, Anthraquinones and Nitroso Compounds, and Inorganic Fluorides Used in Drinking-water and Dental Preparations*, Lyon, pp. 39–61

IARC (1986) *IARC Monographs on the Evaluation of the Carcinogenic Risk of Chemicals to Humans*, Vol. 39, *Some Chemicals Used in Plastics and Elastomers*, Lyon, pp. 347–365

IARC (1987a) *IARC Monographs on the Evaluation of Carcinogenic Risks to Humans*, Suppl. 7, *Overall Evaluations of Carcinogenicity: An Updating of* IARC Monographs *Volumes 1 to 42*, Lyon, pp. 362–363

IARC (1987b) *IARC Monographs on the Evaluation of Carcinogenic Risks to Humans*, Suppl. 7, *Overall Evaluations of Carcinogenicity: An Updating of* IARC Monographs *Volumes 1 to 42*, Lyon, pp. 211–216

IARC (1987c) *IARC Monographs on the Evaluation of Carcinogenic Risks to Humans*, Suppl. 7, *Overall Evaluations of Carcinogenicity: An Updating of* IARC Monographs *Volumes 1 to 42*, Lyon, pp. 99–100

IARC (1987d) *IARC Monographs on the Evaluation of Carcinogenic Risks to Humans*, Suppl. 7, *Overall Evaluations of Carcinogenicity: An Updating of* IARC Monographs *Volumes 1 to 42*, Lyon, p. 248

Ketkar, M.B. & Mohr, U. (1982) The chronic effects of magenta, paramagenta and phenyl-β-naphthylamine in rats after intragastric administration. *Cancer Lett.*, **16**, 203–206

Kornbrust, D.J. & Barfknecht, T.R. (1984) Comparison of rat and hamster hepatocyte primary culture/DNA repair assays. *Environ. Mutag.*, **6**, 1–11

Lawlor, T.E., Haworth, S.R., Lilja, H.S., Cameron, T.P. & Dunkel, V.C. (1987) Detection of mutagenic activity in the urine of rodents treated with *p*-rosaniline. *Environ. Mutag.*, **9**, 69–78

Mitchell, A.D., Rudd, C.J. & Caspary, W.J. (1988) Evaluation of the L5178Y mouse lymphoma cell mutagenesis assay: intralaboratory results for sixty-three coded chemicals tested at SRI International. *Environ. mol. Mutag.*, **12** (Suppl. 13), 37–101

Mortelmans, K., Haworth, S., Lawlor, T., Speck, W., Tainer, B. & Zeiger, E. (1986) *Salmonella* mutagenicity tests. II. Results from the testing of 270 chemicals. *Environ. Mutag.*, **8** (Suppl. 7), 1–119

Myhr, B.C. & Caspary, W.J. (1988) Evaluation of the L5178Y mouse lymphoma cell mutagenesis assay: intralaboratory results with sixty-three coded chemicals tested at Litton Bionetics, Inc. *Environ. Mutag.*, **12** (Suppl. 13), 103–194

Myhr, B.C., McGregor, D., Bowers, L., Riach, C., Brown, A.G., Edwards, I, McBride, D., Martin, R. & Caspary, W.J. (1990) L5178Y mouse lymphoma cell mutation assay results with 41 compounds. *Environ. Mutag.*, **16** (Suppl. 18), 138–167

Pienta, R.J. & Kawalek, J.C. (1981) Transformation of hamster embryo cells by aromatic amines. *Natl Cancer Inst. Monogr.*, **58**, 243–251

Pienta, R.J., Poiley, J.A. & Lebherz, W.B., III (1977) Morphological transformation of early passage golden Syrian hamster embryo cells derived from cryopreserved primary cultures as a reliable in vitro bioassay for identifying diverse carcinogens. *Int. J. Cancer*, **19**, 642–655

Piolatto, G., Negri, E., La Vecchia, C., Pira, E., Decarli, A. & Peto, J. (1991) Bladder cancer mortality of workers exposed to aromatic amines: an updated analysis. *Br. J. Cancer*, **63**, 457–459

Pouchert, C.J. (1981) *The Aldrich Library of Infrared Spectra*, 3rd ed., Milwaukee, WI, Aldrich Chemical Co., pp. 1448, 1483, 1488

Rehn, L. (1895) Bladder tumour in fuchsin workers (Ger.). *Arch. klin. Chir.*, **50**, 588–600

Rosenkranz, H.S. & Poirier, L.A. (1979) Evaluation of the mutagenicity and DNA-modifying activity of carcinogens and noncarcinogens in microbial systems. *J. natl Cancer Inst.*, **62**, 873–892

Rubino, G.F., Scansetti, G., Piolatto, G. & Pira, E. (1982) The carcinogenic effect of aromatic amines: an epidemiological study of the role of *o*-toluidine and 4,4′-methylene bis(2-methylaniline) in inducing bladder cancer in man. *Environ. Res.*, **27**, 241–254

Sadtler Research Laboratories (1980) *Sadtler Standard Spectra. 1980 Cumulative Index*, Philadelphia, PA

Sadtler Research Laboratories (1991) *Sadtler Standard Spectra. 1981–1991 Supplementary Index*, Philadelphia, PA

Simmon, V.F. (1979a) In vitro mutagenicity assays of chemical carcinogens and related compounds with *Salmonella typimurium*. *J. natl Cancer Inst.*, **62**, 893–899

Simmon, V.F. (1979b) In vitro assays for recombinogenic activity of chemical carcinogens and related compounds with *Saccharomyces cerevisiae* D3. *J. natl Cancer Inst.*, **62**, 901–909

Simmon, V.F., Rosenkranz, H.S., Zeiger, E. & Poirier, L.A. (1979) Mutagenic activity of chemical carcinogens and related compounds in the intraperitoneal host-mediated assay. *J. natl Cancer Inst.*, **62**, 911–918

Speck, W.T., Santella, R.M. & Rosenkranz, H.S. (1978) An evaluation of the prophage lambda induction (inductest) for the detection of potential carcinogens. *Mutat. Res.*, **54**, 101–104

US Environmental Protection Agency (1990) *Textile Dye Weighing Monitoring Study* (EPA Reports Nos EPA-560/5-90-009 and EPA-560/5-90-010, Main Report, Supplement and Site Visit Reports), Washington DC, Office of Toxic Substances

US National Library of Medicine (1992a) *Hazardous Substances Data Bank* (HSDB Record Nos. 2952 and 6192), Bethesda, MD

US National Library of Medicine (1992b) *Registry of Toxic Effects of Chemical Substances* (RTECS Nos. CX9850000 and CX9850100), Bethesda, MD

US National Toxicology Program (1986) *Toxicology and Carcinogenesis Studies of CI Basic Red 9 Monohydrochloride (Pararosaniline) (CAS No. 569-61-9) in Fischer F344/N Rats and B6C3F$_1$ Mice (Feed Studies)* (NTP Tech. Rep. No. 285; NIH Publ. No. 86-2541), Research Triangle Park, NC

US Tariff Commission (1922) *Census of Dyes and Other Synthetic Organic Chemicals, 1921* (Tariff Information Series No. 26), Washington DC, US Government Printing Office, p. 66

US Tariff Commission (1965) *Synthetic Organic Chemicals, United States Production and Sales, 1964* (TC Publication 167), Washington DC, US Government Printing Office, pp. 18, 98

Vineis, P. & Magnani, C. (1985) Occupation and bladder cancer in males: a case–control study. *Int. J. Cancer*, **35**, 599–606

Williams, G.M., Laspia, M.F. & Dunkel, V.C. (1982) Reliability of the hepatocyte primary culture/DNA repair test in testing of coded carcinogens and noncarcinogens. *Mutat. Res.*, **97**, 359–370

Williams, G.M., Mori, H. & McQueen, C.A. (1989) Structure–activity relationships in the rat hepatocyte DNA-repair test for 300 chemicals. *Mutat. Res.*, **221**, 263–286

CI DIRECT BLUE 15

1. Exposure Data

1.1 Chemical and physical data

1.1.1 Synonyms, structural and molecular data

Chem. Abstr. Serv. Reg. No.: 2429-74-5; replaces 51568-94-6; 95032-75-0

Chem. Abstr. Name: 3,3'-[(3,3'-Dimethoxy[1,1'-biphenyl]-4,4'-diyl) bis(azo)]bis[5-amino-4-hydroxy-2,7-naphthalenedisulfonic acid], tetrasodium salt

Colour Index No.: 24400

Synonym: Direct Blue 15

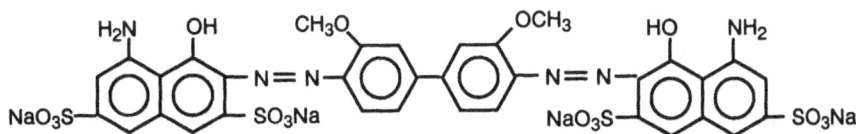

$C_{34}H_{24}N_6O_{16}S_4.4Na$ Mol. wt: 992.85

1.1.2 Chemical and physical properties

(a) *Description*: Dark-blue powder (US National Toxicology Program, 1992)

(b) *Melting-point*: 300 °C (decomposes) (US National Toxicology Program, 1992)

(c) *Spectroscopy data*: Infrared and nuclear magnetic resonance spectral data have been reported (US National Toxicology Program, 1992).

(d) *Solubility*: Soluble in water; insoluble in most organic solvents (Society of Dyers and Colourists, 1971a)

1.1.3 Trade names, technical products and impurities

Some trade names are: Airedale Blue D; Aizen Direct Sky Blue 5B; Aizen Direct Sky Blue 5BH; Amanil Sky Blue; Atlantic Sky Blue A; Atul Direct Sky Blue; Azine Sky Blue 5B; Belamine Sky Blue A; Benzanil Sky Blue; Benzo Sky Blue A-CF; Benzo Sky Blue S; Cartasol Blue 2GF; Chloramine Sky Blue A; Chloramine Sky Blue 4B; Chrome Leather Pure Blue; Cresotine Pure Blue; Diacotton Sky Blue 5B; Diamine Blue 6B; Diamine Sky Blue; Diaphtamine Pure Blue; Diazol Pure Blue 4B; Diphenyl Brilliant Blue; Diphenyl Sky Blue 6B; Direct Blue 10G; Direct Blue HH; Direct Pure Blue; Direct Pure Blue M; Direct Sky

–235–

Blue; Direct Sky Blue A; Direct Sky Blue 5B; Enianil Pure Blue AN; Fenamin Sky Blue; Hispamin Sky Blue 3B; Kayafect Blue Y; Kayaku Direct Sky Blue 5B; Mitsui Direct Sky Blue 5B; Naphtamine Blue 10G; Niagara Blue 4B; Niagara Sky Blue; Nippon Direct Sky Blue; Nippon Sky Blue; Nitto Direct Sky Blue 5B; Oxamine Sky Blue 5B; Paper Blue S; Phenamine Sky Blue A; Pontamine Sky Blue 5BX; Shikiso Direct Sky Blue 5B; Sky Blue 4B; Sky Blue 5B; Tertrodirect Blue F; Vondacel Blue HH.

The raw dye contains about 25% sodium chloride; a desalted preparation (containing ~ 3% salt) contained about 50% CI Direct Blue 15 and about 35 impurities, including 3,3'-dimethoxybenzidine dihydrochloride at 836–1310 ppm (mg/kg). Benzidine was not present at the detection limit of 1 ppm (mg/kg) (US National Toxicology Program, 1992).

CI Direct Blue 15 is available at a purity of 65.5%, containing 15 ppm 3,3'-dimethoxy-benzidine (*ortho*-dianisidine; see IARC, 1974, 1987) (Bowman *et al.*, 1982).

1.1.4 *Analysis*

No data were available to the Working Group.

1.2 Production and use

1.2.1 *Production*

CI Direct Blue 15 was first prepared in 1890 (Society of Dyers and Colourists, 1971a). It is produced by coupling 3,3'-dimethoxybenzidine to 1-amino-8-naphthol-3,6-disulfonic acid under alkaline conditions (US Environmental Protection Agency, 1987).

Approximate US production was 108 tonnes in 1972, 241 tonnes in 1977, 98 tonnes in 1981 and 123 tonnes in 1982 (US International Trade Commission, 1974, 1978, 1982, 1983).

1.2.2 *Use*

CI Direct Blue 15 is used to dye cellulose, leather, paper, cotton, silk and wool and to stain biological materials; it is also used to tint cinematographic film (Society of Dyers and Colourists, 1971b). The use pattern for CI Direct Blue 15 in the USA is 65% in textile dyeing, 30% as a paper colourant and 5% for other uses.

1.3 Occurrence

1.3.1 *Natural occurrence*

CI Direct Blue 15 is not known to occur as a natural product.

1.3.2 *Occupational exposure*

No data were available to the Working Group.

The US Environmental Protection Agency, the American Textile Manufacturers Institute and the Ecological and Toxicological Association of the Dyestuffs Manufacturing Industry conducted a joint survey in 1986–87 to estimate airborne concentrations of dye dust in dye weighing rooms of plants where powder dyes are used in the dyeing and printing of textiles. The survey was based on a sample of 24 sites chosen at random from among textile plants where powder dyes are weighed. Although CI Direct Blue 15 was not included in the survey, the results were considered to be representative of dye dust levels during weighing of this type of powder dye. The mean airborne concentration of total active colourant in the plants monitored was estimated to be 0.085 mg/m^3 (US Environmental Protection Agency, 1990).

On the basis of a survey conducted in the USA between 1981 and 1983, the US National Institute for Occupational Safety and Health estimated that a total of 4527 workers, including 201 women, may have been exposed to CI Direct Blue 15 in seven industries (US National Library of Medicine, 1992).

1.3.3 *Other*

Anaerobic biodegradation of CI Direct Blue 15 gives rise to the amine metabolite, 3,3'-dimethoxybenzidine. Following incubation of 100 mg/l of dyestuff at 35 °C in the presence of anaerobic sludge inoculum, primary degradation was complete within seven days (Brown & Hamburger, 1987).

1.4 Regulations and guidelines

In Germany, derived azo dyes must be handled like the corresponding hypothetical reduction products. CI Direct Blue 15 must therefore be handled like 3,3'-dimethoxybenzidine, which is classified as an A2 compound. Those materials are considered to have been proven to be carcinogenic only in animal experimentation but under conditions comparable to those of possible human exposure at the workplace (Deutsche Forschungsgemeinschaft, 1992).

2. Studies of Cancer in Humans

No data were available to the Working Group.

3. Studies of Cancer in Experimental Animals

3.1 Oral administration

Rat

Groups of 50, 35, 65 and 50 male and 50, 35, 65 and 50 female Fischer 344/N rats, 40–47 days old, were administered 0, 630, 1250 or 2500 mg/l (ppm) CI Direct Blue 15 (purity, ~ 50%; with ~ 35 impurities, including 3,3'-dimethoxybenzidine) in distilled drinking-water for 96 weeks and were necropsied at 103–104 weeks of age. Survival at 22 months was 37/50, 8/35, 11/65 and 2/50 for male rats and 40/50, 13/35, 22/65 and 4/50 for females in the control, low-, mid- and high-dose groups, respectively ($p < 0.001$ for both males and females). The decreased survival in the treated groups was due to development of treatment-related neoplasms. As shown in Table 1, there were increased incidences of benign and malignant tumours of the skin, Zymbal gland, liver, oral cavity and small intestines and of mononuclear-cell leukaemia in male and female rats, of benign and malignant tumours of the large intestine and preputial gland in males and of the clitoral gland and uterus in females (US National Toxicology Program, 1992).

Table 1. Survival and tumour incidences in male and female Fischer 344/N rats administered CI Direct Blue 15 in the drinking-water for 96 weeks

Survival and tumour types[a]	Dose (mg/l [ppm])				p Value[b]
	0	630	1250	2500	
Males					
Survival[c]	37/50	8/35	11/65	2/50	
Skin					
Basal-cell adenoma or carcinoma	2/50	9/35	27/65	28/50	< 0.001
Sebaceous gland adenoma	0/50	1/35	7/65	3/50	= 0.002
Squamous-cell papilloma or carcinoma	2/50	4/35	11/65	19/50	< 0.001
Zymbal gland: adenoma or carcinoma	1/50	5/35	10/65	20/50	< 0.001
Preputial gland: adenoma or carcinoma	8/49	5/35	23/64	9/48	< 0.001[d]
Hepatocellular neoplasms[f]	0/50	6/35	9/65	11/50	< 0.001
Oral cavity: squamous-cell papilloma or carcinoma	1/50	10/35	24/65	17/50	< 0.001
Small intestine: adenocarcinoma	0/50	0/35	0/65	2/50	= 0.078
Large intestine: polyps or adenocarcinoma	0/50	1/35	6/65	8/50	< 0.001
Mononuclear-cell leukaemia	17/50	19/35	28/65	20/50	< 0.001[d]
Females					
Survival	40/50	13/35	22/65	4/50	
Squamous-cell papilloma or carcinoma of the skin	0/50	2/35	6/65	5/50	= 0.001
Zymbal gland: adenoma or carcinoma	0/50	4/35	11/65	17/50	< 0.001
Clitoral gland: adenoma or carcinoma	7/50	11/31	24/64	27/50	< 0.001
Hepatocellular neoplastic nodule or carcinoma	0/50	0/35	2/65	5/50	< 0.001
Oral cavity: squamous-cell papilloma or carcinoma	2/50	4/35	19/65	15/50	< 0.001
Small intestine: adenocarcinoma	0/50	0/35	1/65	3/50	= 0.032
Uterine adenoma or adenocarcinoma	1/50	0/35	1/65	4/50	= 0.004
Mononuclear-cell leukaemia	7/50	13/35	27/65	15/50	< 0.001[d]

From US National Toxicology Program (1992)

[a]Terms used by authors

[b]Logistic regression trend test

[c]At 22 months; reduced survival in exposed groups due to neoplasia

[d]Life-table test

4. Other Relevant Data

4.1 Absorption, distribution, metabolism and excretion

4.1.1 *Humans*

No data were available to the Working Group.

4.1.2 *Experimental systems*

Anaerobic biodegradation of CI Direct Blue 15 gives rise to the amine metabolite, 3,3'-dimethoxybenzidine (Brown & Hamburger, 1987). The dye was cleaved by pure cultures of anaerobic bacteria and by suspensions derived from the intestinal content of rats, with subsequent formation of the amine (Cerniglia *et al.*, 1982).

CI Direct Blue 15 (100 mg/kg) containing 46 ppm (mg/kg) 3,3'-dimethoxybenzidine as an impurity was administered once in the diet to two female mongrel dogs weighing 15 kg, and 48-h urine was analysed for 3,3'-dimethoxybenzidine, the potential metabolic product (Lynn *et al.*, 1980). Excretion was found to be 0.03% of the dose of dye administered, which cannot be attributed to the level of impurity. The same dose was also administered once to four male Sprague-Dawley rats by intragastric intubation; after 72 h, $0.17 \pm 0.18\%$ of the theoretical maximum was excreted as 3,3'-dimethoxybenzidine and the monoacetyl derivative, the latter constituting a substantial fraction.

When [^{14}C-biphenyl]CI Direct Blue 15 was given as a single dose of 12 mg/kg to six-week-old male Fischer 344 rats by gavage, 74.4% of the dose was excreted in the faeces and 18.8% in urine within 192 h. Only 12% of the dose appeared as intact dye in the faeces within 48 h, the remainder being unidentified metabolic products. Excretion of the free diamine, 3,3'-dimethoxybenzidine, and of its mono- and diacetyl derivatives in urine was determined to be 0.22, 0.27 and 0.22% of the dose, respectively. An equivalent dose of ^{14}C-labelled 3,3'-dimethoxybenzidine was administered for comparison: 52% of the dose appeared in the faeces and 35% in the urine, indicating that the free amine is metabolized to a greater extent than the dye. Only 1.5% of the dose in faeces could be attributed to the free amine fraction, including the acetylated metabolites; in urine, 1.18% of the dose was excreted as the parent compound, 0.35% as the monoacetyl derivative and 0.93% as the diacetyl derivative. Radiolabel was found in all tissues examined from rats dosed with ^{14}C-CI Direct Blue 15. The levels peaked at 4 and 8 h and were highest in the gastrointestinal tract, liver, kidney and lung (Bowman *et al.*, 1982).

4.2 Toxic effects

4.2.1 *Humans*

No data were available to the Working Group.

4.2.2 *Experimental animals*

CI Direct Blue 15 binds to albumin, α_1-lipoprotein, β-lipoprotein, haemopexin, pre-albumin and α_1-antichymotrypsin, to alter their mobility in crossed immunoelectrophoresis and to degrade C_3 globulin (Emmet *et al.*, 1985). The importance of these findings *in vivo* remains to be established, as it is not known how much unchanged dye is absorbed and transported within the body.

CI Direct Blue 15 was tested for subchronic toxicity in male and female Fischer 344 rats (Morgan *et al.*, 1989; US National Toxicology Program, 1992). Groups of 10 animals of each sex received the dye in drinking-water for 13 weeks at concentrations of 0, 0.063, 0.125, 0.25, 0.50 and 1.0% for females and 0, 0.125, 0.25, 0.50, 1.0 and 3.0% for males. Seven male rats died in the highest-dose group; the first death occurred after three weeks and the last after 13 weeks. Groups given 1% CI Direct Blue 15 gained 17% less body weight than controls, and males treated with 3% of the dye gained 43% less weight than controls. Absolute and relative kidney weights increased in a dose-related manner in males and females. Changes in haematology and clinical chemistry were not observed. Histopathology showed renal and hepatic toxicity in high-dose males that died before termination of the study. In addition to necrosis of hepatocytes and fatty metamorphosis, blue pigment was observed in Kupffer cells. Focal necrosis occurred in proximal tubular epithelial cells. Mild chronic nephropathy was observed in male and female rats given 1% of dye.

4.3 Reproductive and prenatal effects

No data were available to the Working Group.

4.4 Genetic and related effects

4.4.1 *Humans*

No data were available to the Working Group.

4.4.2 *Experimental systems* (see also Table 2 and Appendices 1 and 2)

Technical-grade CI Direct Blue 15 was not mutagenic to *Salmonella typhimurium* in standard protocols, but it was mutagenic under conditions favouring azo reduction, which would generate 3,3'-dimethoxybenzidine, a known mutagen. CI Direct Blue 15 was reported in an abstract to be mutagenic at the *tk* locus in mouse lymphoma L5178Y cells. It did not induce unscheduled DNA synthesis in rat hepatocytes (abstract) or sister chromatid exchange or chromosomal aberrations in Chinese hamster ovary cells *in vitro*.

Activated *ras* genes were found in 21/34 tumours induced in rats by CI Direct Blue 15 (US National Toxicology Program, 1992) and in 1/38 spontaneous tumours tested (Reynolds *et al.*, 1990; Table 3).

Table 2. Genetic and related effects of CI Direct Blue 15

Test system	Result — Without exogenous metabolic system	Result — With exogenous metabolic system	Dose[a] (LED/HID)	Reference
SAF, *Salmonella typhimurium*, forward mutation (arabinose resistance)	0	+[b,c]	100.0000	Krishna *et al.* (1986)
SA0, *Salmonella typhimurium* TA100, reverse mutation	0	−[d]	250.0000	Elliott & Gregory (1980)
SA0, *Salmonella typhimurium* TA100, reverse mutation	0	+[e]	62.5000	Elliott & Gregory (1980)
SA0, *Salmonella typhimurium* TA100, reverse mutation	0	+[f]	150.0000	Brown & Dietrich (1983)
SA0, *Salmonella typhimurium* TA100, reverse mutation	0	(+)[g]	150.0000	Brown & Dietrich (1983)
SA0, *Salmonella typhimurium* TA100, reverse mutation	−	−	5000.0000	Mortelmans *et al.* (1986)
SA5, *Salmonella typhimurium* TA1535, reverse mutation	−	−	5000.0000	Mortelmans *et al.* (1986)
SA7, *Salmonella typhimurium* TA1537, reverse mutation	−	−	5000.0000	Mortelmans *et al.* (1986)
SA8, *Salmonella typhimurium* TA1538, reverse mutation	0	+[d]	125.0000	Reid *et al.* (1984)
SA9, *Salmonella typhimurium* TA98, reverse mutation	0	+[f]	0.0000	Sugimura *et al.* (1977)
SA9, *Salmonella typhimurium* TA98, reverse mutation	0	(+)[d]	500.0000	Elliott & Gregory (1980)
SA9, *Salmonella typhimurium* TA98, reverse mutation	0	+[e]	62.5000	Elliot & Gregory (1980)
SA9, *Salmonella typhimurium* TA98, reverse mutation	0	+[f]	150.0000	Brown & Dietrich (1983)
SA9, *Salmonella typhimurium* TA98, reverse mutation	0	(+)[g]	150.0000	Brown & Dietrich (1983)
SA9, *Salmonella typhimurium* TA98, reverse mutation	0	+[h]	50.0000	Prival *et al.* (1984)
SA9, *Salmonella typhimurium* TA98, reverse mutation	0	+[b]	100.0000	Krishna *et al.* (1986)
SA9, *Salmonella typhimurium* TA98, reverse mutation	−	−	5000.0000	Mortelmans *et al.* (1986)
URP, Unscheduled DNA synthesis, rat primary hepatocytes *in vitro*	−	0	0.0000	Mirsalis *et al.* (1983); abstr.
GST, Gene mutation, mouse lymphoma L5178Y cells *in vitro*	−	+	0.0000	Rudd *et al.* (1983); abstr.
SIC, Sister chromatid exchange, Chinese hamster ovary cells *in vitro*	−	−	2500.0000	Galloway *et al.* 1987
CIC, Chromosomal aberrations, Chinese hamster ovary cells *in vitro*	−	−	2500.0000	Galloway *et al.* 1987

+, positive; (+), weakly positive; −, negative; 0, not tested

[a] μg/ml; 0.0000, not given

[b] Preincubation with hamster or rat liver S9 and flavin mononucleotide supplementation

[c] Rat liver S9 more effective

[d] Anaerobic preincubation or riboflavin supplementation

[e] Plate incorporation and reduction using sodium dithionite

[f] Aerobic preincubation with riboflavin

[g] Anaerobic preincubation with rat caecal bacterial extract, flavin mononucleotide and liver S9

[h] Preincubation with no shaking and hamster liver S9 with flavin mononucleotide

Table 3. Activating *ras* mutations in tumours induced in Fischer 344 rats by CI Direct Blue 15 and in untreated animals

Tumour type	Frequency	N-ras	H-ras Total	Codon 12		Codon 13		Codon 61		
				GAA	AGA	CGC	GTC	AAA	CTA	CGA
Treated										
Preputial gland adenoma	1/1		1					1		
Preputial gland carcinoma	1/3		1			1				
Clitoral gland carcinoma	8/10	1	7	1		4		2		
Basal-cell carcinoma	5/6	1	4			1	1	1		1
Squamous-cell carcinoma (skin)	6/7		6			2		4		
Mammary fibroadenoma	0/2									
Mammary adenocarcinoma	0/3									
Duodenal adenocarcinoma	0/1									
Subcutaneous fibroma	0/1									
Untreated										
Clitoral gland adenoma	1/2		1							1
Preputial gland carcinoma	0/1									
Mammary gland fibro-adenoma or adenoma	0/11									
Mammary adenocarcinoma	0/2									
Subcutaneous fibroma or fibroadenoma	0/5									
Lipoma	0/1									
Testicular interstitial-cell adenoma	0/5									
Fibrosarcoma	0/2									
Mononuclear-cell leukaemia	0/3									
Adrenal phaeochromocytoma	0/1									
Pancreatic acinar adenoma	0/1									
Pancreatic islet-cell adenoma	0/1									
Pituitary adenoma	0/1									
Splenic haemangiosarcoma	0/1									
Prostatic adenocarcinoma	0/1									

Adapted from Reynolds *et al.* (1990)

5. Summary of Data Reported and Evaluation

5.1 Exposure data

CI Direct Blue 15, a bis-azo dye derived from 3,3'-dimethoxybenzidine, is used mainly for dyeing textiles and paper. The technical grade contains about 50% of pure dye, in addition to inorganic salts and a mixture of about 35 organic compounds, including 3,3'-dimethoxybenzidine.

5.2 Human carcinogenicity data

No data were available to the Working Group.

5.3 Animal carcinogenicity data

Technical-grade CI Direct Blue 15 was tested for carcinogenicity in one study in rats by administration in the drinking-water. It produced benign and malignant tumours of the skin, Zymbal gland, liver, small intestine and oral cavity as well as leukaemia in animals of each sex, of the large intestine and preputial gland in males and of the uterus and clitoral gland in females.

5.4 Other relevant data

CI Direct Blue 15 caused renal and hepatic toxicity in rats. Reductive cleavage of the azo bonds to yield 3,3'-dimethoxybenzidine was demonstrated *in vivo*.

CI Direct Blue 15 induced mutation in bacteria under conditions that favour reduction. Neither sister chromatid exchange nor chromosomal aberrations were induced in cultured mammalian cells.

5.5 Evaluation[1]

There is *inadequate evidence* in humans for the carcinogenicity of CI Direct Blue 15.

There is *sufficient evidence* in experimental animals for the carcinogenicity of technical-grade CI Direct Blue 15.

Overall evaluation

CI Direct Blue 15 is *possibly carcinogenic to humans (Group 2B)*.

6. References

Bowman, M.C., Oller, W.L., Nony, C.R., Rowland, K.L., Billedeau, S.M. & Lowry, L.K. (1982) Metabolism and distribution of two ^{14}C-benzidine-congener-based dyes in rats as determined by GC, HPLC, and radioassays. *J. anal. Toxicol.*, **6**, 164–174

---

[1]For definition of the italicized terms, see Preamble, pp. 26–30.

Brown, J.P. & Dietrich, P.S. (1983) Mutagenicity of selected sulfonated azo dyes in the *Salmonella/*-microsome assay: use of aerobic and anaerobic activation procedures. *Mutat. Res.*, **116**, 305–315

Brown, D. & Hamburger, B. (1987) The degradation of dyestuffs: Part III. Investigations of their ultimate degradability. *Chemosphere*, **16**, 1539–1553

Cerniglia, C.A., Freeman, J.P., Franklin, W. & Pack, L.D. (1982) Metabolism of azo dyes derived from benzidine, 3,3'-dimethylbenzidine and 3,3'-dimethoxybenzidine to potentially carcinogenic aromatic amines by intestinal bacteria. *Carcinogenesis*, **3**, 1255–1260

Deutsche Forschungsgemeinschaft (1992) *MAK and BAT-Values List 1992. Maximum Concentrations at the Workplace (MAK) and Biological Tolerance Values (BAT) for Working Materials* (Report No. 28), Weinheim, VCH Verlagsgesellschaft, pp. 80–81, 87

Elliott, J. & Gregory, A.R. (1980) Mutagenicity of a series of benzidine congener based dyes. *Vet. hum. Toxicol.*, **22**, 413–417

Emmet, M., Cerniglia, C.E. & Crowle, A.J. (1985) Differential serum protein binding of benzidine and benzidine-congener based dyes and their derivatives. *Arch. Toxicol.*, **57**, 130–135

Galloway, S.M., Armstrong, M.J., Reuben, C., Colman, S., Brown, B., Cannon, C., Bloom, A.D., Nakamura, F., Ahmed, M., Duk, S., Rimpo, J., Margolin, B.H., Resnick, M., Anderson, B. & Zeiger, E. (1987) Chromosome aberrations and sister chromatid exchanges in Chinese hamster ovary cells. Evaluations of 108 chemicals. *Environ. Mutag.*, **10** (Suppl. 10), 1–175

IARC (1974) *IARC Monographs on the Evaluation of Carcinogenic Risk of Chemicals to Man*, Vol. 4, *Some Aromatic Amines, Hydrazine and Related Substances, N-Nitroso Compounds and Miscellaneous Alkylating Agents*, Lyon, pp. 41–47

IARC (1987) *IARC Monographs on the Evaluation of Carcinogenic Risks to Humans*, Suppl. 7, *Overall Evaluations of Carcinogenicity: An Updating of* IARC Monographs *Volumes 1 to 42*, Lyon, pp. 198–199

Krishna, G., Xu, J. & Nath, J. (1986) Comparative mutagenicity studies of azo dyes and their reduction products in *Salmonella typhimurium*. *J. Toxicol. environ. Health*, **18**, 111–120

Lynn, R.K., Donielson, D.W., Ilias, A.M., Kennish, J.M., Wong, K. & Matthews, H.B. (1980) Metabolism of bisazobiphenyl dyes derived from benzidine, 3,3'-dimethoxybenzidine or 3,3'-dimethylbenzidine to carcinogenic aromatic amines in the dog and rat. *Toxicol. appl. Pharmacol.*, **56**, 248-258

Mirsalis, J., Tyson, K., Beck, J., Loh, F., Steinmetz, K., Contreras, C., Austere, L., Martin, S. & Spalding, J. (1983) Induction of unscheduled DNA synthesis (UDS) in hepatocytes following *in vitro* and *in vivo* treatment (Abstract No. Ef-5). *Environ. Mutag.*, **5**, 482

Morgan, D.L., Jameson, C.W., Mennear, J.H., Ulland, B.M. & Lemen, J.K. (1989) Thirteen-week toxicity studies of 3,3'-dimethoxybenzidine and CI Direct Blue 15 in the Fischer 344 rat. *Toxicology*, **59**, 297–309

Mortelmans, K., Haworth, S., Lawlor, T., Speck, W., Tainer, B. & Zeiger, E. (1986) *Salmonella* mutagenicity tests. II. Results from the testing of 270 chemicals. *Environ. Mutag.*, **8** (Suppl. 7), 1–119

Prival, M.J., Bell, S.J., Mitchell, V.D., Peiperl, M.D. & Vaughan, V.L. (1984) Mutagenicity of benzidine and benzidine-congener dyes and selected monoazo dyes in a modified *Salmonella* assay. *Mutat. Res.*, **136**, 33–47

Reid, T.M., Morton, K.C., Wang, C.Y. & King, C.M. (1984) Mutagenicity of azo dyes following metabolism by different reductive/oxidative systems. *Environ. Mutag.*, **6**, 705–717

Reynolds, S.H., Patterson, R.M., Mennear, J.H., Maronpot, R.R. & Anderson, M.W. (1990) *ras* Gene activation in rat tumors induced by benzidine congeners and derived dyes. *Cancer Res.*, **50**, 266–272

Rudd, C.J., Mitchell, A.D. & Spalding, J. (1983) L5178Y mouse lymphoma cell mutagenesis assay of coded chemicals incorporating analyses of the colony size distributions (Abstract No. Cd-19). *Environ. Mutag.*, **5**, 419

Society of Dyers and Colourists (1971a) *Colour Index*, 3rd ed., Vol. 4, Bradford, Yorkshire, p. 4208

Society of Dyers and Colourists (1971b) *Colour Index*, 3rd ed., Vol. 2, Bradford, Yorkshire, p. 2226

Sugimura, T., Nagao, M., Kawachi, T., Honda, M., Yahagi, T., Seino, Y., Sato, S., Matsukura, N., Matsushima, T., Shirai, A., Sawamura, M. & Matsumoto, H. (1977) Mutagen–carcinogens in food, with special reference to highly mutagenic pyrolytic products in broiled foods. In: Hiatt, H.H., Watson, J.D. & Winsten, J.A., eds, *Origins of Human Cancer*, Book C, *Human Risk Assessment*, Cold Spring Harbor, NY, CSH Press, pp. 1561–1577

US Environmental Protection Agency (1987) *Health and Environmental Effects Profile for Niagara Blue 4B* (Report No. EPA-600/X-87/389/US NTIS PB89-120273), Cincinnati, OH, Environmental Criteria and Assessment Office

US Environmental Protection Agency (1990) *Textile Dye Weighing Monitoring Study* (EPA Reports Nos EPA-560/5-90-009 and EPA-560/5-90-010; Main Report, Supplement and Site Visit Reports), Washington DC, Office of Toxic Substances

US International Trade Commission (1974) *Synthetic Organic Chemicals, United States Production and Sales, 1972* (USITC Publication No. 681), Washington DC, US Government Printing Office, p. 61

US International Trade Commission (1978) *Synthetic Organic Chemicals, United States Production and Sales, 1977* (USITC Publication No. 920), Washington DC, US Government Printing Office, p. 97

US International Trade Commission (1982) *Synthetic Organic Chemicals, United States Production and Sales, 1981* (USITC Publication No. 1292), Washington DC, US Government Printing Office, p. 59

US International Trade Commission (1983) *Synthetic Organic Chemicals, United States Production and Sales, 1982* (USITC Publication No. 1422), Washington DC, US Government Printing Office, p. 60

US National Library of Medicine (1992) *Registry of Toxic Effects of Chemical Substances* (RTECS No. QJ6420000), Bethesda, MD

US National Toxicology Program (1992) *Toxicology and Carcinogenesis Studies of CI Direct Blue 15 (CAS No. 2429-74-5) in F344/N Rats (Drinking Water Studies)* (NTP TR 397; NIH Publ. No. 92-2852), Research Triangle Park, NC

CI ACID RED 114

1. Exposure Data

1.1 Chemical and physical data

1.1.1 Synonyms, structural and molecular data

Chem. Abstr. Serv. Reg. No.: 6459-94-5

Chem. Abstr. Name: 8-[(3,3'-Dimethyl-4'-[(4-[((4-methylphenyl]sulfonyl)oxy]phenyl)-azo][1,1'-biphenyl]-4-yl)azo]-7-hydroxy-1,3-naphthalenedisulfonic acid, disodium salt

Colour Index No.: 23635

Synonyms: Acid Red 114; CI Acid Red 114, disodium salt

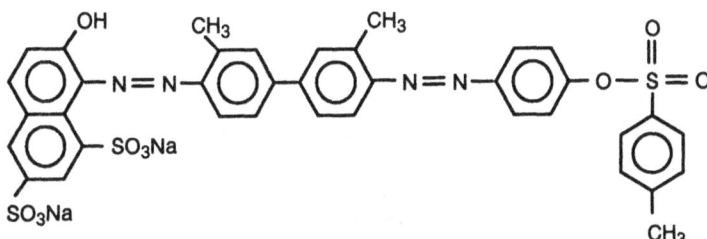

$C_{37}H_{28}N_4O_{10}S_3.2Na$ Mol. wt: 830.84

1.1.2 Chemical and physical properties

(a) *Description*: Deep-maroon powder (Green, 1990); red powder (US National Toxicology Program, 1991)

(b) *Melting-point*: 250–300 °C (decomposes) (US National Toxicology Program, 1991)

(c) *Spectroscopy data*: Infrared, ultraviolet and nuclear magnetic resonance spectral data have been reported (Pouchert, 1981; Sadtler Research Laboratories, 1988; Green, 1990; US National Toxicology Program, 1991).

(d) *Solubility*: Soluble in water (80 g/l at 80 °C) (International Dyestuffs Corp., 1990); very slightly soluble in ethanol (Green, 1990)

1.1.3 Trade names, technical products and impurities

Some trade names are: Acid Leather Red BG; Amacid Milling Red PRS; Benzyl Fast Red BG; Benzyl Red BR; Elcacid Milling Fast Red RS; Erionyl Red RS; Fenafor Red PB; Folan Red B; Intrazone Red BR; Kayanol Milling Red RS; Leather Fast Red B; Levanol Red

GG; Midlon Red PRS; Milling Fast Red B; Milling Red B; Milling Red BB; Milling Red SWB; Polar Red RS; Sandolan Red N-RS; Sella Fast Red RS; Sulphonol Red R; Suminol Milling Red RS; Supranol Fast Red 3G; Supranol Fast Red GG; Supranol Red PBX-CF; Supranol Red R; Telon Fast Red GG; Tertracid Milling Red B; Vondamol Fast Red RS.

Technical-grade CI Acid Red 114 is available in commercial mixtures containing 25–85% pure dye. Other typical ingredients include sodium chloride and mineral oil (see IARC, 1984, 1987) (Crompton & Knowles Corp., 1990; International Dyestuffs Corp., 1990; US National Toxicology Program, 1991; Aldrich Chemical Co., 1992).

1.1.4 *Analysis*

No data were available to the Working Group.

1.2 Production and use

1.2.1 *Production*

CI Acid Red 114, a bright red anionic bisazo dye, is manufactured by converting 3,3'-dimethylbenzidine (*ortho*-tolidine; see IARC, 1972) to the tetraazonium salt, which is then coupled successively to G acid (2-naphthol-6,8-disulfonic acid) and phenol. The phenol hydroxy function is then esterified with *para*-tolylsulfonyl chloride (Green, 1990).

CI Acid Red 114 has been produced commercially since the early 1900s. In the USA, there were six manufacturers and two importers of CI Acid Red 114 in 1977 (US Environmental Protection Agency, 1988). Annual production volume by five manufacturers in 1990 was estimated to be 10–100 tonnes, whereas it was 170 tonnes in 1979 (US International Trade Commission, 1980). In 1980, the USA imported about 7 tonnes of CI Acid Red 114 (US International Trade Commission, 1981).

1.2.2 *Use*

CI Acid Red 114 is used to dye wool (from a weak acid bath), silk (from either a neutral or acetic acid bath), jute and leather. Wool and silk are also printed directly (Green, 1990).

1.3 Occurrence

1.3.1 *Natural occurrence*

CI Acid Red 114 is not known to occur as a natural product.

1.3.2 *Occupational exposure*

No data were available to the Working Group.

The US Environmental Protection Agency, the American Textile Manufacturers Institute and the Ecological and Toxicological Association of the Dyestuffs Manufacturing Industry conducted a joint survey in 1986–87 to estimate airborne concentrations of dye dust in dye weighing rooms of plants where powder dyes are used in the dyeing and printing of textiles. The survey was based on a sample of 24 sites chosen at random from among textile plants where powder dyes are weighed. Although CI Acid Red 114 was not among the dyes included in the survey, the results are considered to be representative of dye dust levels during weighing of this type of powder dye. The mean airborne concentration of total active colourant in the plants monitored was estimated to be 0.085 mg/m^3 (US Environmental Protection Agency, 1990).

On the basis of a survey conducted in the USA between 1981 and 1983, the US National Institute for Occupational Safety and Health estimated that a total of 18 511 workers, including 352 women, may have been exposed to CI Acid Red 114 at 300 textile and leather goods manufacturing plants (US National Library of Medicine, 1992).

1.3.3 Other

Anaerobic biodegradation of CI Acid Red 114 gives rise to the amine metabolites, 3,3′-dimethylbenzidine and 4-methylbenzenesulfonic acid (4′-aminophenyl) ester. Following incubation of 100 mg/l of dyestuff at 35 °C in the presence of anaerobic sludge inoculum, primary degradation was complete within seven days (Brown & Hamburger, 1987).

1.4 Regulations and guidelines

In Germany, CI Acid Red 114 must be handled like the corresponding hypothetical reduction amine, 3,3′-dimethylbenzidine, which is classified as an A_2 compound. Such materials are considered to have been proven to be carcinogenic only in animal experimentation but under conditions comparable to those of possible human exposure at the workplace (Deutsche Forschungsgemeinschaft, 1992).

2. Studies of Cancer in Humans

No data were available to the Working Group.

3. Studies of Cancer in Experimental Animals

3.1 Oral administration

Rat

Groups of 50, 35, 65 and 50 male and 50, 35, 65 and 50 female Fischer 344/N rats, five weeks old, were administered 0, 70, 150 or 300 mg/l (ppm) (males) and 0, 150, 300 or 600 ppm (females) CI Acid Red 114 (purity, 85%; with about 15 organic chemicals of similar structure, including approximately 5 ppm 3,3′-dimethylbenzidine and < 1 ppm benzidine in distilled drinking-water for 104 weeks. Survival at 105 weeks was 24/50, 15/35, 26/65 and 1/50 for male rats and 36/50, 13/35, 6/64 and 0/50 for females in the control, low-, mid- and high-dose groups, respectively ($p < 0.001$ for both males and females). All female rats receiving 600 ppm died by week 89. The decreased survival in the treated groups was due to development of treatment-related neoplasms. As shown in Table 1, there were increased incidences of benign and malignant tumours of the skin, Zymbal gland and liver in male and female rats, and of the clitoral gland, oral cavity, small and large intestine and lung in female rats (US National Toxicology Program, 1991).

Table 1. Survival and tumour incidences in male and female Fischer 344/N rats administered CI Acid Red 114 in the drinking-water for 104 weeks

Survival and tumour types[a]	Dose (mg/l [ppm])				p Value[b]
Males	0	70	150	300	
Females	0	150	300	600	
Males					
Survival[c]	24/50	15/35	26/65	1/50	
Skin					
Basal-cell adenoma or carcinoma	1/50	5/35	28/65	32/50	< 0.001
Sebaceous-cell adenoma or carcinoma	1/50	1/35	5/65	6/50	= 0.007
Squamous-cell papilloma or carcinoma	1/50	2/35	11/65	9/50	= 0.001
Keratoacanthoma	1/50	1/35	4/65	7/50	< 0.001
Zymbal gland adenoma or carcinoma	0/50	0/35	8/65	7/50	= 0.005
Liver neoplasms	2/50	2/35	15/65	20/50	< 0.001
Females					
Survival	36/50	13/35	6/64	0/50	
Basal-cell adenoma or carcinoma of the skin	0/50	4/35	7/65	5/50	= 0.012
Zymbal gland adenoma or carcinoma	0/50	3/35	18/65	19/50	< 0.001
Clitoral gland adenoma or carcinoma	11/48	17/32	28/62	23/50	< 0.001
Liver neoplasms	0/50	0/35	19/64	8/50	< 0.001
Lung adenoma or carcinoma	1/50	2/35	9/65	4/50	= 0.007
Oral cavity squamous-cell papilloma or carcinoma	0/50	3/35	9/65	6/50	= 0.017
Small intestine polyps or adenocarcinoma	0/50	0/35	1/63	2/50	> 0.05
Large intestine polyps or adenocarcinoma	0/50	1/35	0/64	3/50	> 0.05

From US National Toxicology Program (1991)
[a]Terms used by authors
[b]Logistic regression test for trend
[c]At 22 months; reduced survival in exposed groups due to tumour development

4. Other Relevant Data

4.1 Absorption, distribution, metabolism and excretion

4.1.1 *Humans*

No data were available to the Working Group.

4.1.2 *Experimental systems*

CI Acid Red 114 (100 mg/kg) containing less than 1% 3,3'-dimethylbenzidine as an impurity was administered once in the diet to two female mongrel dogs weighing 15 kg, and

48-h urine was analysed for 3,3'-dimethylbenzidine, the potential metabolic product (Lynn *et al.*, 1980). Excretion was found to be 0.04% of the dose of dye administered, which is in excess of what would be expected from the level of impurity; *para*-aminophenyl-*para*-toluenesulfonate was also identified as a urinary metabolite. The same dose of CI Acid Red 114 was also administered once to four male Sprague-Dawley rats by intragastric intubation; after 72 h, only 0.01% of the dose could be identified as 3,3'-dimethylbenzidine.

4.2 Toxic effects

4.2.1 *Humans*

No data were available to the Working Group.

4.2.2 *Experimental animals*

CI Acid Red 114 was tested for toxicity in male and female Fischer 344/N rats in a range-finding study for carcinogenicity testing (US National Toxicology Program, 1991). The purity of the test compound was estimated to be 82–85%; impurities consisted of about 15 organic chemicals of similar structure, with benzidine at less than 1 ppm and 3,3'-dimethylbenzidine at about 5 ppm. In a 13-day study, groups of five rats were dosed with 0, 10 000, 20 000 or 30 000 ppm (mg/l) in drinking-water. Except for one accidental death, all rats survived to the end of the study. Final mean body weights were significantly lower for males in the mid- and high-dose groups (83 and 77%, respectively) and for females in all dose groups (92, 88 and 80%, respectively). Hypocellularity of sternal bone marrow was found in three males and in all females given 20 000 ppm. The marrow was depleted of erythroid and myeloid cells. Lymphocytic depletion of the thymus was observed in four males and one female of the same dose group.

In the 13-week study, groups of 10 rats received 0, 600, 1200, 2500, 5000 or 10 000 ppm (mg/l) CI Acid Red 114 in the drinking-water for 94 days (males) or 95 days (females) (US National Toxicology Program, 1991). All rats survived. Body weights were lower than those in controls in all groups that received 1200 ppm and above (94–85%). Relative liver weights were increased in all dosed males and females; absolute and relative kidney weights were increased in females receiving doses of 1200 ppm and above. Haematocrit, haemoglobin and erythrocyte counts were decreased in dosed females, and the erythrocyte count was reduced at 1500 ppm and above in males. Some enzyme levels were elevated, consistent with mild hepatocellular damage, and minimal-to-mild lesions in liver were seen upon histopatho-logical examination. Kupffer cells in the livers of most treated females contained brown pigment. An increased prevalence of reticulum-cell hyperplasia of the mesenteric lymph node was observed in treated males and females. Tubular regeneration and chronic inflammation of the kidneys occurred more frequently in treated females than in controls. Minimal amounts of brownish pigment were also seen in the tubular epithelial cells of the kidneys.

4.3 Reproductive and prenatal effects

No data were available to the Working Group.

4.4 Genetic and related effects

4.4.1 *Humans*

No data were available to the Working Group.

4.4.2 *Experimental systems* (see also Table 2 and Appendices 1 and 2)

CI Acid Red 114 was mutagenic to *Salmonella typhimurium* strains TA1538 and TA98 under reducing conditions. It did not induce sex-linked recessive lethal mutation in *Drosophila melanogaster* and did not induce unscheduled DNA synthesis in primary cultures of rat hepatocytes (abstract) or sister chromatid exchange or chromosomal aberrations in cultured Chinese hamster ovary cells. It did not induce unscheduled DNA synthesis in the hepatocytes of rats dosed orally (abstract).

Activated *ras* genes were found in 13/16 tumours induced in rats by CI Acid Red 114 (US National Toxicology Program, 1991) and in 1/38 spontaneous tumours tested (a CGA in codon 61 in a clitoral gland adenoma) (Reynolds *et al.*, 1990; Table 3).

5. Summary of Data Reported and Evaluation

5.1 Exposure data

CI Acid Red 114, a bis-azo dye derived from 3,3'-dimethylbenzidine, is used to dye wool, silk, jute and leather.

5.2 Human carcinogenicity data

No data were available to the Working Group.

5.3 Animal carcinogenicity data

CI Acid Red 114 was tested for carcinogenicity in one study in rats by administration in the drinking-water. It increased the incidences of benign and malignant tumours of the skin, Zymbal gland and liver in male and female rats, and of the clitoral gland, lung, oral cavity and small and large intestine in female rats.

5.4 Other relevant data

Reductive cleavage of the azo bonds to yield 3,3'-dimethylbenzidine was demonstrated *in vivo*.

CI Acid Red 114 induced gene mutation in bacteria under reducing conditions. It did not induce gene mutation in insects or sister chromatid exchange or chromosomal aberrations in cultured mammalian cells.

Table 2. Genetic and related effects of CI Acid Red 114

Test system	Result — Without exogenous metabolic system	Result — With exogenous metabolic system	Dose (LED/HID)[a]	Reference
SA0, Salmonella typhimurium TA100, reverse mutation	–	–	500.0000	Venturini & Tamaro (1979)
SA0, Salmonella typhimurium TA100, reverse mutation	0	–[b]	200.0000	Elliot & Gregory (1980)
SA0, Salmonella typhimurium TA100, reverse mutation	0	+[c]	62.5000	Elliot & Gregory (1980)
SA0, Salmonella typhimurium TA100, reverse mutation	–	–	167.0000	Mortelmans et al. (1986)
SA5, Salmonella typhimurium TA1535, reverse mutation	–	–	500.0000	Venturini & Tamaro (1979)
SA5, Salmonella typhimurium TA1535, reverse mutation	–	–	167.0000	Mortelmans et al. (1986)
SA7, Salmonella typhimurium TA1537, reverse mutation	–	–	167.0000	Mortelmans et al. (1986)
SA8, Salmonella typhimurium TA1538, reverse mutation	–	–	500.0000	Venturini & Tamaro (1979)
SA8, Salmonella typhimurium TA1538, reverse mutation	–	+[d]	100.0000	Reid et al. (1984)
SA9, Salmonella typhimurium TA98, reverse mutation	–	–	500.0000	Venturini & Tamaro (1979)
SA9, Salmonella typhimurium TA98, reverse mutation	0	–[b,e]	500.0000	Elliot & Gregory (1980)
SA9, Salmonella typhimurium TA98, reverse mutation	0	+[c]	62.5000	Elliot & Gregory (1980)
SA9, Salmonella typhimurium TA98, reverse mutation	0	+[f]	40.0000	Prival et al. (1984)
SA9, Salmonella typhimurium TA98, reverse mutation	–	(+)[g]	500.0000	Mortelmans et al. (1986)
SA9, Salmonella typhimurium TA98, reverse mutation	0	+[e]	125.0000	Dellarco & Prival (1989)
DMX, Drosophila melanogaster, sex-linked recessive lethal mutations	–		1500.0000	Woodruff et al. (1985)
DMX, Drosophila melanogaster, sex-linked recessive lethal mutations	–		50000.0000 feed	Woodruff et al. (1985)
URP, Unscheduled DNA synthesis, rat primary hepatocytes in vitro	–	0	0.0000	Mirsalis et al. (1983); abstr.
SIC, Sister chromatid exchange, Chinese hamster ovary cells in vitro	–	–	50.0000	US National Toxicology Program (1991)

Table 2 (contd)

Test system	Result		Dose (LED/HID)[a]	Reference
	Without exogenous metabolic system	With exogenous metabolic system		
CIC, Chromosomal aberrations, Chinese hamster ovary cells *in vitro*	–	–	50.0000	US National Toxicology Program (1991)
UPR, Unscheduled DNA synthesis, rat hepatocytes *in vivo*	–		0.0000 po	Mirsalis *et al.* (1983); abstr.

+, positive; (+), weakly positive; –, negative; 0, not tested
[a]In-vitro tests, μg/ml; in-vivo tests, mg/kg bw
[b]Anaerobic preincubation or with riboflavin supplementation
[c]Plate incorporation, with reduction using sodium dithionate
[d]Bacterial caecal reduction
[e]Plate incorporation with or without riboflavin
[f]Preincubation with hamster or rat liver S9 and flavin mononucleotide supplementation, no aeration
[g]Hamster liver S9

Table 3. Activating *ras* mutations in tumours induced in Fischer 344 rats by CI Acid Red 114 and in untreated animals

Tumour type	Frequency	N-*ras*	H-*ras* Total	Codon 12		Codon 13		Codon 61		
				GAA	AGA	CGC	GTC	AAA	CTA	CGA
Treated										
Clitoral gland adenoma	4/4		4			1		1	1	1
Basal-cell adenoma (skin)	4/5	1	3	2	1					
Basal-cell carcinoma (skin)	1/1		1		1					
Squamous–cell carcinoma (skin)	3/3		3					2	1	
Trichoepithelioma (skin)	1/1		1		1					
Fibrosarcoma	0/1									
Mammary fibroadenoma	0/1									
Untreated										
Clitoral gland adenoma	1/2		1							1
Preputial gland carcinoma	0/1									
Mammary gland fibroadenoma or adenoma	0/11									
Mammary adenocarcinoma	0/2									
Subcutaneous fibroma or fibroadenoma	0/5									
Lipoma	0/1									
Testicular interstitial-cell adenoma	0/5									
Fibrosarcoma	0/2									
Mononuclear-cell leukaemia	0/3									
Adrenal phaeochromocytoma	0/1									
Pancreatic acinar adenoma	0/1									
Pancreatic islet-cell adenoma	0/1									
Pituitary adenoma	0/1									
Splenic haemangiosarcoma	0/1									
Prostatic adenocarcinoma	0/1									

Adapted from Reynolds *et al.* (1990)

5.5 Evaluation[1]

There is *inadequate evidence* in humans for the carcinogenicity of CI Acid Red 114.

There is *sufficient evidence* in experimental animals for the carcinogenicity of CI Acid Red 114.

---

[1]For definition of the italicized terms, see Preamble, pp. 26–30.

Overall evaluation

CI Acid Red 114 is *possibly carcinogenic to humans (Group 2B)*.

6. References

Aldrich Chemical Co. (1992) *Aldrich Catalog/Handbook of Fine Chemicals 1992–1993*, Milwaukee, WI, p. 25

Brown, D. & Hamburger, B. (1987) The degradation of dyestuffs: Part III. Investigations of their ultimate degradability. *Chemosphere*, **16**, 1539–1553

Crompton & Knowles Corp. (1990) *Material Safety Data Sheet: Intrazone Red BR (CI Acid Red 114)*, Reading, PA

Dellarco, V.L. & Prival, M.J. (1989) Mutagenicity of nitro compounds in *Salmonella typhimurium* in the presence of flavin mononucleotide in a preincubation asssay. *Environ. Mutag.*, **13**, 116–127

Deutsche Forschungsgemeinschaft (1992) *MAK- and BAT-Values List 1992. Maximum Concentrations at the Workplace (MAK) and Biological Tolerance Values (BAT) for Working Materials* (Report No. 28), Weinheim, VCH Verlagsgesellschaft, pp. 64, 80–81

Elliot, J. & Gregory, A.R. (1980) Mutagenicity of a series of benzidine congener based dyes. *Vet. hum. Toxicol.*, **22**, 413–417

Green, F.J. (1990) *The Sigma-Aldrich Handbook of Stains, Dyes and Indicators*, Milwaukee, WI, Aldrich Chemical Co., p. 38

IARC (1972) *IARC Monographs on the Evaluation of Carcinogenic Risk of Chemicals to Man*, Vol. 1, *Some Inorganic Substances, Chlorinated Hydrocarbons, Aromatic Amines, N-Nitroso Compounds, and Natural Products*, Lyon, pp. 87–91

IARC (1984) *IARC Monographs on the Evaluation of the Carcinogenic Risks of Chemicals to Humans*, Vol. 33, *Polynuclear Aromatic Compounds, Part 2: Carbon Blacks, Mineral Oils and Some Nitroarenes*, Lyon, pp. 87–168

IARC (1987) *IARC Monographs on the Evaluation of Carcinogenic Risks to Humans*, Suppl. 7, *Overall Evaluations of Carcinogenicity: An Updating of* IARC Monographs *Volumes 1 to 42*, Lyon, pp. 252–254

International Dyestuffs Corp. (1990) *Material Safety Data Sheet: Elcacid Milling Fast Red RS (Acid Red 114)*, Clifton, NJ

Lynn, R.K., Donielson, D.W., Ilias, A.M., Kennish, J.M., Wong, K. & Matthews, H.B. (1980) Metabolism of bisazobiphenyl dyes derived from benzidine, 3,3'-dimethylbenzidine or 3,3'-dimethoxybenzidine to carcinogenic aromatic amines in the dog and rat. *Toxicol. appl. Pharmacol.*, **56**, 248–258

Mirsalis, J., Tyson, K., Beck, J., Loh, F., Steinmetz, K., Contreras, C., Austere, L., Martin, S. & Spalding, J. (1983) Induction of unscheduled DNA synthesis (UDS) in hepatocytes following *in vitro* and *in vivo* treatment (Abstract No. Ef-5). *Environ. Mutag.*, **5**, 482

Mortelmans, K., Haworth, S., Lawlor, T., Speck, W., Tainer, B. & Zeiger, E. (1986) *Salmonella* mutagenicity tests. II. Results from the testing of 270 chemicals. *Environ. Mutag.*, **8** (Suppl. 7), 1–119

Pouchert, C.J., ed. (1981) *The Aldrich Library of Infrared Spectra*, 3rd Ed., Milwaukee, WI, Aldrich Chemical Co., p. 1465

Prival, M.J., Bell, S.J., Mitchell, V.D., Peiperl, M.D. & Vaughan, V.L. (1984) Mutagenicity of benzidine and benzidine-congener dyes and selected monoazo dyes in a modified *Salmonella* assay. *Mutat. Res.*, **136**, 33–47

Reid, T.M., Morton, K.C., Wang, C.Y. & King, C.M. (1984) Mutagenicity of azo dyes following metabolism by different reductive/oxidative systems. *Environ. Mutag.*, **6**, 705–717

Reynolds, S.H., Patterson, R.M., Mennear, J.H., Maronpot, R.R. & Anderson, M.W. (1990) *ras* Gene activation in rat tumors induced by benzidine congeners and derived dyes. *Cancer Res.*, **50**, 266–272

Sadtler Research Laboratories (1988) *Sadtler Standard Spectra*, Philadelphia, PA

US Environmental Protection Agency (1988) *Computer Printout (CIS): 1977 Production Statistics for Chemicals in the Non-confidential Initial TSCA Chemical Substances Inventory*, Washington DC, Office of Pesticides and Toxic Substances

US Environmental Protection Agency (1990) *Textile Dye Weighing Monitoring Study* (EPA Report No. EPA-560/5-90-009, Main Report and Site Visit Reports), Washington DC, Office of Toxic Substances

US International Trade Commission (1980) *Synthetic Organic Chemicals, United States Production and Sales, 1979* (USITC Publication No. 1099), Washington DC, US Government Printing Office, p. 65

US International Trade Commission (1981) *Imports of Benzenoid Chemicals and Products, 1980* (USITC Publication No. 1163), Washington DC, US Government Printing Office, p. 47

US National Library of Medicine (1992) *Registry of Toxic Effects of Chemical Substances* (RTECS No. QJ6475500), Bethesda, MD

US National Toxicology Program (1991) *Toxicology and Carcinogenesis Studies of CI Acid Red 114 (CAS No. 6459-94-5) in F344/N Rats (Drinking Water Studies)* (NTP TR 405; NIH Publ. No. 92-3136), Research Triangle Park, NC, US Department of Health and Human Services

Venturini, S. & Tamaro, M. (1979) Mutagenicity of anthraquinone and azo dyes in Ames' *Salmonella typhimurium* test. *Mutat. Res.*, **68**, 307–312

Woodruff, R.C., Mason, J.M., Valencia, R. & Zimmering, S. (1985) Chemical mutagenesis testing in *Drosophila*. V. Results of 53 coded compounds tested for the National Toxicology Program. *Environ. Mutag.*, **7**, 677–702

CI PIGMENT RED 3

1. Exposure Data

1.1 Chemical and physical data

1.1.1 *Synonyms, structural and molecular data*

Chem. Abstr. Serv. Reg. No.: 2425-85-6
Replaces CAS Reg. No.: 12238-48-1; 12240-01-6; 12240-02-7; 39310-30-0
Chem. Abstr. Name: 1-[(4-Methyl-2-nitrophenyl)azo]-2-naphthalenol
Colour Index No.: 12120
Synonyms: D&C Red No. 35; D and C Red No. 35; 1-(4-methyl-2-nitrophenylazo)-2-naphthol; 1-[(2-nitro-4-methylphenyl)azo]-2-naphthol; 1-(*ortho*-nitro-*para*-tolylazo)-2-naphthol; toluidine red

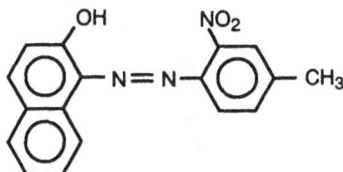

$C_{17}H_{13}N_3O_3$ Mol. wt: 307.31

1.1.2 *Chemical and physical properties*

  (a) *Description*: Dark-red powder (Stubbs, 1973; Green, 1990)
  (b) *Melting-point*: 270–272 °C (Green, 1990)
  (c) *Density*: 1.37–1.50 g/cm^3 (Stubbs, 1973)
  (d) *Spectroscopy data*: Infrared, ultraviolet and nuclear magnetic resonance spectral data have been reported (Pouchert, 1981; Green, 1990; Sadtler Research Laboratories, 1980, 1991; US National Toxicology Program, 1992).
  (e) *Solubility*: Slightly soluble in water (0.8 g/l), ethanol (0.7 g/l), ethylene glycol methyl ether (0.9 g/l), acetone and benzene; very soluble in mineral spirits, aromatic hydrocarbons and plasticizers (Stubbs, 1973; Green, 1990)

1.1.3 *Trade names, technical products and impurities*

Some trade names are: Accosperse Toluidine Red XL; ADC Toluidine Red B; Atlasol Spirit Red 3; CP Toluidine Toner A 2989; CP Toluidine Toner A 2990; CP Toluidine Toner

–259–

Dark RS 3340; CP Toluidine Toner Deep X 1865; CP Toluidine Toner Light RS 3140; CP Toluidine Toner RT 6101; CP Toluidine Toner RT 6104; Calcotone Toluidine Red YP; Carnelio Helio Red; Chromatex Red J; Dainichi Permanent Red 4R; Deep Fastona Red; Duplex Toluidine Red L 20-3140; Eljon Fast Scarlet PV Extra; Eljon Fast Scarlet RN; Enialit Light Red RL; Fast Red A; Fast Red AB; Fast Red J; Fast Red JE; Fast Red R; Fastona Red B; Fastona Scarlet RL; Fastona Scarlet YS; Graphtol Red A 4RL; Hansa Red B; Hansa Red G; Hansa Scarlet RB; Hansa Scarlet RN; Hansa Scarlet RNC; Helio Fast Red BN; Helio Fast Red RL; Helio Fast Red RN; Helio Red RL; Helio Red Toner; Hispalit Fast Scarlet RN; Independence Red; Irgalite Fast Red P 4R; Irgalite Fast Scarlet RND; Irgalite Red PV 2; Irgalite Red RNPX; Irgalite Scarlet RB; Isol Fast Red HB; Isol Fast Red RN 2B; Isol Fast Red RN 2G; Isol Fast Red RNB; Isol Fast Red RNG; Isol Toluidine Red HB; Isol Toluidine Red RN 2B; Isol Toluidine Red RN 2G; Isol Toluidine Red RNB; Isol Toluidine Red RNG; Japan Red 221; Japan Red No. 221; Kromon Helio Fast Red; Kromon Helio Fast Red YS; Lake Red 4R; Lake Red 4RII; Lithol Fast Scarlet RN; Lutetia Fast Red 3R; Lutetia Fast Scarlet RF; Lutetia Fast Scarlet RJN; Monolite Fast Scarlet CA; Monolite Fast Scarlet GSA; Monolite Fast Scarlet RB; Monolite Fast Scarlet RBA; Monolite Fast Scarlet RN; Monolite Fast Scarlet RNA; Monolite Fast Scarlet RNV; Monolite Fast Scarlet RT; No. 2 Forthfast Scarlet; Oralith Red P 4R; Permanent Red 4R; Pigment Red 3; Pigment Red RL; Pigment Scarlet; Pigment Scarlet B; Pigment Scarlet N; Pigment Scarlet R; Polymo Red FGN; Recolite Fast Red RBL; Recolite Fast Red RL; Recolite Fast Red RYL; Sanyo Scarlet Pure; Sanyo Scarlet Pure No. 1000; Scarlet Pigment RN; Segnale Light Red 2B; Segnale Light Red B; Segnale Light Red BR; Segnale Light Red C 4R; Segnale Light Red RL; Seikafast Red 4R4016; Siegle Red 1; Siegle Red B; Siegle Red BB; Silogomma Red RLL; Silosol Red RBN; Silosol Red RN; Siloton Red BRLL; Siloton Red RLL; Symuler Fast Red 4R100; Symuler Fast Scarlet 4R; Syton Fast Scarlet RB; Syton Fast Scarlet RD; Syton Fast Scarlet RN; Tertropigment Red HAB; Tertropigment Scarlet LRN; Toluidine Red 10451; Toluidine Red 3B; Toluidine Red 4R; Toluidine Red BFB; Toluidine Red BFGG; Toluidine Red D 28-3930; Toluidine Red Light; Toluidine Red M 20-3785; Toluidine Red R; Toluidine Red RT 115; Toluidine Red Toner; Toluidine Red XL 20-3050; Toluidine Toner; Toluidine Toner Dark 5040; Toluidine Toner HR-X 2700; Toluidine Toner HR-X 2741; Toluidine Toner Keep HR-X 2742; Toluidine Toner L 20-3300; Toluidine Toner RT 252; Versal Scarlet PRNL; Versal Scarlet RNL; Vulcafor Scarlet A

Technical grades of CI Pigment Red 3 are available commercially with purities ranging up to > 97%. One impurity that has been reported is 1-[(4-methoxy-2-nitrophenyl)azo]-2-naphthalenol (BASF Corp., 1991; Aldrich Chemical Co., 1992; US National Toxicology Program, 1992).

1.1.4 *Analysis*

No data were available to the Working Group.

1.2 Production and use

1.2.1 Production

CI Pigment Red 3 was first prepared in 1905. It is manufactured by diazotization of 2-nitro-*para*-toluidine and coupling the resultant diazonium salt with 2-naphthol (Stubbs, 1973; Society of Dyers and Colourists, 1982; Green, 1990).

Approximate US production of CI Pigment Red 3 was 1430 tonnes in 1950, 930 tonnes in 1960, 780 tonnes in 1970, 754 tonnes in 1975, 460 tonnes in 1980, 380 tonnes in 1985 and 350 tonnes in 1990 (Stubbs, 1973; US International Trade Commission, 1977, 1981, 1986, 1991).

1.2.2 Use

CI Pigment Red 3 is one of the most widely used of all red pigments because of its bright scarlet hue, high tinctorial strength and good stability to acids, alkalis and light. Some limitation is imposed by its relatively poor fastness to organic solvents. It is widely used in paints and printing inks. Other uses have included synthetic resin lacquers and leather finishes, inks for foil and tinplate printing, paper coating and dyeing, wallpaper, linoleum, carbon papers, typewriter ribbons, artists' materials and textile printing. It has been used in rubber, plastics and cement (Society of Dyers and Colourists, 1971; Stubbs, 1973; Green, 1990).

1.3 Occurrence

1.3.1 Natural occurrence

CI Pigment Red 3 is not known to occur as a natural product.

1.3.2 Occupational exposure

No data were available to the Working Group.

The US Environmental Protection Agency, the American Textile Manufacturers Institute and the Ecological and Toxicological Association of the Dyestuffs Manufacturing Industry conducted a joint survey in 1986–87 to estimate airborne concentrations of dye dust in dye weighing rooms of industrial plants where powder dyes are used in the dyeing and printing of textiles. The survey was based on a sample of 24 sites chosen at random from among textile plants where powder dyes are weighed. Although CI Pigment Red 3 was not among the dyes included in the survey, the results are considered to be representative of dye dust levels during weighing of this type of powder dye. The mean airborne concentration of active colourant in the plants monitored was estimated to be 0.085 mg/m^3 (US Environmental Protection Agency, 1990).

On the basis of a survey conducted in the USA between 1981 and 1983, the US National Institute for Occupational Safety and Health estimated that a total of 51 931 workers, including 11 615 women, were potentially exposed to CI Pigment Red 3 in 57 industries (US National Library of Medicine, 1992).

1.4 Regulations and guidelines

CI Pigment Red 3 is allowed for use exclusively in cosmetic products intended to come into contact only briefly with the skin (Commission of the European Communities, 1976, 1986, 1990).

CI Pigment Red 3 (D&C Red No. 35) was cancelled for use in foods, drugs or cosmetics in the USA in 1966 (US Food and Drug Administration, 1992).

2. Studies of Cancer in Humans

No data were available to the Working Group.

3. Studies of Cancer in Experimental Animals

3.1 Oral administration

3.1.1 *Mouse*

Groups of 50 male and 50 female B6C3F$_1$ mice, six weeks old, were fed 0, 12 500, 25 000 or 50 000 mg/kg of diet (ppm) CI Pigment Red 3 (purity > 97%) in the diet for 103 weeks. At the end of the experiment (110 weeks), 33/50 control, 28/50 low-dose, 31/50 mid-dose and 33/50 high-dose males, and 39/50 control, 37/50 low-dose, 31/50 mid-dose and 25/50 high-dose females ($p < 0.001$) were still alive. Renal-cell adenomas occurred at a significantly higher incidence in high-dose male mice than in controls (control, 0/50; low-dose, 0/50; mid-dose, 0/50; high-dose, 6/50; $p = 0.017$, logistic regression test); and follicular-cell adenoma of the thyroid gland occurred with a positive trend in male mice (control, 0/50; low-dose, 0/49; mid-dose, 1/50; high-dose, 5/50; $p = 0.001$, logistic regression trend test) (US National Toxicology Program 1992).

3.1.2 *Rat*

Groups of 50 male and 50 female Fischer 344/N rats, six weeks old, were fed 0, 6000, 12 500 or 25 000 ppm (mg/kg) CI Pigment Red 3 (purity > 97%) in the diet for 103 weeks. At the end of the experiment (110 weeks), 28/50 control, 40/50 low-dose, 28/50 mid-dose and 20/50 high-dose males, and 32/50 control, 41/50 low-dose, 39/50 mid-dose and 40/50 high-dose females were still alive. In male rats, the incidence of benign adrenal phaeochromocytomas was significantly increased in the mid- and high-dose groups compared to controls (control, 22/50; low-dose, 29/50; mid-dose, 35/50; high-dose, 34/50; $p = 0.004$, logistic regression trend test). In female rats, hepatocellular adenomas occurred with a positive trend, with a significantly greater incidence in the high-dose group than in the control group (control, 0/50; low-dose, 0/50; mid-dose, 1/50; high-dose, 10/50; $p = 0.001$, logistic regression test) (US National Toxicology Program, 1992).

4. Other Relevant Data

4.1 Absorption, distribution, metabolism and excretion

4.1.1 *Humans*

No data were available to the Working Group.

4.1.2 *Experimental systems*

The absorption of CI Pigment Red 3 (purity, 94.7 %) was studied in male Fischer 344 rats, seven to eight weeks of age, given the compound once at 11.8 mg/kg bw suspended in corn oil by gavage. Gut contents, faeces and various tissues were extracted 1, 4, 24 and 48 h after dosing and the amount of parent compound present was determined. None was found in blood, liver or kidneys, and it was concluded that the compound is not absorbed from the intestinal tract. Recovery after 48 h was 72.4% of the dose, suggesting that the compound may be partly degraded by intestinal bacteria. [The Working Group noted that absorption of cleavage products or metabolites was not analysed.]

4.2 Toxic effects

4.2.1 *Humans*

CI Pigment Red 3 has been associated with contact dermatitis following cosmetic use (Sugai *et al.*, 1977).

4.2.2 *Experimental systems*

CI Pigment Red 3 (purity greater than 97%) was tested for toxicity in groups of five (14-day study) and 10 male and 10 female Fischer 344 rats and B6C3F$_1$ mice in a range-finding study for carcinogenicity testing (Morgan *et al.*, 1989; US National Toxicology Program, 1992). The compound was mixed into the feed at concentrations of 0, 6000, 12 500, 25 000, 50 000 or 100 000 ppm (mg/kg) and administered for 14 days, or at concentrations of 0, 3000, 6000, 12 500, 25 000 or 50 000 ppm (mg/kg) and administered for 90 days. Female rats gained less weight than controls with all doses in both studies. The liver weight:body weight ratio increased significantly in male and female rats with all doses in both studies, and the kidney weight:body weight ratio in all males except the 6000 ppm group in the 90-day study. Body weight gains of mice treated for 90 days did not differ from those of controls. The haematocrit and haemoglobin concentrations were decreased in a dose-related manner in rats after 14 and 90 days, and reticulocytosis occurred at dose levels of 25 000 and 100 000 after 14 days and at all dose levels after 90 days in both males and females. These changes were observed to a lesser extent in mice. Histological lesions were seen in both species, which consisted of haematopoietic cell proliferation in the bone marrow, spleen, liver and kidney in the 90-day study.

4.3 Reproductive and prenatal effects

No data were available to the Working Group.

4.4 Genetic and related effects

4.4.1 *Humans*

No data were available to the Working Group.

4.4.2 *Experimental systems* (see also Table 1 and Appendices 1 and 2)

CI Pigment Red 3 was not mutagenic to *Salmonella typhimurium*, except in the presence of an exogenous metabolic system from hamster (but not rat) liver, when it was weakly mutagenic at precipitating doses. It did not induce sister chromatid exchange or chromosomal aberrations in cultured Chinese hamster ovary cells.

5. Summary of Data Reported and Evaluation

5.1 Exposure data

CI Pigment Red 3, one of the most widely used red pigments, is found in paints, inks, plastics, rubber and textiles.

5.2 Human carcinogenicity data

No data were available to the Working Group.

5.3 Animal carcinogenicity data

CI Pigment Red 3 was tested for carcinogenicity by administration in the diet in one study in mice and in one study in rats. In male mice, it induced follicular-cell adenomas of the thyroid and renal-cell adenomas. There was an increased incidence of adrenal phaeochromocytomas in male rats and of hepatocellular adenomas in female rats.

5.4 Other relevant data

CI Pigment Red 3 did not induce gene mutation in bacteria or sister chromatid exchange or chromosomal aberrations in cultured mammalian cells.

5.5 Evaluation[1]

There is *inadequate evidence* in humans for the carcinogenicity of CI Pigment Red 3.

There is *limited evidence* in experimental animals for the carcinogenicity of CI Pigment Red 3.

---

[1]For definition of the italicized terms, see Preamble, pp. 26–30.

Table 1. Genetic and related effects of CI Pigment Red 3

Test system	Result		Dose[a] (LED/HID)	Reference
	Without exogenous metabolic system	With exogenous metabolic system		
SA0, *Salmonella typhimurium* TA100, reverse mutation	–	–	500.0000	Miyagoshi *et al.* (1983)
SA0, *Salmonella typhimurium* TA100, reverse mutation	–	–[b]	167.0000[c]	Mortelmans *et al.* (1986)
SA5, *Salmonella typhimurium* TA1535, reverse mutation	–	–	167.0000[c]	Mortelmans *et al.* (1986)
SA7, *Salmonella typhimurium* TA1537, reverse mutation	–	–	167.0000[c]	Mortelmans *et al.* (1986)
SA9, *Salmonella typhimurium* TA98, reverse mutation	–	–	500.0000	Miyagoshi *et al.* (1983)
SA9, *Salmonella typhimurium* TA98, reverse mutation	–	–[b]	167.0000[c]	Mortelmans *et al.* (1986)
SIC, Sister chromatid exchange, Chinese hamster ovary cells *in vitro*	–	–	160.0000	US National Toxicology Program (1992)
CIC, Chromosomal aberrations, Chinese hamster ovary cells *in vitro*	–	–	160.0000	US National Toxicology Program (1992)

–, negative

[a]In-vitro tests, µg/ml; in-vivo tests, mg/kg bw

[b]Negative with rat liver S9, weakly positive with hamster liver S9 at precipitating doses

[c]Higher doses contained precipitate

Overall evaluation

CI Pigment Red 3 *cannot be classified as to its carcinogenicity to humans (Group 3).*

6. References

Aldrich Chemical Co. (1992) *Aldrich Catalog/Handbook of Fine Chemicals 1992–1993*, Milwaukee, WI, p. 1203

BASF Corp. (1991) *Material Safety Data Sheet: SICO Red NB L 3740 (Pigment Red 3)*, Parsippany, NJ

Commission of the European Communities (1976) Council Directive 76/768/EEC of 27 July 1976. *Off. J. Eur. Commun.*, **L262**, 169–200

Commission of the European Communities (1986) Commission Directive 86/179/EEC of 28 February 1986 (Seventh Adaptation to Technical Progress of Council Directive 76/768/EEC of 27 July 1976). *Off. J. Eur. Commun.*, **L138**, 40

Commission of the European Communities (1990) Proposal for a Council Directive on the approximation of the laws of the Member States relating to cosmetic products. *Off. J. Eur. Commun.*, **C322**, 29–77

El Dareer, S.M, Tillery, K.F. & Hill, D.L. (1984) Investigations on the disposition of oral doses of some water-insoluble pigments. *Bull. environ. Contam. Toxicol.*, **32**, 171–174

Green, F.J. (1990) *The Sigma-Aldrich Handbook of Stains, Dyes and Indicators*, Milwaukee, WI, Aldrich Chemical Co., p. 716

Miyagoshi, M., Hayakawa, Y. & Nagayama, T. (1983) Studies on the mutagenicity of cosmetic azo-dyes. *Eisei Kagaku (J. hyg. Chem.)*, **29**, 212–220

Morgan, D.L., Jameson, C.W., Mennear, J.H. & Prejean, J.D. (1989) 14-Day and 90-day toxicity studies of CI Pigment Red 3 in Fischer 344 rats and B6C3F$_1$ mice. *Food Chem. Toxicol.*, **27**, 793–800

Mortelmans, K., Haworth, S., Lawlor, T., Speck, W., Tainer, B. & Zeiger, E. (1986) *Salmonella* mutagenicity tests II. Results from the testing of 270 chemicals. *Environ. Mutag.*, **8** (Suppl. 7), 1–119

Pouchert, C.J. (1981) *The Aldrich Library of Infrared Spectra*, 3rd ed., Milwaukee, WI, Aldrich Chemical Co., p. 1456

Sadtler Research Laboratories (1980) *Sadtler Standard Spectra, 1980 Cumulative Index*, Philadelphia, PA

Sadtler Research Laboratories (1991) *Sadtler Standard Spectra, 1981–1991 Supplementary Index*, Philadelphia, PA

Society of Dyers and Colourists (1971) *Colour Index*, 3rd ed., Vol. 3, Bradford, Yorkshire, pp. 3298–3299

Society of Dyers and Colourists (1982) *Colour Index*, 3rd ed., *Pigments and Solvent Dyes*, Bradford, Yorkshire, p. 284

Stubbs, D.H. (1973) Toluidine, para and chlornitraniline reds. In: Patton, T.C., ed., *Pigment Handbook*, Vol. 1, *Properties and Economics*, New York, John Wiley & Sons, pp. 461–472

Sugai, T., Takahashi, Y. & Takagi, T. (1977) Pigmented cosmetic dermatitis and coal tar dyes. *Contact Derm.*, **3**, 249–256

US Environmental Protection Agency (1990) *Textile Dye Weighing Monitoring Study* (EPA Report No. EPA-560/5-90-009, Main Report and Site Visit Reports), Washington DC, Office of Toxic Substances

US Food and Drug Administration (1992) Cancellation of certificates. *US Code fed. Regul.*, **21**, part 81.30, pp. 366–369

US International Trade Commission (1977) *Synthetic Organic Chemicals, US Production and Sales, 1975* (USITC Publication 804), Washington DC, US Government Printing Office, p. 79

US International Trade Commission (1981) *Synthetic Organic Chemicals, US Production and Sales, 1980* (USITC Publication 1183), Washington DC, US Government Printing Office, p. 103

US International Trade Commission (1986) *Synthetic Organic Chemicals, US Production and Sales, 1985* (USITC Publication 1892), Washington DC, US Government Printing Office, p. 87

US International Trade Commission (1991) *Synthetic Organic Chemicals, US Production and Sales, 1990* (USITC Publication 2470), Washington DC, US Government Printing Office, p. 5-2

US National Library of Medicine (1992) *Registry of Toxic Effects of Chemical Substances* (RTECS No. QK4247000), Bethesda, MD

US National Toxicology Program (1992) *Toxicology and Carcinogenesis Studies of CI Pigment Red 3 (CAS No. 2425-85-6) in F344/N Rats and B6C3F$_1$ Mice (Feed Studies)* (NTP TR 407; NIH Publ. No. 92-3138), Research Triangle Park, NC, US Department of Health and Human Services

AROMATIC AMINES

4,4'-METHYLENEBIS(2-CHLOROANILINE) (MOCA)

This substance was evaluated by previous working groups, in 1973 (IARC, 1974) and 1987 (IARC, 1987a). Since that time, new data have become available, and these have been incorporated into the monograph and taken into consideration in the evaluation.

1. Exposure Data

1.1 Chemical and physical data

1.1.1 *Synonyms, structural and molecular data*

Chem. Abstr. Serv. Reg. No.: 101-14-4; replaces 29371-14-0; 51065-07-7; 78642-65-6
Chem. Abstr. Name: 4,4'-Methylenebis(2-chlorobenzenamine)
IUPAC Systematic Name: 4,4'-Methylenebis(2-chloroaniline)
Synonyms: Bis(4-amino-3-chlorophenyl)methane; bis(3-chloro-4-aminophenyl)methane; 3,3'-dichloro-4,4'-diaminodiphenylmethane; MBOCA; methylenebis(3-chloro-4-aminobenzene); 4,4'-methylenebis(*ortho*-chloroaniline)

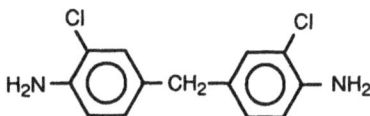

$C_{13}H_{12}Cl_2N_2$ Mol. wt: 267.16

1.1.2 *Chemical and physical properties*

From American Conference of Governmental Industrial Hygienists (1990a), unless otherwise noted

   (a) *Description*: Light-brown (technical material) to colourless crystalline (pure compound) (Anon., 1985) solid with a faint amine-like odour
   (b) *Melting-point*: 100–109 °C
   (c) *Specific gravity*: 1.44 at 4 °C
   (d) *Spectroscopy data*: Infrared, ultraviolet and nuclear magnetic resonance spectral data have been reported (Sadtler Research Laboratories, 1980; Pouchert, 1981; Sadtler Research Laboratories, 1991).
   (e) *Solubility*: Slightly soluble in water (13.9 mg/l) (Voorman & Penner, 1986); very soluble in benzene, diethyl ether and ethanol. It is also soluble in (g/100 ml): trichloroethylene, 4.2; toluene, 7.5; ethoxyethyl acetate, 34.4; methyl ethyl ketone, 43.0; tetrahydrofuran, 55.5; dimethylformamide, 61.7; and dimethyl sulfoxide, 75.0

(f) *Vapour pressure*: 1.3×10^{-5} mm Hg [1.7 mPa] at 60 °C

(g) *Octanol/water partition coefficient (P)*: log P, 3.94 (US National Library of Medicine, 1992)

(h) *Conversion factor*: $mg/m^3 = 10.9 \times ppm$[1]

1.1.3 *Trade names, technical products and impurities*

Some trade names of MOCA are Bisamine S; Bisamine A, Cuamine M; Cuamine MT; Curalin M, Curalon M; Curene 442; Diamet Kh; LD 813; Millionate M; Quodorole

Commercial-grade MOCA was originally offered in flake form, for a short period in the 1960s; it is currently available as granules (prill), pellets (pastilles) and as a liquid mixture premixed with polyhydric alcohols (polyols). It is available at a purity of 99.7–99.8%, with 2-chloroaniline as a typical impurity (0.1–0.3% by weight) (PEDCo Environmental, 1984; Anon, 1985; Palmer Davis Seika, 1992; US National Library of Medicine, 1992; Ihara Chemical Industry Co., undated).

1.1.4 *Analysis*

Several methods for the analysis of MOCA in various matrices are presented in Table 1. The method of the US National Institute for Occupational Safety and Health (1990) for 4,4′-methylenedianiline can also be used for the analysis of MOCA in air.

MOCA is excreted primarily as a heat-labile glucuronide metabolite; very little is eliminated as acetylated metabolites. The latter can be hydrolysed to the parent compound by heating under acidic conditions (Linch *et al.*, 1971; Ward *et al.*, 1986; Cocker *et al.*, 1988, 1990). In order to detect unmetabolized MOCA and the glucuronide conjugate in urine samples, heat hydrolysis should be performed before analysis (Cocker *et al.*, 1990; Lowry & Clapp, 1992). MOCA detected without hydrolysis is referred to as 'free' MOCA.

1.2 Production and use

1.2.1 *Production*

The manufacture of MOCA is based on the reaction of formaldehyde (see IARC, 1982a, 1987b) and 2-chloroaniline (Anon., 1985).

MOCA was developed and marketed in the mid-1950s and was first reported to the US Tariff Commission in 1956 (US Tariff Commission, 1957). It was manufactured by two companies in the USA, both of which had ceased production by 1980. US production started at approximately 500 tonnes per year and was estimated to have reached 1500 tonnes by 1970. Since 1980, all MOCA used in the USA has been imported from Japan (Ward *et al.*, 1987) and Taiwan. There are currently approximately 100 industrial users of MOCA in the USA.

---

[1]Calculated from: $mg/m^3 = $ (molecular weight/24.45) $\times$ ppm, assuming normal temperature (25 °C) and pressure (760 mm Hg [101.3 kPa])

Table 1. Methods for the analysis of MOCA

Sample matrix	Sample preparation	Assay procedure	Limit of detection	Reference
Air	Adsorb on silica gel; desorb with methanol	HPLC/UV	3 μg/m^3	Taylor (1977)
	Collect on glass fibre filter; extract with methanol	HPLC/ECD	100 ng/m^3	Purnell & Warwick (1981)
	Collect on acid-treated glass, extract with toluene; derivatize with heptafluoro-butyric anhydride	GC/ECD	440 ng/m^3	US Occupational Safety and Health Administration (1988)
Prepolymer	Dissolve in a solution of tetrahydrofuran saturated with ammonia or of dioxane	HPLC/UV	NR	Becker et al. (1974)
Polymer	Extract with toluene; concentrate and react with trifluoroacetic anhydride	GC	NR	Becker et al. (1974)
	Extract with toluene	HPLC/UV	NR	Becker et al. (1974)
Soil	Filter aqueous extract; preconcentrate on reverse-phase chromatography column	HPLC/ECD	≤ 1 μg/kg	Rice & Kissinger (1981)
Urine	Adjust pH to > 12; extract with diethyl ether:hexane solution; convert to hepta-fluorobutyryl derivative with heptafluoro-butyric anhydride	GC/ECD	1 μg/l	Eller (1985)
	Adjust pH to 9.5; extract with diethyl ether; wash, dry, concentrate and purify by TLC; extract and convert to trifluoro-acetyl derivative	GC/FID	1 μg/l	Van Roosmalen et al. (1981)
	Clean up sample, extract with dichloro-methane	HPLC/PCD	1 μg/l	Ducos et al. (1985); Lowry & Clapp (1992)
	Extract with acetonitrile; precolumn enrichment	HPLC/UV HPLC/ECD	20 ng 2.2 ng	Trippel-Schulte et al. (1986)
	Alkaline hydrolysis at 95 °C; extract with hexane	HPLC/UV	1 ng (10 μg/l)	McKerrell et al. (1987)
	Hydrolyse at 80 °C; extract with diethyl ether; derivatize with heptafluorobutyryl chloride	GC/MS	NR	Cocker et al. (1990)
	Preserve sample with citric acid; alkalize sample to pH 12; extract with diethyl ether:hexane; derivatize with penta-fluoropropionic anhydride	GC/ECD	1 μg/l	US National Institute for Occupational Safety and Health (1984)
Water	Filter sample; preconcentrate on reverse-phase chromatography column	LC/ECD	≤ 1 μg/l	Rice & Kissinger (1981)

Abbreviations: HPLC/UV, high-performance liquid chromatography/ultraviolet detection; HPLC/ECD, high-performance liquid chromatography/electrochemical detection; GC/ECD, gas chromatography/electron capture detection; NR, not reported; GC/FID, gas chromatography/flame ionization detection; TLC, thin-layer chromatography; HPLC/PCD, high-performance liquid chromatography/photoconductivity detection; GC/MS, gas chromatography/mass spectrometry; LC/ECD, liquid chromatography/elctrochemical detection

Only one firm in the United Kingdom has manufactured MOCA. In 1979, about 100 tonnes of MOCA were used in about 70 factories; by 1983, only 36 industrial users of MOCA had been identified, and the number of workers exposed was about 200 (Locke, 1986). MOCA is no longer manufactured in the United Kingdom.

In 1972, world production was about 3300 tonnes (Will *et al.*, 1981). Currently, there are three major producers in the world: two in Japan and one in Taiwan. In the early 1980s, Japan produced approximately 2000 tonnes of MOCA per year; in the mid-1980s, the level was 3000 tonnes; and by the early 1990s, the level was approximately 3600 tonnes. Japan exports 40–60% of its production, approximately 900–1000 tonnes going to the USA, 450 to Europe and 450 to Southeast Asia, Canada, Brazil, South Africa and Australia. Taiwan currently produces 1000 tonnes per year, with 450 tonnes exported to Japan and 45–90 tonnes to the USA. Small quantities may also be produced in the Republic of Korea and France (Chemical Information Services, 1991).

1.2.2 *Use*

MOCA is used principally as a curing agent for polyurethane prepolymers in the manufacturing of high-performance, specialized, castable urethane rubber products (see IARC, 1982b, 1987c). Mouldings such as industrial tyres and rollers, shock absorption pads and conveyor belting are among the wide variety of uses (Anon., 1985; American Conference of Governmental Industrial Hygienists, 1990a). A use of MOCA that is specific to Japan and the Far East is as a curing agent in roofing and wood sealing.

1.3 Occurrence

1.3.1 *Natural occurrence*

MOCA is not known to occur as a natural product.

1.3.2 *Occupational exposure*

Occupational exposure to MOCA may occur through inhalation, ingestion and skin absorption: because of its low vapour, it can be inhaled as a dust when processed in a dry form; poor personal hygiene can allow contamination of the hands and ingestion while eating or smoking; however, the most likely route of exposure is thought to be by skin absorption after contact with contaminated surfaces (Linch *et al.*, 1971; Clapp *et al.*, 1991; Lowry & Clapp, 1992). Evaluations of sources of exposure have included sampling of air, work surfaces (e.g., wipe) and urine of potentially exposed workers.

Urinary levels as high as 25 000 μg/l were reported when MOCA was first produced in a full-scale commercial manufacturing plant in the USA in 1962; however, the analytical methods used were non-specific. By 1970, more specific analytical methods had been developed that involved acid hydrolysis of initial urine samples, and better work practices and engineering controls had been implemented. The average urinary level in four workers involved in pelletizing and packaging MOCA at the same plant was found by gas chromatography to be 695 μg/l (range, 70–1500 μg/l); personal air levels were generally below the detection limit of 10 μg/m^3, and the workers wore respirators. Average urinary concentrations in workers in MOCA production were 620 µg/l in 1969 and 250 µg/l in 1970, when local ventilation, fresh daily clothing, wash-down of the operating area twice daily and use of butyl rubber gloves were introduced. The authors concluded that inhalation was not the primary route of exposure (Linch *et al.*, 1971).

The extent of exposure to MOCA was determined in 19 factories in France during the early 1980s (Ducos *et al.*, 1985). In more than 340 analyses of urine from 150 workers, MOCA was present at below the detection limit of 0.5 µg/l up to levels of 1600 µg/l. The levels of 'free' MOCA, determined by high-performance liquid chromatography (HPLC) in urine samples in specific factories are presented in Table 2, which shows dramatic decreases in urinary levels after modifications in the handling of MOCA were instituted.

Table 2. Occupational exposure to MOCA in France

Process	Year surveyed	Before or after improvements	No. of samples/ workers	Urinary concentration (µg/l)	
				Mean	Range
Production of crystal MOCA (1 plant)	1982	Before	12 workers	600	
	1983	After	53 samples	46	20–62
Blending of solid MOCA with polyol (1 plant)	1982	Before	4 workers	318	75–940
	1983	After	3 workers	5	1–9
Production of urethane elastomers from solid pellets of MOCA or in solution (2 plants)	1982	Before	22 workers	100	43–156
	1984	After	25 workers	26	18–34

From Ducos *et al.* (1985)

In a plastics manufacturing and processing plant in Germany, 49 urine samples collected randomly from workers were found (using reversed-phase HPLC with ultraviolet detection) to contain between 15 (limit of detection) and 100 µg/l of 'free' MOCA. Concentrations in work place air were not determined (Will *et al.*, 1981).

In the United Kingdom, urine samples were taken from workers in a polyurethane plastics manufacturing company every month during 1978–82 (Thomas & Wilson, 1984). The process involved melting of pelletized MOCA before blending it with liquid polymer. After improvements designed to prevent exposures, urinary concentrations of 50 nmol/mmol creatinine [about 1300 µg/l] of 'free' MOCA were gradually reduced to less than 5 nmol/mmol creatinine [130 µg/l] by 1982.

In Japan, airborne levels and urinary concentrations of MOCA were determined (by HPLC with electrochemical detection) for five workers making polyurethane elastomer products (Ichikawa *et al.*, 1990). Average airborne concentrations of 0.2–0.5 µg/m^3 were measured over one week for four workers who transferred dry MOCA into a mixing vessel and processed elastomer tubes; a worker who poured hot elastomer mix was exposed to an average air concentration of 8.9 µg/m^3. The mean urinary concentrations at the end of each working day were 2.4–64.0 µg/g creatinine [about 4–120 µg/l] for the four workers and 96.6 µg/g creatinine [200 µg/l] for the worker who poured the mix [not specified whether 'free' or hydrolysed]. There was no significant difference between preshift and postshift urinary concentrations. It was estimated that only 0.5–5% of the total exposure was due to inhalation.

Monitoring of 'free' MOCA concentrations in urine, using non-specific thin-layer chromatography, was performed on a voluntary basis by several companies in the USA after 1978 (Lowry & Clapp, 1992); in 1984, the analysis was made more specific by introducing HPLC. Between 1980 and 1983, 3323 urinary samples were analysed from 54 companies: the MOCA levels exceeded 50 µg/l in 16.9% of all samples and exceeded 100 µg/l in 9.2% (Ward et al., 1987). In 1985, the urinary concentration exceeded 50 µg/l in 12% of all samples tested; in 1990, 8% of all samples exceeded that level (Lowry & Clapp, 1992).

In Western Australia, urinary levels of 'free' MOCA were determined by gas chromatography in workers in five of seven companies where MOCA was used in the manufacture of polyurethane polymers from 1984 onwards (Wan et al., 1989). The initial levels were at a geometric mean of 30 µg/l; after a training programme on the safe use of MOCA, the level was reduced to 10 µg/l.

Urinary levels of MOCA were reported at a plant in the USA which made cast polyurethane products (Clapp et al., 1991). Of 77 samples collected and analysed by HPLC, five contained more than 50 µg/l; all were from workers who mixed pelletized MOCA (Table 3). The level of MOCA in 40 samples of personal air was below the limit of detection (~ 0.02 µg/m^3) in 88%; in the remainder, the level was less than 1 µg/m^3.

Table 3. Distribution of urinary levels of MOCA in workers in a cast polyurethane products plant in the USA

Job	No. of workers	No. of samples with mean concentration of MOCA (µg/l urine)[a]					
		ND	< 5	5–50	50–100	> 100	Total
Mixer	2	0	0	5	3	2	10
Moulder	16	10	3	22	0	0	35
Clean-up man	1	1	0	3	0	0	4
Trimmer	3	4	0	0	0	0	4
Supervisor	2	5	0	0	0	0	5
Office employee	7	14	0	0	0	0	14

From Clapp et al. (1991); ND, not detected
[a]Normalized to specific gravity of 1.019; limit of detection, 5 µg/l

In an accidental exposure in the USA, a 30-year old male polyurethane moulder accidentally sprayed molten MOCA (approximately 3 gallons [11.4 l]) over his upper body and extremities, where it remained for several seconds. He was wearing trousers, a shirt with rolled-up sleeves, asbestos gloves, safety glasses and a respirator. He did not ingest any MOCA, and the duration of exposure was limited by removing his clothing, showering and washing gently within approximately 45 min of the initial exposure. Analysis of his urine 4 h after the exposure showed a peak concentration of 1700 µg/l; the urinary level remained above 100 µg/l for four days (Osorio et al., 1990). In a separate accident, a worker was sprayed in the face with hot liquid MOCA, some of which entered his mouth. His eyes and face were washed immediately. The urinary concentration was 3600 μg/l (1400 μg/g creatinine) 5 h after exposure (Hosein & Van Roosmalen, 1978).

A survey of the concentrations of MOCA on work surfaces during various operations in 39 plants representing 10–20% of all the polyurethane plants using MOCA in the USA is summarized in Table 4 (PEDCo Environmental, 1984).

Table 4. Surface contaminations during some processes involving MOCA in the USA

Process	No. of facilities	No. of samples	Mean surface concentration ($\mu g/100\ cm^2$)
Storage and manual transfer of solid MOCA to melting operations	18	37	847
Manual transfer of molten MOCA to mixing operation and mixing	8	9	1 650
Storage and manual transfer of liquid MOCA to mixing with other compounds	8	25	30
Manual mixing of liquid MOCA with other compounds	3	4	15 000

From PEDCo Environmental (1984)

1.3.3 *Water, sediments and soil*

Extensive environmental contamination with MOCA on several hundred hectares of land surrounding a MOCA plant was found in 1979 in Adrian, MI, USA. Levels up to several milligrams per kilogram were found in gardens and community recreation areas. MOCA was also found in the urine of factory workers and of young children living in the contaminated area (Keeslar, 1986). The concentrations in sediment samples collected from the lagoon used by the plant ranged from 1600 to 3800 ppm (mg/kg dry weight). Effluent water from the lagoon had a concentration of 250 ppb (μg/l), deep well-water from under the plant had a concentration of 1.5 ppb, and surface run-off water had a concentration of 1 ppb. Activated sludge from the sewage-treatment plant contained an estimated 18 ppm (mg/kg). MOCA was not detected in sewage-treatment plant influent or effluent water (detection limit, 0.5 ppb (μg/l)) or in the water of a river located near the plant (detection limit, 0.1 ppb) (Parris *et al.*, 1980; Verschueren, 1983; Fishbein, 1984).

MOCA is rapidly bound to the soil matrix and probably exists largely as covalent adducts. Some MOCA was metabolized by oxidation of the methylene bridge to a benzophenone derivative, 4,4'-diamino-3,3'-dichlorobenzophenone, presumably by microbial activity (Voorman & Penner, 1986).

1.4 Regulations and guidelines

Occupational exposure limits and guidelines for MOCA in some countries are presented in Table 5.

Table 5. Occupational exposure limits and guidelines for MOCA

Country	Year	Concentration (mg/m^3)	Interpretation	Classification as carcinogen
Australia		0.22 (s)	TWA	
Belgium		0.22 (s)	TWA	
Denmark				Yes
Finland		0.2 (s)	TWA	
		0.6 (s)	STEL	
France		0.22	TWA	
Germany				Yes
Italy	1978	0.22 (s)	TWA	
Mexico	1983	0.22 (s)	TWA	
Netherlands	1989	0.22 (s)	TWA	
Sweden				Yes
Switzerland	1992	0.02 (s)	TWA	
United Kingdom		0.005 (s)	TWA (MEL)	
USA				
ACGIH	1992	0.11 (s)[a]	TWA (TLV)	
NIOSH	1990	0.003	TWA (REL)	
OSHA	1990	0.22 (s)	TWA (PEL)	
Venezuela	1978	0.22 (s)	TWA	

From National Swedish Board of Occupational Safety and Health (1984); Health and Safety Executive (1985); Cook (1987); American Conference of Governmental Industrial Hygienists (ACGIH) (1990b, 1992); ILO (1991); Caisse Nationale Assurance (1992)

Abbreviations: TWA, time-weighted average; STEL, short-term exposure limit; MEL, maximum exposure level; TLV, threshold limit value; NIOSH, National Institute of Occupational Safety and Health; OSHA, Occupational Safety and Health Administration; REL, recommended exposure level; PEL, permissible exposure level; (s), skin notation

[a]Intended change to 0.11 mg/m^3 for 1992–93, with notation A$_2$, suspected human carcinogen (American Conference of Governmental Industrial Hygienists, 1992)

In the European Economic Community, MOCA is classified as a category 2 carcinogen, substances that should be regarded as if they were carcinogenic to man, and is labelled as R45 (may cause cancer) (Commission of the European Communities, 1967, 1991). Since MOCA may cause cancer, the Council Directive on protection of workers from risks related to exposure to carcinogens at work applies (Commission of the European Communities, 1990), which requires employers to replace carcinogenic agents or to take measures to prevent or reduce exposure.

In Germany, MOCA is classified with A$_2$ compounds, which are considered to have been proven to be carcinogenic only in animal experimentation but under conditions comparable to those of possible human exposure at the workplace (Deutsche Forschungsgemeinschaft, 1992). MOCA has been classified as a carcinogen in Denmark since 1976 (Arbejdstilsynet, 1977) and in the Netherlands since 1989.

The recommended maximum exposure level for MOCA in the United Kingdom was 200 µg/m^3 over 8 h, until 1979, when a control limit of 50 µg/m^3 was recommended. In 1984, after consideration of studies on MOCA, the control limit was lowered to 5 µg/m^3 (Locke, 1986). In Switzerland, the limit value for occupational exposure to MOCA was recently lowered from 0.22 mg/m^3 to 0.02 mg/m^3 (Caisse Nationale Assurance, 1992).

In the USA, the only biological exposure limit for MOCA is that of the State of California, of 100 µg/l in urine (State of California, 1992). The American Conference of Governmental Industrial Hygienists (1992) announced an intended change of the present time-weighted threshold limit value of 0.22 mg/m^3 to 0.11 mg/m^3 in 1992–93.

2. Studies of Cancer in Humans

2.1 Descriptive studies

Up to 1971, a total of 209 employees had had potential contact with MOCA in the Chambers Works, New Jersey, USA, where manufacture began in 1954 (Linch et al., 1971). No case of cancer of the bladder was mentioned in the medical records of the company.

In a review, Cartwright (1983) reported that a cohort study was under way in a plant where MOCA was manufactured and where 13 new cases of bladder cancer had occurred within a period of a few years. The number was stated as being far larger than that which would be expected.

A study was undertaken in a small plant in Michigan, USA, where MOCA had been produced between 1968 and 1979. All 532 workers employed in 1968–79 and an additional 20 workers first employed in 1980 and 1981 who had had possible exposure owing to contamination of the plant site were included (Ward et al., 1988, 1990). The median duration of employment was 3.2 months. The workers may have been heavily exposed, since urinary levels of MOCA several months after production had ceased were reported to have ranged up to 50 000 µg/l. The workers had not been exposed to benzidine or β-naphthylamine. Of the 552 predominantly white (89.5%) workers, 452 participated in a telephone interview in 1981 and 385 participated in a urine screening examination. Three asymptomatic bladder tumours were identified. After a 28-year-old worker was diagnosed with a noninvasive papillary transitional-cell tumour, the screening procedure was supplemented for some workers with cystoscopy. A second worker, aged 29 years, was diagnosed with a papillary bladder neoplasm, and, in a subsequent round of screening, a third, 44-year-old worker was diagnosed with a papillary transitional-cell carcinoma of the bladder. The expected number of bladder tumours could not be calculated, as no valid comparison rates of asymptomatic bladder tumours were available.

3. Studies of Cancer in Experimental Animals

3.1 Oral administration

3.1.1 *Mouse*

Groups of 25 male and 25 female HaM/ICR mice, six to eight weeks old, were fed diets containing 0, 1000 or 2000 mg/kg of diet (ppm) MOCA as the hydrochloride (97% pure) for

18 months. Surviving animals were killed 24 months after the start of the study; about 55% of the control and treated mice were still alive at 20–22 months. The effective numbers of animals at the end of the study were: males—control, 18; low-dose, 13; high-dose, 20; females—control, 20; low-dose, 21; high-dose, 14. Haemangiomas or haemangiosarcomas (mainly subcutaneous) combined occurred in 0/18 control, 3/13 low-dose and 8/20 high-dose male mice. 'Hepatomas' occurred in 0/20 control, 9/21 low-dose and 7/14 high-dose female mice ($p < 0.01$, Fisher exact test). The incidence of lymphosarcomas and reticulum-cell sarcomas was decreased in treated females. The authors stated that the incidence of vascular tumours in the high-dose animals was comparable to that in historical controls of the same strain (Russfield et al., 1975).

3.1.2 Rat

Groups of 25 male and 25 female Wistar rats, 100 days [14 weeks] of age, were fed 0 or 1000 mg/kg of diet (ppm) MOCA [purity unspecified] in a protein-deficient diet [not otherwise specified] for 500 days [71 weeks] [total dose, 27 g/kg bw], followed by an observation period on protein-deficient diet. Animals were killed when moribund; mean survival of treated males and females was 565 days [81 weeks] and 535 days [76 weeks], respectively, and mean survival of male and female controls on a similar diet was 730 days [104 weeks]. Of the 25 treated males, 23 died with tumours; 'hepatomas' occurred in 22/25 [$p < 0.001$, Fisher exact test], and lung tumours (mainly carcinomas) in 8/25 [$p = 0.002$, Fisher exact test]. Among the treated females, 20 rats died with tumours; 'hepatomas' occurred in 18/25 [$p < 0.001$ Fisher exact test], and lung tumours were observed in 5/25 [$p = 0.025$, Fisher exact test]. No 'hepatoma' or lung tumour was observed among control animals (Grundmann & Steinhoff, 1970).

Groups of 25 male Charles River CD-1 rats, six to eight weeks old, were administered diets containing 0, 500 or 1000 mg/kg of diet (ppm) MOCA as the hydrochloride (97% pure) for 18 months. All surviving animals were killed 24 months after the start of the study; about 55% of the control and treated animals were still alive at 20–22 months. The effective numbers were: 22 control, 22 low-dose and 19 high-dose animals. 'Hepatomas' occurred in 0/22 control, 1/22 low-dose and 4/19 high-dose rats [$p < 0.05$, Cochran-Armitage trend test] (Russfield et al., 1975). [The Working Group noted the small number of animals used in the study.]

Groups of 50 males and 50 female Charles River CD rats, 36 days [5 weeks] of age were administered 0 (control) or 1000 mg/kg of diet (ppm) MOCA ($\sim 95\%$ pure) in a standard diet (23% protein) for life. The average duration of the experiment was 560 days [80 weeks] for treated males, 548 days [78 weeks] for treated females, 564 days [80 weeks] for male controls and 628 days [89 weeks] for female controls. Six animals from each group were sacrificed at one year for interim evaluation. Lung adenocarcinomas occurred in 21/44 ($p < 0.05$, χ^2 test) treated males and 27/44 ($p < 0.05$, χ^2 test) treated females. An additional squamous-cell carcinoma of the lung was observed in one treated male and one treated female. No lung tumour was observed among control animals. Lung adenomatosis, considered to be a preneoplastic lesion, developed in 14/44 treated males and 11/44 treated females and in 1/44 male controls and 1/44 female controls ($p < 0.05$). Pleural mesotheliomas occurred in 4/44 treated males and 2/44 treated females; no such tumour was observed among controls.

Hepatocellular adenomas and hepatocellular carcinomas occurred in 3/44 and 3/44 treated males and in 2/44 and 3/44 treated females, respectively, but not in controls. Ingestion of MOCA resulted in a lower incidence of pituitary tumours in treated females than in controls (1/44 *versus* 12/44) (Stula *et al.*, 1975).

In the same study, another 25 males and 25 females were administered 0 (control) or 1000 ppm MOCA ($\sim$ 95% pure) in a low-protein diet (7%) for 16 months. Six animals from each group were sacrificed at one year for interim evaluation. The average duration of the experiment was 400 days [57 weeks] for treated males, 423 days [60 weeks] for treated females, 384 days [55 weeks] for control males and 466 days [66 weeks] for control females. Lung adenocarcinomas occurred in 5/21 treated males ($p < 0.05$, χ^2 test) and 6/21 females ($p < 0.05$, χ^2 test); no such tumour developed in 21 untreated male or female controls. Hepatocellular adenomas occurred in 5/21 treated males ($p < 0.05$, χ^2 test) and 2/21 treated females; hepatocellular carcinomas were observed in 11/21 treated males ($p < 0.05$, χ^2 test) and 1/21 treated females; no hepatocellular tumour was observed among 21 untreated males or females. Fibroadenomas of the mammary gland occurred in 1/21 treated and 7/21 control female rats ($p < 0.05$). Mammary gland adenocarcinomas developed in 6/21 treated female rats and in 0/21 untreated females ($p < 0.05$, χ^2 test) (Stula *et al.*, 1975).

Groups of 100, 100, 75 and 50 male Charles River CD rats, 35 days [5 weeks] of age, were fed either a 'protein-adequate' (27%) diet containing 0, 250, 500 or 1000 mg/kg of diet (ppm) MOCA (industrial grade [purity unspecified]) or a 'protein-deficient' (8%) diet containing 0, 125, 250 and 500 ppm MOCA for 18 months followed by a 32-week observation period. Animals were sacrificed at 104 weeks. Administration of MOCA was associated with decreased survival in both groups: mean survival time (weeks) was: 'protein-adequate' diet: control, 89; low-dose, 87; mid-dose, 80 ($p < 0.01$); high-dose, 65 ($p < 0.001$); 'protein-deficient' diet: control, 87; low-dose, 81; mid-dose, 79; high-dose, 77 ($p < 0.05$). The numbers of rats on the 'protein-adequate' diet still alive at week 104 were: control, 20/100; low-dose, 14/100; mid-dose, 10/75; and high-dose, 0/50 (at 84 weeks, there were six surviving rats). The numbers of animals on the 'protein-deficient' diet still alive at week 104 were: control, 34/100; low-dose, 22/100; mid-dose, 14/75; and high-dose, 5/50. MOCA induced several tumour types in both groups; the incidences of the predominant tumours are shown in Table 6. Dose-related increases in the incidences of lung tumours, mammary adenocarcinomas, Zymbal gland carcinomas and hepatocellular carcinomas were observed in both experiments. The highest tumour incidence was observed in the lung. An increased incidence of haemangiosarcomas was observed only in the group on the 'protein-deficient' diet. In groups given 500 ppm MOCA, tumour incidence was generally lower in those fed 'protein-deficient' diet, but hepatocellular carcinomas and Zymbal gland carcinomas occurred at a higher incidence in this group (18 and 12%) than in the 'protein-adequate' group (4 and 7%). The incidence of pituitary adenomas decreased with increasing concentration of MOCA in the 'protein-adequate' diet, perhaps because of decreased survival in the treated groups (Kommineni *et al.*, 1978).

Table 6. Percentages of male rats with tumours at specific sites after feeding of MOCA in diets with different protein contents

Dietary protein	MOCA (ppm)	No. of rats autopsied	Lung adeno-carcinomas	All lung tumours	Mammary adenocarcinomas	Zymbal gland carcinomas	Hepatocellular carcinomas	Haemangio-sarcomas	Pituitary adenomas[a]
Adequate (27%)	0	100	0	1	1	1	0	2	42
	250	100	14***	23***	5	8*	3	4	36
	500	75	27***	37***	11**	7	4	4	25*
	1000	50	62***	70***	28***	22***	36***	0	4***
Deficient (8%)	0	100	0	0	0	0	0	1	23
	125	100	3	6**	1	0	0	2	16
	250	75	9**	15***	4	5*	0	5	12*
	500	50	16***	26***	6*	12***	18***	8*	20

From Kommineni et al. (1978); *, $p < 0.05$; **, $p < 0.01$; ***, $p < 0.001$

[a]Includes pituitary adenocarcinomas (0–2 per group)

3.1.3 Dog

A group of six female beagle dogs, approximately one year old, were administered a daily dose of 100 mg MOCA ($\sim$ 90%, $\sim$ 10% polyamines with a three-ring structure and $\sim$ 0.9% *ortho*-chloroaniline) by capsule on three days a week for six weeks, then on five days a week for up to nine years. A further group of six females served as untreated controls. One treated dog died early, at 3.4 years of age, because of intercurrent infection; the other animals were killed between 8.3 and nine years. Transitional-cell carcinomas of the urinary bladder occurred in four of five treated dogs, and a composite tumour (transitional-cell carcinoma/adenocarcinoma) of the urethra developed in one dog. No such tumour was observed among six untreated controls ($p < 0.025$, Fisher exact test) (Stula *et al.*, 1977).

3.2 Subcutaneous administration

Rat

In a study reported as a short communication, groups of 17 male and 17 female Wistar rats [age unspecified] were injected subcutaneously with 500 or 1000 mg/kg bw MOCA (94% pure) as a suspension in saline either once a week or at longer time intervals for 620 days [88 weeks] (total dose, 25 g/kg bw). The rats were fed a laboratory diet with a normal protein content. The mean observation period was 778 days [111 weeks]. A total of 22 animals developed 29 malignant tumours. Hepatocellular carcinomas occurred in 9/34 [$p < 0.0042$, Fisher exact test], and malignant lung tumours (six adenocarcinomas, one carcinoma) were observed in 7/34 [$p < 0.016$, Fisher exact test]. A malignant subcutaneous tumour [unspecified] was found in one rat [sex unspecified]. Among 25 male and 25 female untreated controls (mean observation period, 1040 days [148 weeks]), a total of 13 malignant tumours, including one lung tumour, developed; no hepatocellular carcinoma was observed (Steinhoff & Grundmann, 1971). [The Working Group noted the inadequate reporting of the experiment.]

4. Other Relevant Data

4.1 Absorption, distribution, metabolism and excretion

4.1.1 Humans

Biological monitoring of workers exposed to MOCA in factories where polyurethane plastics were manufactured showed levels of MOCA in urine that ranged from 1 to 1000 nmol/mmol creatinine (0.1–110 μM; 27–27 000 μg/l), with averages ranging from 5 to 50 nmol MOCA/mmol creatinine at different sampling periods (Thomas & Wilson, 1984; Cocker *et al.*, 1988; Edwards & Priestly, 1992). Exposure appeared to occur *via* both inhalation and skin absorption (Linch *et al.*, 1971; Ward *et al.*, 1986) (see also section 1.3.2). Assuming that MOCA levels in urine represent about 1% of the total absorbed and that spot urine sampling is indicative of 24-h urine collection (1.3 l urine per day), the calculated internal dose corresponding to 100 μg/l urine is 13 mg per day (Ward *et al.*, 1986); the internal doses of workers therefore range from 3.5 to 3500 mg per day [calculated by the Working Group from the data given above]. Studies on percutaneous absorption of MOCA through cultured neonatal foreskin showed rapid, time-dependent absorption (Chin *et al.*, 1983).

In the individual who was sprayed accidentally with molten MOCA (see p. 276), pharma-cokinetic analyses (one-compartment model) indicated a biological half-time of 23 h, with 94% elimination from the body in four days; 35% of the parent MOCA present in the urine was excreted as conjugates (Osorio *et al.*, 1990). High levels of MOCA (3.6 mg/l [13 μM]) were also found in the urine of another worker accidentally sprayed with MOCA (Hosein & Van Roosmalen, 1978; see pp. 276–277) 4 and 11 h after exposure. By 17 and 20 h, the levels had decreased to 0.03–0.06 mg/l [0.1–0.2 μM].

Urinary metabolites of MOCA detected in humans (Cocker *et al.*, 1990) include its *N*-acetyl derivative (1–9% of urinary MOCA in 10/23 individuals) (Cocker *et al.*, 1988) and its *N*-glucuronide (levels two- to three-fold higher than those of MOCA) (Cocker *et al.*, 1990). Urinary thioethers were not detected (Edwards & Priestly, 1992).

4.1.2 *Experimental systems*

Oxidative metabolism of [methylene-^{14}C]- and [aniline-^{14}C]MOCA (58 and 10.9 mCi/mmol, respectively [radiochemical purity unspecified]), by human liver microsomes has been demonstrated *in vitro*, resulting in the formation of its *N*-hydroxy(4-amino-4'-hydroxyl-amino-3,3'-dichlorodiphenylmethane), 6-hydroxy(5-hydroxy-4,4'-diamino-3,3'-dichlorodi-phenyl methane) and [methylene or C$^{4,4'}$]hydroxy(4,4'-diamino-3,3'-dichlorobenzhydrol) derivatives (see Fig. 1) (Morton *et al.*, 1988). In a survey of liver microsomes from 22 indivi-duals, the rate of *N*-oxidation of [methylene-^{14}C]MOCA (57 mCi/mmol; radiochemical purity, > 95%) varied by eight fold; *N*-hydroxy-MOCA was always the major metabolite, accounting for 81–94% of all the oxidation products (Butler *et al.*, 1989). Using antibodies and other inhibitors, substrate–activity correlations and purified or recombinant enzymes, cytochrome P450 3A4 was identified as the major enzyme that catalyses MOCA *N*-oxidation in human liver; a minor role for cytochrome P450 2A6 was shown (Yun *et al.*, 1992). It has been suggested that human and dog urinary bladder explant cultures metabolize MOCA, on the basis of the apparent covalent binding of ^{3}H-MOCA (30 Ci/mmol; radiochemical purity, 97%) to DNA (Shivapurkar *et al.*, 1987).

In male beagle-type mongrel dogs, ^{14}C-MOCA (58 mCi/mmol [radiochemical purity unspecified]) was applied to 25 cm^2 of shaved skin in 0.5 ml acetone or was injected intravenously in 0.5 ml propylene glycol at total doses of 10 mg per dog. By 24 h, urine collected through surgically implanted catheters contained 1.3% of the administered percutaneous dose (0.4% of which was unchanged MOCA) and 45% of the intravenous dose (0.54% of which was unchanged MOCA). Following intravenous injection, the time-course of disappearance of MOCA from the blood was rapid, with an apparent volume of distri-bution of 244 l and biphasic half-times of 0.09 and 0.70 h. After skin application, no radiolabel was measured in blood up to 24 h later. Biliary excretion was 0.62% of the dose after percutaneous administration and 32% after intravenous injection; none was unchanged MOCA. Tissue distribution was 10–20 times greater after intravenous dosing and was highest in liver, kidney, fat and lung tissues (Manis *et al.*, 1984). As with other carcinogenic aromatic amines, the major urinary metabolite of MOCA in dogs, accounting for 75% of the

Fig. 1. Oxidative metabolism of MOCA by liver microsomes

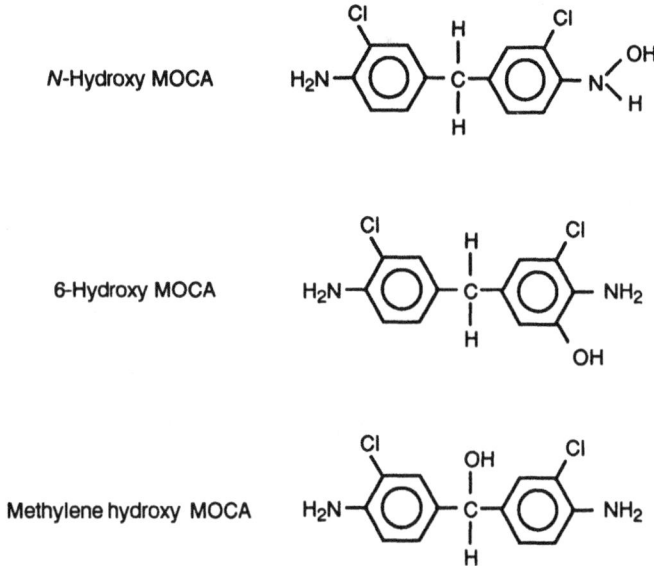

N-Hydroxy MOCA

6-Hydroxy MOCA

Methylene hydroxy MOCA

From Chen *et al.* (1989)

urinary radiolabel, was the sulfate conjugate of the *ortho*-hydroxy metabolite, 6-hydroxy-MOCA (5-hydroxy-3,3'-dichloro-4,4'-diaminodiphenyl methane-5-sulfate) (Manis & Braselton, 1984). The same major metabolite was detected in dog liver and kidney slices incubated with ^{14}C-MOCA [58 mCi/mmol, methylene-labelled; 10.9 mCi/mmol, aniline-labelled; radiochemical purity, > 99%]. An unknown glucoside and three glucuronide metabolites were also observed; and apparent covalent binding to DNA was measured, which was greater in liver than kidney (Manis & Braselton, 1986).

In female LAC:Porton rats, [methylene-^{14}C]MOCA (8.3 mCi/mmol [radiochemical purity unspecified]) was mixed with unlabelled MOCA in solutions of glycerol formol–arachis oil and given by intraperitoneal (1, 13 or 100 mg/kg bw) or oral administration (10 mg/kg bw). The urine contained 23–41% of the radiolabel after 48 h, of which 1–2% was unchanged MOCA, while faeces contained 60–69% of the administered dose. At least nine metabolites were observed in the urine. Tissue distribution of radiolabel after 48 h was highest in the liver, then fat > kidney, small intestine (Farmer *et al.*, 1981).

^{14}C-MOCA (58 mCi/mmol; radiochemical purity, > 98%) was injected intravenously to female Sprague-Dawley rats at a dose of 0.5 mg/kg bw in ethanol:Tween 80:water. After 48 h, 21 and 73% of the dose was excreted in urine and faeces, respectively. The levels of radiolabel were highest in liver, then in lung, kidney, fat and adrenal gland (Tobes *et al.*, 1983).

Male Sprague-Dawley rats given [methylene-^{14}C]MOCA (58 mCi/mmol; radiochemical purity, 96%) by gavage (11–12 mg/kg bw in propylene glycol) excreted 16.5% of the dose in the urine (0.25% as unchanged MOCA) and 70% in faeces after 72 h. Up to 2.54% was excreted in urine (0.008% as unchanged MOCA) and 2.11% in faeces after application of 2.5 mg MOCA in acetone to shaved skin (Groth et al., 1984). In 30-day old male Charles River CD rats, administration of [methylene-^{14}C]MOCA (4–7 mCi/mmol; radiochemical purity, ~ 93%) by gavage in dimethyl sulfoxide:water (60:40) at a dose of 5.5–5.6 mg per rat resulted in 16–27% of the label being excreted into urine (≤ 0.2% as unchanged MOCA) and 32–50% in faeces after 24 h. The major biliary metabolite was identified as MOCA N-glucuronide (Morton et al., 1988). Male Wistar rats given unlabelled recrystallized MOCA at a dose of 125 or 250 mg/kg intraperitoneally in peanut oil daily for five days excreted 'free' MOCA at a level of 1–6.5 μmol/mmol creatinine in urine 24 h after the last dose (Edwards & Priestly, 1992).

The half-times of MOCA in whole blood, lymphocytes, urinary bladder and liver of male Sprague-Dawley rats ranged from 4 to 17 days after a single oral dose (281 μmol [75 mg/kg bw]) of [methylene-^{14}C]MOCA (42.4 μCi/ml; radiochemical purity, > 99.5%) in corn oil. The order of covalent binding to DNA was liver > bladder > lymphocytes. Similar results were obtained after dermal application, except that adduct formation was approximately 100-fold less (Cheever et al., 1988, 1990). Multiple oral doses of 7.5 mg/kg bw for up to 28 days induced a linear increase in globin binding and half-times that were comparable to those seen after a single oral dose of 75 mg/kg; tissue levels of MOCA were highest in the liver, kidney and lung. Induction of cytochromes P450 by phenobarbital resulted in a three-fold increase in globin binding but a slight decrease in binding to liver. Intraperitoneal treatment resulted in three-fold higher binding levels in liver, globin and whole blood (Cheever et al., 1991). In a similar study with male Sprague-Dawley rats and English guinea-pigs, intraperitoneal injection of ^{14}C-MOCA (58 mCi/mmol [radiochemical purity unspecified]) in propylene glycol:dimethyl sulfoxide:saline (4:4:2) at 0.5–50 mg/kg to rats and subcutaneous injection of 5–500 mg/kg to rats and 4–100 mg/kg to guinea-pigs resulted in a nearly linear, dose-related increase in haemoglobin binding. β-Naphthoflavone but not phenobarbital pretreatment of rats was found to increase MOCA–haemoglobin adduct formation in vivo (Chen et al., 1991). In female Wistar rats dosed orally with 1, 3.8, 4.3, 66 and 134 mg/kg [aniline-^{14}C]MOCA (58 mCi/mmol; radiochemical purity, > 95%) or unlabelled MOCA in ethanol:propylene glycol (1:4), MOCA was bound in decreasing amounts to DNA, RNA and protein of lung, liver and kidney; 0.19% of the dose was bound to haemoglobin and 0.026% to serum albumin after 24 h. Alkaline hydrolysis of MOCA-bound haemoglobin released free MOCA (Sabbioni & Neumann, 1990), indicating the presence of a sulfinamide adduct derived from N-hydroxy-MOCA in the circulation and its oxidative conversion to a nitroso derivative in the erythrocytes. This assumption was confirmed by reactions of haemoglobin with either N-hydroxy-MOCA or its nitroso derivative in vitro and by the observation of high levels of haemoglobin binding after intravenous administration of N-hydroxy-MOCA (Chen et al., 1991).

Oxidative metabolism of [methylene-^{14}C]- and [aniline-^{14}C]MOCA (58 and 10.9 mCi/-mmol; radiochemical purity, > 99% (Chen et al., 1989) [or radiochemical purity unspecified (Morton et al., 1988)]) by rat, dog and guinea-pig liver microsomes has been demonstrated in vitro, resulting in formation of the N-hydroxy and 6-hydroxy derivatives. In rat and guinea-pig liver microsomes, N-hydroxy-MOCA appeared to be the major metabolite, whereas 6-

hydroxy-MOCA was predominant in dog liver microsomes. In rats, a methylene-hydroxy derivative was also found.

Using inducers, specific inhibitors and purified enzymes, cytochromes P450 2B1 (P450$_{PB-B}$) and P450 2B2 (P450$_{PB-D}$) were identified as the major enzymes that catalyse MOCA N-oxidation in rat liver; a minor role for cytochromes P450 1A2 (P450$_{ISF-G}$), P450 2C11 (P450$_{UT-A}$) and P450 1A1 (P450$_{BNF-B}$) was shown (Butler et al., 1989).

N-Glucuronidation of MOCA has been demonstrated in vitro with uridine diphosphoglucuronic acid-fortified liver microsomes from polychlorinated biphenyl-induced rats (Cocker et al., 1990). MOCA was metabolized rapidly by Bacillus megaterium and a Nocardiopsis species to N-acetyl, N,N'-diacetyl, N-hydroxy-N-acetyl and N-hydroxy-N,N'-diacetyl metabolites (Yoneyama & Matsumura, 1984) (see Fig. 2).

4.2 Toxic effects

4.2.1 Humans

Medical surveillance of workers with known exposure to MOCA revealed no acute toxicity; the methaemoglobinaemia syndrome, seen with exposures to other aromatic amines, was not observed (Linch et al., 1971). The individual who was sprayed with three gallons of molten MOCA (see p. 276) had an initial 'mild sunburn' sensation on the arms, but no further symptom was found in a two-week follow-up period. Renal and liver function tests were normal, and methaemoglobinemia, haematuria and proteinuria were not observed (Osorio et al., 1990). The initial responses in the worker sprayed in the face with MOCA (see pp. 276–277) were conjunctivitis, a burning sensation in the eyes and face and nausea (Hosein & Van Roosmalen, 1978).

4.2.2 Experimental systems

In a nine-year chronic study in dogs (Stula et al., 1977; see p. 283), elevated levels of plasma glutamic-pyruvic transaminase were noted during the first and last two years of treatment, accompanied by urinary changes indicative of genitourinary cancer after seven years.

MOCA also induces enzymes involved in drug metabolism and cell proliferation. Single intraperitoneal injections of technical-grade MOCA (purity, 90–100%) to male Sprague-Dawley rats at doses of 0.4–100 mg/kg bw in dimethyl sulfoxide resulted in dose-dependent increases in the levels of microsomal epoxide hydratase, ethoxyresorufin O-deethylase, ethoxycoumarin O-deethylase and glutathione S-transferase, but a decrease in aldrin epoxidase activity (Wu et al., 1989a). Ornithine decarboxylase, which regulates polyamine synthesis and cell division and is increased by tumour promoters, was strongly induced in male Sprague-Dawley rats 12 h after intraperitoneal injection of 75 mg/kg bw MOCA in corn oil; the level returned to control values after 42 h (Savage et al., 1992).

In primary cultures of rat hepatocytes, MOCA induced dose-dependent leakage of two intracellular enzymes, lactate dehydrogenase and glutamic-oxaloacetic transaminase (McQueen & Williams, 1982).

Fig. 2. Microbial metabolism of MOCA

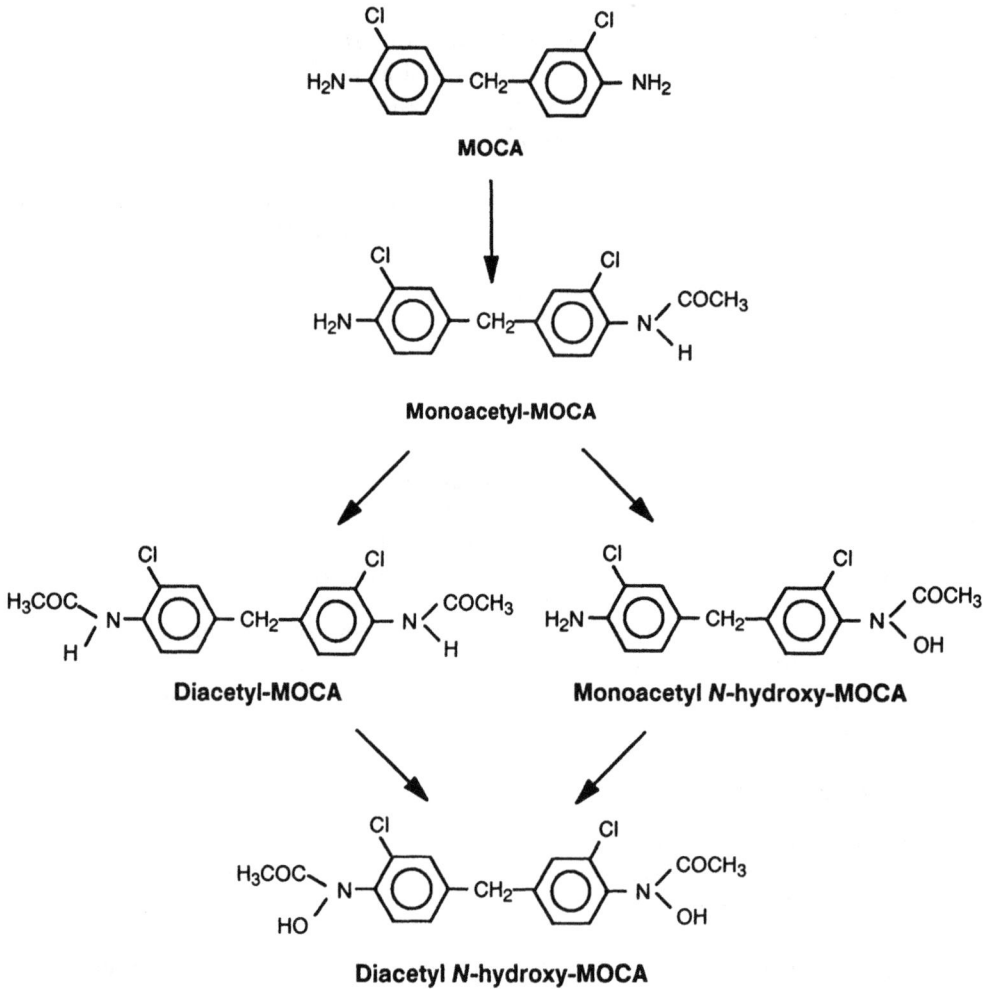

From Yoneyama and Matsumura (1984)

4.3 Reproductive and prenatal effects

No data were available to the Working Group.

4.4 Genetic and related effects

4.4.1 *Humans*

Exfoliated urothelial cells recovered from urine samples (Osorio *et al.*, 1990) provided by the worker accidentally sprayed with molten MOCA (see p. 276) at different times following exposure (up to 430 h) had a single, major DNA adduct, shown by ^{32}P-post-labelling and thin-layer chromatography to co-chromatograph with the known major N-hydroxy-MOCA–DNA adduct, N-(deoxyadenosine-8-yl)-4-amino-3-chlorobenzyl alcohol. The adduct was detected in cells from urine collected up to 98 h after initial exposure, but not thereafter (Kaderlik *et al.*, 1993). This finding is in agreement with the calculated biological half-time for MOCA in urine, 23 h, and the prediction that 94% of an initial dose will be eliminated within 96 h (Osorio *et al.*, 1990).

An increased frequency of sister chromatid exchange was seen in peripheral lymphocytes from a small number of workers exposed to MOCA in polyurethane manufacture (Edwards & Priestly, 1992).

4.4.2 *Experimental systems* (see also Table 7 and Appendices 1 and 2)

MOCA caused prophage induction in *Escherichia coli* and differential toxicity in *Bacillus subtilis rec*-deficient strains. It was mutagenic to *Salmonella typhimurium*, *Escherichia coli* and at the *tk* locus in mouse lymphoma L5178Y cells, but not to *Saccharomyces cerevisiae*. MOCA caused aneuploidy in *S. cerevisiae* but gave equivocal results with regard to gene conversion and did not induce mitotic crossing over in the same organism. It induced mutation in *Drosophila melanogaster* and unscheduled DNA synthesis in primary cultures of hepatocytes from mice, rats and Syrian hamsters. Sister chromatid exchange but not chromosomal aberration was induced in Chinese hamster ovary cells; and neither sister chromatid exchange nor chromosomal aberration was induced in human cells (abstract). MOCA induced cell transformation in mammalian cells and inhibited gap-junctional intercellular communication in cultured rat liver cells.

MOCA induced sister chromatid exchange in lymphocytes of rats treated *in vivo*. It formed adducts with DNA in cultured canine and human bladder cells, in the livers of rats treated topically or by intraperitoneal administration *in vivo* and in lung, liver and kidney following oral administration to rats. One of three HPLC peaks of an enzymatic digest of DNA derived from rats treated *in vivo* was identified tentatively as N-(deoxyadenosin-8-yl)-4-amino-3-chlorobenzyl alcohol (Silk *et al.*, 1989). Reaction of N-hydroxy[methylene-^{14}C]MOCA with DNA *in vitro* resulted in the formation of two major adducts, which were identified by mass spectroscopy as N-(deoxyadenosin-8-yl)-4-amino-3-chlorobenzyl alcohol and N-(deoxyadenosin-8-yl)-4-amino-3-chlorotoluene. The same adducts were formed *in vivo*: In rats given a single dose of 95 μmol/kg bw [methylene-^{14}C]MOCA by gavage, DNA adducts were found after 24 h at 7 pmol/mg DNA in liver, 2 pmol/mg in lung and 0.5 pmol/mg in kidney (Segerbäck & Kadlubar, 1992). MOCA also binds to RNA and proteins, including haemoglobin, in rats treated *in vivo*.

N-Hydroxy-MOCA was mutagenic to *S. typhimurium* TA98 and TA100 in the absence of an exogenous metabolic activation system but did not inhibit intercellular communication in cultured WB-F344 rat liver epithelial cells. Other MOCA metabolites, *ortho*-hydroxy-MOCA, 4-amino-3,3'-dichloro-4'-nitrosodiphenylmethane (mononitroso derivative) and di(3-chloro-4-nitrosophenyl)methane (dinitroso derivative), were not mutagenic to *S. typhimurium* TA98 or TA100. The mutagenic activity of the mononitroso derivative towards TA100, however, appeared to be masked by its toxicity (Kuslikis *et al.*, 1991).

Table 7. Genetic and related effects of MOCA

Test system	Result		Dose[a] (LED/HID)	Reference
	Without exogenous metabolic system	Wirh exogenous metabolic system		
PRB, Prophage λ induction, *Escherichia coli*	0	+	1000.0000	Thomson (1981)
BSD, *Bacillus subtilis rec* strains, differential toxicity	+	+	1000.0000	Kada (1981)
SAF, *Salmonella typhimurium*, forward mutation	0	+	50.0000	Bridges *et al.* (1981)
SA0, *Salmonella typhimurium* TA100, reverse mutation	0	+	50.0000	McCann *et al.* (1975)
SA0, *Salmonella typhimurium* TA100, reverse mutation	–	+	16.0000	Baker & Bonin (1981)
SA0, *Salmonella typhimurium* TA100, reverse mutation	–	+	12.5000	Brooks & Dean (1981)
SA0, *Salmonella typhimurium* TA100, reverse mutation	–	+	0.0000	Garner *et al.* (1981)
SA0, *Salmonella typhimurium* TA100, reverse mutation	–	+	10.0000	Hubbard *et al.* (1981)
SA0, *Salmonella typhimurium* TA100, reverse mutation	–	+	0.0000	Ichinotsubo *et al.* (1981)
SA0, *Salmonella typhimurium* TA100, reverse mutation	–	+	25.0000	MacDonald (1981)
SA0, *Salmonella typhimurium* TA100, reverse mutation	–	+	12.5000	Martire *et al.* (1981)
SA0, *Salmonella typhimurium* TA100, reverse mutation	–	+	25.0000	Nagao & Takahashi (1981)
SA0, *Salmonella typhimurium* TA100, reverse mutation	–	+	25.0000	Simmon & Shepherd (1981)
SA0, *Salmonella typhimurium* TA100, reverse mutation	–	+	25.0000	Venitt & Crofton-Sleigh (1981)
SA0, *Salmonella typhimurium* TA100, reverse mutation	–	+	17.0000[b]	Haworth *et al.* (1983)
SA0, *Salmonella typhimurium* TA100, reverse mutation	–	+	25.0000	Cocker *et al.* (1985)
SA0, *Salmonella typhimurium* TA100, reverse mutation	–	+	12.5000	Hesbert *et al.* (1985)
SA0, *Salmonella typhimurium* TA100, reverse mutation	–	+	6.7000	Cocker *et al.* (1986)
SA0, *Salmonella typhimurium* TA100, reverse mutation	0	+	3.3000	Kugler-Steigmeier *et al.* (1989)
SA0, *Salmonella typhimurium* TA100, reverse mutation	0	+	12.5000	Wu *et al.* (1989b)
SA0, *Salmonella typhimurium* TA100, reverse mutation	–	–	500.0000	Richold & Jones (1981)
SA0, *Salmonella typhimurium* TA100, reverse mutation	–	+	6.3000	Rowland & Severn (1981)
SA0, *Salmonella typhimurium* TA100, reverse mutation	0	?	0.0000	Trueman (1981)
SA5, *Salmonella typhimurium* TA1535, reverse mutation	–	–	0.0000	Baker & Bonin (1981)
SA5, *Salmonella typhimurium* TA1535, reverse mutation	–	–	1000.0000	Brooks & Dean (1981)
SA5, *Salmonella typhimurium* TA1535, reverse mutation	–	–	500.0000	Richold & Jones (1981)
SA5, *Salmonella typhimurium* TA1535, reverse mutation	–	–	1000.0000	Rowland & Severn (1981)
SA5, *Salmonella typhimurium* TA1535, reverse mutation	–	–	0.0000	Simmon & Shepherd (1981)
SA5, *Salmonella typhimurium* TA1535, reverse mutation	0	+	0.0000	Trueman (1981)

Table 7 (contd)

Test system	Result		Dose[a] (LED/HID)	Reference
	Without exogenous metabolic system	Wirh exogenous metabolic system		
SA5, *Salmonella typhimurium* TA1535, reverse mutation	–	–	167.0000	Haworth *et al.* (1983)
SA7, *Salmonella typhimurium* TA1537, reverse mutation	–	–	0.0000	Baker & Bonin (1981)
SA7, *Salmonella typhimurium* TA1537, reverse mutation	–	–	1000.0000	Brooks & Dean (1981)
SA7, *Salmonella typhimurium* TA1537, reverse mutation	–	–	0.0000	Martire *et al.* (1981)
SA7, *Salmonella typhimurium* TA1537, reverse mutation	–	–	0.0000	Nagao & Takahashi (1981)
SA7, *Salmonella typhimurium* TA1537, reverse mutation	–	–	500.0000	Richold & Jones (1981)
SA7, *Salmonella typhimurium* TA1537, reverse mutation	–	–	167.0000	Haworth *et al.* (1983)
SA7, *Salmonella typhimurium* TA1537, reverse mutation	–	–	1000.0000	Rowland & Severn (1981)
SA7, *Salmonella typhimurium* TA1537, reverse mutation	–	–	0.0000	Simmon & Shepherd (1981)
SA7, *Salmonella typhimurium* TA1537, reverse mutation	0	–	1250.0000	Trueman (1981)
SA8, *Salmonella typhimurium* TA1538, reverse mutation	–	–	0.0000	Simmon & Shepherd (1981)
SA8, *Salmonella typhimurium* TA1538, reverse mutation	–	–	0.0000	Baker & Bonin (1981)
SA8, *Salmonella typhimurium* TA1538, reverse mutation	–	–	1000.0000	Brooks & Dean (1981)
SA8, *Salmonella typhimurium* TA1538, reverse mutation	–	–	500.0000	Richold & Jones (1981)
SA8, *Salmonella typhimurium* TA1538, reverse mutation	0	–	1250.0000	Trueman (1981)
SA8, *Salmonella typhimurium* TA1538, reverse mutation	–	+	40.0000	Gatehouse (1981)
SA9, *Salmonella typhimurium* TA98, reverse mutation	–	+	0.0000	Baker & Bonin (1981)
SA9, *Salmonella typhimurium* TA98, reverse mutation	–	+	0.0000	Brooks & Dean (1981)
SA9, *Salmonella typhimurium* TA98, reverse mutation	–	+	0.0000	Garner *et al.* (1981)
SA9, *Salmonella typhimurium* TA98, reverse mutation	–	–	0.0000	Hubbard *et al.* (1981)
SA9, *Salmonella typhimurium* TA98, reverse mutation	–	–	0.0000	Ichinotsubo *et al.* (1981)
SA9, *Salmonella typhimurium* TA98, reverse mutation	–	+	25.0000	MacDonald (1981)
SA9, *Salmonella typhimurium* TA98, reverse mutation	–	+	0.0000	Martire *et al.* (1981)
SA9, *Salmonella typhimurium* TA98, reverse mutation	–	+	0.0000	Nagao & Takahashi (1981)
SA9, *Salmonella typhimurium* TA98, reverse mutation	–	–	500.0000	Richold & Jones (1981)
SA9, *Salmonella typhimurium* TA98, reverse mutation	–	–	1000.0000	Rowland & Severn (1981)
SA9, *Salmonella typhimurium* TA98, reverse mutation	–	+	0.0000	Simmon & Shepherd (1981)
SA9, *Salmonella typhimurium* TA98, reverse mutation	0	+	0.0000	Trueman (1981)
SA9, *Salmonella typhimurium* TA98, reverse mutation	–	+	25.0000	Venitt & Crofton–Sleigh (1981)

Table 7 (contd)

Test system	Result		Dose[a] (LED/HID)	Reference
	Without exogenous metabolic system	With exogenous metabolic system		
SA9, *Salmonella typhimurium* TA98, reverse mutation	0	+	0.0000	Rao et al. (1982)
SA9, *Salmonella typhimurium* TA98, reverse mutation	-	+	50.0000	Haworth et al. (1983)
SA9, *Salmonella typhimurium* TA98, reverse mutation	0	+	167.0000	Kugler–Steigmeier et al. (1989)
SA9, *Salmonella typhimurium* TA98, reverse mutation	0	+	25.0000	Wu et al. (1989b)
EC2, *Escherichia coli* WP2, reverse mutation	0	-	0.0000	Matsushima et al. (1981)
ECW, *Escherichia coli* WP2 uvrA, reverse mutation	-	-	250.0000	Matsushima et al. (1981)
ECR, *Escherichia coli* WP2 uvrA (pKM101), reverse mutation	-	+	10.0000	Matsushima et al. (1981)
ECW, *Escherichia coli* WP2 uvrA, reverse mutation	-	-	0.0000	Gatehouse (1981)
ECW, *Escherichia coli* WP2 uvrA, reverse mutation	-	+	25.0000	Venitt & Crofton–Sleigh (1981)
SCG, *Saccharomyces cerevisiae*, gene conversion	-	-	167.0000	Jagannath et al. (1981)
SCG, *Saccharomyces cerevisiae*, gene conversion	+	0	100.0000	Sharp & Parry (1981)
SCH, *Saccharomyces cerevisiae*, homozygosis	-	-	100.0000	Kassinova et al. (1981)
SCR, *Saccharomyces cerevisiae*, reverse mutation	-	-	889.0000	Mehta & von Borstel (1981)
SCN, *Saccharomyces cerevisiae*, aneuploidy	+	0	50.0000	Parry & Sharp (1981)
DMM, *Drosophila melanogaster*, somatic mutation	(+)[c]		1335.0000	Kugler–Steigmeier et al. (1989)
URP, Unscheduled DNA synthesis, rat primary hepatocytes	+	0	2.6700	McQueen et al. (1981)
URP, Unscheduled DNA synthesis, rat primary hepatocytes	+	0	100.0000	Williams et al. (1982)
URP, Unscheduled DNA synthesis, rat primary hepatocytes	+	0	2.6700	Mori et al. (1988)
UIA, Unscheduled DNA synthesis, mouse primary hepatocytes	+	0	13.3500	McQueen et al. (1981)
UIA, Unscheduled DNA synthesis, Syrian hamster primary hepatocytes	+	0	2.6700	McQueen et al. (1981)
G5T, Gene mutation, mouse lymphoma L5178Y cells *in vitro*	-	+	42.0000	Mitchell et al. (1988)
G5T, Gene mutation, mouse lymphoma L5178Y cells *in vitro*	-	+	5.0000	Myhr & Caspary (1988)
SIC, Sister chromatid exchange, Chinese hamster ovary cells *in vitro*	-	-	10.0000	Perry & Thomson (1981)
SIC, Sister chromatid exchange, Chinese hamster ovary cells *in vitro*	+[c]	(+)[c]	50.0000	Galloway et al. (1985)
CIC, Chromosomal aberrations, Chinese hamster ovary cells *in vitro*	-[d]	-[d]	300.0000	Galloway et al. (1985)

Table 7 (contd)

Test system	Result Without exogenous metabolic system	With exogenous metabolic system	Dose[a] (LED/HID)	Reference
SHL, Sister chromatid exchanges, human leukocytes	–	–	0.0000	Ho et al. (1979); abstr.
CHL, Chromosomal aberrations, human leukocytes	–	–	0.0000	Ho et al. (1979); abstr.
TCS, Cell transformation in Syrian hamster kidney BHK cells	+	+	13.7000	Daniel & Dehnel (1981)
TCS, Cell transformation in Syrian hamster kidney BHK cells	0	+	2.5000	Styles (1981)
TRR, Cell transformation, RLV/Fischer rat embryo cells	+	0	1.0000	Dunkel et al. (1981)
TBM, Cell transformation in BALB/c 3T3 mouse cells	+	0	0.2000	Dunkel et al. (1981)
SVA, Sister chromatid exchange, rat lymphocytes in vivo	+		125.0000 × 6 mg/kg, ip	Edwards & Priestly (1992)
MVM, Micronucleus test, mouse bone marrow in vivo	+		32.0000 × 2 ip	Salamone et al. (1981)
BID, Binding (covalent) to DNA in human bladder cells in vitro (^{32}P post-labelling)	+	0	0.0300	Stoner et al. (1988)
BID, Binding (covalent) to DNA in dog bladder cells in vitro (^{32}P post-labelling)	+	0	0.0300	Stoner et al. (1988)
BVD, Binding (covalent) to rat liver DNA in vivo (tritium label)	+		24.0000 × 1 ip	Silk et al. (1989)
BVD, Binding (covalent) to rat lung, liver and kidney DNA in vivo (^{14}C-label)	+		25.0000 × 1 po	Segerbäck & Kadlubar (1992)
BVD, Binding (covalent) to rat liver DNA in vivo (^{14}C-label)	+		75.0000 × 1 po	Cheever et al. (1990)
BVD, Binding (covalent) to rat liver DNA in vivo (^{14}C-label)	+		75.0000 skin	Cheever et al. (1990)
BVD, Binding (covalent) to rat liver DNA in vivo	+		1.4300 × po	Kugler–Steigmeier et al. (1989)
BVD, Binding (covalent) to rat lung DNA in vivo	+		1.4300 × po	Kugler–Steigmeier et al. (1989)
BVP, Binding (covalent) to rat globin in vivo (^{14}C-label)	+		75.0000 × 1 po	Cheever et al. (1990)
BVP, Binding (covalent) to rat lung, liver and kidney RNA and protein in vivo	+		1.0000 × 1 po	Sabbioni & Neumann (1990)
ICR, Inhibition of cell–cell communication in WB-F344 rat liver epithelial cells in vitro	+	0	2.0000	Kuslikis et al. (1991)

+, positive; (+), weakly positive; –, negative; 0, not tested
[a] In-vitro tests, μg/ml; in-vivo tests, mg/kg bw; 0.0000, not given
[b] Positive in two laboratories; in a third laboratory, negative with rat S9, weakly positive with hamster S9
[c] Positive in one laboratory; negative in another
[d] Tested in two laboratories

5. Summary of Data Reported and Evaluation

5.1 Exposure data

4,4'-Methylenebis(2-chloroaniline) (MOCA) was introduced in the mid-1950s in the production of high-performance polyurethane mouldings. It is used in many countries, with a total worldwide production of several thousand tonnes per year; it is used as a curing agent for roofing and wood sealing in Japan and the Far East. There was considerable occupational exposure by cutaneous absorption in the early years of use of MOCA, as revealed by urine analysis, but exposure has decreased with the implementation of control measures. Extensive environmental contamination is known to have occurred in a large area surrounding at least one factory, prior to the introduction of controls.

5.2 Human carcinogenicity data

Three asymptomatic cases of cancer of the urinary bladder (two in men under the age of 30 among 552 workers) were identified in a factory where MOCA was produced and where screening for this cancer was undertaken in a subgroup. Although this finding suggests an excess, expected numbers could not be calculated.

5.3 Animal carcinogenicity data

MOCA was tested for carcinogenicity by oral administration in the diet in mice in one study, in rats of each sex in two studies, in male rats in a further two studies using normal and low-protein diets and in capsules in female dogs. It was also tested by subcutaneous administration to rats in one study. Oral administration of MOCA increased the incidence of liver tumours in female mice. In a series of experiments in which rats were fed either standard or low-protein diets, it induced liver-cell tumours and malignant lung tumours in males and females in one study, a few liver-cell tumours in male rats in another, lung adenocarcinomas and hepatocellular tumours in males and females in a third and malignant lung tumours, mammary gland adenocarcinomas, Zymbal gland carcinomas and hepatocellular carcinomas in a fourth. Oral administration of MOCA to female beagle dogs produced transitional-cell carcinomas of the urinary bladder and urethra. Subcutaneous administration to rats produced hepatocellular carcinomas and malignant lung tumours.

5.4 Other relevant data

MOCA forms adducts with DNA, both *in vitro* and *in vivo*. One of the two major adducts, *N*-(deoxyadenosin-8-yl)-4-amino-3-chlorobenzyl alcohol, was found in rat tissues; it also co-chromatographed with a DNA adduct from urothelial cells recovered from the urine of a worker in the polyurethane industry who was accidentally exposed to a high dose of MOCA. An increased frequency of sister chromatid exchange was seen in a small number of workers exposed to MOCA.

MOCA induced DNA damage in prokaryotes, cultured mammalian and human cells and in animals treated *in vivo*. Gene mutation was induced in bacteria and cultured mammalian cells, but not in yeast. Equivocal results for mitotic recombination were obtained in yeasts. Aneuploidy was induced in yeast and sister chromatid exchange, transformation and inhibition of intercellular communication in cultured mammalian cells. Micronuclei were induced in the bone marrow of mice treated *in vivo*, and sister chromatid exchange was induced in the bone marrow of rats treated *in vivo*.

MOCA is comprehensively genotoxic. Furthermore, (i) rats, dogs and humans metabolize MOCA to *N*-hydroxy-MOCA by hepatic cytochromes P450; (ii) DNA adducts are formed by reaction with *N*-hydroxy-MOCA, and MOCA is genotoxic in bacteria and mammalian cells; (iii) the same major MOCA–DNA adduct is formed in the target tissues for carcinogenicity in animals (rat liver and lung; dog urinary bladder) as that found in urothelial cells from a man with known occupational exposure to MOCA.

5.5 Evaluation[1]

There is *inadequate evidence* in humans for the carcinogenicity of 4,4'-methylenebis(2-chloroaniline) (MOCA).

There is *sufficient evidence* in experimental animals for the carcinogenicity of 4,4'-methylenebis(2-chloroaniline) (MOCA).

Overall evaluation[2]

4,4'-Methylenebis(2-chloroaniline) (MOCA) is *probably carcinogenic to humans (Group 2A)*.

6. References

American Conference of Governmental Industrial Hygienists (1990a) Notice of intended changes—4,4'-methylenebis(2-chloroaniline), perfluoroiso-butylene, and triethanolamine. *Appl. occup. environ. Hyg.*, 5, 798–804

American Conference of Governmental Industrial Hygienists (1990b) *Guide to Occupational Exposure Values—1990*, Cincinnati, OH, p. 12

American Conference of Governmental Industrial Hygienists (1992) *Annual Reports of the Committees on Threshold Limit Values and Biological Exposure Indices*, Cincinnati, OH, p. 1

Anon. (1985) International toxicity update. *Dangerous Prop. ind. Mater. Rep.*, 5, 30–36

Arbejdstilsynet (Labor Inspection) (1977) *Liste over Hygiejniske Graensevaerdier 1977* (List of limit values 1977), Copenhagen

Baker, R.S.U. & Bonin, A.M. (1981) Study of 42 coded compounds with the *Salmonella*/mammalian microsome assay. *Prog. Mutat. Res.*, 1, 249–260

---

[1]For definition of the italicized terms, see Preamble, pp. 26–30.
[2]Overall evaluation 2A and not 2B on the basis of supporting evidence from other relevant data

Becker, J.W., Blackwell, J., Caruso, P.P., Pugh, T.L. & Yeager, F.W. (1974) Determination of unreacted 'MOCA' in polyether-based polyurethane systems. *Rubber World*, **170**, 57–62, 80

Bridges, B.A., MacGregor, D., Zeiger, E., Bonin, A., Dean, B.J., Lorenzo, F., Garner, R.C., Gatehouse, D., Hubbard, S., Ichinotsubo, D., MacDonald, D., Martire, G., Matsushima, T., Mohn, G., Nagao, M., Richold, M., Rowland, I., Simmon, V., Skopek, T., Truman, R. & Venitt, S. (1981) Summary report on the performance of bacterial mutation assays. *Prog. Mutat. Res.*, **1**, 49–67

Brooks, T.M. & Dean, B.J. (1981) Mutagenic activity of 42 coded compounds in the *Salmonella/*-microsome assay with preincubation. *Prog. Mutat. Res.*, **1**, 261–270

Butler, M.A., Guengerich, F.P. & Kadlubar, F.F. (1989) Metabolic oxidation of the carcinogens 4-aminobiphenyl and 4,4'-methylene-bis(2-chloroaniline) by human hepatic microsomes and by purified rat hepatic cytochrome P-450 monooxygenases. *Cancer Res.*, **49**, 25–31

Caisse Nationale Assurance (1992) *Valeurs Limites d'Exposition aux postes de travail 1992*, Lucerne, Division Médecine du Travail

Cartwright, R.A. (1983) Historical and modern epidemiological studies on populations exposed to *N*-substituted aryl compounds. *Environ. Health Perspectives*, **49**, 13–19

Cheever, K.L., Richards, D.E., Weigel, W.W., Begley, K.B., Savage, R.E., Jr & Daniel, F.B. (1988) Macromolecular adduct formation by 4,4'-methylene-bis(2-chloroaniline) in adult male rat. *Scand. J. Work Environ. Health*, **14** (Suppl. 1), 57–59

Cheever, K.L., Richards, D.E., Weigel, W.W., Begley, K.B., DeBord, D.G., Swearengin, T.F. & Savage, R.E., Jr (1990) 4,4'-Methylene-bis(2-chloroaniline)(MOCA): comparison of macromolecular adduct formation after oral or dermal administration in the rat. *Fundam. appl. Toxicol.*, **14**, 273–283

Cheever, K.L., DeBord, D.G. & Swearengin, T.F. (1991) 4,4'-Methylene bis(2-chloroaniline) (MOCA): the effect of multiple oral administration, route, and phenobarbital induction on macromolecular adduct formation in the rat. *Fundam. appl. Toxicol.*, **16**, 71–80

Chemical Information Services (1991) *Directory of World Chemical Producers 1992/93*, Dallas, TX, p. 79

Chen, T.H., Kuslikis, B.I. & Braselton, W.E., Jr (1989) Hydroxylation of 4,4'-methylenebis(2-chloro-aniline) by canine, guinea pig, and rat liver microsomes. *Drug Metab. Disposition*, **17**, 406–413

Chen, T.H., Kuslikis, B.I. & Braselton, W.E., Jr (1991) Unlabeled hemoglobin adducts of 4,4'-methylenebis(2-chloroaniline) in rats and guinea pigs. *Arch. Toxicol.*, **65**, 177–185

Chin, B., Tobes, M.C. & Han, S.S. (1983) Absorption of 4,4'-methylenebis[2-chloroaniline] by human skin. *Environ. Res.*, **32**, 167–178

Clapp, D.E., Piacitelli, G.M., Zaebst, D.D. & Ward, E. (1991) Assessing exposure to 4,4'-methylene bis(2-chloroaniline) (MBOCA) in the workplace *Appl. occup. environ. Hyg.*, **6**, 125–130

Cocker, J., Boobis, A.R., Gibson, J.F. & Davies, D.S. (1985) The metabolic activation of 4,4'-methylenebis(2-chlorobenzeneamine) to a bacterial mutagenic by hepatic postmitochondrial supernatant from human and other species. *Environ. Mutag.*, **7**, 501–509

Cocker, J., Boobis, A.R. & Davies, D.S. (1986) Routes of activation of 4,4'-methylenebis(2-chloro-aniline) and 4,4'-methylenedianiline to bacterial mutagens. *Food chem. Toxicol.*, **24**, 755–756

Cocker, J., Boobis, A.R. & Davies, D.S. (1988) Determination of the *N*-acetyl metabolites of 4,4'-methylene dianiline and 4,4'-methylene-bis(2-chloroaniline) in urine. *Biomed. environ. Mass Spectrom.*, **17**, 161–167

Cocker, J., Boobis, A.R., Wilson, H.K. & Gompertz, D. (1990) Evidence that a β-N-glucuronide of 4,4'-methylenebis (2-chloroaniline) (MbOCA) is a major urinary metabolite in man: implications for biological monitoring. *Br. J. ind. Med.*, **47**, 154–161

Commission of the European Communities (1967) Council Directive of 16 August 1967 on the approximation of the laws, regulations and administrative provisions relating to the classification, packaging and labelling of dangerous substances. *Off. J. Eur. Commun.*, **L196**, 1

Commission of the European Communities (1990) Council Directive of 28 June 1990 on the protection of workers from the risks related to exposure to carcinogens at work (6th individual Directive within the meaning of Article 16 of Directive 89/391/EEC). *Off. J. Eur. Commun.*, **L196**, 1–7

Commission of the European Communities (1991) Twelfth Adaptation to Technical Progress of Council Directive 67/548/EEC of 16 August 1967. *Off. J. Eur. Commun.*, **L180A**, 918

Cook, W.A. (1987) *Occupational Exposure Limits—Worldwide*, Akron, OH, American Industrial Hygiene Association, pp. 146, 199

Daniel, M.R. & Dehnel, J.M. (1981) Cell transformation test with baby hamster kidney cells. *Prog. Mutat. Res.*, **1**, 626–637

Deutsche Forschungsgemeinschaft (1992) *MAK- and BAT-Values List 1992. Maximum Concentrations at the Workplace (MAK) and Biological Tolerance Values (BAT) for Working Materials* (Report No. 28), Weinheim, VCH Verlagsgesellschaft, p. 49

Ducos, P., Maire, C. & Gaudin, R. (1985) Assessment of occupational exposure to 4,4'-methylene-bis(2-chloroanilione) 'MOCA' by a new sensitive method for biological monitoring. *Int. Arch. occup. environ. Health*, **55**, 159–167

Dunkel, V.C., Pienta, R.J., Sivak, A. & Traul, K.A. (1981) Comparative neoplastic transformation responses of BALB/3T3 cells, Syrian hamster embryo cells, and Rauscher murine leukemia virus-infected Fischer 344 rat embryo cells to chemical carcinogens. *J. natl Cancer Inst.*, **67**, 1303–1315

Edwards, J.W. & Priestly, B.G. (1992) Biological and biological-effect monitoring of workers exposed to 4,4'-methylene-bis(2-chloroaniline). *Hum. exp. Toxicol.*, **11**, 229–236

Eller, P.M., ed. (1985) *NIOSH Manual of Analytical Methods*, 3rd ed., Suppl. 1 (DHHS (NIOSH) Publ. No. 84-100), Washington DC, US Government Printing Office, pp. 8302-1—8302-4

Farmer, P.B., Rickard, J. & Robertson, S. (1981) The metabolism and distribution of 4,4'-methylene-bis(2-chloroaniline) (MBOCA) in rats. *J. appl. Toxicol.*, **1**, 317–322

Fishbein, L. (1984) Aromatic amines. In: Hutzinger, O., ed., *The Handbook of Environmental Chemistry*, Vol. 3, Part C, Berlin, Springer-Verlag, pp. 1–40

Galloway, S.M., Bloom, A.D., Resnick, M., Margolin, B.H., Nakamura, F., Archer, P. & Zeiger, E. (1985) Development of a standard protocol for in vitro cytogenetic testing with Chinese hamster ovary cells: comparison of results for 22 compounds in two laboratories. *Environ. Mutag.*, **7**, 1–51

Garner, R.C., Welch, A. & Pickering, C. (1981) Mutagenic activity of 42 coded compounds in the *Salmonella*/microsome assay. *Prog. Mutat. Res.*, **1**, 280–284

Gatehouse, D. (1981) Mutagenic activity of 42 coded compounds in the 'microtiter' fluctuation test. *Prog. Mutat. Res.*, **1**, 376–386

Groth, D.H., Weigel, W.W., Tolos, W.P., Brewer, D.E., Cheever, K.L. & Burg, J.R. (1984) 4,4'-Methylene-bis-*ortho*-chloro-aniline (MBOCA): absorption and excretion after skin application and gavage. *Environ. Res.*, **34**, 38–54

Grundmann, E. & Steinhoff, D. (1970) Liver and lung tumours after administration of 3,3'-dichloro-4,4'-diaminodiphenylmethane to rats (Ger.). *Z. Krebsforsch.*, **74**, 28–39

Haworth, S., Lawlor, T., Mortelmans, K., Speck, W. & Zeiger, E. (1983) *Salmonella* mutagenicity test results for 250 chemicals. *Environ. Mutag.*, **1**, 3–142

Health and Safety Executive (1985) *Occupational Exposure Limits 1987*, London, Her Majesty's Stationery Office

Hesbert, A., Bottin, M.C. & De Ceaurriz, J. (1985) Mutagenicity of 4,4′-methylene-bis(2-chloroaniline) 'MOCA' and its *N*-acetyl derivatives in *S. typhimurium*. *Int. Arch. occup. environ. Health*, **55**, 169–174

Ho, T., Hardigree, A.A., Larimer, F.W., Nix, C.E., Rao, T.K., Tipton, S.C. & Epler, J.L. (1979) Comparative mutagenicity study of potentially carcinogenic industrial compounds (Abstract Ea-10). *Environ. Mutag.*, **1**, 167–168

Hosein, H.R. & Van Roosmalen, P.B. (1978) Acute exposure to methylene-bis-ortho chloroaniline (MOCA). *Am. ind. Hyg. Assoc. J.*, **39**, 496–497

Hubbard, S.A., Green, M.H.L., Bridges, B.A., Wain, A.J. & Bridges, J.W. (1981) Fluctuation test with S9 and hepatocyte activation. *Prog. Mutat. Res.*, **1**, 361–370

IARC (1974) *IARC Monographs on the Evaluation of Carcinogenic Risk of Chemicals to Humans, Vol. 4, Some Aromatic Amines, Hydrazine and Related Substances, N-Nitroso Compounds and Miscellaneous Alkylating Agents*, Lyon, pp. 65–71

IARC (1982a) *IARC Monographs on the Evaluation of the Carcinogenic Risk of Chemicals to Humans, Vol. 29, Some Industrial Chemicals and Dyestuffs*, Lyon, pp. 345–389

IARC (1982b) *IARC Monographs on the Evaluation of the Carcinogenic Risk of Chemicals to Humans, Vol. 28, The Rubber Industry*, Lyon

IARC (1987a) *IARC Monographs on the Evaluation of Carcinogenic Risks to Humans*, Suppl. 7, *Overall Evaluations of Carcinogenicity: An Updating of* IARC Monographs *Volumes 1 to 42*, Lyon, pp. 246–247

IARC (1987b) *IARC Monographs on the Evaluation of Carcinogenic Risks to Humans*, Suppl. 7, *Overall Evaluations of Carcinogenicity: An Updating of* IARC Monographs *Volumes 1 to 42*, Lyon, pp. 211–216

IARC (1987c) *IARC Monographs on the Evaluation of Carcinogenic Risks to Humans*, Suppl. 7, *Overall Evaluations of Carcinogenicity: An Updating of* IARC Monographs *Volumes 1 to 42*, Lyon, pp. 332–334

Ichikawa, Y., Yoshida, M., Okayama, A., Hara, I. & Morimoto, K. (1990) Biological monitoring for workers exposed to 4,4′-methylenebis (2-chloroaniline). *Am. ind. Hyg. Assoc. J.*, **51**, 5–7

Ichinotsubo, D., Mower, H. & Mandel, M. (1981) Mutagen testing of a series of paired compounds with the Ames *Salmonella* testing system. *Prog. Mutat. Res.*, **1**, 298–301

Ihara Chemical Industry Co. (undated) *Data Sheet: Cuamine-M (4,4′-Methylene bis(2-chloroaniline))*, Tokyo

ILO (1991) *Occupational Exposure Limits for Airborne Toxic Substances*, 3rd ed. (Occupational Safety and Health Series No. 37), Geneva, International Labour Office, pp. 128–129

Jagannath, D.R., Vultaggio, D.M. & Brusick, D.J. (1981) Genetic activity of 42 coded compounds in the mitotic gene conversion assay using *Saccharomyces cerevisiae* strain D4. *Prog. Mutat. Res.*, **1**, 456–467

Kada, T. (1981) The DNA-damaging activity of 42 coded compounds in the rec-assay. *Prog. Mutat. Res.*, **1**, 175–182

Kaderlik, K.R., Talaska, G., DeBord, D.G., Osorio, A.M. & Kadlubar, F.F. (1993) 4,4′-Methylene-bis(2-chloroaniline)–DNA adduct analysis in human exfoliated urothelial cells by ^{32}P-postlabelling. *Cancer Epidemiol. Biomarkers Prev.*, **2**, 63–69

Kassinova, G.V., Kovaltsova, S.V., Marfin, S.V. & Zakharov, I.A. (1981) Activity of 40 coded compounds in differential inhibition and mitotic crossing-over assays in yeast. *Prog. Mutat. Res.*, **1**, 434–455

Keeslar, F.L. (1986) The removal and control of methylene bis orthochloroaniline in residential and industrial areas of Adrian, Michigan. In: *1986 Hazardous Material Spills—Conference Proceedings. Preparedness, Prevention, Control and Cleanup of Releases, May 5–8, 1986, St Louis, Missouri* (NIOSH-00165082), Cincinatti, OH, National Institute for Occupational Safety and Health

Kommineni, C., Groth, D.H., Frockt, I.J., Voelker, R.W. & Stanovick, R.P. (1978) Determination of the tumorigenic potential of methylene-bis-orthochloroaniline. *J. environ. Pathol. Toxicol.*, **2**, 149–171

Kugler-Steigmeier, M.E., Friederich, U., Graf, U., Lutz, W.K., Maier, P. & Schlatter, C. (1989) Genotoxicity of aniline derivatives in various short-term tests. *Mutat. Res.*, **211**, 279–289

Kuslikis, B.I., Trosko, J.E. & Braselton, W.E., Jr (1991) Mutagenicity and effect on gap-junctional intercellular communication of 4,4′-methylenebis(2-chloroaniline) and its oxidized metabolites. *Mutagenesis*, **6**, 19–24

Linch, A.L., O'Connor, G.B., Barnes, J.R., Killian, A.S., Jr & Neeld, W.E., Jr (1971) Methylene-bis-*ortho*-chloroaniline (MOCA): evaluation of hazards and exposure control. *Am. ind. Hyg. Assoc. J.*, **32**, 802–819

Locke, J. (1986) Fixing exposure limits for toxic chemicals in the UK—some case studies. *Sci. total Environ.*, **51**, 237–260

Lowry, L.K. & Clapp, D.E. (1992) Urinary 4,4′-methylenebis(2-chloroaniline) (MBOCA): a case study for biological monitoring. *Appl. occup. environ. Hyg.*, **7**, 1–6

MacDonald, D.J. (1981) *Salmonella*/microsome tests on 42 coded chemicals. *Prog. Mutat. Res.*, **1**, 285–297

Manis, M.O. & Braselton, W.E., Jr (1984) Structure elucidation and in vitro reactivity of the major metabolite of 4,4′-methylenebis(2-chloroaniline) (MBOCA) in canine urine. *Fundam. appl. Toxicol.*, **4**, 1000–1008

Manis, M.O. & Braselton, W.E., Jr (1986) Metabolism of 4,4′-methylenebis(2-chloroaniline) by canine liver and kidney slices. *Drug Metab. Disposition*, **14**, 166-174

Manis, M.O., Williams, D.E., McCormack, K.M., Schock, R.J., Lepper, L.F., Ng, Y.-C. & Braselton, W.E. (1984) Percutaneous absorption, disposition, and excretion of 4,4′-methylenebis(2-chloroaniline) in dogs. *Environ. Res.*, **33**, 234–245

Martire, G., Vricella, G., Perfumo, A.M. & De Lorenzo, F. (1981) Evaluation of the mutagenic activity of coded compounds in the *Salmonella* test. *Prog. Mutat. Res.*, **1**, 271–279

Matsushima, T., Takamoto, Y., Shirai, A., Sawamura, M. & Sugimura, T. (1981) Reverse mutation test on 42 coded compounds with the *E. coli* WP2 system. *Prog. Mutat. Res.*, **1**, 387–395

McCann, J., Choi, E., Yamasaki, E. & Ames, B.N. (1975) Detection of carcinogens as mutagens in the *Salmonella*/microsome test: assay of 300 chemicals. *Proc. natl Acad. Sci. USA*, **72**, 5135–5139

McKerrell, P.J., Saunders, G.A. & Geyer, R. (1987) Determination of 4,4′-methylenebis(2-chloroaniline) in urine by high-performance liquid chromatography. *J. Chromatogr.*, **408**, 399–401

McQueen, C.A. & Williams, G.M. (1982) Cytotoxicity of xenobiotics in adult rat hepatocytes in primary culture. *Fundam. appl. Toxicol.*, **2**, 139–144

McQueen, C.A., Maslansky, C.J., Crescenzi, S.B. & Williams, G.M. (1981) The genotoxicity of 4,4′-methylenebis-2-chloroaniline in rat, mouse and hamster hepatocytes. *Toxicol. appl. Pharmacol.*, **58**, 231–235

Mehta, R.D. & von Borstel, R.C. (1981) Mutagenic activity of 42 encoded compounds in the haploid yeast reversion assay, strain XV185-14C. *Prog. Mutat. Res.*, **1**, 414–423

Mitchell, A.D., Rudd, C.J. & Caspary, W.J. (1988) Evaluation of the L5178Y mouse lymphoma cell mutagenesis assay: intralaboratory results for sixty-three coded chemicals tested at SRI International. *Environ. mol. Mutag.*, **12** (Suppl. 13), 37–101

Mori, H., Yoshimi, N., Sugie, S., Iwata, H., Kawai, K., Mashizu, N. & Shimizu, H. (1988) Genotoxicity of epoxy resin hardeners in the hepatocyte primary culture/DNA repair test. *Mutat. Res.*, **204**, 683–688

Morton, K.C., Lee, M.-S., Siedlik, P. & Chapman, R. (1988) Metabolism of 4,4'-methylenebis-2-chloroaniline (MOCA) by rats *in vivo* and formation of N-hydroxy MOCA by rat and human liver microsomes. *Carcinogenesis*, **9**, 131–139

Myhr, B.C. & Caspary, W.J. (1988) Evaluation of the L5178Y mouse lymphoma cell mutagenesis system: intralaboratory results for 63 coded chemicals tested at Litton Bionetics, Inc. *Environ. mol. Mutag.*, **12** (Suppl. 13), 103–194

Nagao, M. & Takahashi, Y. (1981) Mutagenic activity of 42 coded compounds in the *Salmonella*/microsome assay. *Prog. Mutat. Res.*, **1**, 302–313

National Swedish Board of Occupational Safety and Health (1984) *Hygieniska Gränsvärden* (Hygiene limit values), Stockholm, p. 32

Osorio, A.M., Clapp, D., Ward, E., Wilson, H.K. & Cocker, J. (1990) Biological monitoring of a worker acutely exposed to MBOCA. *Am. J. ind. Med.*, **18**, 577–589

Palmer Davis Seika (1992) *Material Safety Data Sheet: Bis Amine A (4,4'-Methylene-bis(2-chloro-aniline))*, Fort Washington, NY

Parris, G.E., Diachenko, G.W., Entz, R.C., Poppiti, J.A., Lombardo, P., Rohrer, T.K. & Hesse, J.L. (1980) Waterborne methylene bis(2-chloroaniline) and 2-chloroaniline contamination around Adrian, Michigan. *Bull. environ. Contam. Toxicol.*, **24**, 497–503

Parry, J.M. & Sharp, D. (1981) Induction of mitotic aneuploidy in the yeast strain D6 by 42 coded compounds. *Prog. Mutat. Res.*, **1**, 468–480

PEDCo Environmental (1984) *Analysis of Workplace Monitoring Data for MOCA* (Contract No. 68-02-3935), Washington DC, US Environmental Protection Agency, Office of Pesticides and Toxic Substances

Perry, P.E. & Thomson, E.J. (1981) Evaluation of the sister chromatid exchange method in mammalian cells as a screening system for carcinogens. *Prog. Mutat. Res.*, **1**, 560–569

Pouchert, C.J. (1981) *The Aldrich Library of Infrared Spectra*, 3rd ed., Milwaukee, WI, Aldrich Chemical Co., p. 730

Purnell, C.J. & Warwick, C.J. (1981) Method 3—Analysis of 3,3'-dichloro- 4,4'-diaminodiphenyl-methane (MOCA) and 2-chloroaniline (OCA) in air. In: Egan, H., Fishbein, L., Castegnaro, M., O'Neill, I.K. & Bartsch, H., eds, *Environmental Carcinogens: Selected Methods of Analysis, Vol. 4, Some Aromatic Amines and Azo Dyes in the General and Industrial Environment* (IARC Scientific Publications No. 40), Lyon, IARC, pp. 133–140

Rao, T.K., Dorsey, G.F., Allen, B.E. & Epler, J.L. (1982) Mutagenicity of 4,4'-methylenedianiline derivatives in the *Salmonella* histidine reversion assay. *Arch. Toxicol.*, **49**, 185–190

Rice, J.R. & Kissinger, P.T. (1981) Method 4—Determination of benzidine, 3,3'-dimethoxybenzidine, 4-aminobiphenyl, 3,3'-dichlorobenzidine and 4,4'-methylene-bis(2-chloroaniline) [MOCA] in soil samples, surface water and groundwater by liquid chromatography with electrochemical detection. In: Egan, H., Fishbein, L., Castegnaro, M., O'Neill, I.K. & Bartsch, H., eds, *Environmental Carcinogens Selected Methods of Analysis*, Vol. 4, *Some Aromatic Amines and Azo Dyes in the General and Industrial Environment* (IARC Scientific Publications No. 40), Lyon, IARC, pp. 141–151

Richold, M. & Jones, E. (1981) Mutagenic activity of 42 coded compounds in the *Salmonella*/-microsome assay. *Prog. Mutat. Res.*, 1, 314–322

Rowland, I. & Severn, B. (1981) Mutagenicity of carcinogens and noncarcinogens in the *Salmonella*/-microsome test. *Prog. Mutat. Res.*, 1, 323–332

Russfield, A.B., Homburger, F., Boger, E., Van Dongen, C.G., Weisburger, E.K. & Weisburger, J.H. (1975) The carcinogenic effect of 4,4'-methylene-bis(2-chloroaniline) in mice and rats. *Toxicol. appl. Pharmacol.*, 31, 47–54

Sabbioni, G. & Neumann, H.-G. (1990) Quantification of haemoglobin binding of 4,4'-methylenebis-(2-chloroaniline) (MOCA) in rats. *Arch. Toxicol.*, 64, 451–458

Sadtler Research Laboratories (1980) *Sadtler Standard Spectra, 1980 Cumulative Index*, Philadelphia, PA

Sadtler Research Laboratories (1991) *Sadtler Standard Spectra, 1981–1991 Supplementary Index*, Philadelphia, PA

Salamone, M.F., Heddle, J.A. & Katz, M. (1981) Mutagenic activity of 41 compounds in the in vivo micronucleus assay. *Prog. Mutat. Res.*, 1, 686–697

Savage, R.E., Jr, Weigel, W.W. & Krieg, E.F., Jr (1992) Induction of ornithine decarboxylase activity by 4,4'-methylene bis(2-chloroaniline) in the rat. *Cancer Lett.*, 62, 63–68

Segerbäck, D. & Kadlubar, F.F. (1992) Characterization of 4,4'-methylenebis(2-chloroaniline)–DNA adducts formed in vivo and in vitro. *Carcinogenesis*, 13, 1587–1592

Sharp, D.C. & Parry, J.M. (1981) Induction of mitotic gene conversion by 41 coded compounds using the yeast culture JD1. *Prog. Mutat. Res.*, 1, 491–501

Shivapurkar, N., Lehman, T.A., Schut, H.A.J. & Stoner, G.D. (1987) DNA binding of 4,4'-methylene-bis(2-chloroaniline) (MOCA) in explant cultures of human and dog bladder. *Cancer Lett.*, 38, 41–48

Silk, N.A., Lay, J.O., Jr & Martin, C.N. (1989) Covalent binding of 4,4'-methylenebis(2-chloroaniline) to rat liver DNA in vivo and of its *N*-hydroxylated derivative to DNA in vitro. *Biochem. Pharmacol.*, 38, 279–287

Simmon, V.F. & Shepherd, G.F. (1981) Mutagenic activity of 42 coded compounds in the *Salmonella*/-microsome assay. *Prog. Mutat. Res.*, 1, 333–342

State of California (1992) *General Industry Safety Orders*, Title 8, No. 5215, *4,4'-Methylenebis(2-chloroaniline)*, Sacramento, CA, pp. 886–890

Steinhoff, D. & Grundmann, E. (971) Carcinogenic effect of 3,3'-dichloro-4,4'-diaminodiphenyl-methane in rats (Ger.). *Naturwissenschaften*, 58, 578

Stoner, G.D., Shivapurkar, N.M., Schut, H.A.J. & Lehman, T.A. (1988) DNA binding and adduct formation of 4,4'-methylene-bis(2-chloroaniline) (MOCA) in explant cultures of human and dog bladder. In: King, C.M., Romano, L.J. & Schuetzle, D., eds, *Carcinogenic and Mutagenic Responses to Aromatic Amines and Nitroarenes*, Amsterdam, Elsevier, pp. 237–240

Stula, E.F., Sherman, H., Zapp, J.A., Jr & Clayton, J.W., Jr (1975) Experimental neoplasia in rats from · oral administration of 3,3'-dichlorobenzidine, 4,4'-methylene-bis(2-chloroaniline), and 4,4'-methylene-bis(2-methylaniline). *Toxicol. appl. Pharmacol.*, **31**, 159–176

Stula, E.F., Barnes, J.R., Sherman, H., Reinhardt, C.F. & Zapp, Z.A., Jr (1977) Urinary bladder tumors in dogs from 4,4'-methylene-bis(2-chloroaniline) (MOCA®). *J. environ. Pathol. Toxicol.*, **1**, 31–50

Styles, J.A. (1981) Activity of 42 coded compounds in the BHK-21 cell transformation test. *Prog. Mutat. Res.*, **1**, 638–646

Taylor, D.G. (1977) *NIOSH Manual of Analytical Methods*, 2nd ed., Vol. 1, Cincinnati, OH, National Institute for Occupational Safety and Health, pp. 236-1—236-9

Thomas, J.D. & Wilson, H.K. (1984) Biological monitoring of workers exposed to 4,4'-methylenebis (2-chloroaniline) (MOCA). *Br. J. ind. Med.*, **41**, 547–551

Thomson, J.A. (1981) Mutagenic activity of 42 coded compounds in the lambda induction assay. *Prog. Mutat. Res.*, **1**, 224–235

Tobes, M.C., Brown, L.E., Chin, B. & Marsh, D.D. (1983) Kinetics of tissue distribution and elimination of 4,4'-methylene bis(2-chloroaniline) in rats. *Toxicol. Lett.*, **17**, 69–75

Trippel-Schulte, P., Zeiske, J. & Kettrup, A. (1986) Track analysis of selected benzidine and diamino-diphenylmethane derivatives in urine by means of liquid chromatography using precolumn sample preconcentration, UV and electrochemical detection. *Chromatographia*, **22**, 138–146

Trueman, R.W. (1981) Activity of 42 coded compounds in the *Salmonella* reverse mutation test. *Prog. Mutat. Res.*, **1**, 343–350

US National Institute for Occupational Safety and Health (1984) *Manual of Analytical Methods*, 3rd ed., *Method 8302* (NIOSH (HEW) Pub. No. 84-100), Cincinatti, OH, pp. 8302-1—8302-4

US National Institute for Occupational Safety and Health (1990) *Manual of Analytical Methods*, 4th ed., *Method 5029* (NIOSH (HEW) Pub. No. 90-100), Cincinatti, OH, pp. 5029-1—5029-5

US National Library of Medicine (1992) *Hazardous Substances Data Bank* (HSDB No. 2629), Bethesda, MD

US Occupational Safety and Health Administration (1988) *o-Dianisidine; 4,4'-Methylenebis(2-chloro-aniline) (MOCA); o-Tolidine (Method No. 71)* Salt Lake City, UT

US Tariff Commission (1957) *Synthetic Organic Chemicals, United States Production and Sales, 1956* (Report No. 200, Second Series), Washington DC, US Government Printing Office, p. 74

Van Roosmalen, P.B., Klein, A.L. & Drummond, I. (1981) Method 8—Determination of 3,3'-dichloro-4,4'-diaminodiphenylmethane (MOCA) in urine. In: Egan, H., Fishbein, L., Castegnaro, M., O'Neill, I.K. & Bartsch, H., eds, *Environmental Carcinogens Selected Methods of Analysis*, Vol. 4, *Some Aromatic Amines and Azo Dyes in the General and Industrial Environment* (IARC Scientific Publications No. 40), Lyon, IARC, pp. 183–191

Venitt, S. & Crofton-Sleigh, C. (1981) Mutagenicity of 42 coded compounds in a bacterial assay using *Escherichia coli* and *Salmonella typhimurium*. *Prog. Mutat. Res.*, **1**, 351–360

Verschueren, K. (1983) *Handbook of Environmental Data on Organic Chemicals*, 2nd ed., New York, Van Nostrand Reinhold, p. 846

Voorman, R. & Penner, D. (1986) Fate of MBOCA [4,4'-methylene-bis(2-chloro- aniline)] in soil. *Arch. environ. Contam. Toxicol.*, **15**, 595–602

Wan, K.C., Dare, B.R. & Street, N.R. (1989) Biomedical surveillance of workers exposed to 4,4'-methylene-bis(2-chloroaniline) (MBOCA) in Perth, Western Australia. *J. R. Soc. Health*, **5**, 159–167

Ward, E., Clapp, D., Tolos, W. & Groth, D. (1986) Efficacy of urinary monitoring for 4,4'-methylene-bis(2-chloroaniline). *J. occup. Med.*, **28**, 637–642

Ward, E., Smith, A.B. & Halperin, W. (1987) 4,4'-Methylenebis (2-chloroaniline): an unregulated carcinogen. *Am. J. ind. Med.*, **12**, 537–549

Ward, E., Halperin, W., Thun, M., Grossman, H.B., Fink, B., Koss, L., Osorio, A.M. & Schulte, P. (1988) Bladder tumors in two young males occupationally exposed to MBOCA. *Am. J. ind. Med.*, **14**, 267–272

Ward, E., Halperin, W., Thun, M., Grossman, H.B., Fink, B., Koss, L., Osorio, A.M. & Schulte, P. (1990) Screening workers exposed to 4,4'-methylene bis(2-chloroaniline) for bladder cancer by cystoscopy. *J. occup. Med.*, **32**, 865–868

Will, W., Gossler, K., Raithel, H.J. & Schaller, K.H. (1981) Quantitative determination of 4,4'-methylene-bis(2-chloraniline) (MOCA®) in the urine by high-pressure liquid chromatography. *Arbeitsmed. Sozialmed. Praventivmed.*, **16**, 201–203

Williams, G.M., Laspia, M.F. & Dunkel, V.C. (1982) Reliability of the hepatocyte primary culture/DNA repair test in testing of coded carcinogens and noncarcinogens. *Mutat. Res.*, **97**, 359–370

Wu, K., Leslie, C.L. & Stacey, N.H. (1989a) Effects of mutagenic and non-mutagenic aniline derivatives on rat liver drug-metabolizing enzymes. *Xenobiotica*, **19**, 1275–1283

Wu, K., Bonin, A.M., Leslie, C.L., Baker, R.S.U. & Stacey, N.H. (1989b) Genotoxity and effects on rat liver drug-metabolizing enzymes by possible substitutes for 4,4'-methylene bis(2-chloroaniline). *Carcinogenesis*, **10**, 2119–2122

Yoneyama, K. & Matsumura, F. (1984) Microbial metabolism of 4,4'-methylene- bis(2-chloroaniline). *Arch. environ. Contam. Toxicol.*, **13**, 501–507

Yun, C.-H., Shimada, T. & Guengerich, F.P. (1992) Contributions of human liver cytochrome P450 enzymes to the *N*-oxidation of 4,4'-methylene-bis(2-chloroaniline). *Carcinogenesis*, **13**, 217–222

para-CHLOROANILINE

1. Exposure Data

1.1 Chemical and physical data

1.1.1 *Synonyms, structural and molecular data*

Chem. Abstr. Serv. Reg. No.: 106-47-8

Chem. Abstr. Name: 4-Chlorobenzenamine

IUPAC Systematic Name: *para*-Chloroaniline

Synonyms: 4-Aminochlorobenzene; *para*-aminochlorobenzene; 1-amino-4-chloroben-zene; 4-amino-1-chlorobenzene; 4-chloro-1-aminobenzene; 4-chloroaniline; 4-chloro-phenylamine; *para*-chlorophenylamine

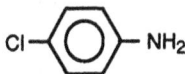

$$Cl-\!\!\bigcirc\!\!-NH_2$$

C_6H_6ClN Mol. wt: 127.57

1.1.2 *Chemical and physical properties of the pure substance*

(a) *Description*: Rhombic prisms (Lide, 1991); technical material: crystalline, colourless to light-amber; flakes, light-yellow to tan (DuPont Co., 1991a,b)

(b) *Boiling-point*: 232 °C (Lide, 1991)

(c) *Melting-point*: 72.5 °C (Lide, 1991)

(d) *Density*: 1.429 at 19 °C/4 °C (Lide, 1991)

(e) *Spectroscopy data*: Infrared, ultraviolet, nuclear magnetic resonance and mass spectral data have been reported (Pouchert, 1981, 1983; Sadtler Research Labora-tories, 1980, 1991; Weast & Astle, 1985).

(f) *Solubility*: Slightly soluble in water (0.237 wt%), acetone, ethanol and diethyl ether (Lide, 1991; DuPont Co., 1991a,b)

(g) *Volatility*: Vapour pressure, 0.15 mm Hg [20 Pa] at 25 °C (technical material); relative vapour density (air = 1), 4.4 (DuPont Co., 1991a,b)

(h) *Octanol/water partition coefficient (P)*: log P, 1.83 (Hansch & Leo, 1979)

(i) *Conversion factor*: mg/m^3 = 5.22 × ppm[1]

---

[1]Calculated from: mg/m^3 = (molecular weight/24.45) × ppm, assuming normal temperature (25 °C) and pressure (760 mm Hg [101.3 kPa])

1.1.3 *Trade names, technical products and impurities*

para-Chloroaniline is commercially available as a technical-grade product with the following specifications: purity, 98.5–99.0% min.; water, 0.10% max.; aniline (see IARC, 1982a, 1987a), 0.1% max.; and isomeric chloroanilines, 0.5% max. (DuPont Co., 1991a; Hoechst Celanese Corp., 1989). It is also available in research quantities at purities ranging from 98 to > 99% (Janssen Chimica, 1990; Riedel-de-Haen, 1990; Heraeus, 1991; Lancaster Synthesis, 1991; TCI America, 1991; Aldrich Chemical Co., 1992; Fluka Chemie AG, 1993).

1.1.4 *Analysis*

A simple gas chromatographic method was developed which provides sensitivity and specificity for the analysis of complex mixtures of common herbicide metabolites, including *para*-chloroaniline, in aqueous solution. The anilines were converted to N-acetyl,N-trifluoroacetyl derivatives and analysed by gas chromatography with electron capture detection (Hargesheimer *et al.*, 1981).

A thin-layer chromatographic method was reported for the analysis of primary aromatic amines, including *para*-chloroaniline, in mixtures with a low-nanogram detection level. Thin-layer chromatograms are developed by diazotization of the amines with nitrogen oxide vapour, followed by coupling with N-(1-naphthyl)ethylenediamine dihydrochloride to produce sharp spots with distinctly different colours (Narang *et al.*, 1982).

In order to assess the applicability of methods developed by the US Environmental Protection Agency and similar survey methods for the determination of a broad range of principal organic hazardous constituents, James *et al.* (1983) evaluated gas chromatography with flame ionization detection and with mass spectrometry for the analysis of complex mixtures containing *para*-chloroaniline. The limit of detection for this compound was 0.20 ng by the first method and 1.9 ng by the second.

A macroporous cation exchanger in the hydrogen form was developed to retain organic bases, including *para*-chloroaniline, as cations from aqueous samples. Neutral organic compounds are removed by washing with methanol and ethyl ether, and the protonated bases are converted to their free base forms with ammonia. After evaporation, the individual bases are separated by gas chromatography with flame ionization detection (Kaczvinsky *et al.*, 1983).

Different adsorption–desorption techniques were compared, including capillary gas chromatography with flame ionization and/or electrochemical detection and a reverse-osmosis technique using reverse-phase high-performance liquid chromatography, for the analysis of selected organic pollutants, including *para*-chloroaniline (Malaiyandi *et al.*, 1987).

Polar aniline derivatives, including *para*-chloroaniline, were determined in aqueous environmental samples by on-line liquid chromatographic preconcentration techniques. The limit of detection using ultraviolet absorption at 235 nm or electrochemical detection was 10 ppt (Hennion *et al.*, 1991).

Fourier transform-infrared techniques were applied to environmental samples to allow identification of trace components at a nanogram level. The precision of the techniques was shown to be comparable to that obtainable by gas chromatography–mass spectrometry (Gurka *et al.*, 1991).

1.2 Production and use

1.2.1 *Production*

para-Chloroaniline is prepared primarily by the reduction of *para*-nitrochlorobenzene (Dunlap, 1981). It has also been produced by the reaction of 1,4-dichlorobenzene (*para*-dichlorobenzene; see IARC, 1982b, 1987b) with ammonia (US National Library of Medicine, 1992).

Production of *para*-chloroaniline in the USA has been estimated to be 45–450 tonnes per year. The compound (or its hydrochloride salt) is produced by one company each in India, Japan, the United Kingdom and the USA and by two companies in Germany (Chemical Information Services, 1991).

1.2.2 *Use*

para-Chloroaniline is used as an intermediate in the manufacture of dyes (Vat Red 32; Azoic Coupling Agents 5 and 10) and pigments (Pigment Green 10) and as an intermediate in the production of some pharmaceuticals and agricultural chemicals (urea herbicides, e.g., monuron; see IARC, 1976) (US National Library of Medicine, 1992).

1.3 Occurrence

1.3.1 *Natural occurrence*

para-Chloroaniline is not known to occur as a natural product.

1.3.2 *Occupational exposure*

No data were available to the Working Group.

1.3.3 *Water and sediments*

Aniline and chlorinated anilines enter the estuarine environment by various routes, since they are formed during the microbial degradation of phenylcarbamate, phenylurea and acylanilide herbicides and nitroaniline fungicides. They can also enter as waste effluents from dye manufacturing plants. In laboratory studies, photolysis was shown to be an important degradation route for *para*-chloroaniline in estuarine water. There was no microbial degradation of chloroanilines during short-term (up to three days) incubations; however, there was rapid microbial degradation of chloroaniline and aniline photoproducts (Schaefer *et al.*, 1980; Sakagami *et al.*, 1986; Huang *et al.*, 1987; Mutanen *et al.*, 1988).

During 1976–78, the water of the Rhine River contained about 0.1 μg/l *para*-chloroaniline. Following bank or dune filtration of the water, the levels were 0.03–0.1 μg/l or < 0.01 μg/l *para*-chloroaniline, respectively. The half-life of the compound in water was estimated to be 0.3–3 days in river water and 30–300 days in groundwater (Zoeteman *et al.*, 1980).

In 1979, the mean concentration of *para*-chloroaniline in the Rhine River at Lobith, the Netherlands, was 0.22 µg/l (max., 0.74). Mean concentrations in the Rhine tributaries, Boven Merwede and Ijssel, were 0.14 (max., 0.24) and 0.13 (max., 0.29) µg/l, respectively. *para*-Chloroaniline was frequently detected in the Meuse River at Eijsden and Lith, but the mean concentrations were only 0.02 (max., 0.08) and 0.03 (max., 0.12) µg/l, respectively (Wegman & De Korte, 1981).

para-Chloroaniline was not detected in two tap-water samples from municipal sources in the Lake Ontario region (Kingston and Trenton), Canada; the estimated detection threshold was 20–30 pg (Malaiyandi *et al.*, 1987).

1.3.4 *Soil*

In soil, *para*-chloroaniline binds to humic materials and is slowly degraded by aerobic and anaerobic processes (Hargesheimer *et al.*, 1981; Freitag *et al.*, 1984; Dao *et al.*, 1986). Residues of *para*-chloroaniline were detected in soil up to 12 years after application of the herbicide buturon (Reiml *et al.*, 1989).

1.3.5 *Other*

Levels of *para*-chloroaniline were determined in goldfish (*Carassius auratus*) after experimental pond water had been treated to maintain a *para*-chloroaniline concentration of 50 ppb (µg/l) for four to six weeks. The highest levels after 10 weeks were found in fat (about 7 mg/kg) (Gebefuegi *et al.*, 1988).

1.4 Regulations and guidelines

Occupational exposure limits have been set in several countries: Bulgaria, 0.3 mg/m^3 (time-weighted average, TWA) with a notation that the compound may irritate skin; Romania, 5 mg/m^3 (average), 10 mg/m^3 (max.), with skin irritation notation; the former USSR, 0.3 mg/m^3 (maximal acceptable concentration) with a skin irritation notation; and the former Yugoslavia, 0.05 mg/m^3 (TWA) (Cook, 1987).

DuPont Co. (1991b) proposed an acceptable exposure limit of 0.5 mg/m^3 for an 8-h TWA and 0.3 mg/m^3 for a 12-h TWA, with a skin irritation notation.

2. Studies of Cancer in Humans

No data were available to the Working Group.

3. Studies of Cancer in Experimental Animals

3.1 Oral administration

3.1.1 *Mouse*

Groups of 50 male and 50 female B6C3F$_1$ mice, six weeks of age, were fed a diet containing 2500 or 5000 mg/kg (ppm) *para*-chloroaniline (technical grade [purity unspecified], melting-point, 68–71 °C) for 78 weeks, followed by a 13-week observation period. A group of 20 male and 20 female controls received the diet alone. Decreased body weight gain was observed in both treated males and females relative to that of controls. The numbers of surviving animals at 91 weeks were: males—control, 18/20; low-dose, 44/50; high-dose, 44/50; females—control, 20/20; low-dose, 41/50; high-dose, 39/50. Haemangio-sarcomas occurred in different organs (subcutaneous tissue, spleen, liver, kidney) in 2/20 control, 9/50 low-dose and 14/50 high dose males; one haemangioma was observed in the low-dose group. The increased incidence of all vascular tumours was significant [$p < 0.025$, Cochran-Armitage trend test]. Among females, haemangiosarcomas occurred at all of the sites in 0/18 control, 3/49 low-dose and 7/42 high-dose animals; one haemangioma was observed in the high-dose group. The increased incidence of combined vascular tumours in females was significant ($p = 0.012$, Cochran-Armitage trend test) (US National Cancer Institute, 1979).

Groups of 50 male and 50 female B6C3F$_1$ mice, seven to eight weeks old, were admi-nistered 3, 10 or 30 mg/kg bw *para*-chloroaniline (99.1% pure) in aqueous hydrochloric acid (molar equivalents) by gavage on five days a week for 103 weeks. Controls received deionized water at a volume of 5 ml/kg. Survival at 104 weeks was: males—controls, 43/50; low-dose, 36/50; mid-dose, 29/50 ($p = 0.005$); high-dose 35/50; females—controls, 39/50; low-dose, 42/50, mid-dose; 44/50, high-dose, 41/50. Hepatocellular adenomas were observed in male mice: controls, 9/50; low-dose, 15/49; mid-dose, 10/50; high-dose, 4/50; and hepatocellular carcinomas occurred with a significantly positive trend: controls, 3/50; low-dose, 7/49; mid-dose, 11/50; high-dose, 17/50 ($p < 0.001$, logistic regression trend test). The incidence in males of hepatocellular adenomas and carcinomas combined was: controls, 11/50; low-dose, 21/49 ($p = 0.019$, logistic regression test); mid-dose, 20/50 ($p = 0.045$, logistic regression test); high-dose, 21/50 ($p = 0.027$, logistic regression test). The incidence of haemangiosarcomas of liver and spleen combined was 4/50 controls, 4/49 low-dose, 1/50 mid-dose and 10/50 high-dose male mice ($p = 0.014$, logistic regression trend test). No significant increase in the incidence of such tumours occurred in females (US National Toxicology Program, 1989; Chhabra *et al.*, 1991).

3.1.2 *Rat*

Groups of 50 male and 50 female Fischer 344 rats, six weeks of age, were fed diets containing 250 or 500 ppm (mg/kg) *para*-chloroaniline (technical grade [purity unspecified]) for 78 weeks. A group of 20 male and 20 female controls received the diet alone. Following a 24-week observation period, the surviving animals were sacrificed. There was no difference in body weight gain in the treated animals compared to the controls. Survival at week 102 was: males—controls, 18/20; low-dose, 46/50; high-dose, 38/50; females—controls, 18/20; low-dose, 49/50; high-dose, 45/50. Mesenchymal tumours (fibroma, fibrosarcoma, haeman-giosarcoma, osteosarcoma, sarcoma not otherwise specified) of the spleen or splenic capsule occurred in 0/20 control, 0/49 low-dose and 10/49 high-dose male rats ($p = 0.001$, Cochran-Armitage trend test) and in 0/18 control, 2/49 low-dose and 5/42 high-dose females (US National Cancer Institute, 1979; Goodman *et al.*, 1984).

Groups of 50 male and 50 female Fischer 344 rats, eight to nine weeks old, were administered 2, 6 or 18 mg/kg bw *para*-chloroaniline (99.1% pure) in aqueous hydrochloric acid (molar equivalents) by gavage on five days per week for 103 weeks. A group of 50 male and 50 female controls received deionized water at 5 ml/kg. Survival at 105 weeks in low-dose and mid-dose males was significantly greater than that in the control group: controls, 18/50; low-dose, 32/50 (p = 0.007); mid-dose, 32/50 (p = 0.005); high-dose 21/50; as was that of high-dose females: controls, 27/50; low-dose, 39/50; mid-dose, 36/50; high-dose, 37/50 (p = 0.043). The incidences of proliferative mesenchymal lesions and fatty metamorphosis of the spleen were increased in high-dose males and females. The incidences of fibromas and sarcomas in males are shown in Table 1. Adrenal phaeochromocytomas, including a few malignant phaeochromocytomas, were observed in 13/49 controls, 14/48 low-dose, 15/48 mid-dose and 26/49 high-dose male rats (p = 0.001, logistic regression trend test). The incidence of mononuclear cell leukaemias was decreased in all treated groups: males—controls, 21/49; low-dose, 3/50; mid-dose, 2/50; high-dose, 3/50; females—controls, 10/50; low-dose, 2/50; mid-dose, 1/50; high-dose, 1/50 (US National Toxicology Program, 1989; Chhabra et al., 1991).

Table 1. Incidences of tumours of the spleen in male rats treated with *para*-chloroaniline

Tumour	Control	Low-dose	Mid-dose	High-dose
Fibroma	0/49	0/50	0/50	2/50
Fibrosarcoma	0/49	1/50	2/50	17/50**
Osteosarcoma	0/49	0/50	1/50	19/50**
Haemangiosarcoma	0/49	0/50	0/50	4/50*
Sarcomas,combined	0/49	1/50	3/50	38/50**

From US National Toxicology Program (1989); *, p = 0.07, logistic regression pair-wise comparison; **, p < 0.001, logistic regression trend test

4. Other Relevant Data

4.1 Absorption, distribution, metabolism and excretion

4.1.1 *Humans*

In a patient suffering from acute poisoning by *para*-chloroaniline, conjugates of the parent compound and 2-hydroxy-4-chloroaniline (2-amino-5-chlorophenol) were detected as major urinary metabolites (Yoshida et al. 1992).

Other evidence for the metabolism of *para*-chloroaniline in humans is indirect and is derived from studies on the anticancer drug, sulofenur [*N*-(5-indanesulfonyl)-*N'*-(4-chlorophenyl)urea]. 4-Chloroaniline-2-sulfate (2-amino-5-chlorophenyl sulfate) and *para*-chloro-oxanilic acid, which are major and minor metabolites, respectively, of *para*-chloroaniline in experimental animals, were identified together with free *para*-chloroaniline as minor urinary metabolites of sulofenur after administration of an oral dose of [^{14}C-*para*-chlorophenyl]-sulofenur (31 mg/kg bw; 91.7 µCi; radiochemical purity, > 99%) to a patient who had previously received the same dose of unlabelled drug daily for six days (Ehlhardt, 1991).

4.1.2 *Experimental systems*

Metabolism of *para*-chloroaniline *in vitro* by human granulocyte myeloperoxidase has been reported, resulting in at least 10 unknown peroxidation products (Bakkenist *et al.*, 1981).

The pharmacokinetics and metabolism of *para*-chloroaniline have been studied extensively in Fischer 344 rats. In male rats administered ^{14}C-labelled compound (5 mCi/mmol [0.04 mCi/mg] [radiochemical purity unspecified]) at 0.3–30 mg/kg bw by gavage in 0.01 N hydrochloric acid, 75–85% of the dose was excreted in urine and 8–12% in faeces by 24 h; only 4% was excreted as unchanged amine in urine, 2.5% in bile and 1% in faeces. At seven days, appreciable radiolabel was still present in blood cells, accounting for 1–2% of the dose. After an intravenous dose of 3.0 mg/kg bw in ethanol:propylene glycol:water (1:1:8), 60% of the dose was excreted in urine after 4 h, 25% was excreted in bile after 6 h, and 90% was eliminated in urine and faeces by 8 h. Initial levels in tissues were highest in muscle > fat > skin > liver > blood; and the kinetics of elimination was biphasic, with an initial half-time of 8 min and terminal half-times of 3–4 h in most tissues, except small intestine and fat (23–29 h). *para*-Chloroacetanilide was detected as a metabolite in bile and in blood, but not in urine or faeces, indicating further metabolism prior to excretion (US National Toxicology Program, 1989).

Additional studies of the metabolism of ^{14}C-*para*-chloroaniline (133 μCi/mg [17 mCi/mmol]; radiochemical purity, > 98%) were carried out in male Fischer 344 rats, female C3H mice and male rhesus monkeys. The compound was given by oral intubation at a dose of 20 mg/kg bw in an aqueous solution adjusted to pH 5 with hydrochloric acid. In rats, mice and monkeys, respectively, the urine contained 90, 82 and 67–74%, and the faeces contained 8, 5 and 1% of the dose after 48 h. The major urinary metabolite in all three species was 4-chloroaniline-2-sulfate; in rats and monkeys, its *N*-acetyl derivative was also detected as a minor urinary metabolite. In rats and to a lesser extent in mice, two additional metabolites, *para*-chloro-oxanilic acid and *para*-chloroglycolanilide, were observed as major and minor urinary metabolites, respectively. In monkeys, *para*-chloroacetanilide, which was not detected in urine or faeces, and 4-chloroaniline-2-sulfate were the major metabolites found in plasma (Ehlhardt & Howbert, 1991).

After oral dosing of female Wistar rats with *para*-chloroaniline [purity unspecified] in propylene glycol at 0.6 mmol [77 mg]/kg bw by gavage, higher levels of haemoglobin binding (569 mmol bound/mol haemoglobin per (mmol compound/kg bw)) were observed than with 12 other monocyclic aromatic amines. The release of free *para*-chloroaniline after alkaline hydrolysis is consistent with the presence of a circulating *N*-hydroxy-*para*-chloroaniline metabolite that enters erythrocytes, is oxidized to *para*-chloronitrosobenzene and forms a sulfinamide adduct with haemoglobin (Birner & Neumann, 1988). These data are also consistent with the observation that at seven days radiolabel persisted in blood cells of Fischer 344 rats treated with radiolabelled *para*-chloroaniline (US National Toxicology Program, 1989).

N-Hydroxylation of *para*-chloroaniline has been demonstrated *in vitro* and shown to be catalysed by hepatic microsomal cytochromes P450 in a wide variety of species, including rats, mice, hamsters, guinea-pigs, rabbits, rainbow trout and red-winged blackbirds. In mammals, multiple isozymes appear to be involved in the catalysis, since enzymes are induced by both phenobarbital- and 3-methylcholanthrene-type inducers (for reviews, see Golly & Hlavica, 1987; Dady *et al.*, 1991). Peroxidative metabolism of *para*-chloroaniline has also been shown to be mediated by horseradish peroxidase, fungal chloroperoxidases, ram seminal vesicle prostaglandin synthase, rabbit liver microsomal lipid peroxides and by rabbit haemoglobin in the presence of erythrocyte reductases. These results indicate that the *N*-hydroxy derivative may be the initial product but that it is further oxidized enzymatically or non-enzymatically to *para*-chloronitrosobenzene. Several dimeric or halogen-containing oxidation products have also been detected (Kaufman *et al.*, 1973; Corbett *et al.*, 1978, 1980; Golly & Hlavica, 1983; Golly *et al.*, 1984; Golly & Hlavica, 1985; Doerge & Corbett, 1991).

4.2 Toxic effects

4.2.1 *Humans*

Methaemoglobinaemia, which is also consistent with the presence of a circulating *N*-hydroxy-*para*-chloroaniline metabolite, has been reported in workers exposed to *para*-chloroaniline and in neonates inadvertently exposed in incubators to chlorhexidine gluconate, which is known to decompose spontaneously to *para*-chloroaniline (Faivre *et al.*, 1971; Linch, 1974; van der Vorst *et al.*, 1990). Methaemoglobinaemia and haemolytic anaemia have also been observed (Hainsworth *et al.*, 1989; Taylor *et al.*, 1989) in phase I clinical trials after high doses of sulofenur (Ehlhardt, 1991).

4.2.2 *Experimental systems*

High levels of methaemoglobinaemia have been demonstrated after oral treatment of female Wistar rats with *para*-chloroaniline [purity unspecified] in propylene glycol at 0.6 mmol [77 mg]/kg bw; of male and female Fischer 344 rats with *para*-chloroaniline hydrochloride (purity, > 99%) in water at 5–80 mg/kg, five days per week for 13 weeks; of male and female B6C3F$_1$ mice with *para*-chloroaniline hydrochloride (purity, > 99%) in water at 7.5–120 mg/kg, five days per week for 13 weeks; and of cats with *para*-chloroaniline [purity and vehicle unspecified] at 0.0625 mmol [8 mg]/kg bw (McLean *et al.*, 1969; Birner & Neumann, 1988; Chhabra *et al.*, 1990). Fischer rats given 80 mg/kg for a further 13 weeks had lowered body weights; and both rats and mice showed dose-related decreases in erythrocyte haemoglobin and increases in spleen weight. Numerous lesions indicative of haemolytic anaemia and methaemoglobinaemia were observed, including haemosiderosis in the kidney, liver and spleen and increased haematopoiesis in the liver and spleen in mice and rats; bone-marrow hyperplasia was seen only in rats (Chhabra *et al.*, 1990). Nephrotoxicity was also reported in male Fischer 344 rats given a single intraperitoneal dose of *para*-chloroaniline [purity unspecified] at 1.5 mmol [191 mg]/kg bw in saline, which induced decreased urine volume, haematuria, elevated blood urea nitrogen and decreased renal cortical uptake of *para*-aminohippurate (Rankin *et al.*, 1986).

LD$_{50}$ values for *para*-chloroaniline [purity and vehicle unspecified] were estimated to be 200–480 mg/kg bw after single gavage doses to male Carworth-Wistar rats and 360 mg/kg bw after dermal administration to male New Zealand rabbits (Smyth *et al.*, 1962).

In the 103-week carcinogenicity study described on p. 309, several treatment-related non-neoplastic lesions were observed, including haemolytic anaemia, methaemoglobinaemia and fibrosis and fatty metaplasia of the spleen (US National Toxicology Program, 1989; Chhabra *et al.*, 1991).

4.3 Reproductive and developmental effects

4.3.1 *Humans*

No data were available to the Working Group.

4.3.2 *Experimental systems*

In a study conducted in Germany, zebrafish (*Brachydanio rerio*) were kept in tap-water to which 0, 0.04, 0.2 or 1.0 mg/l *para*-chloroaniline (technical grade; purity, > 99%) had been added (Bresch *et al.*, 1990). The concentrations in the aquaria were analysed weekly by high-performance liquid chromatography. No adverse effect was noted in the F_0 fish or on the numbers and viability of eggs produced. Eggs collected during the 22nd week of exposure were allowed to develop with continuing exposure to 4-chloroaniline. Mortality was not increased, but, at sexual maturity, over 90% of the F_1 fish raised in 1.0 mg/l had spinal abnormalities and abnormal abdominal swellings. Significantly fewer eggs were produced by F_1 fish in all three exposed groups, and the viability of eggs was reduced in the 1.0 mg/l group. An F_2 generation exhibited the same effects: morphological abnormalities, reduced egg counts and reduced viability of eggs at 1.0 mg/l, and reduced egg counts at 0.04 and 0.2 mg/l.

4.4 Genetic and related effects

4.4.1 *Humans*

No data were available to the Working Group.

4.4.2 *Experimental systems* (see also Table 2 and Appendices 1 and 2)

para-Chloroaniline preferentially killed the pol A⁻ strain in the *Escherichia coli* pol A⁻/pol A⁺ assay, both in the presence and absence of an exogenous metabolic system. It was not mutagenic to *Salmonella typhimurium*, except to strain TA98, for which conflicting data were obtained. It induced mutations in *Aspergillus nidulans* and in mouse lymphoma L5178Y cells at the *tk* locus. it did not induce mitotic recombination in *Saccharomyces cerevisiae*. *para*-Chloroaniline transformed primary cultures of Syrian hamster embryo cells, only in the later of two studies from the same laboratory. It induced sister chromatid exchange and chromosomal aberrations in Chinese hamster ovary cells *in vitro*.

5. Summary of Data Reported and Evaluation

5.1 Exposure data

para-Chloroaniline is used as an intermediate in the manufacture of dyes, pigments, agricultural chemicals and pharmaceuticals. It is a persistent environmental degradation product of some herbicides and fungicides.

Table 2. Genetic and related effects of *para*-chloroaniline

Test system	Result		Dose[a] (LED/HID)	Reference
	Without exogenous metabolic system	With exogenous metabolic system		
ECL, *Escherichia coli* pol A/N3110-P3478, differential toxicity	+	+	5.0000	Rosenkranz & Poirier (1979)
ECW, *Escherichia coli*, differential toxicity WP2 *uvrA*	-	-	1667.0000	Dunkel et al. (1985)
SA0, *Salmonella typhimurium* TA100, reverse mutation	-	-	500.0000	Simmon (1979a)
SA0, *Salmonella typhimurium* TA100, reverse mutation	0	-	0.0000	Zimmer et al. (1980)
SA0, *Salmonella typhimurium* TA100, reverse mutation	-	-	1667.0000	Dunkel et al. (1985)
SA0, *Salmonella typhimurium* TA100, reverse mutation	-	-	500.0000	Mortelmans et al. (1986)
SA5, *Salmonella typhimurium* TA1535, reverse mutation	-	-	125.0000	Rosenkranz & Poirier (1979)
SA5, *Salmonella typhimurium* TA1535, reverse mutation	-	-	500.0000	Simmon (1979a)
SA5, *Salmonella typhimurium* TA1535, reverse mutation	-	-	1667.0000	Dunkel et al. (1985)
SA5, *Salmonella typhimurium* TA1535, reverse mutation	-	-	1667.0000	Mortelmans et al. (1986)
SA7, *Salmonella typhimurium* TA1537, reverse mutation	-	-	500.0000	Simmon (1979a)
SA7, *Salmonella typhimurium* TA1537, reverse mutation	-	-	1667.0000	Dunkel et al. (1985)
SA7, *Salmonella typhimurium* TA1537, reverse mutation	-	-	500.0000	Mortelmans et al. (1986)
SA&, *Salmonella typhimurium* TA1537, reverse mutation	0	0	0.0000	Zimmer et al. (1980)
SA8, *Salmonella typhimurium* TA1538, reverse mutation	-	-	125.0000	Rosenkranz & Poirier (1979)
SA8, *Salmonella typhimurium* TA1538, reverse mutation	-	-	500.0000	Simmon (1979a)
SA8, *Salmonella typhimurium* TA1538, reverse mutation	-	-	1667.0000	Dunkel et al. (1985)
SA9, *Salmonella typhimurium* TA98, reverse mutation	-	-	500.0000	Simmon (1979a)
SA9, *Salmonella typhimurium* TA98, reverse mutation	-	+	333.0000	Dunkel & Simmon (1980)
SA9, *Salmonella typhimurium* TA98, reverse mutation	-	+[b]	500.0000	Dunkel et al. (1985)
SA9, *Salmonella typhimurium* TA98, reverse mutation	-	+[c]	333.0000	Mortelmans et al. (1986)
SA9, *Salmonella typhimurium* TA98, reverse mutation	0	-	0.0000	Zimmer et al. (1980)
SCH, *Saccharomyces cerevisiae*, mitotic recombination	-	-	2000.0000	Simmon (1979b)
ANR, *Aspergillus nidulans*, reverse mutation	+	0	200.0000	Prasad (1970)
GST, Gene mutation, mouse lymphoma L5178Y cells, *tk* locus	+	(+)	16.0000	Mitchell et al. (1988)
GST, Gene mutation, mouse lymphoma L5178Y cells, *tk* locus	(+)	+	16.0000	Myhr & Caspary (1988)

Table 2 (contd)

Test system	Result		Dose[a] (LED/HID)	Reference
	Without exogenous metabolic system	With exogenous metabolic system		
G5T, Gene mutation, mouse lymphoma L5178Y cells, *tk* locus	+	+	25.0000	Myhr *et al.* (1990)
TCS, Cell transformation, Syrian hamster embryo cells, clonal assay	+	0	0.0100	Pienta & Kawalek (1981)
TCS, Cell transformation, Syrian hamster embryo cells, clonal assay	–	0	100.0000	Pienta *et al.* (1977)
CIC, Chromosomal aberrations, CHO cells *in vitro*	+[c]	+[c]	500.0000	Anderson *et al.* (1990)

+, positive; (+), weakly positive; –, negative; 0, not tested

[a] In-vitro tests, μg/ml; in-vivo tests, mg/kg bw

[b] Positive in three of four laboratories

[c] Positive in one of two laboratories

5.2 Human carcinogenicity data

No data were available to the Working Group.

5.3 Animal carcinogenicity data

para-Chloroaniline was tested for carcinogenicity in mice and rats by administration in the diet and by gavage. It produced haemangiosarcomas in male and female mice in different organs after administration in the diet. It induced haemangiosarcomas of the spleen and liver and hepatocellular adenomas and carcinomas in male mice after administration by gavage. It induced sarcomas of the spleen and splenic capsule in male rats in both studies.

5.4 Other relevant data

para-Chloroaniline causes methaemoglobinaemia and is metabolized similarly in humans and experimental animals.

para-Chloroaniline induced DNA damage in bacteria, but conflicting results were obtained for gene mutation. Gene mutation but not mitotic recombination was induced in fungi. Gene mutation, sister chromatid exchange and chromosomal aberrations were induced in cultured mammalian cells, while conflicting data were obtained for cell transformation.

5.5 Evaluation[1]

There is *inadequate evidence* in humans for the carcinogenicity of *para*-chloroaniline.

There is *sufficient evidence* in experimental animals for the carcinogenicity of *para*-chloroaniline.

Overall evaluation

para-Chloroaniline is *possibly carcinogenic to humans (Group 2B)*.

6. References

Aldrich Chemical Co. (1992) *Aldrich Catalog/Handbook of Fine Chemicals 1992–1993*, Milwaukee, WI, p. 269

Anderson, B.E., Zeiger, E., Shelby, M.D., Resnick, M.A., Gulati, D.K., Ivett, J.L. & Loveday, K.S. (1990) Chromosome aberration and sister chromatid exchange test results with 42 chemicals. *Environ. Mol. Mutag.*, **16** (Suppl. 18), 55–137

Bakkenist, A.R.J., Plat, H. & Wever, R. (1981) Oxidation of 4-chloro-aniline catalyzed by human myeloperoxidase. *Bioorg. Chem.*, **10**, 324–328

---

[1]For definition of the italicized terms, see Preamble, pp. 26–30.

Birner, G. & Neumann, H.-G. (1988) Biomonitoring of aromatic amines. II: Hemoglobin binding of some monocyclic aromatic amines. *Arch. Toxicol.*, **62**, 110–115

Bresch, H., Beck, H., Ehlermanmn, D., Schlaszus, H. & Urbanek, M. (1990) A long-term toxicity test comprising reproduction and growth of zebrafish with 4-chloroaniline. *Arch. environ. Contam. Toxicol.*, **19**, 419–427

Chhabra, R.S., Thompson, M., Elwell, M.R. & Gerken, D.K. (1990) Toxicity of *p*-chloroaniline in rats and mice. *Food chem. Toxicol.*, **28**, 717–722

Chhabra, R.S., Huff, J.E., Haseman, J.K., Elwell, M.R. & Peters, A.C. (1991) Carcinogenicity of *p*-chloroaniline in rats and mice. *Food chem. Toxicol.*, **29**, 119–124

Chemical Information Services (1991) *Directory of World Chemical Producers 1992/1993 Edition*, Dallas, TX, p. 135

Cook, W.A. (1987) *Occupational Exposure Limits—Worldwide*, Akron, OH, American Industrial Hygiene Association, pp. 132, 171

Corbett, M.D., Chipko, B.R. & Baden, D.G. (1978) Chloroperoxidase-catalysed oxidation of 4-chloro-aniline to 4-chloronitrosobenzene. *Biochem. J.*, **175**, 353–360

Corbett, M.D., Chipko, B.R. & Batchelor, A.O. (1980) The action of chloride peroxidase on 4-chloro-aniline. *Biochem. J.*, **187**, 893–903

Dady, J.M., Bradbury, S.P., Hoffman, A.D., Voit, M.M. & Olson, D.L. (1991) Hepatic microsomal *N*-hydroxylation of aniline and 4-chloroaniline by rainbow trout (*Onchorhyncus mykiss*). *Xeno-biotica*, **21**, 1605–1620

Dao, T.H., Bouchard, D., Mattice, J. & Lavy, T.L. (1986) Soil sorption of aniline and chloroanilines: direct and indirect concentration measurements of the adsorbed phase. *Soil Sci.*, **141**, 26–30

Doerge, D.R. & Corbett, M.D. (1991) Peroxygenation mechanisms for chloroperoxidase-catalyzed *N*-oxidation of arylamines. *Chem. Res. Toxicol.*, **4**, 556–560

Dunkel, V.C. & Simmon, V.F. (1980) Mutagenic activity of chemicals previously tested for carcino-genicity in the National Cancer Institute Bioassay Program. In: Montesano, R., Bartsch, H. & Tomatis, L., eds, *Molecular and Cellular Aspects of Carcinogen Screening Tests* (IARC Scientific Publications No. 27), Lyon, IARC, pp. 283–302

Dunkel, V.C., Zeiger, E., Brusick, D., McCoy, E., McGregor, D., Mortelmans, K., Rosenkranz, H.S. & Simmon, V.F. (1985) Reproducibility of microbial mutagenicity assays: II. Testing of carcinogens and noncarcinogens in *Salmonella* typhimurium and *Escherichia coli*. *Environ. Mutag.*, **7** (Suppl. 5), 1–248

Dunlap, K.L. (1981) Nitrobenzene and nitrotoluenes. In: Mark, H.F., Othmer, D.F., Overberger, C.G., Seaborg, G.T. & Grayson, N., eds, *Kirk-Othmer Encyclopedia of Chemical Technology*, 3rd ed., Vol. 15, New York, John Wiley & Sons, pp. 916–932

DuPont Co. (1991a) *Material Safety Data Sheet: p-Chloroaniline*, Wilmington, DE

DuPont Co. (1991b) *Product Specification Sheet: p-Chloroaniline Tech*, Wilmington, DE

Ehlhardt, W.J. (1991) Metabolism and disposition of the anticancer agent sulofenur in mouse, rat, monkey, and human. *Drug Metab. Disposition*, **19**, 370–375

Ehlhardt, W.J. & Howbert, J.J. (1991) Metabolism and disposition of *p*-chloroaniline in rat, mouse, and monkey. *Drug Metab. Disposition*, **19**, 366–369

Faivre, M., Armand, J., Évreux, J.-C., Duverneuil, G. & Colin, C. (1971) Toxic methaemoglobinaemia due to aniline derivatives: *para*-chloroaniline and *para*-toluidine (Fr.). *Arch. Mal. prof.*, **32**, 575–577

Fluka Chemie AG (1993) *Fluka Chemika-BioChemika*, Buchs, p. 304

Freitag, D., Scheunert, I., Klein, W. & Korte, F. (1984) Long-term fate of 4-chloroaniline-^{14}C in soil and plants under outdoor conditions. A contribution to terrestrial ecotoxicology of chemicals. *J. agric. Food Chem.*, **32**, 203–207

Gebefuegi, I., Lay, J.-P. & Korte, F. (1988) *Influence of Environmental Chemicals in the Aquatic Environment* (NBS Special Publication 740), Washington DC, National Bureau of Standards, Program for Environmental Specimen Banking, pp. 31–39

Golly, I. & Hlavica, P. (1983) The role of hemoglobin in the *N*-oxidation of 4-chloroaniline. *Biochim. biophys. Acta*, **760**, 69–76

Golly, I. & Hlavica, P. (1985) *N*-Oxidation of 4-chloroaniline by prostaglandin synthase. Redox cycling of radical intermediates. *Biochem. J.*, **260**, 803–809

Golly, I. & Hlavica, P. (1987) Regulative mechanisms in NADH- and NADPH-supported *N*-oxidation of 4-chloroaniline catalyzed by cytochrome b_5-enriched rabbit liver microsomal fractions. *Biochim. biophys. Acta*, **913**, 219–227

Golly, I., Hlavica, P. & Wolf, J. (1984) The role of lipid peroxidation in the *N*-oxidation of 4-chloroaniline. *Biochem. J.*, **224**, 415–421

Goodman, D.G., Ward, J.M. & Reichardt, W.D. (1984) Splenic fibrosis and sarcomas in F344 rats fed diets containing aniline hydrochloride, *p*-chloroaniline, azobenzene, *o*-toluidine hydrochloride, 4,4'-sulfonyldianiline, or D & R Red No. 9. *J. natl Cancer Inst.*, **73**, 256–273

Gurka, D.F., Pyle, S.M., Farnham, I. & Titus, R. (1991) Application of hyphenated Fourier transform–infrared techniques to environmental analysis. *J. chromatogr. Sci.*, **29**, 339–344

Hainsworth, J.D., Hande, K.R., Satterlee, W.G., Kuttesch, J., Johnson, D.H., Grindey, G., Jackson, L.E. & Greco, F.A. (1989) Phase I clinical study of *N*-[(4-chlorophenyl)amino]carbonyl-2,3-dihydro-1H-indene-5-sulfonamide (LY186641). *Cancer Res.*, **49**, 5217–5220

Hansch, C. & Leo, A. (1979) *Substituent Constants for Correlation Analysis in Chemistry and Biology*, New York, John Wiley & Sons, p. 201

Hargesheimer, E.E., Coutts, R.T. & Pasutto, F.M. (1981) Gas–liquid chromatographic determination of aniline metabolites of substituted urea and carbamate herbicides in aqueous solution. *J. Assoc. off. anal. Chem.*, **64**, 833–840

Hennion, M.-C., Subra, P., Coquart, V. & Rosset, R. (1991) Determination of polar aniline derivatives in aqueous environmental samples using on-line liquid chromatographic preconcentration techniques. *Fresenius J. anal. Chem.*, **339**, 488–493

Heraeus (1991) *Feinchemikalien und Forschungsbedarf*, Karlsruhe, p. 166

Hoechst Celanese Corp. (1989) *Hoechst Chemicals—Product Information—Sales Department Fine Chemicals*, Charlotte, NC

Huang, H.-M., Hodson, R.E. & Lee, R.F. (1987) Degradation of aniline and chloroanilines by sunlight and microbes in estuarine water. *Water Res.*, **21**, 309–316

IARC (1976) *IARC Monographs on the Evaluation of Carcinogenic Risk of Chemicals to Man*, Vol. 12, *Some Carbamates, Thiocarbamates and Carbazides*, Lyon, pp. 167–176

IARC (1982a) *IARC Monographs on the Evaluation of the Carcinogenic Risk of Chemicals to Humans*, Vol. 27, *Some Aromatic Amines, Anthraquinones and Nitroso Compounds, and Inorganic Fluorides Used in Drinking-water and Dental Preparations*, Lyon, pp. 39–61

IARC (1982b) *IARC Monographs on the Evaluation of the Carcinogenic Risk of Chemicals to Humans*, Vol. 29, *Some Industrial Chemicals and Dyestuffs*, Lyon, pp. 213–238

IARC (1987a) *IARC Monographs on the Evaluation of Carcinogenic Risks to Humans*, Suppl. 7, *Overall Evaluations of Carcinogenicity: An Updating of* IARC Monographs *Volumes 1 to 42*, Lyon, pp. 99–100

IARC (1987b) *IARC Monographs on the Evaluation of Carcinogenic Risks to Humans*, Suppl. 7, *Overall Evaluations of Carcinogenicity: An Updating of* IARC Monographs *Volumes 1 to 42*, Lyon, pp. 192–193

James, R.H., Dillon, H.K. & Miller, H.C. (1983) Survey methods for the determination of principal organic hazardous constituents (POHCs). I. Methods for laboratory analysis. In: *Proceedings of the 8th Annual Research Symposium on Incineration Treatment and Hazardous Waste* (Report No. EPA-600/9-83-003; US NTIS PB83-210450), Washington DC, US Environmental Protection Agency, Office of Research and Development, pp. 159–173

Janssen Chimica (1990) *1991 Catalog Handbook of Fine Chemicals*, Beerse, p. 251

Kaczvinsky, J.R., Jr, Saitoh, K. & Fritz, J.S. (1983) Cation-exchange concentration of basic organic compounds from aqueous solution. *Anal. Chem.*, **55**, 1210–1215

Kaufman, D.D., Plimmer, J.R. & Klingebiel, U.I. (1973) Microbial oxidation of 4-chloroaniline. *J. agric. Food Chem.*, **21**, 127–132

Lancaster Synthesis (1991) *MTM Research Chemicals/Lancaster Catalogue 1991/92*, Windham, NH, MTM Plc, p. 275

Lide, D.R., ed. (1991) *CRC Handbook of Chemistry and Physics*, 72nd ed., Boca Raton, FL, CRC Press, p. C-68

Linch, A.L. (1974) Biological monitoring for industrial exposure to cyanogenic aromatic nitro and amino compounds. *Am. ind. Hyg. Assoc. J.*, **7**, 426–432

Malaiyandi, M., Wightman, R.H. & LaFerriere, C. (1987) Concentration of selected organic pollutants: comparison of adsorption and reverse-osmosis techniques. *Adv. Chem. Ser.*, **214**, 163–179

McLean, S., Starmer, G.A. & Thomas, J. (1969) Methaemoglobin formation by aromatic amines. *J. Pharm. Pharmacol.*, **21**, 441–450

Mitchell, A.D., Rudd, C.J. & Caspary, W.J. (1988) Evaluation of the L5178Y mouse lymphoma cell mutagenesis assay: intralaboratory results for sixty-three coded chemicals tested at SRI International. *Environ. mol. Mutag.*, **12** (Suppl. 13), 37–101

Mortelmans, K., Haworth, S., Lawlor, T., Speck, W., Tainer, B. & Zeiger, E. (1986) *Salmonella* mutagenicity tests: II. Results from the testing of 270 chemicals. *Environ. Mutag.*, **8** (Suppl. 7), 1–119

Mutanen, R.M., Siltanen, H.T., Kuukka, V.P., Annila, E.A. & Varama, M.M.O. (1988) Residues of diflubenzuron and two of its metabolites in a forest ecosystem after control of the pine looper moth, *Bupalus piniarius* L. *Pestic. Sci.*, **23**, 131–140

Myhr, B.C. & Caspary, W.J. (1988) Evaluation of the L5178Y mouse lymphoma cell mutagenesis assay: intralaboratory results for 63 coded chemicals tested within Litton Bionetics, Inc. *Environ. mol. Mutag.*, **12** (Suppl. 13), 103–194

Myhr, B., McGregor, D., Bowers, L., Riach, C., Brown, A.G., Edwards, I., McBride, D., Martin, R. & Caspary, W.J. (1990) L5178Y Mouse lymphoma cell mutation assay results with 41 compounds. *Environ. mol. Mutag.*, **16** (Suppl. 18), 138–167

Narang, A.S., Choudhury, D.R. & Richards, A. (1982) Separation of aromatic amines by thin-layer and high-performance liquid chromatography. *J. chromatogr. Sci.*, **20**, 235–237

Pienta, R.J. & Kawalek, J.C. (1981) Transformation of hamster embryo cells by aromatic amines. *Natl Cancer Inst. Monogr.*, **58**, 243–251

Pienta, R.J., Poiley, J.A. & Lebherz, W.B., III (1977) Morphological transformation of early passage golden Syrian hamster embryo cells derived from cryopreserved primary cultures as a reliable in vitro bioassay for identifying diverse carcinogens. *Int. J. Cancer*, **19**, 642–655

Pouchert, C.J. (1981) *The Aldrich Library of Infrared Spectra*, 3rd ed., Milwaukee, WI, Aldrich Chemical Co., p. 723

Pouchert, C.J. (1983) *The Aldrich Library of NMR Spectra*, 2nd ed., Vol. 1, Milwaukee, WI, Aldrich Chemical Co., p. 1010

Prasad, I. (1970) Mutagenic effects of the herbicide 3',4'-dichloropropionanilide and its degradation products. *Can. J. Microbiol.*, **16**, 369–372

Rankin, G.O., Yang, D.J., Cressey-Veneziano, K., Casto, S., Wang, R.T. & Brown, P.I. (1986) In vivo and in vitro nephrotoxicity of aniline and its monochlorophenyl derivatives in the Fischer 344 rat. *Toxicology*, **38**, 269–283

Reiml, D., Scheunert, I. & Korte, F. (1989) Leaching of conversion products of [^{14}C]buturon from soil during 12 years after application. *J. agric. Food Chem.*, **37**, 244–248

Riedel-de-Haen (1990) *Laboratory Chemicals 1990*, Seelze, p. 299

Rosenkranz, H.S. & Poirier, L.A. (1979) Evaluation of the mutagenicity and DNA-modifying activity of carcinogens and noncarcinogens in microbial systems. *J. natl Cancer Inst.*, **62**, 873–892

Sadtler Research Laboratories (1980) *Sadtler Standard Spectra, 1980, Cumulative Index*, Philadelphia, PA

Sadtler Research Laboratories (1991) *Sadtler Standard Spectra, 1981–1991*, Philadelphia, PA

Sakagami, Y., Yokoyama, H. & Ose, Y. (1986) Degradation of disinfectants by *Pseudomonas aeruginosa* isolated from activated sludge—identification of degradation products. *J. Hyg. Chem.*, **32**, 427–432

Schaefer, C.H., Colwell, A.E. & Dupras, E.F., Jr (1980) The occurrence of *p*-chloroaniline and *p*-chlorophenylurea from the degradation of diflubenzuron in water and fish. In: Grant, C.D. & Washino, R.K., eds, *Proceedings and Papers of the 48th Annual Conference of the California Mosquito and Vector Control Association (CMVCA), Inc.*, Visalia, CA, CMVCA Press, pp. 84–89

Simmon, V.F. (1979a) *In vitro* mutagenicity assays of chemical carcinogens and related compounds with *Salmonella typhimurium*. *J. natl Cancer Inst.*, **62**, 893–899

Simmon, V.F. (1979b) In vitro assays for recombinogenic activity of chemical carcinogens and related compounds with *Saccharomyces cerevisiae* D3. *J. natl Cancer Inst.*, **62**, 901–909

Smyth, H.F., Jr, Carpenter, C.P., Weil, C.S., Pozzani, U.C. & Striegel, J.A. (1962) Range-finding toxicity data: list VI. *Am. ind. Hyg. Assoc. J.*, **23**, 95–107

Taylor, C.W., Alberts, D.S., Ketcham, M.A., Satterlee, W.G., Holdsworth, M.T., Plezia, P.M., Peng, Y.-M., McCloskey, T.M., Roe, D.J., Hamilton, M. & Salmon, S.E. (1989) Clinical pharmacology of a novel diarylsulfonylurea anticancer agent. *J. clin. Oncol.*, 7, 1733–1740

TCI America (1991) *Organic Chemicals 91/92 Catalog*, Portland, OR, p. 270

US National Cancer Institute (1979) *Bioassay of p-Chloroaniline for Possible Carcinogenicity (CAS No. 106-47-8)* (NCI-CG-TR-189; DHEW Publ. No. (NIH) 79-1745), Bethesda, MD

US National Library of Medicine (1992) *Hazardous Substances Data Bank* (HSDB No. 2047), Bethesda, MD

US National Toxicology Program (1989) *Toxicology and Carcinogenesis Studies of para-Chloroaniline Hydrochloride (CAS No. 20265-96-7) in F344/N Rats and B6C3F₁ Mice (Gavage Studies)* (NTP Technical Report 351; NIH Publication No. 89-2806), Research Triangle Park, NC

van der Vorst, M.M.J., Tamminga, P., Wijburg, F.A. & Schutgens, R.B.H. (1990) Severe methaemoglobinaemia due to *para*-chloroaniline intoxication in premature neonates. *Eur. J. Pediatr.*, **150**, 72–73

Weast, R.C. & Astle, M.J., eds (1985) *CRC Handbook of Data on Organic Compounds*, Vol. 2, Boca Raton, FL, CRC Press, Inc., p. 463

Wegman, R.C.C. & De Korte, G.A.L. (1981) Aromatic amines in surface waters of the Netherlands. *Water Res.*, **15**, 391–394

Yoshida, T., Mamoru, H., Takeo, T., Keiko, M. & Katashi, A. (1992) Amounts of urinary metabolites of p-chloroaniline and their half lives in a patient with acute poisoning (Jpn.). *Sangyo Igaku*, **34**, 126–130

Zimmer, D., Mazurek, J., Petzold, G. & Bhuyan, B.K. (1980) Bacterial mutagenicity and mammalian cell DNA damage by several substituted anilines. *Mutat. Res.*, **77**, 317–326

Zoeteman, B.C.J., Harmsen, K., Linders, J.B.H.J., Morra, C.F.H. & Slooff, W. (1980) Persistent organic pollutants in river water and ground water of the Netherlands. *Chemosphere*, **9**, 231–249

2,6-DIMETHYLANILINE (2,6-XYLIDINE)

1. Exposure Data

1.1 Chemical and physical data

1.1.1 *Synonyms, structural and molecular data*

Chem. Abstr. Serv. Reg. No.: 87-62-7
Chem. Abstr. Name: 2,6-Dimethylbenzenamine
IUPAC Systematic Name: 2,6-Xylidine
Synonyms: 1-Amino-2,6-dimethylbenzene; 2-amino-1,3-dimethylbenzene; 2-amino-1,3-xylene; 2-amino-*meta*-xylene; 2,6-dimethylphenylamine; *ortho*-xylidine; 2,6-*meta*-xylidine; 2,6-xylylamine

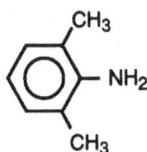

$C_8H_{11}N$ Mol. wt: 121.18

1.1.2 *Chemical and physical properties of the pure substance*

(a) *Description*: Clear liquid (Ethyl Corp., 1990); pungent odour (Ethyl Corp., 1991)
(b) *Boiling-point*: 214 °C at 739 mm Hg [98.5 kPa] (Lide, 1991)
(c) *Melting-point*: 11.2 °C (Lide, 1991)
(d) *Density*: 0.9842 at 20 °C (Lide, 1991)
(e) *Spectroscopy data*: Infrared, ultraviolet and nuclear magnetic resonance spectral data have been reported (Sadtler Research Laboratories, 1980; Pouchert, 1981, 1983; Sadtler Research Laboratories, 1991).
(f) *Solubility*: Slightly soluble in water (7.5 g/l at 20 °C); soluble in ethanol and diethyl ether (Hoechst Celanese Corp., 1989; Lide, 1991)
(g) *Volatility*: Vapour pressure, 0.125 mm Hg [17 Pa] at 25 °C; 1 mm Hg [133 Pa] at 44 °C (Chao *et al.*, 1983; Lide, 1991)
(h) *Stability*: Sensitive to air oxidation and light; inflammable (Hoechst Celanese Corp., 1989)

(*i*) *Conversion factor*: mg/m^3 = 5.0 × ppm[1]

1.1.3 *Trade names, technical products and impurities*

2,6-Dimethylaniline is available commercially at purities ranging from 98 to 99.6%, with xylenol as a typical impurity (Hoechst Celanese Corp., 1989; Ethyl Corp., 1991). It is also available in research quantities at purities in the same order of magnitude (Janssen Chimica, 1990; Riedel-de Haen, 1990; Heraeus, 1991; Lancaster Synthesis, 1991; TCI America, 1991; Aldrich Chemical Co., 1992; Fluka Chemie AG, 1993).

1.1.4 *Analysis*

Amines can be liberated during the manufacture of rubber, especially by vulcanization and other other thermal degradations. A method was described for the determination of free aromatic amines, including 2,6-dimethylaniline, using high-temperature glass-capillary gas chromatography and nitrogen-selective detection (thermionic specific detector), with detection limits of 10–20 pg (Dalene & Skarping, 1985).

Combined gas chromatography–mass spectrometry and –Fourier transform–infrared spectrometry have been used for the identification of a large number of aromatic compounds, including 2,6-dimethylaniline. Use of infrared spectrometry often allowed unambiguous differentiation of isomers (Chiu *et al.*, 1984).

An isocratic on-line liquid chromatographic preconcentration system with ultraviolet absorbance detection at 230 nm has been developed for the determination in tap-water of polar pollutants, including 2,6-dimethylaniline, with widely varying characteristics. The detection limit for 2,6-dimethylaniline was 0.4 µg/l (Brouwer *et al.*, 1991).

A procedure has been described for the detection of 2,6-disubstituted anilines, including 2,6-dimethylaniline, in the low-nanogram range in blood. The aromatic anilines were extracted from blood with ethyl acetate, converted to the corresponding *N*-heptafluorobutyramides and analysed by gas chromatography with electron capture detection; identities were confirmed by gas chromatrography–mass spectrometry (DeLeon *et al.*, 1983).

1.2 Production and use

1.2.1 *Production*

2,6-Dimethylaninile is prepared by nitration of xylene and reduction, followed by removal of the 2,4-isomer by formation of the acetate salt, removal of the 2,5-isomer by formation of the hydrochloride salt, and recovery of the 2,6-isomer by sublimation (US National Library of Medicine, 1992a).

2,6-Dimethylaniline is produced by one company each in Japan, Switzerland and the USA and by three companies in Germany (Chemical Information Services, 1991).

---

[1]Calculated from: mg/m^3 = (molecular weight/24.45) × ppm, assuming normal temperature (25 °C) and pressure (760 mm Hg [101.3 kPa])

1.2.2 *Use*

2,6-Dimethylaniline is used as a chemical intermediate in the manufacture of pesticides, dyestuffs, antioxidants, pharmaceuticals, synthetic resins, fragrances and other products (Ethyl Corp., 1990; Kuney, 1991).

1.3 Occurrence

1.3.1 *Natural occurrence*

2,6-Dimethylaniline is one of many amino compounds occurring naturally in Latakia tobacco leaves (Irvine & Saxby, 1969).

1.3.2 *Occupational exposure*

No data were available to the Working Group.

On the basis of a survey conducted in the USA between 1981 and 1983, the US National Institute for Occupational Safety and Health estimated that a total of 4354 workers, including 729 women, may have been exposed to 2,6-dimethylaniline in five occupations (US National Library of Medicine, 1992b).

1.3.3 *Water and sediments*

2,6-Dimethylaniline was identified in a sample from a shallow aquifer contaminated by coal-tar wastes. The site, in St Louis Park, MN, USA, had been used as a waste disposal site by a coal-tar distillation (see IARC, 1984, 1985, 1987a) and wood-preserving facility from 1918 through 1972 (Pereira *et al.*, 1983).

1.3.4 *Other*

Xylidine metabolites are released from drugs, and particularly the xylidine group of local anaesthetics. 2,6-Dimethylaniline was identified as a metabolite in the urine of rats, guinea-pigs, dogs and humans administered lidocaine orally (Keenaghan & Boyes, 1972). 2,6-Dimethylaniline may also enter the environment through the degradation of certain pesticides (US National Toxicology Program, 1990). It was detected in stack effluents from an incinerator burning hazardous wastes (James *et al.*, 1985) and has been detected in tobacco smoke (Irvine & Saxby, 1969; Patrianakos & Hoffman, 1979; Florin *et al.*, 1980; Pettersson *et al.*, 1980; Thelestam *et al.*, 1980; see IARC, 1986, 1987b).

1.4 Regulatory status and guidelines

Occupational exposure limits and guidelines for all isomers of xylidine, including 2,6-dimethylaniline, in some countries are presented in Table 1.

2. Studies of Cancer in Humans

No data were available to the Working Group.

Table 1. Occupational exposure limits and guidelines for xylidine (all isomers)

Country	Year	Concentration (mg/m^3)	Skin irritant notation	Interpretation
Australia		10	Yes	TWA
Austria		25	Yes	TWA
Belgium		10	Yes	TWA
ex-Czechoslovakia		5	No	TWA
Denmark	1988	10	Yes	TWA
Finland		25	Yes	TWA
		50	No	STEL
France		10	Yes	TWA
Germany	1992	25	Yes	TWA
Hungary		5	Yes	TWA
		10	No	STEL
Indonesia	1978	25	Yes	TWA
Italy	1978	10	Yes	TWA
Mexico	1983	25	Yes	TWA
Netherlands	1989	25	Yes	TWA
Poland	1984	5	No	TWA
Romania	1975	1	Yes	TWA
		2	Yes	STEL
Switzerland		10	Yes	TWA
United Kingdom	1990	10	Yes	TWA
		50	No	STEL
USA				
ACGIH	1992	2.5	Yes[a]	TWA
OSHA	1989	10	Yes	TWA
ex-USSR		3	Yes	STEL
Venezuela	1978	25	Yes	TWA
		25	Yes	Ceiling
ex-Yugoslavia	1971	3	No	TWA

From Cook (1987); ACGIH (1991); ILO (1991); Deutsche Forschungsgemeinschaft (1992); TWA, time-weighted average; STEL, short-term exposure limit
[a] A$_2$, suspected human carcinogen

3. Studies of Cancer in Experimental Animals

Pre- and postnatal administration in the diet

Rat

Groups of 28 male and 56 female Charles River CD rats, five weeks of age, were administered 0, 300, 1000 or 3000 ppm (mg/kg) of diet 2,6-dimethylaniline (99.06% pure). At 16 weeks of age, they were mated, and the pregnant females were allowed to deliver naturally over a two-week period (F_0 generation). F_0 females continued to receive treatment or control diet during pregnancy and lactation. Progeny (F_1) were weaned at 21 days of age, and groups of 56 males and 56 females received the same diet as their parents for 102 weeks. Mean body weight gains relative to those of controls were reduced for high-dose male and mid-dose and high-dose female rats (by > 10%). Survival at 105 weeks was: males—control, 43/56; low-dose 40/56; mid-dose 33/56; high-dose, 14/56 (p < 0.001); females—control, 33/56; low-dose 25/56; mid-dose, 32/56; high-dose, 24/56. In males, papillary adenomas of the nasal cavity occurred in 0/56 control, 0/56 low-dose, 2/56 mid-dose and 10/56 high-dose rats (p = 0.001, incidental tumour test). Carcinomas [not otherwise specified] of the nasal cavity were observed only in high-dose males (26/56; p < 0.001, life table test); two adenocarcinomas were also observed in high-dose male rats. In females, nasal adenomas occurred in 0/56 control, 0/56 low-dose, 1/56 mid-dose and 6/56 high-dose rats (p = 0.02, incidental tumour test). Carcinomas of the nasal cavity occurred in 0/56 control, 0/56 low-dose, 1/56 mid-dose and 24/56 high-dose females (p < 0.001, life table test). Unusual tumours of the nasal cavity also occurred among high-dose males and females: one undifferentiated sarcoma was present in a female, rhabomyosarcomas occurred in two males and two females, and malignant mixed tumours (features of adenocarcinomas and rhabdo-myosarcomas) were observed in one male and one female rat. Subcutaneous fibromas and fibrosarcomas combined occurred in 0/56 control, 2/56 low-dose, 2/56 mid-dose and 5/56 high-dose male rats (p = 0.001, life table test; p < 0.001 life table trend test); and in 1/56 control, 2/56 low-dose, 2/56 mid-dose and 6/56 high-dose female rats (p = 0.01, life table trend test). Neoplastic nodules of the liver occurred in female rats with a significant positive trend: control, 0/56; low-dose, 1/56; mid-dose, 2/56; high-dose, 4/55 (p = 0.03, incidental test; p = 0.012, incidental trend test). Hepatocellular carcinomas occurred in 1/56 control, 0/56 low-dose, 1/56 mid-dose and 1/55 high-dose female rats (US National Toxicology Program, 1990). [The Working Group noted that no data were provided on the parent generation.]

4. Other Relevant Data

4.1 Absorption, distribution, metabolism and excretion

4.1.1 *Humans*

Evidence for the metabolism of 2,6-dimethylaniline in humans is derived from studies on cigarette smokers and nonsmokers and on patients receiving the anaesthetic and cardiac drug, lidocaine, which is known to be metabolized principally to 2,6-dimethylaniline. Using capillary gas chromatography–mass spectrometry, haemoglobin adducts of 2,6-dimethyl-aniline were found to be present at high levels in nonsmokers with no known exposure to this compound; moreover, adduct levels were appreciably lower in cigarette smokers. In contrast, 2,6-dimethylaniline–haemoglobin adduct levels were elevated substantially in patients receiving lidocaine treatment. These results are indicative of environmental and iatrogenic exposure to 2,6-dimethylaniline, and of its biotransformation to a circulating N-hydroxy-2,6-dimethylaniline metabolite in humans, which enters erythrocytes, is oxidized to 2,6-dimethyl-nitrosobenzene and forms a sulfinamide adduct with haemoglobin (Bryant et al., 1988, 1992 (abstract)).

On the basis of the haemoglobin binding index determined in rats, the levels of 2,6-di-methylaniline–haemoglobin adducts found in nonsmokers correspond to an estimated daily exposure of 23 μg (Sabbioni, 1992). 2,6-Dimethylaniline has also been found as a human urinary metabolite of two other drugs, etidocaine and lidamidine hydrochloride (US National Toxicology Program, 1990).

4.1.2 *Experimental systems*

Since free 2,6-dimethylaniline may be formed by intestinal metabolism of 2,6-dimethyl-aniline-based azo dyes, its absorption into the circulation from the small intestine was studied. Male Wistar rats were instilled with 10 mg 2,6-dimethylaniline ('pure') in 10 ml phosphate-buffered saline pH 6 into the intestine. Since the absorption half-time was rapid (14.4 min), metabolism of azo dyes by intestinal microflora would be expected to result in complete absorption of the resulting 2,6-dimethylaniline by the body (Plá-Delfina *et al.*, 1972).

The metabolism of 2,6-dimethylaniline was examined qualitatively in male Osborne-Mendel rats given the hydrochloride salt [purity unspecified] by gavage in water at 200 mg/kg bw. 4-Hydroxy-2,6-dimethylaniline and 3-methyl-2-aminobenzoic acid were identified as major and minor urinary metabolites, respectively. The unchanged amine could be detected chromatographically, but only after acidic urine hydrolysis, suggesting the presence of urinary *N*-conjugates (Lindstrom *et al.*, 1963). These data were confirmed by enzymatic hydrolysis in male Fischer 344 rats given 2,6-dimethylaniline (> 99% pure) by gavage in corn oil at a daily dose of 262.5 mg/kg bw for 10 days. Levels of the 4-hydroxy metabolite were further increased by pretreatment with 3-methylcholanthrene, but not by pretreatment with phenobarbital. Oral administration to male beagle dogs (25 mg/kg bw per day for 10 days) resulted in the same major metabolite; 3-methyl-2-aminobenzoic acid and its glycine conjugate were minor components in the urine. Evidence was also provided for the presence of two potentially reactive metabolites, 2,6-dimethyl-4-nitrosobenzene, which may arise from *N*-hydroxy-2,6-dimethylaniline, and 2,6- or 3,5-dimethyl-4-iminoquinone, neither of which was detectable in rats (Short *et al.*, 1989a).

Haemoglobin adduct levels were determined in female Wistar rats given 0.5 mmol [61 mg]/kg bw 2,6-dimethylaniline (purity, > 98%) by gavage in propylene glycol and found to be significant but relatively low [haemoglobin binding index = 1.1 mmol compound/mol haemoglobin per (mmol compound/kg bw)], in comparison with levels of adducts of other aromatic amines (Sabbioni, 1992).

4.2 Toxic effects

4.2.1 *Humans*

Methaemoglobinaemia has been reported following lidocaine treatment of human subjects (Burne & Doughty, 1964; Weiss *et al.*, 1987). Like haemoglobin adduct formation, it can be attributed to a circulating *N*-hydroxy metabolite.

4.2.2 *Experimental systems*

Methaemoglobinaemia has been reported in cats but not dogs following an intravenous dose of 30 mg/kg bw 2,6-dimethylaniline [purity unspecified] in a pH 5.5 saline vehicle. Lidocaine also caused methaemoglobinaemia in cats after intravenous treatment at 47 mg/kg bw (McLean *et al.*, 1967, 1969).

LD_{50} values have been determined in several rodent strains. In male Osborne-Mendel rats given the hydrochloride [purity unspecified] in water by gavage, the LD_{50} was 2042 mg/kg bw (Lindstrom *et al.*, 1969). The LD_{50} of 2,6-dimethylaniline [purity and vehicle unspecified] administered by gavage was estimated as 840 mg/kg bw (Jacobson, 1972) and 1230 mg/kg for male Sprague-Dawley rats and 710 mg/kg for male CF_1 mice (Vernot *et al.*, 1977). An LD_{50} of 630 mg/kg was reported (Short *et al.*, 1983) for male Fischer 344 rats administered 2,6-dimethylaniline [purity unspecified] by gavage without a vehicle. The LD_{50} for female Fischer 344 rats given the compound (> 99% pure) by gavage in corn oil was calculated to be 1160 mg/kg; and LD_{50} values of 1270–1310 mg/kg were estimated for male and female Charles River CD rats after a single gavage dose (purity, > 99%) in corn oil (US National Toxicology Program, 1990).

In rats, only splenic haemosiderosis was observed in male Fischer 344 animals administered 2,6-dimethylaniline [purity unspecified] by gavage without a vehicle at daily doses of 157.5 mg/kg bw for 5–20 days (Short *et al.*, 1983). In male and female Sprague-Dawley rats given 400–700 mg/kg by gavage [purity not specified] daily for four weeks, however, decreased weight gain, lowered haemoglobin values and liver enlargement were observed, with increases in the levels of microsomal glucuronyltransferase in males and females and of aniline hydroxylase in females (Magnusson *et al.*, 1971, 1979). Similarly, in male and female Fischer 344 rats given the compound (> 99% pure) by gavage in corn oil at doses up to 310 mg/kg for five days a week for 13 weeks, increased liver weight, decreased body weight and decreases in erythrocyte, haemoglobin and haematocrit levels were observed (US National Toxicology Program, 1990). In male Osborne-Mendel rats given up to 10 000 ppm 2,6-dimethylaniline in the diet for three to six months, 25% weight retardation, anaemia, liver enlargement (no microscopic change), splenic congestion and kidney damage that included depressed scar formation, tubular atrophy, interstitial fibrosis, chronic inflammation, papillary oedema and necrosis, and cystic dilation of tubular segments were observed, predominantly at the high dose (Lindstrom *et al.*, 1963). In the 104-week carcinogenicity study described on pp. 326–327, male and female Charles River CD rats developed non-neoplastic changes including dose-related decreases in body weight gain and inflammation, hyperplasia and squamous metaplasia of the nasal mucosa (US National Toxicology Program, 1990).

Chronic dosing of male and female beagle dogs with oral doses (in capsules) of 50 mg/kg bw 2,6-dimethylaniline for four weeks resulted in decreased body weight, hyperbilirubinaemia, hypoproteinaemia and, in contrast to rats, marked fatty degenerative changes in the liver (Magnusson *et al.*, 1971).

4.3 Reproductive and prenatal effects

No data were available to the Working Group.

4.4 Genetic and related effects

4.4.1 *Humans*

No data were available to the Working Group.

4.4.2 *Experimental systems* (see also Table 2 and Appendices 1 and 2)

Reports on the mutagenicity of 2,6-dimethylaniline in *Salmonella typhimurium* are conflicting. In the most detailed report, two of three participating laboratories reproducibly demonstrated weak activity in the presence of an exogenous metabolic system from hamster, but not rat, liver. 2,6-Dimethylaniline was reported to induce mutation in mouse lymphoma cells at the *tk* locus (abstract), and it induced both sister chromatid exchange and chromosomal aberrations in Chinese hamster ovary cells.

It did not induce micronuclei in the bone marrow of mice treated *in vivo* by oral administration. Unlabelled 2,6-dimethylaniline bound covalently to the DNA of the ethmoid turbinates and liver of rats after oral pretreatment.

5. Summary of Data Reported and Evaluation

5.1 Exposure data

2,6-Dimethylaniline is used as a chemical intermediate in the manufacture of pesticides, dyestuffs, antioxidants, pharmaceuticals and other products. It is a metabolite of the xylidine group of anaesthetics, including, for example, lidocaine, and is produced by the reduction of certain azo dyes by intestinal microflora. It may also enter the environment through degradation of certain pesticides.

5.2 Human carcinogenicity data

No data were available to the Working Group.

5.3 Animal carcinogenicity data

2,6-Dimethylaniline was tested for carcinogenicity in one study in rats by pre- and postnatal administration in the diet. It induced adenomas and carcinomas as well as several sarcomas in the nasal cavity. It also produced subcutaneous fibromas and fibrosarcomas in both males and females and increased the incidence of neoplastic nodules in the livers of female rats.

5.4 Other relevant data

Methaemoglobinaemia has been observed in humans and animals exposed to 2,6-dimethylaniline. The metabolism of 2,6-dimethylaniline in humans and rats appears to be similar and gives rise to a characteristic haemoglobin adduct in both species.

Table 2. Genetic and related effects of 2,6-dimethylaniline

Test system	Result		Dose[a] (LED/HID)	Reference
	Without exogenous metabolic system	With exogenous metabolic system		
SA0, *Salmonella typhimurium* TA100, reverse mutation	–[b]	–[b]	363.0000	Florin et al. (1980)
SA0, *Salmonella typhimurium* TA100, reverse mutation	0	–	0.0000	Zimmer et al. (1980)
SA0, *Salmonella typhimurium* TA100, reverse mutation	–	(+)[c]	167.0000	Zeiger et al. (1988)
SA0, *Salmonella typhimurium* TA100, reverse mutation	0	–	2000.0000	Kugler–Steigmeier et al. (1989)
SA5, *Salmonella typhimurium* TA1535, reverse mutation	–	–	1815.0000	Florin et al. (1980)
SA5, *Salmonella typhimurium* TA1535, reverse mutation	–	–	1667.0000	Zeiger et al. (1988)
SA7, *Salmonella typhimurium* TA1537, reverse mutation	–	–	1815.0000	Florin et al. (1980)
SA7, *Salmonella typhimurium* TA1537, reverse mutation	–	–	1667.0000	Zeiger et al. (1988)
SA7, *Salmonella typhimurium* TA1537, reverse mutation	0	–	0.0000	Zimmer et al. (1980)
SA9, *Salmonella typhimurium* TA98, reverse mutation	–[b]	–[b]	363.0000	Florin et al. (1980)
SA9, *Salmonella typhimurium* TA98, reverse mutation	–	–	1667.0000	Zeiger et al. (1988)
SA9, *Salmonella typhimurium* TA98, reverse mutation	0	–	0.0000	Zimmer et al. (1980)
G5T, Gene mutation, mouse lymphoma L5178Y cells, *tk* locus	+	+	0.0000	Rudd et al. (1983); abstr.
SIC, Sister chromatid exchange, Chinese hamster ovary (CHO) cells *in vitro*	+	+	301.0000	Galloway et al. (1987)
CIC, Chromosomal aberrations, Chinese hamster ovary (CHO) cells *in vitro*	+	+	1200.0000	Galloway et al. (1987)
MVM, Micronucleus test, ICR mouse bone marrow *in vivo*	–		350 mg/kg po × 1	Parton et al. (1988)
MVM, Micronucleus test, ICR mouse bone marrow *in vivo*	–		375 mg/kg po × 3	Parton et al. (1990)
BVD, Binding (covalent) to DNA, rats *in vivo*	+		4 mg/kg ip[d] × 1	Short et al. (1989b)

+, positive; (+), weakly positive; –, negative; 0, not tested
[a]In-vitro tests, μg/ml; in-vivo tests, mg/kg bw
[b]Spot tests only
[c]Weakly positive in two of three laboratories, negative in the other one
[d]Pretreatment with unlabelled 262.5 mg/kg 2,6-dimethylaniline daily for nine days

2,6-Dimethylaniline gave conflicting results for gene mutation in bacteria. Sister chromatid exchange and chromosomal aberrations were induced in cultured mammalian cells. The compound bound covalently to DNA in rat tissues but did not induce micronuclei in the bone marrow of mice treated *in vivo*.

5.5 Evaluation[1]

There is *inadequate evidence* in humans for the carcinogenicity of 2,6-dimethylaniline. There is *sufficient evidence* in experimental animals for the carcinogenicity of 2,6-dimethylaniline.

Overall evaluation

2,6-Dimethylaniline is *possibly carcinogenic to humans (Group 2B)*.

6. References

Aldrich Chemical Co. (1992) *Aldrich Catalog/Handbook of Fine Chemicals 1992–1993*, Milwaukee, WI, p. 491

American Conference of Governmental Industrial Hygienists (1991) *1991–1992 Threshold Limit Values for Chemical Substances and Physical Agents and Biological Exposure Indices*, Cincinnati, OH, p. 38

Brouwer, E.R., Liska, I., Geerdink, R.B., Frintrop, P.C.M., Mulder, W.H., Lingeman, H. & Brinkman, U.A.T. (1991) Determination of polar pollutants in water using an on-line liquid chromatographic preconcentration system. *Chromatographia*, **32**, 445–452

Bryant, M.S., Vineis, P., Skipper, P.L. & Tannenbaum, S.R. (1988) Hemoglobin adducts of aromatic amines: associations with smoking status and type of tobacco. *Proc. natl Acad. Sci. USA*, **85**, 9788–9791

Bryant, M.S., Simmons, H.F., Harrell, R.E. & Hinson, J.A. (1992) Hemoglobin adducts of 2,6-dimethylaniline in cardiac patients administered lidocaine (Abstract No. 878). *Proc. Am. Assoc. Cancer Res.*, **33**, 146

Burne, D. & Doughty, A. (1964) Methaemoglobinaemia following lignocaine (Letter to the Editor). *Lancet*, **ii**, 971

Chao, J., Lin, C.T. & Chung, T.H. (1983) Vapor pressure of coal chemicals. *J. phys. chem. Ref. Data*, **12**, 1033–1063

Chemical Information Services Ltd (1991) *Directory of World Chemical Producers 1992/93 Edition*, Dallas, TX, p. 598

Chiu, K.S., Biemann, K., Krishnan, K. & Hill, S.L. (1984) Structural characterization of polycyclic aromatic compounds by combined gas chromatography/mass spectrometry and gas chromatography/Fourier transform infrared spectrometry. *Anal. Chem.*, **56**, 1610–1615

Cook, W.A. (1987) *Occupational Exposure Limits—Worldwide*, Akron, OH, American Industrial Hygiene Association, pp. 126, 157, 224

---

[1]For definition of the italicized terms, see Preamble, pp. 26–30.

Dalene, M. & Skarping, G. (1985) Trace analysis of amines and isocyanates using glass capillary gas chromatography and selection detection. IV. Determination of free aromatic amines using nitrogen-selective detection. *J. Chromatogr.*, **331**, 321–330

DeLeon, I.R., Brown, N.J., Cocchiara, J.P., Cruz, S.G. & Laseter, J.L. (1983) Trace analysis of 2,6-disubstituted anilines in blood by capillary gas chromatography. *J. anal. Toxicol.*, **7**, 185-187

Deutsche Forschungsgemeinschaft (1992) *MAK and BAT-Values List 1992. Maximum Concentrations at the Workplace (MAK) and Biological Tolerance Values (BAT) for Working Materials* (Report No. 28), Weinheim, VCH Verlagsgesellschaft, p. 68

Ethyl Corp. (1990) *Orthoalkylated Anilines—2,6-Dimethylaniline (DMA)*, Baton Rouge, LA

Ethyl Corp. (1991) *Material Safety Data Sheet: DMA (2,6-Dimethylaniline)*, Baton Rouge, LA

Florin, I., Rutberg, L., Curvall, M. & Enzell, C.R. (1980) Screening of tobacco smoke constituents for mutagenicity using the Ames' test. *Toxicology*, **15**, 219–232

Fluka Chemie AG (1993) *Fluka Chemika-BioChemika*, Buchs, p. 514

Galloway, S.M., Armstrong, M.J,. Reuben, C., Colman, S., Brown, B., Cannon, C., Bloom, A.D., Nakamura, F., Ahmed, N., Duk, S., Rimpo, J., Margolin, B.H., Resnick, M.A., Anderson, B. & Zeiger, E. (1987) Chromosome aberrations and sister chromatid exchanges in Chinese hamster ovary cells: evaluations of 108 chemicals. *Environ. mol. Mutag.*, **10** (Suppl. 10), 1-175

Heraeus (1991) *Feinchemikalien und Forschungsbedarf*, Karlsruhe, p. 280

Hoechst Celanese Corp. (1989) *Hoechst Chemicals—Product Information—Sales Department Fine Chemicals*, Charlotte, NC

IARC (1984) *IARC Monographs on the Evaluation of the Carcinogenic Risk of Chemicals to Humans*, Vol. 34, *Polynuclear Aromatic Compounds, Part 3: Industrial Exposures in Aluminium Production, Coal Gasification, Coke Production, and Iron and Steel Founding*, Lyon, pp. 65–69, 101–131

IARC (1985) *IARC Monographs on the Evaluation of the Carcinogenic Risk of Chemicals to Humans*, Vol. 35, *Polynuclear Aromatic Compounds, Part 4: Bitumens, Coal-tars and Derived Products, Shale-oils and Soots*, Lyon, pp. 83–159

IARC (1986) *IARC Monographs on the Evaluation of the Carcinogenic Risk of Chemicals to Humans*, Vol. 38, *Tobacco Smoking*, Lyon

IARC (1987a) *IARC Monographs on the Evaluation of Carcinogenic Risks to Humans*, Suppl. 7, *Overall Evaluations of Carcinogenicity: An Updating of* IARC Monographs *Volumes 1 to 42*, Lyon, pp. 175–176

IARC (1987b) *IARC Monographs on the Evaluation of Carcinogenic Risks to Humans*, Suppl. 7, *Overall Evaluations of Carcinogenicity: An Updating of* IARC Monographs *Volumes 1 to 42*, Lyon, pp. 359–362

ILO (1991) *Occupational Exposure Limits for Airborne Toxic Substances*, 3rd ed. (Occupational Safety and Health Series 37), Geneva, International Labour Office, pp. 420–423

Irvine, W.J. & Saxby, M.J. (1969) Steam volatile amines of Latakia tobacco leaf. *Phytochemistry*, **8**, 473-476

Jacobson, K.H. (1972) Acute oral toxicity of mono- and di-alkyl ring-substituted derivatives of aniline. *Toxicol. appl. Pharmacol.*, **22**, 153-154

James, R.H., Adams, R.E., Finkel, J.M., Miller, H.C. & Johnson, L.D. (1985) Evaluation of analytical methods for the determination of POHC (principal organic hazardous constituents) in combustion products. *J. Air Pollut. Control Assoc.*, **35**, 959–969

Janssen Chimica (1990) *1991 Catalog Handbook of Fine Chemicals*, Beerse, p. 477

Keenaghan, J.B. & Boyes, R.N. (1972) The tissue distribution, metabolism and excretion of lidocaine in rats, guinea pigs, dogs and man. *J. Pharmacol. exp. Ther.*, **180**, 454–463

Kugler-Steigmeier, M.E., Friederich, U., Graf, U., Lutz, W.K., Maier, P. & Schlatter, C. (1989) Genotoxicity of aniline derivatives in various short-term tests. *Mutat. Res.*, **211**, 279–289

Kuney, J.H., ed. (1991) *Chemcyclopedia 92—The Manual of Commercially Available Chemicals*, Washington DC, American Chemical Society, p. 64

Lancaster Synthesis (1991) *MTM Research Chemicals/Lancaster Catalogue 1991/92*, Windham, NH, MTM Plc, p. 535

Lide, D.R., ed. (1991) *CRC Handbook of Chemistry and Physics*, 72nd ed., Boca Raton, FL, CRC Press, pp. 3–41, 6–76

Lindstrom, H.V., Hansen, W.H., Nelson, A.A. & Fitzhugh, O.G. (1963) The metabolism of FD&C Red No. 1. II. The fate of 2,5-*para*-xylidine and 2,6-*meta*-xylidine in rats and observations of the toxicity of xylidine isomers. *J. Pharmacol. exp. Ther.*, **142**, 257–264

Lindstrom, H.V., Bowie, W.C., Wallace, W.C., Nelson, A.A. & Fitzhugh, O.G. (1969) The toxicity and metabolism of mesidine and pseudocumidine in rats. *J. Pharmacol. exp. Ther.*, **167**, 223–234

Magnusson, G., Bodin, N.-O. & Hansson, E. (1971) Hepatic changes in dogs and rats induced by xylidine isomers. *Acta pathol. microbiol. scand.*, **79**, 639–648

Magnusson, G., Majeed, S.K., Down, W.H., Sacharin, R.M. & Jorgeson, W. (1979) Hepatic effects of xylidine isomers in rats. *Toxicology*, **12**, 63–74

McLean, S., Murphy, B.P., Starmer, G.A. & Thomas, J. (1967) Methaemoglobin formation induced by aromatic amines and amides. *J. Pharm. Pharmacol.*, **19**, 146–154

McLean, S., Starmer, G.A. & Thomas, J. (1969) Methaemoglobin formation by aromatic amines. *J. Pharm. Pharmacol.*, **21**, 441–450

Parton, J.W., Probst, G.S. & Garriott, M.L. (1988) The in vivo effect of 2,6-xylidine on induction of micronuclei in mouse bone marrow cells. *Mutat. Res.*, **206**, 281–283

Parton, J.W., Beyers, J.E., Garriott, M.L. & Tamura, R.N. (1990) The evaluation of multiple dosing protocol for the mouse bone-marrow micronucleus assay using benzidine and 2,6-xylidine. *Mutat. Res.*, **234**, 165–168

Patrianakos, C. & Hoffman, D. (1979) Chemical studies of tobacco smoke. LXIV. On the analysis of aromatic amines in cigarette smoke. *J. anal. Toxicol.*, **3**, 150–154

Pereira, W.E., Rostad, C.E., Garbarino, J.R. & Hult, M.F. (1983) Groundwater contamination by organic bases derived from coal-tar wastes. *Environ. Toxicol. Chem.*, **2**, 283–294

Pettersson, B., Curvall, M. & Enzell, C.R. (1980) Effects of tobacco smoke compounds on the noradrenaline induced oxidative metabolism in isolated brown fat cells. *Toxicology*, **18**, 1–15

Plá-Delfina, J.M., del Poso, A., Martín, A. & Alvarez, J.L. (1972) Absorption, distribution and elimination of aromatic amines: application of these pharmacokinetic parameters to chronic toxicity studies (Span.) *Cienc. ind. farm.*, **4**, 47–53

Pouchert, C.J. (1981) *The Aldrich Library of Infrared Spectra*, 3rd ed., Milwaukee, WI, Aldrich Chemical Co., p. 727

Pouchert, C.J. (1983) *The Aldrich Library of NMR Spectra*, 2nd ed., Vol. 1, Milwaukee, WI, Aldrich Chemical Co., p. 1018

Riedel-de Haen (1990) *Laboratory Chemicals 1990*, Seelze, p. 494

Rudd, C.J., Mitchell, A.D. & Spalding, J. (1983) L5178Y Mouse lymphoma cell mutagenesis assay of coded chemicals incorporating analyses of the colony size distributions (Abstract No. Cd-19). *Environ. Mutag.*, **5**, 419

Sabbioni, G. (1992) Hemoglobin binding of monocyclic aromatic amines: molecular dosimetry and quantitative structure activity relationships for the *N*-oxidation. *Chem.-biol. Interactions*, **81**, 91–117

Sadtler Research Laboratories (1980) *Sadtler Standard Spectra. 1980 Cumulative Index*, Philadelphia, PA

Sadtler Research Laboratories (1991) *Sadtler Standard Spectra. 1981–1991 Supplementary Index*, Philadelphia, PA

Short, C.R., King, C., Sistrunk, P.W. & Kerr, K.M. (1983) Subacute toxicity of several ring-substituted dialkylanilines in the rat. *Fundam. appl. Toxicol.*, **3**, 285–292

Short, C.R., Hardy, M.L. & Barker, S.A. (1989a) The in vivo oxidative metabolism of 2,4- and 2,6-dimethylaniline in the dog and rat. *Toxicology*, **57**, 45–58

Short, C.R., Joseph, M. & Hardy, M.L. (1989b) Covalent binding of [^{14}C]-2,6-dimethylaniline to DNA of rat liver and ethmoid turbinate. *J. Toxicol. environ. Health*, **27**, 85–94

TCI America (1991) *Organic Chemials 91/92 Catalog*, Portland, OR, p. 1279

Thelestam, M., Curvall, M. & Enzell, C.R. (1980) Effects of tobacco smoke compounds on the plasma membranes of cultured human lung fibroblasts. *Toxicology*, **15**, 203–217

US National Library of Medicine (1992a) *Hazardous Substances Data Bank* (HSDB No. 2094), Bethesda, MD

US National Library of Medicine (1992b) *Registry of Toxic Effects of Chemical Substances* (RTECS No. ZE9275000), Bethesda, MD

US National Toxicology Program (1990) *Toxicology and Carcinogenesis Studies of 2,6-Xylidine (2,6-Dimethylaniline) (CAS No. 87-62-7) in Charles River CD Rats (Feed Studies)* (NTP Technical Report 278; NIH Publication No. 90-2534), Research Triangle Park

Vernot, E.H., MacEwen, J.D., Haun, C.C. & Kinkead, E.R. (1977) Acute toxicity and skin corrosion data for some organic and inorganic compounds and aqueous solutions. *Toxicol. appl. Pharmacol.*, **42**, 417–423

Weiss, L.D., Generalovich, T., Heller, M.B., Paris, P.M., Stewart, R.D., Kaplan, R.M. & Thompson, D.R. (1987) Methemoglobin levels following intravenous lidocaine administration. *Ann. Emerg. Med.*, **16**, 323–325

Zeiger, E., Anderson, B., Haworth, S., Lawlor, T. & Mortelmans, K. (1988) *Salmonella* mutagenicity tests: IV. Results from the testing of 300 chemicals. *Environ. mol. Mutag.*, **11** (Suppl. 12), 1–158

Zimmer, D., Mazurek, J., Petzold, G. & Bhuyan, B.K. (1980) Bacterial mutagenicity and mammalian cell DNA damage by several substituted anilines. *Mutat. Res.*, **77**, 317–326

N,*N*-DIMETHYLANILINE

1. Exposure Data

1.1 Chemical and physical data

1.1.1 *Synonyms, structural and molecular data*

Chem. Abstr. Serv. Reg. No.: 121-69-7

Chem. Abstr. Name: *N*,*N*-Dimethylbenzenamine

IUPAC Systematic Name: *N*,*N*-Dimethylaniline

Synonyms: (Dimethylamino)benzene; *N*,*N*-dimethylaminobenzene; dimethylaniline; dimethylphenylamine; *N*,*N*-dimethylphenylamine

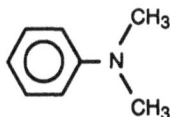

$C_8H_{11}N$ Mol. wt: 121.18

1.1.2 *Chemical and physical properties*

(a) *Description*: Yellowish to brownish oily liquid (Sax & Lewis, 1987)

(b) *Boiling-point*: 192–194 °C (Eller, 1985; Lide, 1991)

(c) *Melting-point*: 2–2.45 °C (Eller, 1985; Lide, 1991)

(d) *Density*: 0.956 g/ml at 20 °C (Eller, 1985)

(e) *Spectroscopy data*: Infrared, ultraviolet and nuclear magnetic resonance spectral data have been reported (Sadtler Research Laboratories, 1980; Pouchert, 1981, 1983; US National Toxicology Program, 1989; Sadtler Research Laboratories, 1991).

(f) *Solubility*: Insoluble in water (2–14 g/l at 25 °C). Since *N*,*N*-dimethylaniline is a basic compound, its solubility is dependent on the pH of the aqueous medium: its solubility in water at pH > 7 is lower than that in water of pH < 5. The data on aqueous solubility reported in the literature thus vary widely (US Environmental Protection Agency, 1986). Soluble in acetone, benzene, chloroform, diethyl ether and ethanol (Amoore & Hautala, 1983; Dragun & Helling, 1985; Sax & Lewis, 1987; Lide, 1991)

(g) *Volatility*: Vapour pressure, 1 mm Hg [133 Pa] at 29.5 °C (Lide, 1991)

(h) *Stability*: Slowly oxidizes and darkens in air; can react with nitrous acid to form ring-substituted nitroso compounds (US Environmental Protection Agency, 1986)

(i) *Octanol/water partition coefficient (P)*: 2.31 (Hansch & Leo, 1979)

(j) *Conversion factor*: mg/m^3 = 4.95 × ppm[1]

1.1.3 *Trade names, technical products and impurities*

N,N-Dimethylaniline is available commercially at a minimum purity of 99.7%, with aniline (see IARC, 1982a, 1987a) (0.05% max.) and *N*-methylaniline (0.3% max.) as impurities (Buffalo Color Corp., 1987, 1992). It is also available in research quantities at purities in the same order of magnitude (Janssen Chimica, 1990; Riedel-de Haen, 1990; Heraeus, 1991; Lancaster Synthesis, 1991; Aldrich Chemical Co., 1992; Fluka Chemie AG, 1993).

1.1.4 *Analysis*

N,N-Dimethylaniline can be detected in air by adsorption on silica gel, desorption with ethanol and analysis by gas chromatography and flame ionization detection. The limit of detection is 10 μg/sample (Campbell *et al.*, 1981; Eller, 1985).

Amines can be liberated during the manufacture of rubber, especially by vulcanization and by other thermal degradations. A method was described for the determination of free aromatic amines, including *N,N*-dimethylaniline, using high-temperature glass-capillary gas chromatography and nitrogen-selective detection (thermionic specific detector), with detection limits of 10–20 pg (Dalene & Skarping, 1985).

A gas chromatographic procedure for the determination of residual *N,N*-dimethylaniline as a contaminant in commercial antibiotics has been described, which involves dissolution of the sample in aqueous alkali, extraction of *N,N*-dimethylaniline with cyclohexane and analysis by gas chromatrography–flame ionization detection (Margosis, 1977).

1.2 Production and use

1.2.1 *Production*

N,N-Dimethylaniline is produced commercially by heating aniline at 300 °C with methanol in the presence of a catalyst at high pressure; sulfuric acid, phosphoric acid or alumina can be used as the catalyst (Northcott, 1978; Rosenwald, 1978; Budavari, 1989).

N,N-Dimethylaniline is produced by one company each in France, Germany, Hungary, Mexico, Poland, the Republic of Korea, Spain and the USA, by two companies in Japan and the United Kingdom and by four companies in India (Chemical Information Services, 1991).

US production was estimated to be 6000 tonnes in 1976 (US Environmental Protection Agency, 1986) and between 1000 and 10 000 tonnes in 1988 (US National Toxicology Program, 1989). In 1987, approximately 500 tonnes were imported into the USA (US International Trade Commission, 1988).

---

[1]Calculated from: mg/m^3 = (molecular weight/24.45) × ppm, assuming normal temperature (25°C) and pressure (760 mm Hg [101.3 kPa])

1.2.2 *Use*

N,N-Dimethylaniline is used as an intermediate in the manufacture of dyes, Michler's ketone and vanillin. It is also used as a specialty industrial solvent, a rubber vulcanizing agent (see IARC, 1982b, 1987b), a stabilizer and an acid scavenger (Northcott, 1978; Sax & Lewis, 1987; Budavari, 1989; US National Toxicology Program, 1989).

1.3 Occurrence

1.3.1 *Natural occurrence*

N,N-Dimethylaniline is not known to occur as a natural product.

1.3.2 *Occupational exposure*

N,N-Dimethylaniline was reported in the air of coal liquefaction plants (Harris *et al.*, 1980) and in the air of a plant for the manufacture of fibre glass-reinforced plastic pipes (Markel & Wilcox, 1981), at levels below the standard of the US Occupational Safety and Health Administration (see below) (US Environmental Protection Agency, 1986). Concentrations of *N,N*-dimethylaniline in 23 workplace air samples from two pilot coal liquefaction plants in Canada were consistently below the analytical detection limit of 0.05 mg/m^3 (Leach *et al.*, 1987).

On the basis of a survey conducted in the USA between 1981 and 1983, the US National Institute for Occupational Safety and Health estimated that a total of 30 480 workers, including 7448 women, were potentially exposed to *N,N*-dimethylaniline in 15 industries at 1428 sites (US National Library of Medicine, 1992).

1.3.3 *Water and soils*

N,N-Dimethylaniline has been detected in Lake Ontario (US Environmental Protection Agency, 1986) and in river water in Spain (Rivera *et al.*, 1987). River water near effluent sources of industrial dyestuff wastes in the Netherlands showed concentrations of up to 3.6 µg/l (Meijers & van der Leer, 1976; Zoeteman *et al.*, 1980). *N,N*-Dimethylaniline was found in soil samples near a dye manufacturing plant in the USA at a concentration of up to 40 mg/kg (Nelson & Hites, 1980).

1.3.4 *Other*

N,N-Dimethylaniline is used as an acid scavenger in the synthesis of penicillins and cephalosporins and has been reported as a contaminant of commercial preparations of those antibiotics at levels of up to 1500 ppm (Margosis, 1977; Quercia *et al.*, 1980).

1.4 Regulations and guidelines

Occupational exposure limits and guidelines for *N,N*-dimethylaniline in some countries are presented in Table 1.

Table 1. Occupational exposure limits and guidelines for N,N-dimethylaniline

Country	Year	Concentration (mg/m^3)	Interpretation
Australia		25	TWA
		50	STEL
Austria	1982	25	TWA
Belgium		25	TWA
		50	STEL
China	1979	5	TWA
Denmark	1988	25	TWA
Finland		25	TWA
		50	STEL
France		25	TWA
Germany	1992	25	TWA
Hungary		5	TWA
		10	STEL
Indonesia	1978	25	TWA
Mexico	1983	25	TWA
Netherlands	1989	25	TWA
Norway	1984	25	TWA
Poland		5	TWA
Romania	1975	10	TWA
		20	STEL
Switzerland		25	TWA
		50	STEL
United Kingdom	1990	25	TWA
		50	STEL
USA			
ACGIH	1992	25	TWA
		50	STEL
NIOSH	1990	10	TWA
		50	STEL
OSHA	1989	25	TWA
		50	STEL
Venezuela	1978	25	TWA
		60	STEL

From Cook (1987); US Occupational Safety and Health Administration (OSHA) (1989); American Conference of Governmental Industrial Hygienists (ACGIH) (1990, 1992); ILO (1991); Deutsche Forschungsgemeinschaft (1992); TWA, time-weighted average; STEL, short-term exposure limit

All countries have a notation that the compound may be a skin irritant.

2. Studies of Cancer in Humans

No data were available to the Working Group.

3. Studies of Cancer in Experimental Animals

3.1 Oral administration

3.1.1 *Mouse*

Groups of 50 male and 50 female B6C3F$_1$ mice, eight weeks old, were administered 0 (controls), 15 or 30 mg/kg bw *N,N*-dimethylaniline (> 98% pure) in 10 ml/kg bw corn oil by gavage on five days a week for 103 weeks. Survival at week 104 was: males—controls, 34/50; low-dose, 30/50; high-dose, 34/50; females—controls, 35/50; low-dose, 39/50; high-dose, 33/50. In females, epithelial hyperplasia of forestomach occurred in 8/50 controls, 11/19 low-dose and 13/50 high-dose; and squamous-cell papillomas of the forestomach were found in 2/50 controls, 2/19 low-dose and 8/50 high-dose animals (p = 0.042, incidental tumour test) (US National Toxicology Program, 1989). [The Working Group noted that only 19 forestomachs from females in the low-dose group were examined microscopically and that the high dose used may not have reached the maximal tolerable dose].

3.1.2 *Rat*

Groups of 50 male and 50 female Fischer 344 rats, seven weeks old, were administered 0 (controls), 3 or 30 mg/kg bw *N,N*-dimethylaniline (> 98% pure) in 5 ml/kg bw corn oil by gavage on five days a week for 103 weeks. Survival at 104 weeks was: males—controls, 29/50; low-dose, 32/50; high-dose, 28/50; females—controls, 21/50; low-dose, 32/50; high-dose, 36/50. Sarcomas of the spleen occurred in 0/49 controls, 0/49 low-dose and 3/50 high-dose male rats; one osteosarcoma of the spleen was observed in a high-dose male. Although the proportion of high-dose male rats with splenic sarcomas or osteosarcomas (4/50, 8%) was not significantly greater than that in controls (0/50), it exceeded the historical control incidence (study laboratory, 1/148 (0.7 ± 1%); all National Toxicology Program laboratories, 3/2081 (0.1 ± 0.5%)). The severity of haematopoiesis and haemosiderosis of the spleen was increased in high-dose rats of each sex, and an increased incidence of fibrosis and fatty metamorphosis of the spleen occurred in high-dose males. The incidence of mononuclear cell leukaemias was significantly decreased in high-dose rats: males—controls, 13/50; low-dose, 4/50; high-dose, 3/50 (p = 0.017, incidental tumour test); females—controls, 11/50; low-dose, 7/50; high-dose, 0/50 (p = 0.005, incidental tumour test) (Abdo *et al.*, 1989 (abstract); US National Toxicology Program, 1989).

4. Other Relevant Data

4.1 Absorption, distribution, metabolism and excretion

4.1.1 *Humans*

No data were available to the Working Group.

4.1.2 *Experimental systems*

The metabolism of *N,N*-dimethylaniline has been studied in adult and fetal human tissues *in vitro*. In adult liver microsomes, both *N*-oxidation and oxidative *N*-demethylation were shown to occur, resulting in the formation of *N,N*-dimethylaniline *N*-oxide and of *N*-methylaniline and formaldehyde, respectively. The *N*-oxide was found to be metabolized further to formaldehyde and *N*-methylaniline (Kitada *et al.*, 1974). *N*-Oxidation has also been demonstrated in fetal liver microsomes, adult kidney microsomes and adult liver homogenates (Ziegler & Gold, 1971; Rane, 1974; Lemoine *et al.*, 1990). In experiments with enzyme inhibitors, antibodies and enzyme thermal stability, it was concluded that the flavin-containing mono-oxygenases are primarily responsible for *N*-oxidation (McManus *et al.*, 1987), while cytochrome(s) P450 appears to catalyse the *N*-demethylation reactions (Lemoine *et al.*, 1990).

The metabolism of *N,N*-dimethylaniline was studied in mongrel dogs given a dose of 40 mg/kg [purity unspecified] by intravenous injection; blood samples were collected over 4 h and urine samples over 48 h. Aniline was detected in blood but not in urine, while *N*-methylaniline, 2- and 4-aminophenol, *N*-methyl-4-aminophenol, *N,N*-dimethyl-2-amino-phenol and *N,N*-dimethyl-4-aminophenol were isolated from urine after enzymatic deconjugation with glucuronidase/sulfatase and were characterized by spectral and chromatographic criteria; *N,N*-dimethylaniline *N*-oxide was not detected. *N,N*-Dimethyl-4-amino-phenol and *N*-methyl-4-aminophenol were recovered as urinary metabolites in rabbits; and rats were found to excrete *N,N*-dimethyl-4-aminophenyl sulfate and 4-aminophenyl sulfate (reviewed by Kiese & Renner, 1974). Incubation of isolated rat hepatocytes with *N,N*-di-methylaniline resulted in the formation of *N*-methylaniline, aniline, *N,N*-dimethylaniline *N*-oxide and *N*-methylaniline *N*-glucuronide (Sherratt & Damani, 1989).

The metabolism of N,N-dimethylaniline has been studied in a wide variety of tissues and species *in vitro*, including the livers of rats, mice, hamsters, rabbits, guinea-pigs, cats, cows, pigs, squirrels, bats, armadillos, opossums, raccoons and several avian, fish, amphibian and reptile species; extrahepatic tissues (notably lung, kidney, nasal mucosa, adrenals and intestine) of rats, pigs and rabbits; and even in a protozoan (Machinist *et al.*, 1968; Pan *et al.*, 1975; Hlavica & Kehl, 1976; Gorrod & Gooderham, 1981; McNulty *et al.*, 1983; Ohmiya & Mehendale, 1983; Agosin & Ankley, 1987). The major reactions are *N*-oxidation of *N,N*-di-methylaniline to form *N,N*-dimethylaniline *N*-oxide and oxidative *N*-demethylation of *N,N*-dimethylaniline and its *N*-oxide to form *N*-methylaniline and formaldehyde. Aryl ring-hydroxylation is a minor reaction and results in the formation of *N,N*-dimethyl-4-amino-phenol and its non-enzymatic decomposition product, *N*-methyl-4-aminophenol. The latter reaction is of interest as it appears to proceed through a reactive quinoneimine intermediate (Gooderham & Gorrod, 1981). Further *N*-demethylation of *N*-methylaniline to aniline and ring- and *N*-hydroxylation to 4-aminophenol and phenylhydroxylamine (Holzer & Kiese, 1960) have also been reported *in vitro*. On the basis of several studies using inhibitors, antibodies, inducers and purified enzymes, *N,N*-dimethylaniline *N*-oxidation has been shown to be catalysed selectively by the flavin-containing mono-oxygenases, while *N*-demethylation and ring-hydroxylation are catalysed primarily by cytochromes P450 (principally the PB, BNF and ISF families) (Devereux & Fouts, 1974; Ziegler & Pettit, 1964; Hlavica &

Hülsmann, 1979; Gorrod & Gooderham, 1981; Akhrem *et al.*, 1982; Hamill & Cooper, 1984; MacDonald *et al.*, 1989; Pandey *et al.*, 1989). The demethylation of *N,N*-dimethylaniline can also be catalysed by peroxidative mechanisms involving ram seminal vesicle prostaglandin synthase (Sivarajah *et al.*, 1982) and fungal chloroperoxidase (Kedderis & Hollenberg, 1984).

4.2 Toxic effects

4.2.1 *Humans*

No data were available to the Working Group.

4.2.2 *Experimental systems*

The LD_{50} values for *N,N*-dimethylaniline [purity and vehicle unspecified] were estimated to be 1350 mg/kg bw after single gavage doses to male Carworth-Wistar rats and 1690 mg/kg bw after dermal administration to male New Zealand rabbits (Smyth *et al.*, 1962).

Exposure of rats to *N,N*-dimethylaniline by inhalation (0.0055 and 0.3 mg/m^3 continuously for 100 days) resulted in methaemoglobinaemia, lowered erythrocyte haemoglobin, leukopenia and reticulocytosis, and reduced muscle chronaxy. Exposure to *N*-methylaniline (0.03 and 0.04 mg/m^3 only) under the same conditions resulted in lesser toxicity but included methaemoglobinaemia (Markosyan, 1969). Intravenous injection of 25 mg/kg bw *N,N*-dimethylaniline to cats increased the levels of haemoglobulin (Holzer & Kiese, (1960).

In chronic studies in which male and female Fischer 344 rats and B6C3F$_1$ mice were given the compound (98.2% pure) by gavage in corn oil at doses of up to 500 mg/kg for five days per week for 13 weeks, dose-related decreases in body weight gain were observed in male rats and cyanosis and decreased motor activity in both species of each sex, as well as splenomegaly and haemosiderosis in the spleen, liver, kidney and testes. Bone marrow hyperplasia was seen in rats and increased haematopoiesis in the liver in mice and in the spleen in mice and rats (Abdo *et al.*, 1990). Rats were generally more sensitive than mice to these toxic effects, all of which could be attributed to chronic methaemoglobinaemia, erythrocyte destruction and erythrophagocytosis.

In the 103-week carcinogenicity study described on p. 341, dose-related, non-neoplastic changes observed in rats involved fibrosis, haemosiderosis, fatty metamorphosis of the spleen and chronic focal inflammation of the liver (US National Toxicology Program, 1989).

After oral dosing of female Wistar rats with *N,N*-dimethylaniline [purity unspecified] in propylene glycol at 73 mg/kg bw, 11.4 mmol [1.4 g] compound/kg bw was bound to haemoglobin (Birner & Neumann, 1988).

4.3 Reproductive and developmental effects

4.3.1 *Humans*

No data were available to the Working Group.

4.3.2 *Experimental systems*

Pregnant CD-1 mice were administered *N,N*-dimethylaniline in corn oil at 365 mg/kg bw per day by gavage on gestation days 6–13 and allowed to deliver litters (Hardin *et al.*,

1987). Live pups were counted and weighed within one-half day after birth and again on the third day after birth. The dose killed 6% of treated females but did not significantly affect maternal body weight gain, number of viable litters (at least one live pup) produced, body weight or number of liveborn pups per litter, or body weight gain or survival of pups up to three days of age.

4.4 Genetic and related effects

4.4.1 *Humans*

No data were available to the Working Group.

4.4.2 *Experimental systems* (see also Table 2 and Appendices 1 and 2)

N,N-Dimethylaniline did not induce mutation in *Salmonella typhimurium* but was mutagenic at the *tk* locus of mouse lymphoma L5178Y cells. It induced both sister chromatid exchange and chromosomal aberrations in Chinese hamster ovary cells but did not induce unscheduled DNA synthesis in rat primary hepatocyte cultures.

5. Summary of Data Reported and Evaluation

5.1 Exposure data

N,N-Dimethylaniline is used as an intermediate in the manufacture of dyes and other products and as a solvent for special purposes, a rubber vulcanizing agent and a stabilizer. It has been detected in ambient water and soil in the vicinity of industrial facilities.

5.2 Human carcinogenicity data

No data were available to the Working Group.

5.3 Animal carcinogenicity data

N,N-Dimethylaniline was tested for carcinogenicity in one study in mice and in one study in rats by gavage. It increased the incidence of forestomach papillomas in female mice. A few splenic sarcomas were observed in treated male rats.

5.4 Other relevant data

The metabolism of *N,N*-dimethylaniline has been studied in many species and in human tissues. It involves enzymatic *N*-demethylation, *N*-oxidation and ring hydroxylation. Aniline is a major metabolite. Chronic methaemoglobinaemia and erythrocyte haemolysis, with concomitant splenomegaly and other pathological lesions characteristic of aniline, were observed in mice and rats treated with *N,N*-dimethylaniline.

Table 2. Genetic and related effects of N,N-dimethylaniline

Test system	Result		Dose[a] (LED/HID)	Reference
	Without exogenous metabolic system	With exogenous metabolic system		
SA0, *Salmonella typhimurium* TA100, reverse mutation	–	–	60.0000	Mori et al. (1980)
SA0, *Salmonella typhimurium* TA100, reverse mutation	–	–	167.0000	Mortelmans et al. (1986)
SA5, *Salmonella typhimurium* TA1535, reverse mutation	–	–	167.0000	Mortelmans et al. (1986)
SA7, *Salmonella typhimurium* TA1537, reverse mutation	–	–	167.0000	Mortelmans et al. (1986)
SA9, *Salmonella typhimurium* TA98, reverse mutation	–	–	60.0000	Mori et al. (1980)
SA9, *Salmonella typhimurium* TA98, reverse mutation	0	–	25.0000	Ho et al. (1981)
SA9, *Salmonella typhimurium* TA98, reverse mutation	–	–	167.0000	Mortelmans et al. (1986)
URP, Unscheduled DNA synthesis, rat primary hepatocytes	–	0	121.2000	Yoshimi et al. (1988)
G5T, Gene mutation, mouse lymphoma L5178Y cells, *tk* locus	+	+	19.0000	US National Toxicology Program (1989)
SIC, Sister chromatid exchange, Chinese hamster (CHO) ovary cells *in vitro*	–	+	30.0000	Loveday et al. (1989)
CIC, Chromosomal aberrations, Chinese hamster (CHO) ovary cells *in vitro*	(+)	+	83.0000	Loveday et al. (1989)

+, positive; (+), weakly positive; –, negative; 0, not tested
[a]In-vitro tests, μg/ml; in-vivo tests, mg/kg bw

N,N-Dimethylaniline did not induce gene mutation in bacteria or DNA damage in cultured mammalian cells. It induced gene mutation, sister chromatid exchange and chromosomal aberrations in cultured mammalian cells.

5.5 Evaluation[1]

There is *inadequate evidence* in humans for the carcinogenicity of N,N-dimethylaniline. There is *limited evidence* in experimental animals for the carcinogenicity of N,N-dimethylaniline.

Overall evaluation

N,N-Dimethylaniline *is not classifiable as to its carcinogenicity to humans (Group 3).*

6. References

Abdo, K.M., Bucher, J., Haseman, J.K., Eustis, S.L. & Huff, J.E. (1989) Induction of splenic sarcomas in F344/N rats given N,N-dimethylaniline (Abstract No. 703). *Proc. Am. Assoc. Cancer Res.*, **30**, 177

Abdo, K.M., Jokinen, M.P. & Hiles, R. (1990) Subchronic (13-week) toxicity studies of N,N-dimethylaniline administered to Fischer 344 rats and $B6C3F_1$ mice. *J. Toxicol. environ. Health*, **29**, 77–88

Agosin, M. & Ankley, G.T. (1987) Conversion of N,N-dimethylaniline to N,N-dimethylaniline-N-oxide by a cytosolic flavin-containing enzyme from *Trypanosoma cruzi. Drug Metab. Disposition*, **15**, 200–203

Akhrem, A.A., Khatyleva, S.Y., Shkumatov, V.M., Chashchin, V.L. & Kiselev, P.A. (1982) Cumene hydroperoxide supported demethylation of N,N-dimethylaniline by cytochrome P-450 from adrenal cortex mitochondria. *Acta biol. med. germ.*, **11**, 1019–1028

Aldrich Chemical Co. (1992) *Aldrich Catalog/Handbook of Fine Chemicals 1992–1993*, Milwaukee, WI, p. 490

American Conference of Governmental Industrial Hygienists (1990) *Guide to Occupational Exposure Values—1990*, Cincinnati, OH, p. 42

American Conference of Governmental Industrial Hygienists (1992) *1992–1993 Threshold Limit Values for Chemical Substances and Physical Agents and Biological Exposure Indices*, Cincinnati, OH, p. 19

Amoore, J.E. & Hautala, E. (1983) Odor as an aid to chemical safety: odor thresholds compared with threshold limit values and volatilities for 214 industrial chemicals in air and water dilution. *J. appl. Toxicol.*, **3**, 272–290

Birner, G. & Neumann, H.-G. (1988) Biomonitoring of aromatic amines. II. Hemoglobin binding of some monocyclic aromatic amines. *Arch. Toxicol.*, **62**, 110–115

Budavari, S., ed. (1989) *The Merck Index*, 11th ed., Rahway, NJ, Merck & Co., p. 510

Buffalo Color Corp. (1987) *Specification Sheet: N,N-dimethylaniline*, Parsippany, NJ

---

[1]For definition of the italicized terms, see Preamble, pp. 26–30.

Buffalo Color Corp. (1992) *Material Safety Data Sheet: Dimethylaniline*, Parsippany, NJ

Campbell, E.E., Wood, G.O. & Anderson, R.G. (1981) Method 1—Gas chromatographic analysis of aromatic amines in air. In: Egan, H., Fishbein, L., Castegnaro, M., O'Neill, I.K. & Bartsch, H., eds, *Environmental Carcinogens: Selected Methods of Analysis*, Vol. 4, *Some Aromatic Amines and Azo Dyes in the General and Industrial Environment* (IARC Scientific Publications No. 40), Lyon, IARC, pp. 109–118

Chemical Information Services Ltd (1991) *Directory of World Chemical Producers 1992/93 Edition*, Dallas, TX, p. 234

Cook, W.A. (1987) *Occupational Exposure Limits—Worldwide*, Akron, OH, American Industrial Hygiene Association, pp. 120, 137, 183

Dalene, M. & Skarping, G. (1985) Trace analysis of amines and isocyanates using glass capillary gas chromatography and selective detection. IV. Determination of free aromatic amines using nitrogen-selective detection. *J. Chromatogr.*, **331**, 321–330

Deutsche Forschungsgemeinschaft (1992) *MAK- and BAT-Values List 1992. Maximum Concentrations at the Workplace (MAK) and Biological Tolerance Values (BAT) for Working Materials* (Report No. 28), Weinheim, VCH Verlagsgesellschaft, p. 36

Devereux, T.R. & Fouts, J.R. (1974) *N*-Oxidation and demethylation of *N,N*-dimethylaniline by rabbit liver and lung microsomes. Effects of age and metals. *Chem.-biol. Interactions*, **8**, 91–105

Dragun, J. & Helling, C.S. (1985) Physicochemical and structural relationships of organic chemicals undergoing soil- and clay-catalyzed free-radical oxidation. *Soil Sci.*, **139**, 100–111

Eller, P.M., ed. (1985) *NIOSH Manual of Analytical Methods*, 3rd ed., Suppl. 1, (DHHS (NIOSH) Publ. No. 84-100), Washington DC, US Government Printing Office, pp. 2002-1—2002-6

Fluka Chemie AG (1993) *Fluka Chemika-BioChemika*, Buchs, p. 513

Gooderham, N.J. & Gorrod, J.W. (1981) Routes to the formation of *N*-methyl-4-aminophenol, a metabolite of *N,N*-dimethylaniline. *Adv. exp. Med. Biol.*, **136B**, 1109–1120

Gorrod, J.W. & Gooderham, N.J. (1981) The in vitro metabolism of *N,N*-dimethylaniline by guinea pig and rabbit tissue preparations. *Eur. J. Drug Metab. Pharmacol.*, **6**, 195–206

Hamill, S. & Cooper, D.Y. (1984) The role of cytochrome P-450 in the dual pathways of *N*-demethylation of *N,N*-dimethylaniline by hepatic microsomes. *Xenobiotica*, **14**, 139–149

Hansch, C. & Leo, A. (1979) *Substituent Constants for Correlation Analysis in Chemistry and Biology*, New York, John Wiley & Sons, p. 235

Hardin, B.D., Schuler, R.L., Burg, J.R., Booth, G.M., Hazelden, K.P., MacKenzie, K.M., Piccirillo, V.J. & Smith, K.N. (1987) Evaluation of 60 chemicals in a preliminary developmental toxicity test. *Teratog. Carcinog. Mutag.*, **7**, 29–48

Harris, L.R., Gideon, J.A., Berardinelli, S., Reed, L.D. & Dobbin, R.D. (1980) *Coal Liquefaction: Recent Findings in Occupational Safety and Health* (NIOSH-80-122/US NTIS PB81-223422), Cincinnati, OH, National Institute for Occupational Safety and Health

Heraeus (1991) *Feinchemikalien und Forschungsbedarf*, Karlsruhe, p. 280

Hlavica, P. & Hülsmann, S. (1979) Studies on the mechanism of hepatic microsomal *N*-oxide formation. *Biochem. J.*, **182**, 109–116

Hlavica, P. & Kehl, M. (1976) Comparative studies on the *N*-oxidation of aniline and *N,N*-dimethylaniline by rabbit liver microsomes. *Xenobiotica*, **11**, 679–689

Ho, C.-H., Clark, B.R., Guerin, M.R., Barkenbus, F.D., Rao, T.K. & Epler, J.L. (1981) Analytical and biological analyses of test materials from the synthetic fuel technologies. IV. Studies of chemical structure–mutagenic activity relationships of aromatic nitrogen compounds relevant to synfuels. *Mutat. Res.*, **85**, 335–345

Holzer, N. & Kiese, M. (1960) Formation of nitrosobenzene, aniline and haemoglobin in cats and dogs after intravenous injection of N-alkylanilines (Ger.). *Naunyn-Schmiedeberg's Arch. exp. Pathol. Pharmakol.*, **238**, 546–556

IARC (1982a) *IARC Monographs on the Evaluation of the Carcinogenic Risk of Chemicals to Humans*, Vol. 27, *Some Aromatic Amines, Anthraquinones, and Nitroso Compounds, and Inorganic Fluorides Used in Drinking-water and Dental Preparations*, Lyon, pp. 39–61

IARC (1982b) *IARC Monographs on the Evaluation of the Carcinogenic Risk of Chemicals to Humans*, Vol. 28, *The Rubber Industry*, Lyon

IARC (1987a) *IARC Monographs on the Evaluation of Carcinogenic Risks to Humans*, Suppl. 7, *Overall Evaluations of Carcinogenicity: An Updating of* IARC Monographs *Volumes 1 to 42*, Lyon, pp. 99–100

IARC (1987b) *IARC Monographs on the Evaluation of Carcinogenic Risks to Humans*, Suppl. 7, *Overall Evaluations of Carcinogenicity: An Updating of* IARC Monographs *Volumes 1 to 42*, Lyon, pp. 332–334

ILO (1991) *Occupational Exposure Limits for Airborne Toxic Substances*, 3rd ed. (Occupational Safety and Health Series No. 37), Geneva, International Labour Office, pp. 164–167

Janssen Chimica (1990) *1991 Catalog Handbook of Fine Chemicals*, Beerse, p. 477

Kedderis, G.L. & Hollenberg, P.F. (1984) pH Kinetic studies of the N-demethylation of N,N-dimethylaniline catalyzed by chloroperoxidase. *Arch. Biochem. Biophys.*, **233**, 315–321

Kiese, M. & Renner, G. (1974) Urinary metabolites of N,N-dimethylaniline produced by dogs. *Arch. Pharmacol.*, **283**, 143–150

Kitada, M., Kamataki, T. & Kitagawa, H. (1974) Comparison of N-oxidation and N-demethylation of dimethylamine in human liver. *Jpn. J. Pharmacol.*, **24**, 644–647

Lancaster Synthesis (1991) *MTM Research Chemicals/Lancaster Catalogue 1991/92*, Windham, NH, MTM Plc, pp. 534–535

Leach, J.M., Otson, R. & Armstrong, V. (1987) Airborne contaminants in two small Canadian coal liquefaction pilot plants. *Am. ind. Hyg. Assoc. J.*, **48**, 693–697

Lemoine, A., Johann, M. & Cresteil, T. (1990) Evidence for the presence of distinct flavin-containing monooxygenases in human tissues. *Arch. Biochem. Biophys.*, **276**, 336–342

Lide, D.R., ed. (1991) *CRC Handbook of Chemistry and Physics*, 72nd ed., Boca Raton, FL, CRC Press, pp. 3–40, 6–76

Loveday, K.S., Lugo, M.H., Resnick, M.A., Anderson, B.E. & Zeiger, E. (1989) Chromosome aberration and sister chromatid exchange tests in Chinese hamster ovary cells *in vitro*: II. Results with 20 chemicals. *Environ. mol. Mutag.*, **13**, 60–94

MacDonald, T.L., Gutheim, W.G., Martin, R.B. & Guengerich, F.P. (1989) Oxidation of substituted N,N-dimethylanilines by cytochrome P-450: estimation of the effective oxidation–reduction potential of cytochrome P-450. *Biochemistry*, **28**, 2071–2077

Machinist, J.M., Dehner, E.W. & Ziegler, D.M. (1968) Microsomal oxidases. III. Comparison of species and organ distribution of dialkylarylamine N-oxide and dealkylase and dialkylarylamine N-oxidase. *Arch. Biochem. Biophys.*, **125**, 858–864

Markel, H., Jr & Wilcox, T. (1981) *Health Hazard Evaluation Report No. HHE- 79-104-838. A.O. Smith-Inland, Inc., Little Rock, AR* (US NTIS PB82-182429), Cincinnati, OH, National Institute for Occupational Safety and Health

Margosis, M. (1977) GLC determination of N,N-dimethylaniline in penicillins. *J. pharmacol. Sci.*, **66**, 1634–1636

Markosyan, T.M. (1969) Comparative toxicity of monomethylaniline and dimethylaniline in chronic test (Russ.). *Gig. Sanit.*, **34**, 7–11

McManus, M.E., Stupans, I., Burgess, W., Koenig, J.A., Hall, P.delaM. & Birkett, D.J. (1987) Flavin-containing monooxygenase activity in human liver microsomes. *Drug Metab. Disposition*, **15**, 256–261

McNulty, M.J., Casanova-Schmitz, M. & Heck, H.d'A. (1983) Metabolism of dimethylamine in the nasal mucosa of the Fischer 344 rat. *Drug Metab. Disposition*, **11**, 421–425

Meijers, A.P. & van der Leer, R.C. (1976) The occurrence of organic micropollutants in the River Rhine and the River Maas in 1974. *Water Res.*, **10**, 597–604

Mori, Y., Niwa, T., Hori, T. & Toyoshi, K. (1980) Mutagenicity of 3′-methyl-N,N-dimethyl-4-amino azobenzene metabolites and related compounds. *Carcinogenesis*, **1**, 121–127

Mortelmans, K., Haworth, S., Lawlor, T., Speck, W., Tainer, B. & Zeiger, E. (1986) *Salmonella* muta-genicity tests: II. Results from the testing of 270 chemicals. *Environ. mol. Mutag.*, **8** (Suppl. 7), 1–119

Nelson, C.R. & Hites, R.A. (1980) Aromatic amines in and near Buffalo River. *Environ. Sci. Technol.*, **14**, 1147–1149

Northcott, J. (1978) Aniline and its derivatives. In: Mark, H.F., Othmer, D.F., Overberger, C.G., Seaborg, G.T. & Grayson, N., eds, *Kirk-Othmer Encyclopedia of Chemical Technology*, 3rd ed., Vol. 2, New York, John Wiley & Sons, pp. 309–321

Ohmiya, Y. & Mehendale, H.M. (1983) *N*-Oxidation of *N,N*-dimethylaniline in the rabbit and rat lung. *Biochem. Pharmacol.*, **32**, 1281–1285

Pan, H.P., Fouts, J.R. & Devereux, T.R. (1975) Hepatic microsomal *N*-oxidation and *N*-demethylation of *N,N*-dimethylaniline in red-winged blackbird compared with rat and other birds. *Life Sci.*, **17**, 819–826

Pandey, R.N., Armstrong, A.P. & Hollenberg, P.F. (1989) Oxidative *N*-demethylation of N,N-dimethyl-aniline by purified isozymes of cytochrome P-450. *Biochem. Pharmacol.*, **38**, 2181–2185

Pouchert, C.J. (1981) *The Aldrich Library of Infrared Spectra*, 3rd ed., Milwaukee, WI, Aldrich Chemical Co., p. 715

Pouchert, C.J. (1983) *The Aldrich Library of NMR Spectra*, 2nd ed., Vol. 1, Milwaukee, WI, Aldrich Chemical Co., p. 990

Quercia, V., De Sena, C., Iela, G., Pagnozzi, G. & Pierini, N. (1980) Determination of the content of *N,N*-dimethylaniline in some antibiotics (Ital.). *Boll. chim. farm.*, **119**, 619–622

Rane, A. (1974) *N*-Oxidation of a tertiary amine (*N,N*-dimethylaniline) by human fetal liver micro-somes. *Clin. Pharmacol. Ther.*, **15**, 32–38

Riedel-de Haen (1990) *Laboratory Chemicals 1990*, Seelze, p. 493

Rivera, J., Ventura, F., Caixach, J., De Torres, M. & Figueras, A. (1987) GC/MS, HPLC and FAB mass spectrometric analysis of organic micropollutants in Barcelona's water supply. *Int. J. environ. anal. Chem.*, **29**, 15–35

Rosenwald, R.H. (1978) Alkylation. In: Mark, H.F., Othmer, D.F., Overberger, C.G., Seaborg, G.T. & Grayson, N., eds, *Kirk-Othmer Encyclopedia of Chemical Technology*, 3rd ed., Vol. 2, New York, John Wiley & Sons, p. 67

Sadtler Research Laboratories (1980) *Sadtler Standard Spectra. 1980 Cumulative Index*, Philadelphia, PA

Sadtler Research Laboratories (1991) *Sadtler Standard Spectra. 1981–1991 Supplementary Index*, Philadelphia, PA

Sax, N.I. & Lewis, R.J. (1987) *Hawley's Condensed Chemical Dictionary*, 11th ed., New York, Van Nostrand Reinhold Co., p. 411

Sherratt, A.J. & Damani, L.A. (1989) The metabolism of *N,N*-dimethylaniline by isolated rat hepatocytes: identification of a novel *N*-conjugate. *Xenobiotica*, **19**, 379–388

Sivarajah, K., Lasker, J.M., Eling, T.E. & Abou-Donia, M.B. (1982) Metabolism of *N*-alkyl compounds during the biosynthesis of prostaglandins. *N*-Dealkylation during prostaglandin biosynthesis. *Mol. Pharmacol.*, **21**, 133–141

Smyth, H.F., Jr, Carpenter, C.P., Weil, C.S., Pozzani, U.C. & Striegel, J.A. (1962) Range-finding toxicity data: list VI. *Am. ind. Hyg. Assoc. J.*, **23**, 95–107

US Environmental Protection Agency (1986) *Health and Environmental Effects Profile for N,N-Dimethylaniline* (Report No. EPA-600/X-87-052/US NTIS PB89-123038), Cincinnati, OH, Environmental Criteria and Assessment Office

US International Trade Commission (1988) *US Imports for Consumption and General Imports* (FT 246/Annual 1987), Washington DC, US Department of Commerce

US National Library of Medicine (1992) *Registry of Toxic Effects of Chemical Substances* (RTECS No. BX4725000), Bethesda, MD

US National Toxicology Program (1989) *Toxicology and Carcinogenesis Studies of N,N-Dimethylaniline (CAS No. 121-69-7) in F344/N Rats and B6C3F1 Mice (Gavage Studies)* (NTP TR 360; NIH Publ. No. 90-2815), Research Triangle Park, NC, US Department of Health and Human Services

US Occupational Safety and Health Administration (1989) Air contaminants—permissible exposure limits. *US Code fed. Regul.*, Part 1910.1000, **Title 29**, p. 602

Yoshimi, N., Sugie, S., Iwata, H., Niwa, K., Mori, H., Hashida, C. & Shimizu, H. (1988) The genotoxicity of a variety of aniline derivatives in a DNA repair test with primary cultured rat hepatocytes. *Mutat. Res.*, **206**, 183–191

Ziegler, D.M. & Gold, M.S. (1971) Oxidative metabolism of tertiary amine drugs by human liver tissue. *Xenobiotica*, **1**, 325–326

Ziegler, D.M. & Pettit, F.H. (1964) Formation of an intermediate *N*-oxide in the oxidative demethylation of *N,N*-dimethylaniline catalyzed by liver microsomes. *Biochem. biophys. Res. Commun.*, **15**, 188–193

Zoeteman, B.C.J., Harmsen, K., Linders, J.B.H.J., Morra, C.F.H. & Slooff, W. (1980) Persistent organic pollutants in river water and groundwater of the Netherlands. *Chemosphere*, **9**, 231–249

SUMMARY OF FINAL EVALUATIONS

Agent	Degree of evidence of carcinogenicity		Overall evaluation of carcinogenicity to humans
	Human	Animal	
2-Amino-4-nitrophenol	Inadequate[a]	Limited	3
2-Amino-5-nitrophenol	Inadequate[a]	Limited	3
para-Chloroaniline	Inadequate[a]	Sufficient	2B
CI Acid Orange 3	Inadequate[a]	Limited	3
CI Acid Red 114	Inadequate[a]	Sufficient	2B
CI Direct Blue 15	Inadequate[a]	Sufficient (technical-grade)	2B
CI Pigment Red 3	Inadequate[a]	Limited	3
D&C Red No. 9 (CI Pigment Red 53:1)	Inadequate[a]	Limited	3
1,4-Diamino-2-nitrobenzene (2-Nitro-para-phenylenediamine)	Inadequate[a]	Limited	3
2,6-Dimethylaniline (2,6-Xylidine)	Inadequate[a]	Sufficient	2B
N,N-Dimethylaniline	Inadequate[a]	Limited	3
Hair colourants, personal use of	Inadequate		3
Hairdresser or barber, occupational exposures as	Limited		2A
HC Blue No. 1	Inadequate[a]	Sufficient	2B
HC Blue No. 2	Inadequate[a]	Inadequate	3
HC Red No. 3	Inadequate[a]	Inadequate	3
HC Yellow No. 4	Inadequate[a]	Inadequate	3
Magenta (containing CI Basic Red 9)	Inadequate		2B
Magenta		Inadequate	
CI Basic Red 9	Inadequate	Sufficient	2B
Manufacture of magenta	Sufficient		1
4,4'-Methylenebis(2-chloroaniline) (MOCA)	Inadequate	Sufficient	2A[b]

[a] No data

[b] Overall evaluation 2A and not 2B on the basis of supporting evidence from other relevant data

APPENDIX 1

SUMMARY TABLES OF
GENETIC AND RELATED EFFECTS

Summary table of genetic and related effects of CI Acid Orange 3

Nonmammalian systems													Mammalian systems																				
Proka-ryotes		Lower eukaryotes				Plants		Insects					In vitro													In vivo								
													Animal cells							Human cells						Animals							Humans					
D	G	D	R	G	A	D	G	C	R	G	C	A	D	G	S	M	C	A	T	I	D	G	S	M	C	DL	A	D	G	S	M	C	A	D	S	M	C	A
+¹																																						

A, aneuploidy; C, chromosomal aberrations; D, DNA damage; DL, dominant lethal mutation; G, gene mutation; I, inhibition of intercellular communication; M, micronuclei; R, mitotic recombination and gene conversion; S, sister chromatid exchange; T, cell transformation

In completing the tables, the following symbols indicate the consensus of the Working Group with regard to the results for each endpoint:

+   considered to be positive for the specific endpoint and level of biological complexity

+¹   considered to be positive, but only one valid study was available to the Working Group

–   considered to be negative

–¹   considered to be negative, but only one valid study was available to the Working Group

?   considered to be equivocal or inconclusive (e.g., there were contradictory results from different laboratories; there were confounding exposures; the results were equivocal)

Summary table of genetic and related effects of HC Blue No. 1 (purified samples)

Nonmammalian systems														Mammalian systems																					
Proka- ryotes		Lower eukaryotes				Plants		Insects					*In vitro*															*In vivo*								
													Animal cells								Human cells						Animals						Humans		
D	G	D	R	G	A	D	G	C	R	G	C	A	D	G	S	M	C	A	T	I	D	G	S	M	C		D	G	S	M	C	DL	A	D	S	M	C	A
–¹	–			–¹	–¹					–¹			+	+¹	+¹					–¹					–¹						+¹							

A, aneuploidy; C, chromosomal aberrations; D, DNA damage; DL, dominant lethal mutation; G, gene mutation; I, inhibition of intercellular communication; M, micronuclei; R, mitotic recombination and gene conversion; S, sister chromatid exchange; T, cell transformation

In completing the tables, the following symbols indicate the consensus of the Working Group with regard to the results for each end-point:

+   considered to be positive for the specific endpoint and level of biological complexity

+¹ considered to be positive, but only one valid study was available to the Working Group

–   considered to be negative

–¹ considered to be negative, but only one valid study was available to the Working Group

?   considered to be equivocal or inconclusive (e.g., there were contradictory results from different laboratories; there were confounding exposures; the results were equivocal)

Summary table of genetic and related effects of HC Blue No. 1 (commercial samples)

Nonmammalian systems													Mammalian systems																										
Proka-ryotes		Lower eukaryotes				Plants		Insects					In vitro															In vivo												
													Animal cells							Human cells								Animals							Humans					
D	G	D	R	G	A	D	G	C	R	G	C	A	D	G	S	M	C	A	T	D	G	S	M	C	A	T	I	D	G	S	M	C	DL	A	D	S	M	C	A
$+^1$	+												+	+	+	+	$-^1$	+					$-^1$			$+^1$													

A, aneuploidy; C, chromosomal aberrations; D, DNA damage; DL, dominant lethal mutation; G, gene mutation; I, inhibition of intercellular communication; M, micronuclei; R, mitotic recombination and gene conversion; S, sister chromatid exchange; T, cell transformation

In completing the tables, the following symbols indicate the consensus of the Working Group with regard to the results for each end-point:

+ considered to be positive for the specific endpoint and level of biological complexity

$+^1$ considered to be positive, but only one valid study was available to the Working Group

$-$ considered to be negative

$-^1$ considered to be negative, but only one valid study was available to the Working Group

? considered to be equivocal or inconclusive (e.g., there were contradictory results from different laboratories; there were confounding exposures; the results were equivocal)

Summary table of genetic and related effects of HC Blue No. 2

Nonmammalian systems												Mammalian systems																														
Prokaryotes		Lower eukaryotes				Plants		Insects				In vitro																			In vivo												
												Animal cells									Human cells									Animals								Humans					
D	G	R	G	A	D	G	C	R	G	C	A	D	G	S	M	C	A	T	I		D	G	S	M	C	A	T	I		D	G	S	M	C	DL	A		D	S	M	C	A
+													+	+	+					−									−								−						

A, aneuploidy; C, chromosomal aberrations; D, DNA damage; DL, dominant lethal mutation; G, gene mutation; I, inhibition of intercellular communication; M, micronuclei; R, mitotic recombination and gene conversion; S, sister chromatid exchange; T, cell transformation

In completing the tables, the following symbols indicate the consensus of the Working Group with regard to the results for each end-point:

+   considered to be positive for the specific endpoint and level of biological complexity

+¹ considered to be positive, but only one valid study was available to the Working Group

–   considered to be negative

–¹ considered to be negative, but only one valid study was available to the Working Group

?   considered to be equivocal or inconclusive (e.g., there were contradictory results from different laboratories; there were confounding exposures; the results were equivocal)

Summary table of genetic and related effects of HC Red No. 3

Nonmammalian systems											Mammalian systems																					
Proka-ryotes		Lower eukaryotes				Plants			Insects		In vitro														In vivo								
											Animal cells						Human cells							Animals						Humans		
D	G	D	R	G	C	A	D	G	C	R	G	C	A	D	G	S	M	C	A	T	I	D	G	S	M	C	A	T	I	D	G	S	M	C	DL	A	D	G	S	M	C	A

+¹

A, aneuploidy; C, chromosomal aberrations; D, DNA damage; DL, dominant lethal mutation; G, gene mutation; I, inhibition of intercellular communication; M, micronuclei; R, mitotic recombination and gene conversion; S, sister chromatid exchange; T, cell transformation

In completing the tables, the following symbols indicate the consensus of the Working Group with regard to the results for each end-point:

+   considered to be positive for the specific endpoint and level of biological complexity

+¹   considered to be positive, but only one valid study was available to the Working Group

–   considered to be negative

–¹   considered to be negative, but only one valid study was available to the Working Group

?   considered to be equivocal or inconclusive (e.g., there were contradictory results from different laboratories; there were confounding exposures; the results were equivocal)

Summary table of genetic and related effects of HC Yellow No. 4

Nonmammalian systems				Mammalian systems			
Proka-ryotes	Lower eukaryotes	Plants	Insects	In vitro		In vivo	
				Animal cells	Human cells	Animals	Humans
D G	D R G A	D G C	R G	C A D G S M C A T I	D G S M C A T I	D G S M C DL A	D S M C A
+¹			+¹ —¹	+¹ ?			

A, aneuploidy; C, chromosomal aberrations; D, DNA damage; DL, dominant lethal mutation; G, gene mutation; I, inhibition of intercellular communication; M, micronuclei; R, mitotic recombination and gene conversion; S, sister chromatid exchange; T, cell transformation

In completing the tables, the following symbols indicate the consensus of the Working Group with regard to the results for each end-point:

+   considered to be positive for the specific endpoint and level of biological complexity
+¹   considered to be positive, but only one valid study was available to the Working Group
–   considered to be negative
–¹   considered to be negative, but only one valid study was available to the Working Group
?   considered to be equivocal or inconclusive (e.g., there were contradictory results from different laboratories; there were confounding exposures; the results were equivocal)

Summary table of genetic and related effects of 2-amino-4-nitrophenol

Nonmammalian systems										Mammalian systems																											
Proka-ryotes		Lower eukaryotes			Plants			Insects		In vitro																	In vivo											
										Animal cells											Human cells								Animals						Humans					
D	G	D	G	R	A	D	G	C	R	G	C	A	D	G	S	M	C	A	T	I	D	G	S	M	C	A	T	I	D	G	S	M	C	DL	A	D	S	M	C	A
+			+1												+1	+1			+1												–1	–1			–1				–1	

A, aneuploidy; C, chromosomal aberrations; D, DNA damage; DL, dominant lethal mutation; G, gene mutation; I, inhibition of intercellular communication; M, micronuclei; R, mitotic recombination and gene conversion; S, sister chromatid exchange; T, cell transformation

In completing the tables, the following symbols indicate the consensus of the Working Group with regard to the results for each end-point:

+ considered to be positive for the specific endpoint and level of biological complexity

+1 considered to be positive, but only one valid study was available to the Working Group

– considered to be negative

–1 considered to be negative, but only one valid study was available to the Working Group

? considered to be equivocal or inconclusive (e.g., there were contradictory results from different laboratories; there were confounding exposures; the results were equivocal)

Summary table of genetic and related effects of 2-amino-5-nitrophenol

Nonmammalian systems				Mammalian systems			
Proka-ryotes	Lower eukaryotes	Plants	Insects	In vitro		In vivo	
				Animal cells	Human cells	Animals	Humans
D G R	A D G C R	G C R A	G C A	D G S M C A T	D G S M C A T I	D G S M C DL A	D S M C A
+				+¹ +¹ +¹		–¹	

A, aneuploidy; C, chromosomal aberrations; D, DNA damage; DL, dominant lethal mutation; G, gene mutation; I, inhibition of intercellular communication; M, micronuclei; R, mitotic recombination and gene conversion; S, sister chromatid exchange; T, cell transformation

In completing the tables, the following symbols indicate the consensus of the Working Group with regard to the results for each end-point:

+   considered to be positive for the specific endpoint and level of biological complexity

+¹   considered to be positive, but only one valid study was available to the Working Group

–   considered to be negative

–¹   considered to be negative, but only one valid study was available to the Working Group

?   considered to be equivocal or inconclusive (e.g., there were contradictory results from different laboratories; there were confounding exposures; the results were equivocal)

Summary table of genetic and related effects of 1,4-diamino-2-nitrobenzene

Nonmammalian systems											Mammalian systems																										
Proka-ryotes		Lower eukaryotes			Plants			Insects			In vitro																In vivo											
											Animal cells									Human cells							Animals							Humans				
D	G	D	G	R	A	D	G	C	R	G	A	D	G	S	M	C	A	T	I	D	G	S	M	C	A	T	I	D	G	S	M	C	DL	A	D	S	M	C	A
+		–¹	–¹								?	+	+¹	+	+	+					+¹							–¹	–	–								

A, aneuploidy; C, chromosomal aberrations; D, DNA damage; DL, dominant lethal mutation; G, gene mutation; I, inhibition of intercellular communication; M, micronuclei; R, mitotic recombination and gene conversion; S, sister chromatid exchange; T, cell transformation

In completing the tables, the following symbols indicate the consensus of the Working Group with regard to the results for each end-point:

+   considered to be positive for the specific endpoint and level of biological complexity

+¹ considered to be positive, but only one valid study was available to the Working Group

–   considered to be negative

–¹ considered to be negative, but only one valid study was available to the Working Group

?   considered to be equivocal or inconclusive (e.g. there were contradictory results from different laboratories; there were confounding exposures; the results were equivocal)

Summary table of genetic and related effects of D&C Red No. 9

Column groups — Nonmammalian systems: Prokaryotes, Lower eukaryotes, Plants, Insects. Mammalian systems: In vitro (Animal cells, Human cells); In vivo (Animals, Humans).

Prokaryotes		Lower eukaryotes			Plants			Insects			Animal cells (in vitro)								Human cells (in vitro)								Animals (in vivo)							Humans (in vivo)				
D	G	D	R	G	A	D	G	C	R	G	D	G	S	M	C	A	T	I	D	G	S	M	C	A	T	I	D	G	S	M	C	DL	A	D	S	M	C	A
–											–¹	–¹	–¹						–¹								–	–¹										

A, aneuploidy; C, chromosomal aberrations; D, DNA damage; DL, dominant lethal mutation; G, gene mutation; I, inhibition of intercellular communication; M, micronuclei; R, mitotic recombination and gene conversion; S, sister chromatid exchange; T, cell transformation

In completing the tables, the following symbols indicate the consensus of the Working Group with regard to the results for each end-point:

+ considered to be positive for the specific endpoint and level of biological complexity

+¹ considered to be positive, but only one valid study was available to the Working Group

– considered to be negative

–¹ considered to be negative, but only one valid study was available to the Working Group

? considered to be equivocal or inconclusive (e.g., there were contradictory results from different laboratories; there were confounding exposures; the results were equivocal)

Summary table of genetic and related effects of CI Basic Red 9

Nonmammalian systems													Mammalian systems																											
Prokaryotes		Lower eukaryotes				Plants		Insects					In vitro[a]																In vivo[b]												
													Animal cells								Human cells								Animals							Humans					
D	G	D	R	G	A	D	G	C	R	G	C	A	D	G	S	M	C	A	T	I	D	G	S	M	C	A	T	I	D	G	S	M	C	DL	A	D	S	M	C	A
+	?				-¹								+		-¹	-¹			+											-						-¹					

A, aneuploidy; C, chromosomal aberrations; D, DNA damage; DL, dominant lethal mutation; G, gene mutation; I, inhibition of intercellular communication; M, micronuclei; R, mitotic recombination and gene conversion; S, sister chromatid exchange; T, cell transformation

In completing the table, the following symbols indicate the consensus of the Working Group with regard to the results for each end-point:

+   considered to be positive for the specific endpoint and level of biological complexity

+¹ considered to be positive, but only one valid study was available to the Working Group

−   considered to be negative

−¹ considered to be negative, but only one valid study was available to the Working Group

?   considered to be equivocal or inconclusive (e.g., there were contradictory results from different laboratories; there were confounding exposures; the results were equivocal)

[a] Mutagenic in a body fluid assay

[b] Host-mediated assays in mouse

Summary table of genetic and related effects of CI Direct Blue 15

Nonmammalian systems											Mammalian systems																													
Proka-ryotes	Lower eukaryotes			Plants				Insects			In vitro																In vivo															
											Animal cells						Human cells									Animals										Humans					
D	G	D	R	A	D	G	C	R	G	C	A	D	G	S	M	C	A	T	I	D	G	S	M	C		A	T	I	D	G	S	M	C	DL	A	D	S	M	C	A
+a														−1								−1																			

A, aneuploidy; C, chromosomal aberrations; D, DNA damage; DL, dominant lethal mutation; G, gene mutation; I, inhibition of intercellular communication; M, micronuclei; R, mitotic recombination and gene conversion; S, sister chromatid exchange; T, cell transformation

In completing the tables, the following symbols indicate the consensus of the Working Group with regard to the results for each end-point:

+   considered to be positive for the specific endpoint and level of biological complexity

+1 considered to be positive, but only one valid study was available to the Working Group

−   considered to be negative

−1 considered to be negative, but only one valid study was available to the Working Group

?   considered to be equivocal or inconclusive (e.g., there were contradictory results from different laboratories; there were confounding exposures; the results were equivocal)

a Positive with reduction, negative without

Summary table of genetic and related effects of CI Acid Red 114

Nonmammalian systems												Mammalian systems																										
Proka-ryotes	Lower eukaryotes			Plants				Insects				In vitro															In vivo											
												Animal cells								Human cells							Animals							Humans				
D	D	G	R	A	D	G	C	R	G	C	A	D	G	S	M	C	A	T	I	D	G	S	M	C	A	T	D	G	S	M	C	DL	A	D	S	M	C	A
+ᵃ					−									−¹								−¹																

A, aneuploidy; C, chromosomal aberrations; D, DNA damage; DL, dominant lethal mutation; G, gene mutation; I, inhibition of intercellular communication; M, micronuclei; R, mitotic recombination and gene conversion; S, sister chromatid exchange; T, cell transformation

In completing the tables, the following symbols indicate the consensus of the Working Group with regard to the results for each end-point:

+   considered to be positive for the specific endpoint and level of biological complexity

+¹   considered to be positive, but only one valid study was available to the Working Group

−   considered to be negative

−¹   considered to be negative, but only one valid study was available to the Working Group

?   considered to be equivocal or inconclusive (e.g. there were contradictory results from different laboratories; there were confounding exposures; the results were equivocal)

ᵃ Positive with reduction, negative without

Summary table of genetic and related effects of CI Pigment Red No. 3

Nonmammalian systems													Mammalian systems																						
Proka-ryotes		Lower eukaryotes				Plants				Insects			In vitro														In vivo								
													Animal cells							Human cells								Animals							Humans				
D	G	D	R	G	A	D	G	C	R	G	C	A	D	G	S	M	C	A	T	D	G	S	M	C	A	T	I	D	G	S	M	C	DL	A	D	S	M	C	A
–																																							

A, aneuploidy; C, chromosomal aberrations; D, DNA damage; DL, dominant lethal mutation; G, gene mutation; I, inhibition of intercellular communication; M, micronuclei; R, mitotic recombination and gene conversion; S, sister chromatid exchange; T, cell transformation

In completing the tables, the following symbols indicate the consensus of the Working Group with regard to the results for each end-point:

+   considered to be positive for the specific endpoint and level of biological complexity

$+^1$ considered to be positive, but only one valid study was available to the Working Group

–   considered to be negative

$-^1$ considered to be negative, but only one valid study was available to the Working Group

?   considered to be equivocal or inconclusive (e.g., there were contradictory results from different laboratories; there were confounding exposures; the results were equivocal)

Summary table of genetic and related effects of 4,4'-methylene bis(2-chloroaniline) (MOCA)

Nonmammalian systems												Mammalian systems																							
Proka-ryotes		Lower eukaryotes			Plants			Insects			In vitro															In vivo										
											Animal cells							Human cells							Animals							Humans			
D	G	D	R	G	A	D	G	C	R	G	D	G	S	M	C	A	T	I	D	G	S	M	C	A	T	I	D	G	S	M	C	DL	A	D	S	M	C	A
+	+	?	⁻¹	+¹						+	+	+	+¹		⁻¹		+	+¹			+¹	+¹					+			+¹	+¹				+¹	+¹		

A, aneuploidy; C, chromosomal aberrations; D, DNA damage; DL, dominant lethal mutation; G, gene mutation; I, inhibition of intercellular communication; M, micronuclei; R, mitotic recombination and gene conversion; S, sister chromatid exchange; T, cell transformation

In completing the tables, the following symbols indicate the consensus of the Working Group with regard to the results for each end-point:

+   considered to be positive for the specific endpoint and level of biological complexity

+¹   considered to be positive, but only one valid study was available to the Working Group

⁻   considered to be negative

⁻¹   considered to be negative, but only one valid study was available to the Working Group

?   considered to be equivocal or inconclusive (e.g., there were contradictory results from different laboratories; there were confounding exposures; the results were equivocal)

Summary table of genetic and related effects of *para*-chloroaniline

Nonmammalian systems											Mammalian systems																										
Prokaryotes			Lower eukaryotes			Plants			Insects		In vitro																In vivo											
											Animal cells							Human cells								Animals							Humans				
D	G	R	A	D	G	C	R	G	C	A	D	G	S	M	C	A	T	D	G	S	M	C	A	T	I	D	G	S	M	C	DL	A	D	S	M	C	A
+¹	?			–¹	+¹								+					?		+					+¹							+¹					

A, aneuploidy; C, chromosomal aberrations; D, DNA damage; DL, dominant lethal mutation; G, gene mutation; I, inhibition of intercellular communication; M, micronuclei; R, mitotic recombination and gene conversion; S, sister chromatid exchange; T, cell transformation

In completing the tables, the following symbols indicate the consensus of the Working Group with regard to the results for each end-point:

+ considered to be positive for the specific endpoint and level of biological complexity
+¹ considered to be positive, but only one valid study was available to the Working Group
– considered to be negative
–¹ considered to be negative, but only one valid study was available to the Working Group
? considered to be equivocal or inconclusive (e.g. there were contradictory results from different laboratories; there were confounding exposures; the results were equivocal)

Summary table of genetic and related effects of 2,6-dimethylaniline

Nonmammalian systems											Mammalian systems																										
Proka-ryotes		Lower eukaryotes				Plants				Insects			In vitro															In vivo										
													Animal cells								Human cells							Animals							Humans				
D	G	A	D	G	R	G	C	R		G	C	A	D	G	S	M	C	A	T	I	D	G	S	M	C	A	T	D	G	S	M	C	DL	A	D	S	M	C	A
	?														+I									+I						+I									-

A, aneuploidy; C, chromosomal aberrations; D, DNA damage; DL, dominant lethal mutation; G, gene mutation; I, inhibition of intercellular communication; M, micronuclei; R, mitotic recombination and gene conversion; S, sister chromatid exchange; T, cell transformation

In completing the tables, the following symbols indicate the consensus of the Working Group with regard to the results for each end-point:

+   considered to be positive for the specific endpoint and level of biological complexity

+I   considered to be positive, but only one valid study was available to the Working Group

–   considered to be negative

–I   considered to be negative, but only one valid study was available to the Working Group

?   considered to be equivocal or inconclusive (e.g., there were confounding exposures; the results were contradictory results from different laboratories; there were confounding exposures; the results were equivocal)

Summary table of genetic and related effects of N,N-dimethylaniline

Nonmammalian systems													Mammalian systems																									
Proka-ryotes			Lower eukaryotes			Plants				Insects				In vitro													In vivo												
													Animal cells								Human cells						Animals									Humans				
D	G	R	D	G	A	D	G	C	R	G	C	A	D	G	S	M	C	A	T	I	D	G	S	M	C	A	D	G	S	M	C	DL	A	D	S	M	C	A
–														+¹	+¹		+¹						–¹															

A, aneuploidy; C, chromosomal aberrations; D, DNA damage; DL, dominant lethal mutation; G, gene mutation; I, inhibition of intercellular communication; M, micronuclei; R, mitotic recombination and gene conversion; S, sister chromatid exchange; T, cell transformation

In completing the tables, the following symbols indicate the consensus of the Working Group with regard to the results for each end-point:

+   considered to be positive for the specific endpoint and level of biological complexity
+¹   considered to be positive, but only one valid study was available to the Working Group
–   considered to be negative
–¹   considered to be negative, but only one valid study was available to the Working Group
?   considered to be equivocal or inconclusive (e.g., there were contradictory results from different laboratories; there were confounding exposures; the results were equivocal)

APPENDIX 2

ACTIVITY PROFILES FOR
GENETIC AND RELATED EFFECTS

APPENDIX 2

ACTIVITY PROFILES FOR
GENETIC AND RELATED EFFECTS

Methods

The x-axis of the activity profile (Waters *et al.*, 1987, 1988) represents the bioassays in phylogenetic sequence by endpoint, and the values on the y-axis represent the logarithmically transformed lowest effective doses (LED) and highest ineffective doses (HID) tested. The term 'dose', as used in this report, does not take into consideration length of treatment or exposure and may therefore be considered synonymous with concentration. In practice, the concentrations used in all the in-vitro tests were converted to µg/ml, and those for in-vivo tests were expressed as mg/kg bw. Because dose units are plotted on a log scale, differences in molecular weights of compounds do not, in most cases, greatly influence comparisons of their activity profiles. Conventions for dose conversions are given below.

Profile-line height (the magnitude of each bar) is a function of the LED or HID, which is associated with the characteristics of each individual test system—such as population size, cell-cycle kinetics and metabolic competence. Thus, the detection limit of each test system is different, and, across a given activity profile, responses will vary substantially. No attempt is made to adjust or relate responses in one test system to those of another.

Line heights are derived as follows: for negative test results, the highest dose tested without appreciable toxicity is defined as the HID. If there was evidence of extreme toxicity, the next highest dose is used. A single dose tested with a negative result is considered to be equivalent to the HID. Similarly, for positive results, the LED is recorded. If the original data were analysed statistically by the author, the dose recorded is that at which the response was significant ($p < 0.05$). If the available data were not analysed statistically, the dose required to produce an effect is estimated as follows: when a dose-related positive response is observed with two or more doses, the lower of the doses is taken as the LED; a single dose resulting in a positive response is considered to be equivalent to the LED.

In order to accommodate both the wide range of doses encountered and positive and negative responses on a continuous scale, doses are transformed logarithmically, so that effective (LED) and ineffective (HID) doses are represented by positive and negative numbers, respectively. The response, or logarithmic dose unit (LDU_{ij}), for a given test system i and chemical j is represented by the expressions

$LDU_{ij} = -\log_{10}$ (dose), for HID values; $LDU \leq 0$

and   (1)

$LDU_{ij} = -\log_{10}$ (dose $\times$ 10^{-5}), for LED values; $LDU \geq 0$.

These simple relationships define a dose range of 0 to –5 logarithmic units for ineffective doses (1–100 000 µg/ml or mg/kg bw) and 0 to +8 logarithmic units for effective doses (100 000–0.001 µg/ml or mg/kg bw). A scale illustrating the LDU values is shown in Figure 1. Negative responses at doses less than 1 µg/ml (mg/kg bw) are set equal to 1. Effectively, an LED value $\geq$100 000 or an HID value $\leq$1 produces an LDU = 0; no quantitative information is gained from such extreme values. The dotted lines at the levels of log dose units 1 and –1 define a 'zone of uncertainty' in which positive results are reported at such high doses (between 10 000 and 100 000 µg/ml or mg/kg bw) or negative results are reported at such low dose levels (1 to 10 µg/ml or mg/kg bw) as to call into question the adequacy of the test.

Fig. 1. Scale of log dose units used on the y-axis of activity profiles

Positive (µg/ml or mg/kg bw)		Log dose units	
0.001	....	8	——
0.01	....	7	—
0.1	....	6	—
1.0	....	5	—
10	....	4	—
100	....	3	—
1000	....	2	—
10 000	....	1	—
100 000	.... 1	0	——
	.... 10	–1	—
	.... 100	–2	—
	.... 1000	–3	—
	.... 10 000	–4	—
	.... 100 000	–5	——

Negative
(µg/ml or mg/kg bw)

LED and HID are expressed as µg/ml or mg/kg bw.

In practice, an activity profile is computer generated. A data entry programme is used to store abstracted data from published reports. A sequential file (in ASCII) is created for each compound, and a record within that file consists of the name and Chemical Abstracts Service number of the compound, a three-letter code for the test system (see below), the qualitative test result (with and without an exogenous metabolic system), dose (LED or HID), citation number and additional source information. An abbreviated citation for each publication is stored in a segment of a record accessing both the test data file and the citation file. During processing of the data file, an average of the logarithmic values of the data subset is calculated, and the length of the profile line represents this average value. All dose values are plotted for each profile line, regardless of whether results are positive or negative. Results obtained in the absence of an exogenous metabolic system are indicated by a bar (–), and results obtained in the presence of an exogenous metabolic system are indicated by an upward-directed arrow (↑). When all results for a given assay are either positive or negative, the mean of the LDU values is plotted as a solid line; when conflicting data are reported for the same assay (i.e., both positive and negative results), the majority data are shown by a solid line and the minority data by a dashed line (drawn to the extreme conflicting response). In the few cases in which the numbers of positive and negative results are equal, the solid line is drawn in the positive direction and the maximal negative response is indicated with a dashed line.

Profile lines are identified by three-letter code words representing the commonly used tests. Code words for most of the test systems in current use in genetic toxicology were defined for the US Environmental Protection Agency's GENE-TOX Program (Waters, 1979; Waters & Auletta, 1981). For *IARC Monographs* Supplement 6, Volume 44 and subsequent volumes, including this publication, codes were redefined in a manner that should facilitate inclusion of additional tests. Naming conventions are described below.

Data listings are presented in the text and include endpoint and test codes, a short test code definition, results [either with (M) or without (NM) an exogenous activation system], the associated LED or HID value and a short citation. Test codes are organized phylogenetically and by endpoint from left to right across each activity profile and from top to bottom of the corresponding data listing. Endpoints are defined as follows: A, aneuploidy; C, chromosomal aberrations; D, DNA damage; F, assays of body fluids; G, gene mutation; H, host-mediated assays; I, inhibition of intercellular communication; M, micronuclei; P, sperm morphology; R, mitotic recombination or gene conversion; S, sister chromatid exchange; and T, cell transformation.

Dose conversions for activity profiles

Doses are converted to µg/ml for in-vitro tests and to mg/kg bw per day for in-vivo experiments.

1. In-vitro test systems

   (a) Weight/volume converts directly to µg/ml.

   (b) Molar (M) concentration × molecular weight = mg/ml = 10^3 µg/ml; mM concentration × molecular weight = µg/ml.

   (c) Soluble solids expressed as % concentration are assumed to be in units of mass per volume (i.e., 1% = 0.01 g/ml = 10 000 µg/ml; also, 1 ppm = 1 µg/ml).

   (d) Liquids and gases expressed as % concentration are assumed to be given in units of volume per volume. Liquids are converted to weight per volume using the density (D) of the solution (D = g/ml). Gases are converted from volume to mass using the ideal gas law, PV = nRT. For exposure at 20–37°C at standard atmospheric pressure, 1% (v/v) = 0.4 µg/ml × molecular weight of the gas. Also, 1 ppm (v/v) = 4×10^{-5} µg/ml × molecular weight.

(e) In microbial plate tests, it is usual for the doses to be reported as weight/plate, whereas concentrations are required to enter data on the activity profile chart. While remaining cognisant of the errors involved in the process, it is assumed that a 2-ml volume of top agar is delivered to each plate and that the test substance remains in solution within it; concentrations are derived from the reported weight/-plate values by dividing by this arbitrary volume. For spot tests, a 1-ml volume is used in the calculation.

(f) Conversion of particulate concentrations given in $\mu g/cm^2$ are based on the area (A) of the dish and the volume of medium per dish; i.e., for a 100-mm dish: $A = \pi R^2 = \pi \times (5\ cm)^2 = 78.5\ cm^2$. If the volume of medium is 10 ml, then $78.5\ cm^2 = 10$ ml and $1\ cm^2 = 0.13$ ml.

2.   In-vitro systems using in-vivo activation

For the body fluid–urine (BF–) test, the concentration used is the dose (in mg/kg bw) of the compound administered to test animals or patients.

3.   In-vivo test systems

(a) Doses are converted to mg/kg bw per day of exposure, assuming 100% absorption. Standard values are used for each sex and species of rodent, including body weight and average intake per day, as reported by Gold et al. (1984). For example, in a test using male mice fed 50 ppm of the agent in the diet, the standard food intake per day is 12% of body weight, and the conversion is dose $= 50\ ppm \times 12\% = 6$ mg/kg bw per day.

Standard values used for humans are: weight—males, 70 kg; females, 55 kg; surface area, 1.7 m^2; inhalation rate, 20 l/min for light work, 30 l/min for mild exercise.

(b) When reported, the dose at the target site is used. For example, doses given in studies of lymphocytes of humans exposed in vivo are the measured blood concentrations in $\mu g/ml$.

Codes for test systems

For specific nonmammalian test systems, the first two letters of the three-symbol code word define the test organism (e.g., SA– for Salmonella typhimurium, EC– for Escherichia coli). If the species is not known, the convention used is –S–. The third symbol may be used to define the tester strain (e.g., SA8 for S. typhimurium TA1538, ECW for E. coli WP2uvrA). When strain designation is not indicated, the third letter is used to define the specific genetic endpoint under investigation (e.g., ––D for differential toxicity, ––F for forward mutation, ––G for gene conversion or genetic crossing-over, ––N for aneuploidy, ––R for reverse mutation, ––U for unscheduled DNA synthesis). The third letter may also be used to define the general endpoint under investigation when a more complete definition is not possible or relevant (e.g., ––M for mutation, ––C for chromosomal aberration).

For mammalian test systems, the first letter of the three–letter code word defines the genetic endpoint under investigation: A–– for aneuploidy, B–– for binding, C–– for chromosomal aberration, D–– for DNA strand breaks, G–– for gene mutation, I–– for inhibition of intercellular communication, M–– for micronucleus formation, R–– for DNA repair, S–– for sister chromatid exchange, T–– for cell transformation and U–– for unscheduled DNA synthesis.

For animal (i.e., non-human) test systems *in vitro*, when the cell type is not specified, the code letters –IA are used. For such assays *in vivo*, when the animal species is not specified, the code letters –VA are used. Commonly used animal species are identified by the third letter (e.g., ––C for Chinese hamster, ––M for mouse, ––R for rat, ––S for Syrian hamster).

For test systems using human cells *in vitro*, when the cell type is not specified, the code letters –IH are used. For assays on humans *in vivo*, when the cell type is not specified, the code letters –VH are used. Otherwise, the second letter specifies the cell type under investigation (e.g., –BH for bone marrow, –LH for lymphocytes).

Some other specific coding conventions used for mammalian systems are as follows: BF– for body fluids, HM– for host-mediated, ––L for leukocytes or lymphocytes *in vitro* (–AL, animals; –HL, humans), –L– for leukocytes *in vivo* (–LA, animals; –LH, humans), ––T for transformed cells.

Note that these are examples of major conventions used to define the assay code words. The alphabetized listing of codes must be examined to confirm a specific code word. As might be expected from the limitation to three symbols, some codes do not fit the naming conventions precisely. In a few cases, test systems are defined by first-letter code words, for example: MST, mouse spot test; SLP, mouse specific locus test, postspermatogonia; SLO, mouse specific locus test, other stages; DLM, dominant lethal test in mice; DLR, dominant lethal test in rats; MHT, mouse heritable translocation test.

The genetic activity profiles and listings were prepared in collaboration with Environmental Health Research and Testing Inc. (EHRT) under contract to the US Environmental Protection Agency; EHRT also determined the doses used. The references cited in each genetic activity profile listing can be found in the list of references in the appropriate monograph.

References

Garrett, N.E., Stack, H.F., Gross, M.R. & Waters, M.D. (1984) An analysis of the spectra of genetic activity produced by known or suspected human carcinogens. *Mutat. Res., 134*, 89–111

Gold, L.S., Sawyer, C.B., Magaw, R., Backman, G.M., de Veciana, M., Levinson, R., Hooper, N.K., Havender, W.R., Bernstein, L., Peto, R., Pike, M.C. & Ames, B.N. (1984) A carcinogenic potency database of the standardized results of animal bioassays. *Environ. Health Perspect., 58*, 9–319

Waters, M.D. (1979) *The GENE-TOX program*. In: Hsie, A.W., O'Neill, J.P. & McElheny, V.K., eds, *Mammalian Cell Mutagenesis: The Maturation of Test Systems* (Banbury Report 2), Cold Spring Harbor, NY, CSH Press, pp. 449–467

Waters, M.D. & Auletta, A. (1981) The GENE-TOX program: genetic activity evaluation. *J. chem. Inf. comput. Sci., 21*, 35–38

Waters, M.D., Stack, H.F., Brady, A.L., Lohman, P.H.M., Haroun, L. & Vainio, H. (1987) Appendix 1: Activity profiles for genetic and related tests. In: *IARC Monographs on the Evaluation of the Carcinogenic Risk of Chemicals to Humans*, Suppl. 6, *Genetic and Related Effects: An Updating of Selected* IARC Monographs *from Volumes 1 to 42*, Lyon, IARC, pp. 687–696

Waters, M.D., Stack, H.F., Brady, A.L., Lohman, P.H.M., Haroun, L. & Vainio, H. (1988) Use of computerized data listings and activity profiles of genetic and related effects in the review of 195 compounds. *Mutat. Res.*, *205*, 295–312

CI ACID ORANGE 3

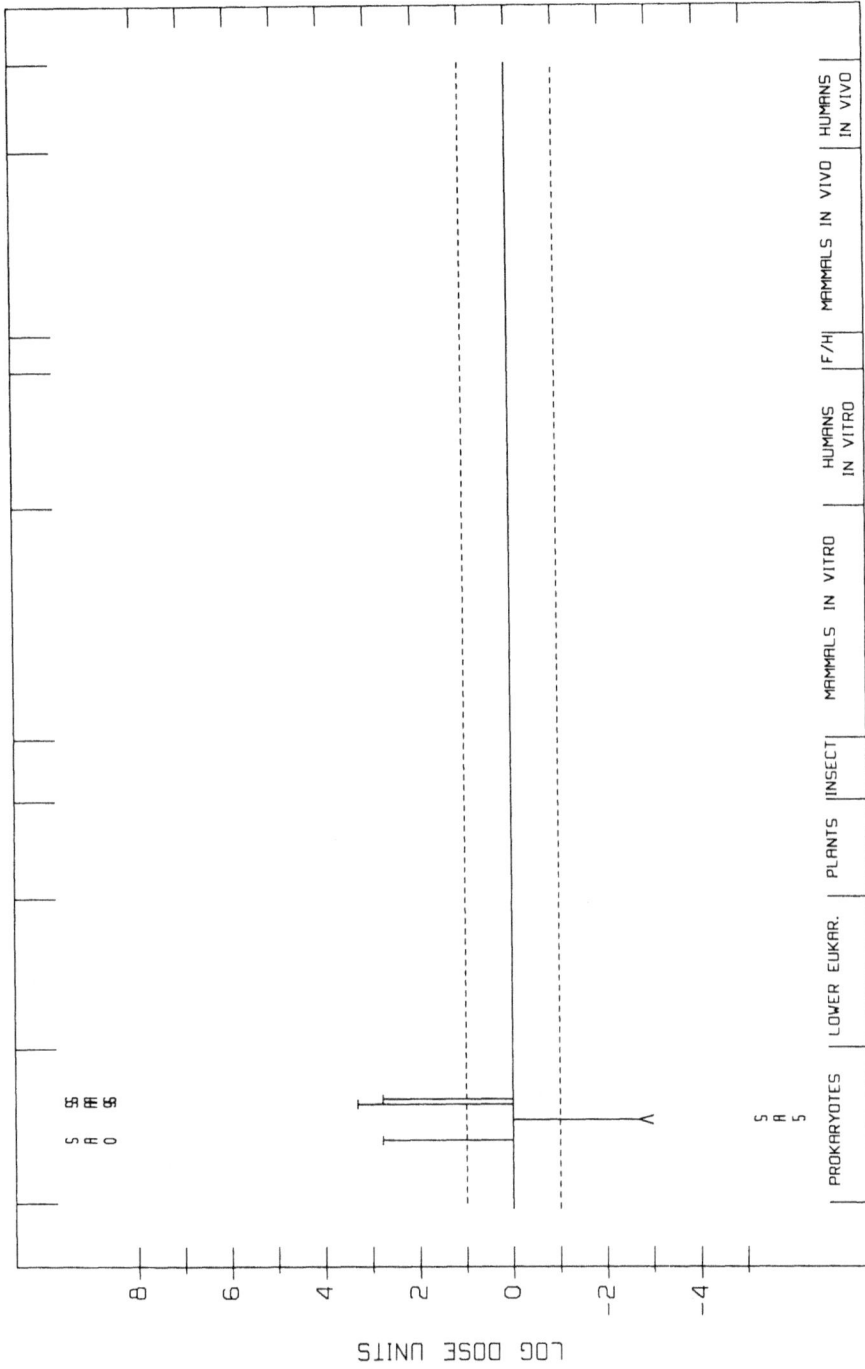

6373-74-6

PROKARYOTES | LOWER EUKAR. | PLANTS | INSECT | MAMMALS IN VITRO | HUMANS IN VITRO | F/H | MAMMALS IN VIVO | HUMANS IN VIVO

LOG DOSE UNITS

8 6 4 2 0 -2 -4

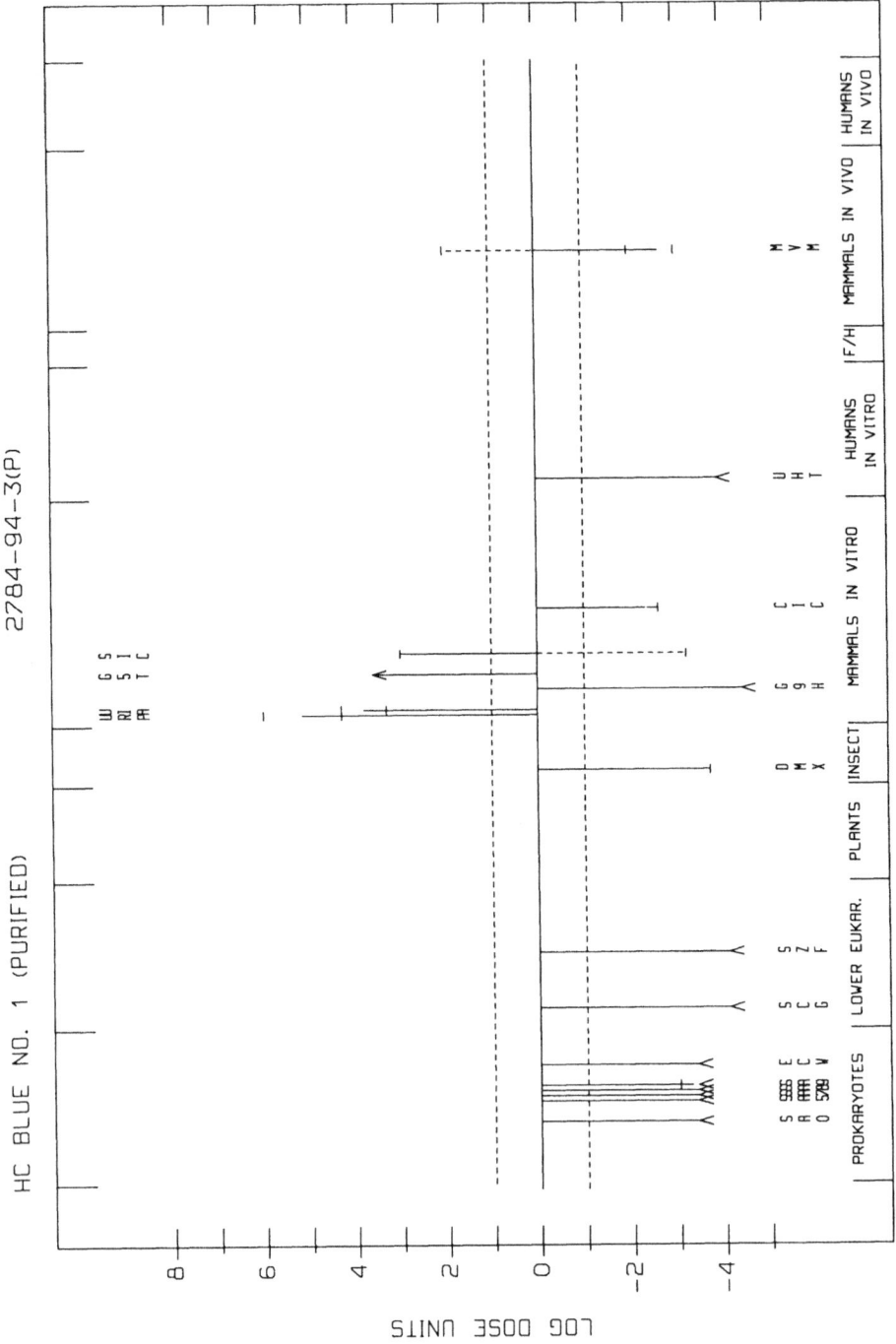

HC BLUE NO. 1 (PURIFIED)

2784-94-3(P)

LOG DOSE UNITS

PROKARYOTES | LOWER EUKAR. | PLANTS | INSECT | MAMMALS IN VITRO | HUMANS IN VITRO | F/H | MAMMALS IN VIVO | HUMANS IN VIVO

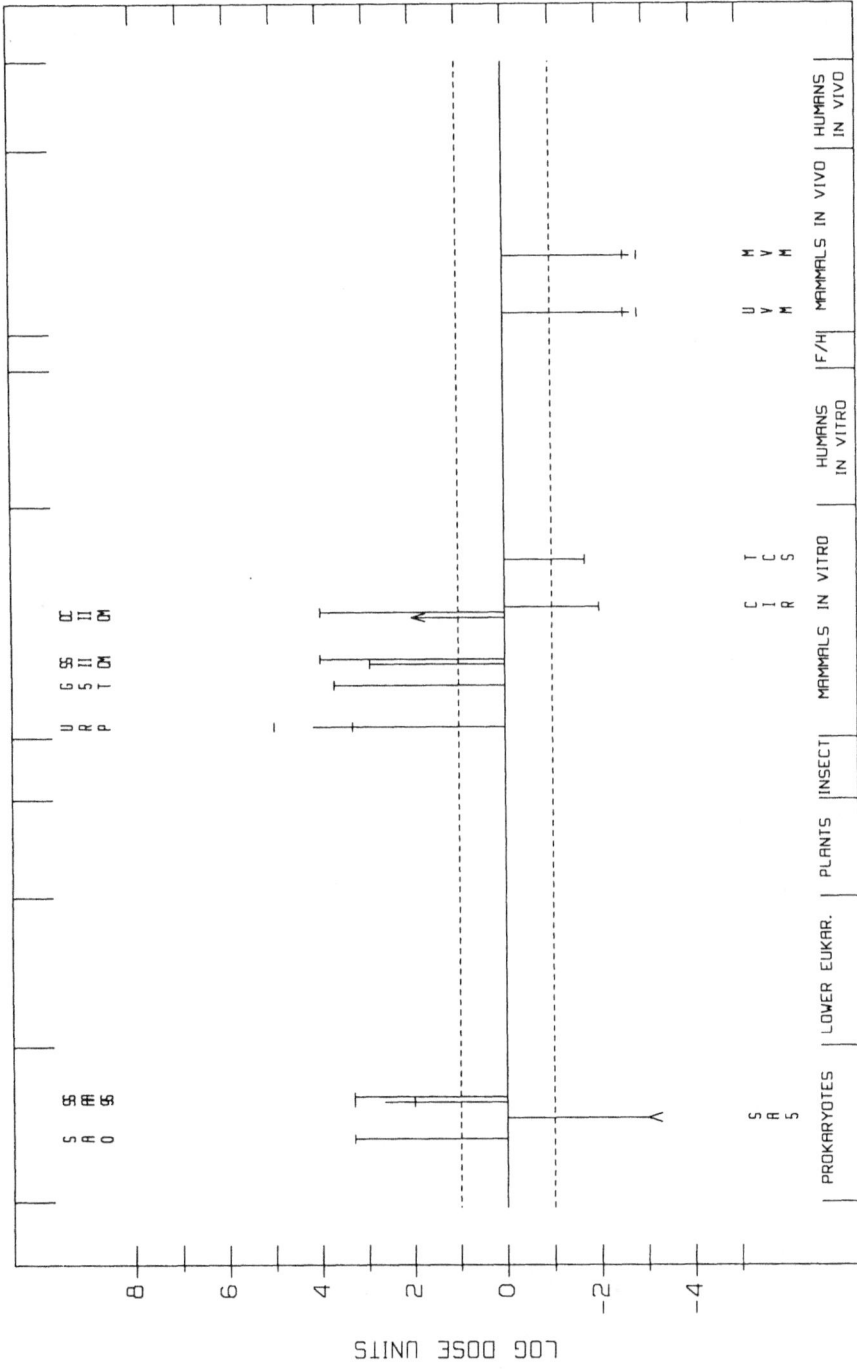

HC BLUE NO. 1 (COMMERCIAL)

2784-94-3(C)

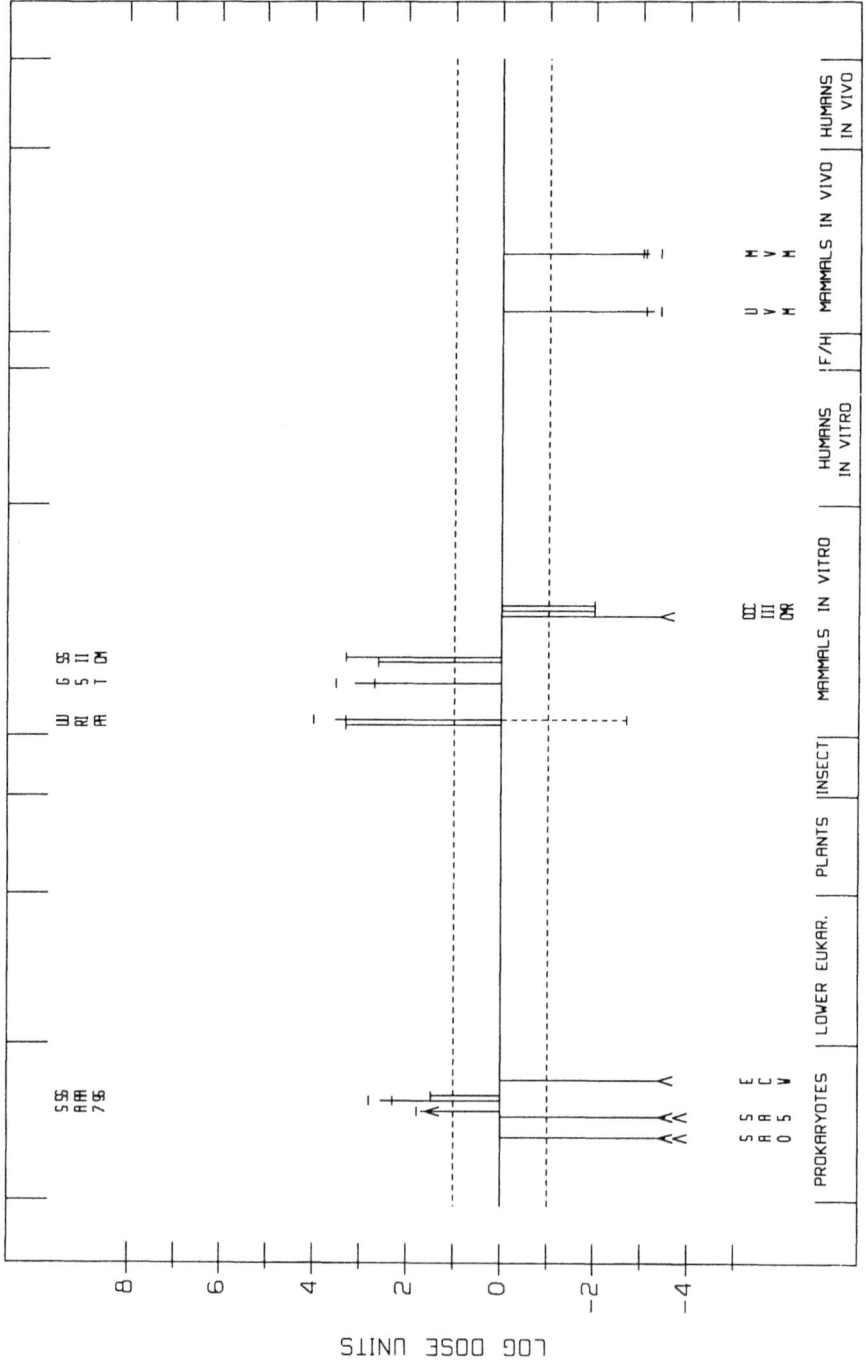

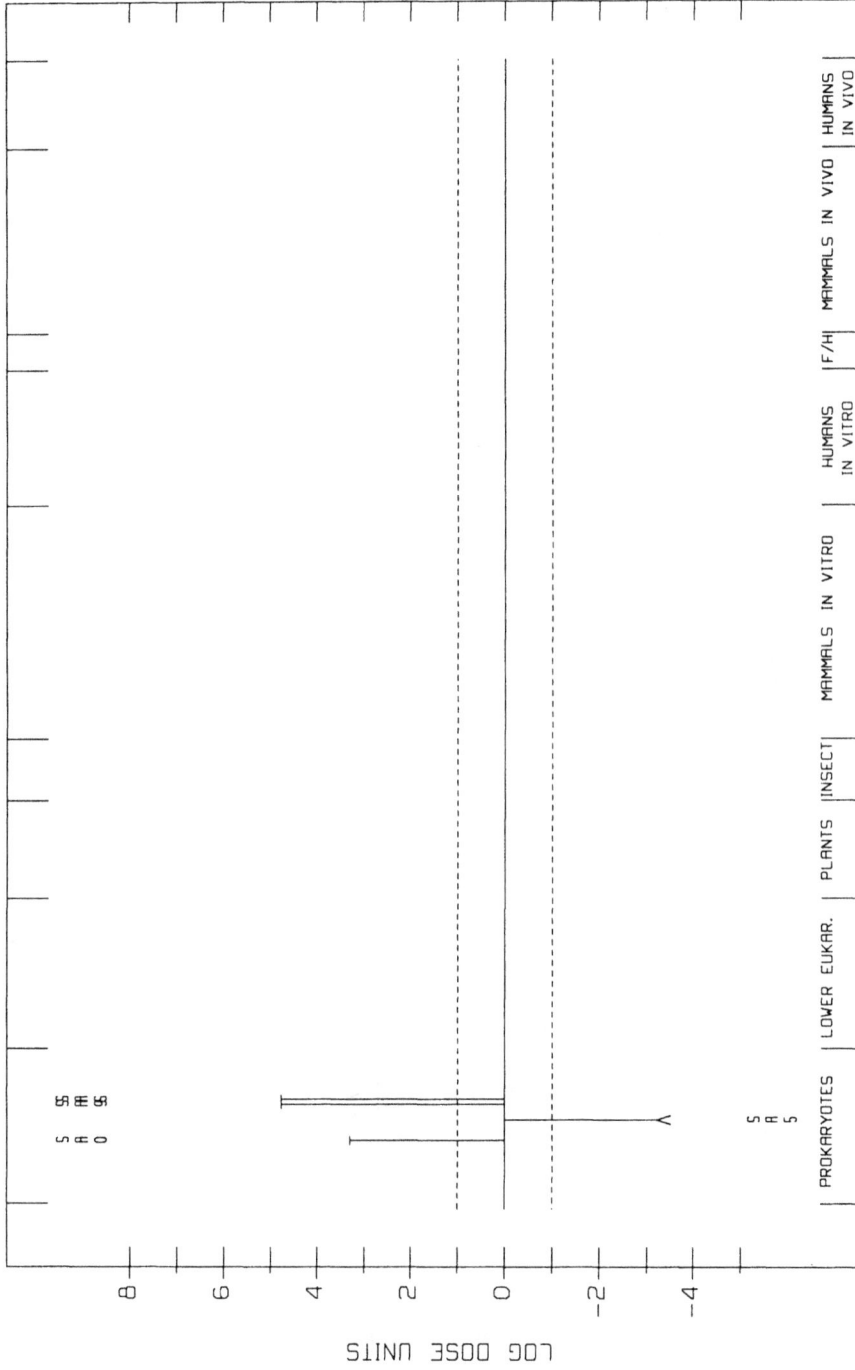

HC RED NO. 3

2871-01-4

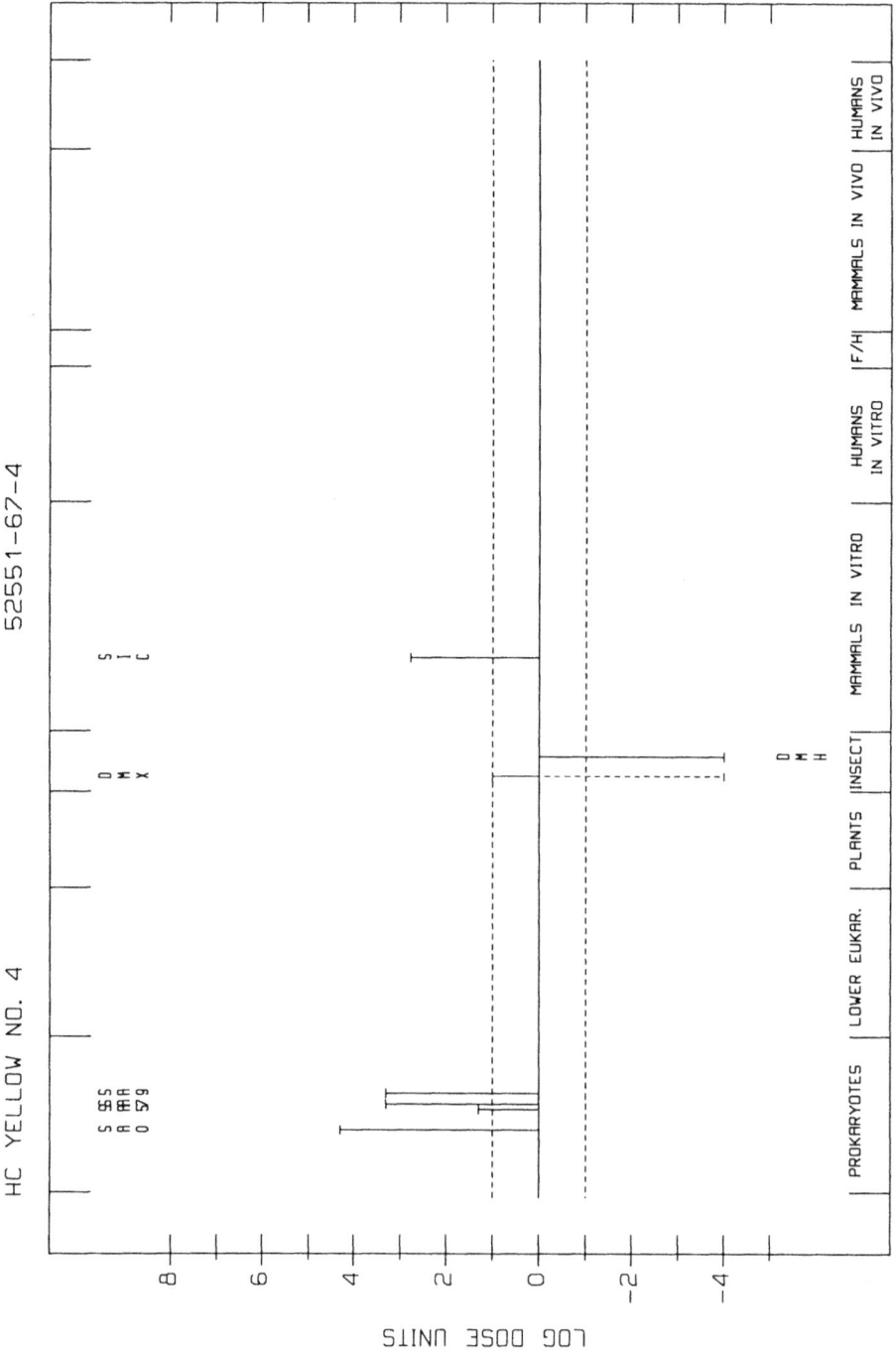

HC YELLOW NO. 4   52551-67-4

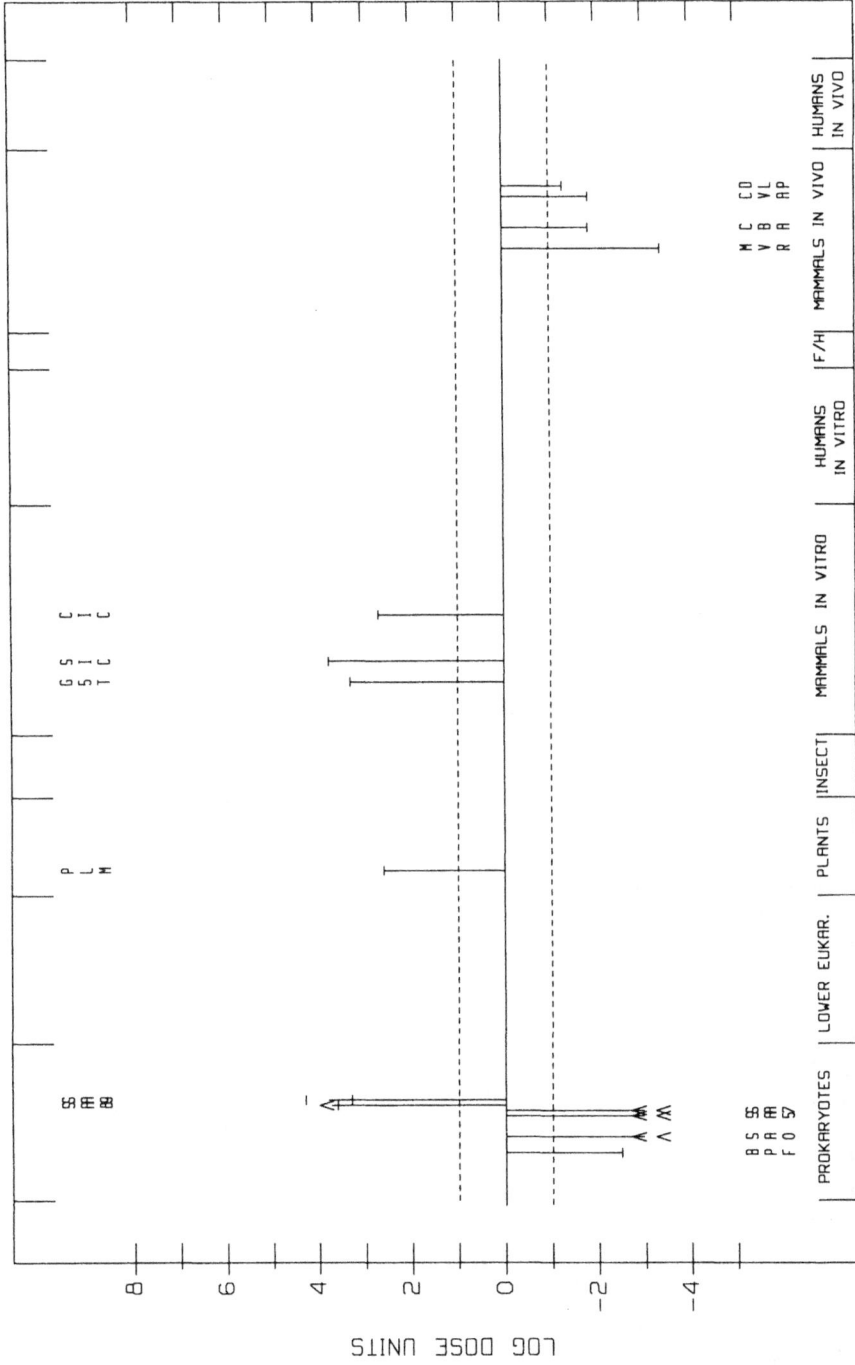

AMINO-4-NITROPHENOL, 2- 99-57-0

AMINO-5-NITROPHENOL, 2-   121-88-0

LOG DOSE UNITS

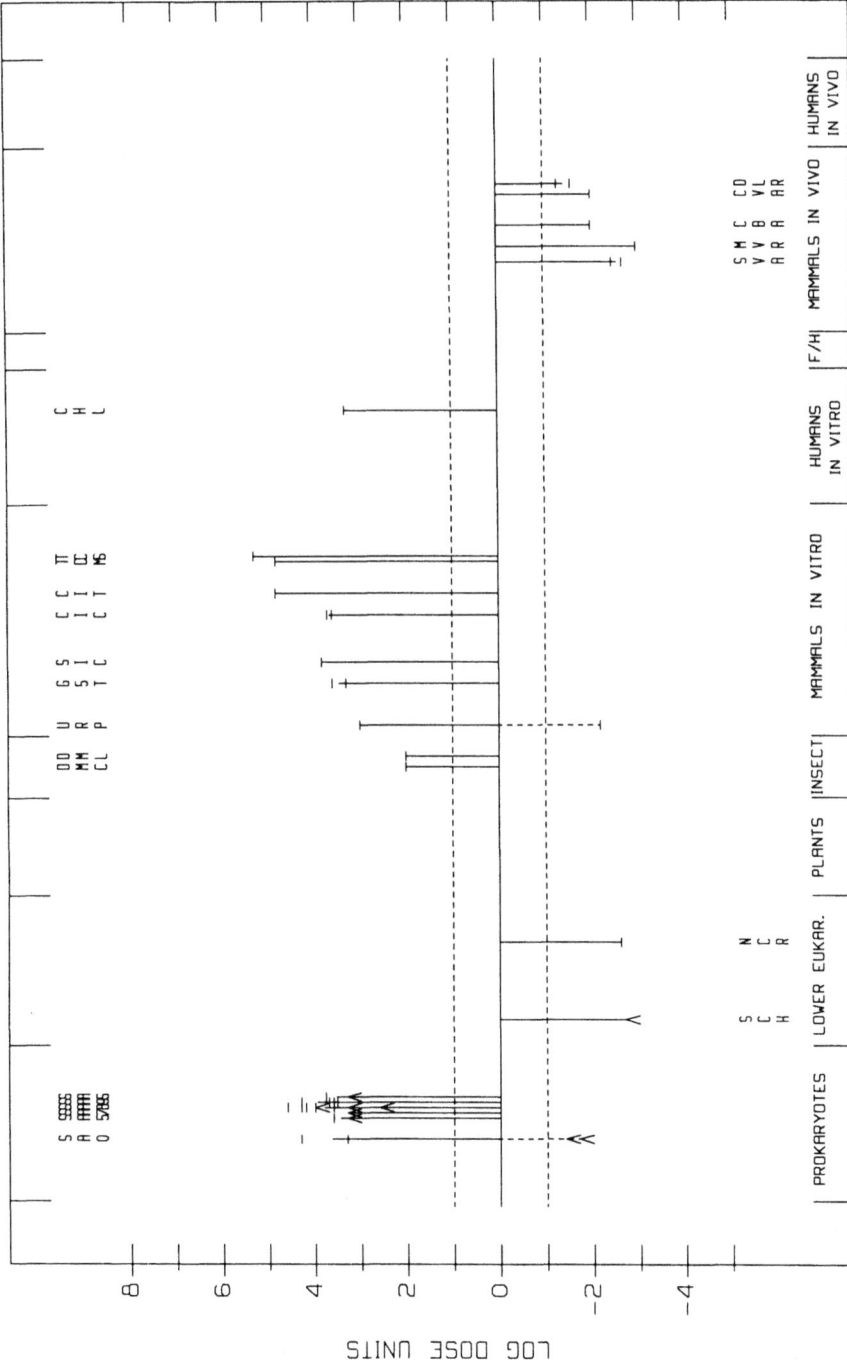

DIAMINO-2-NITROBENZENE, 1,4-   5307-14-2

LOG DOSE UNITS

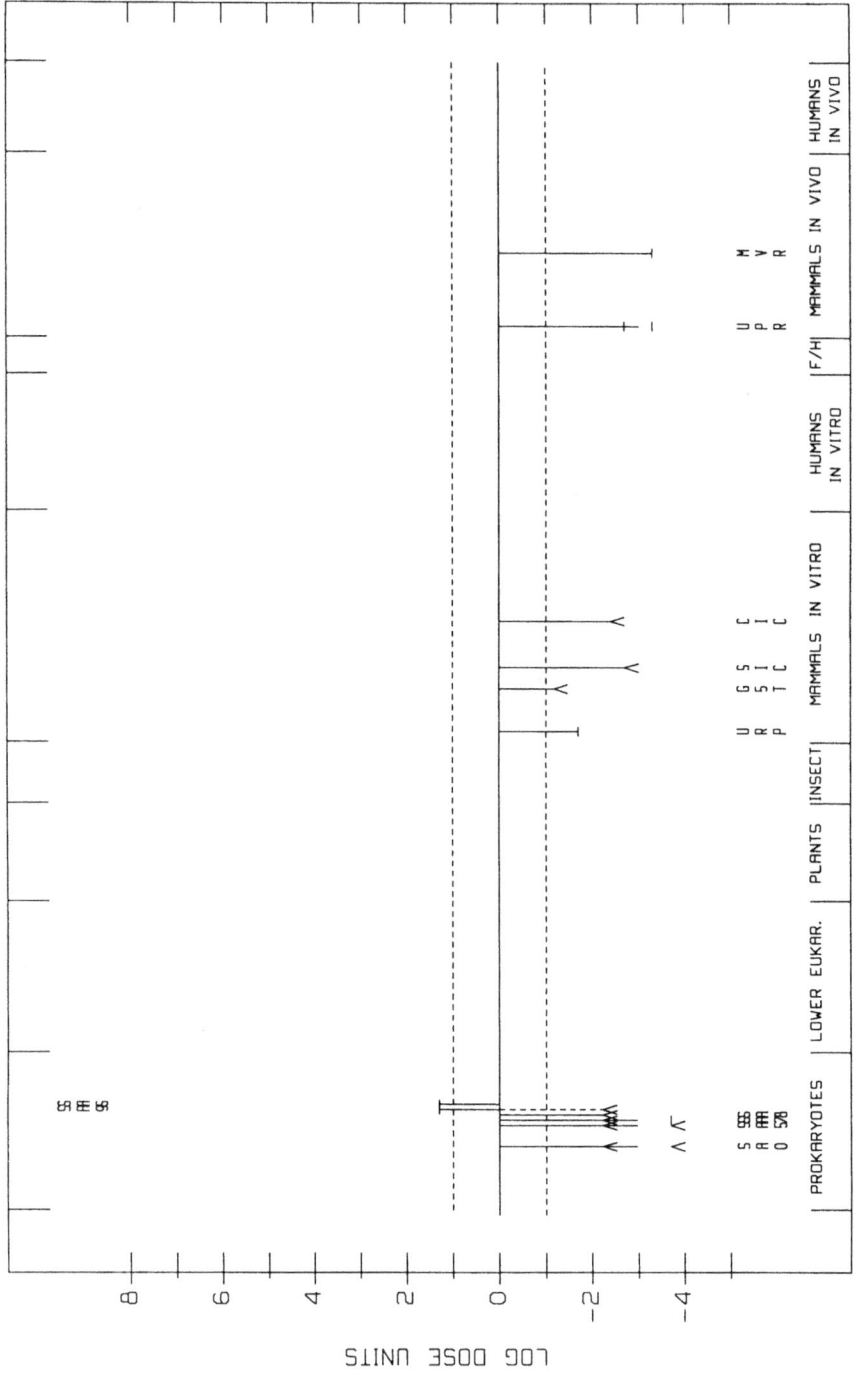

D & C RED NO. 9

5160-02-1

LOG DOSE UNITS

8 6 4 2 0 -2 -4

PROKARYOTES | LOWER EUKAR. | PLANTS | INSECT | MAMMALS IN VITRO | HUMANS IN VITRO | F/H | MAMMALS IN VIVO | HUMANS IN VIVO

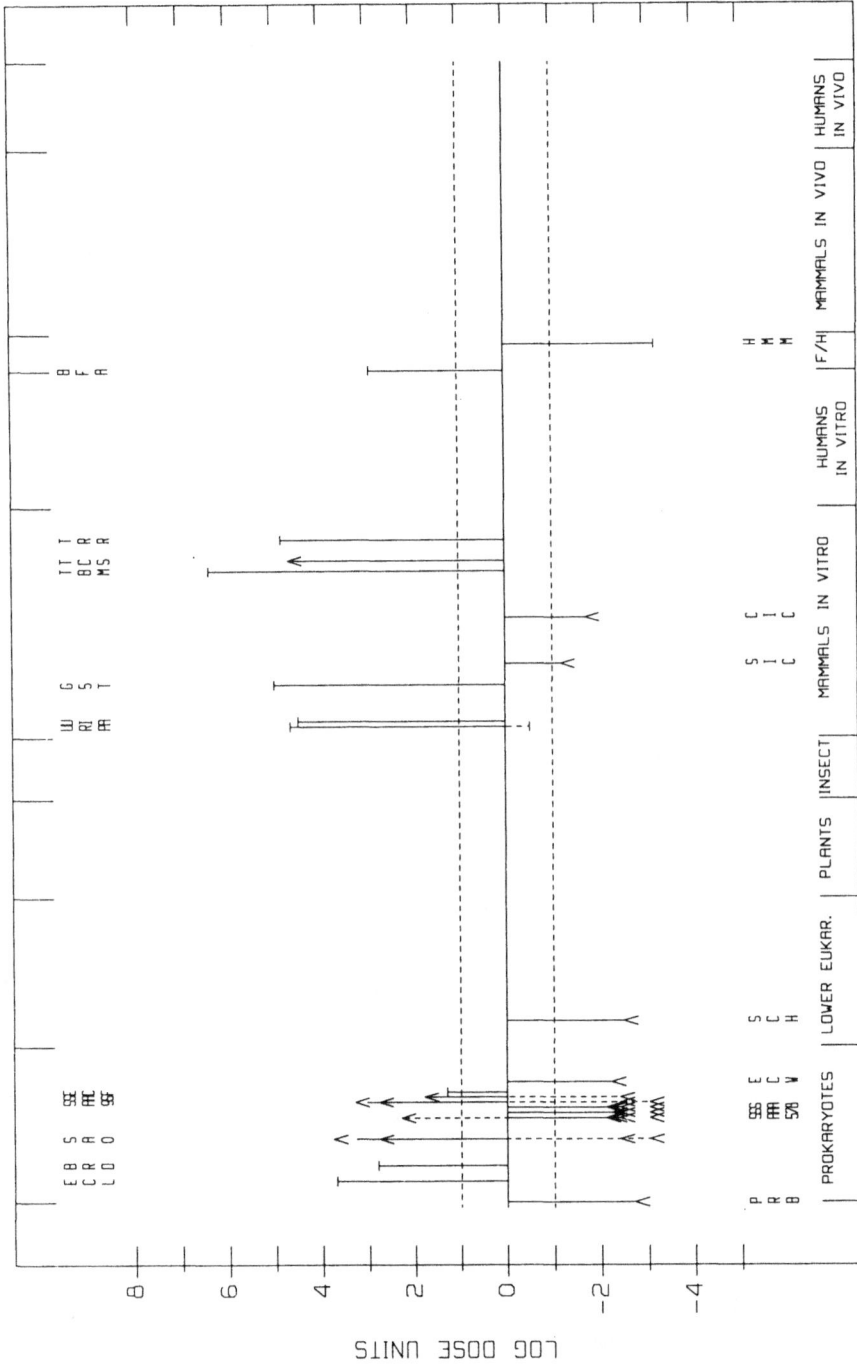

CI BASIC RED 9

569-61-9

LOG DOSE UNITS

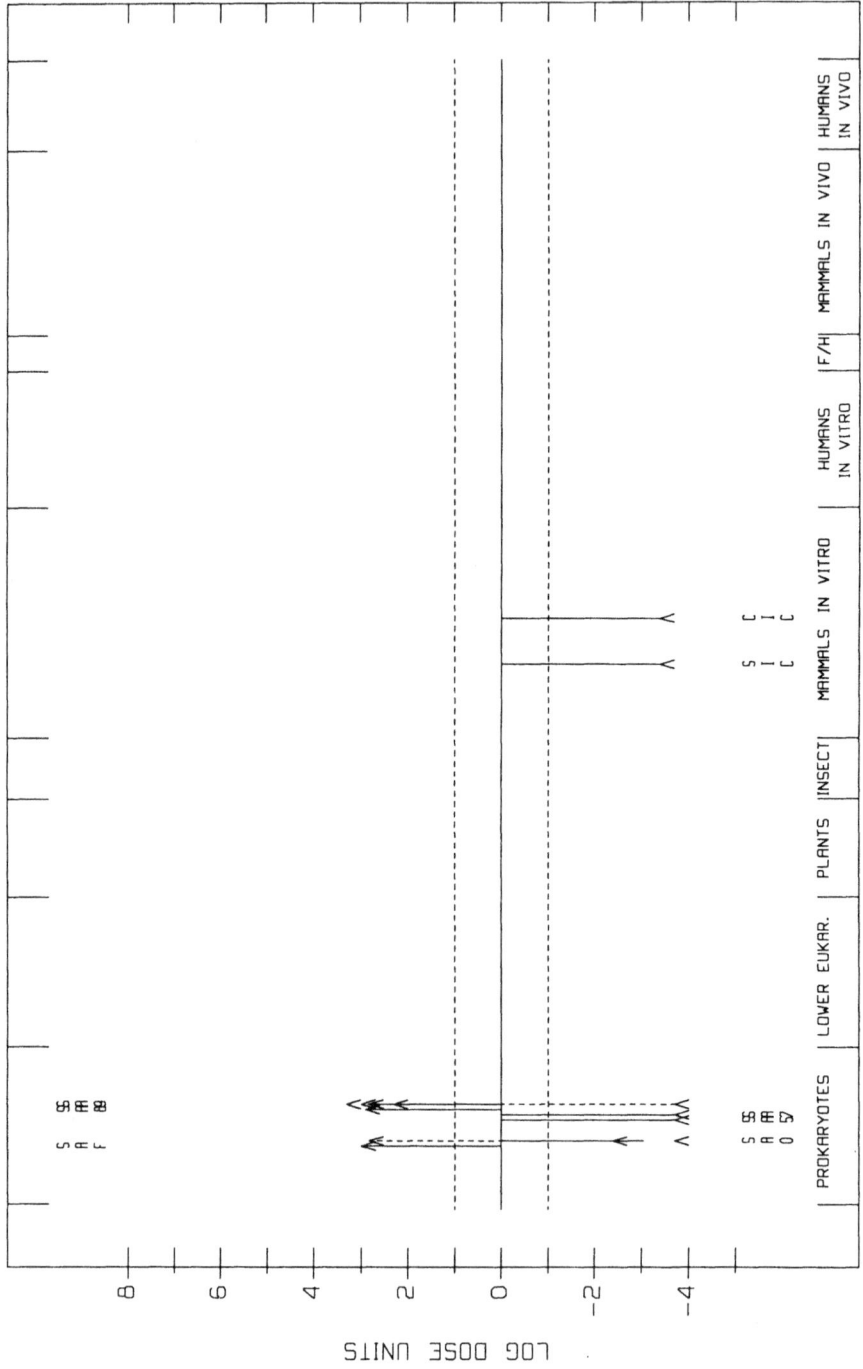

CI DIRECT BLUE 15

2429-74-5

LOG DOSE UNITS

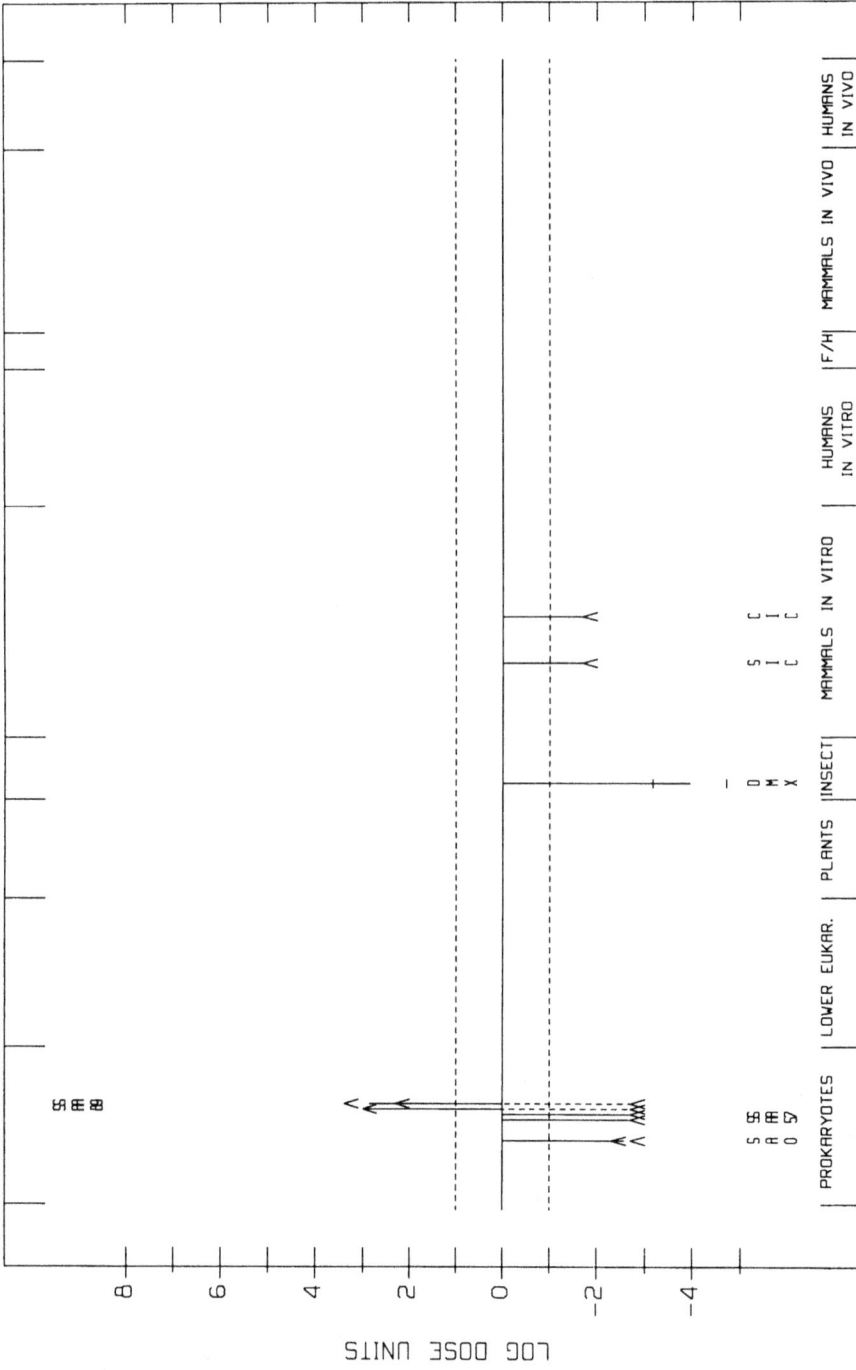

CI ACID RED 114

6459-94-5

LOG DOSE UNITS

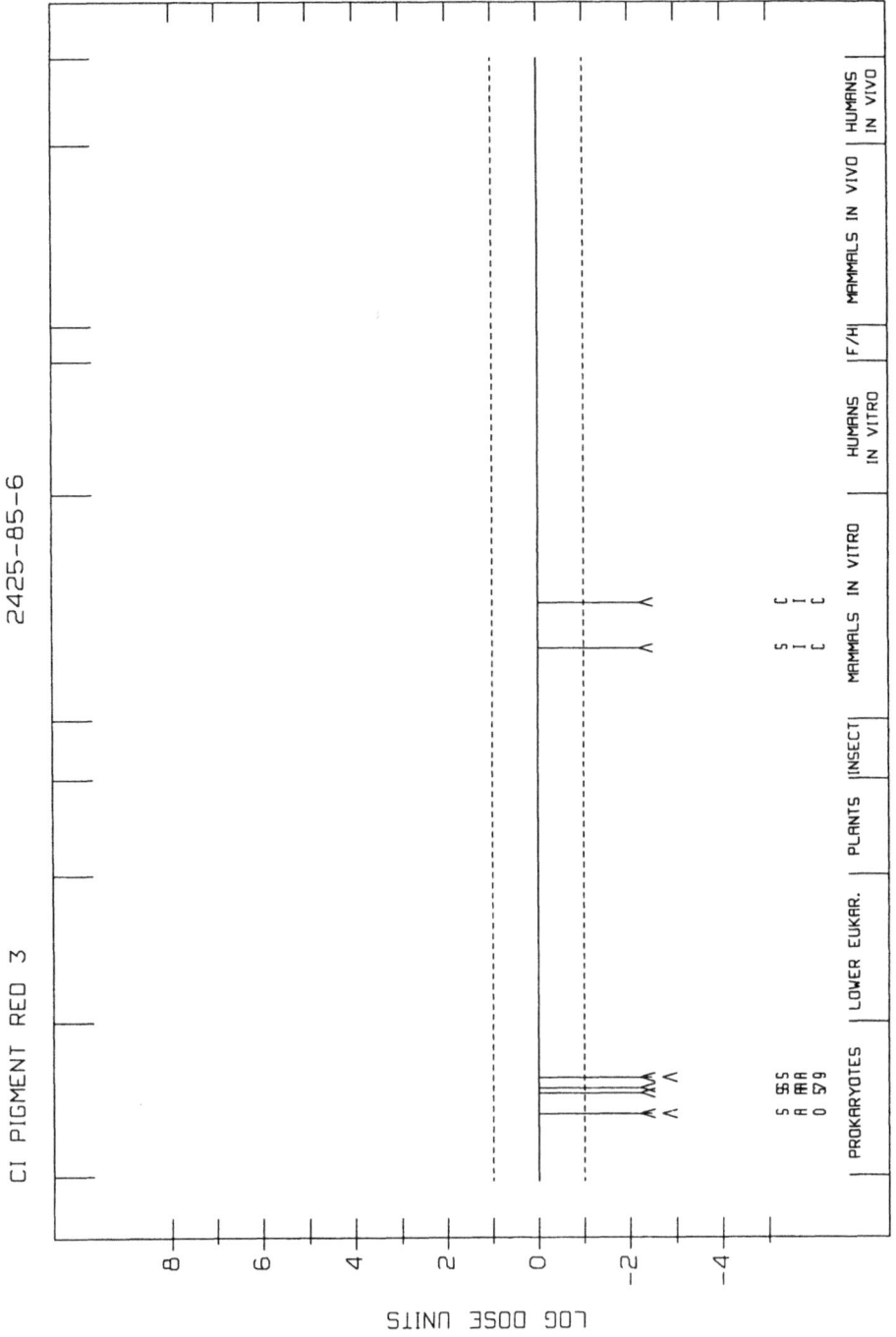

CI PIGMENT RED 3

2425-85-6

PROKARYOTES | LOWER EUKAR. | PLANTS | INSECT | MAMMALS IN VITRO | HUMANS IN VITRO | F/H | MAMMALS IN VIVO | HUMANS IN VIVO

LOG DOSE UNITS

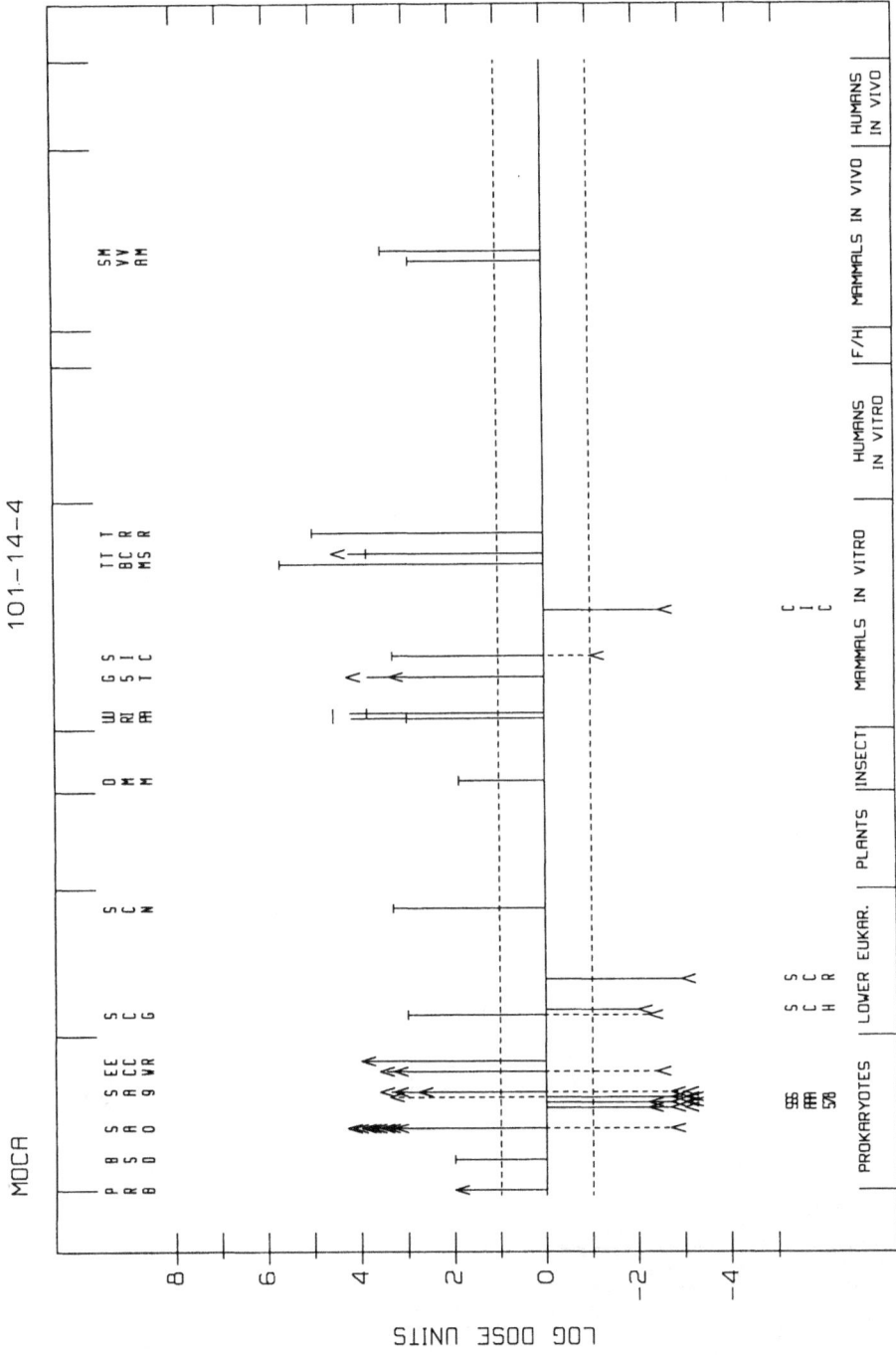

MOCA

101-14-4

LOG DOSE UNITS

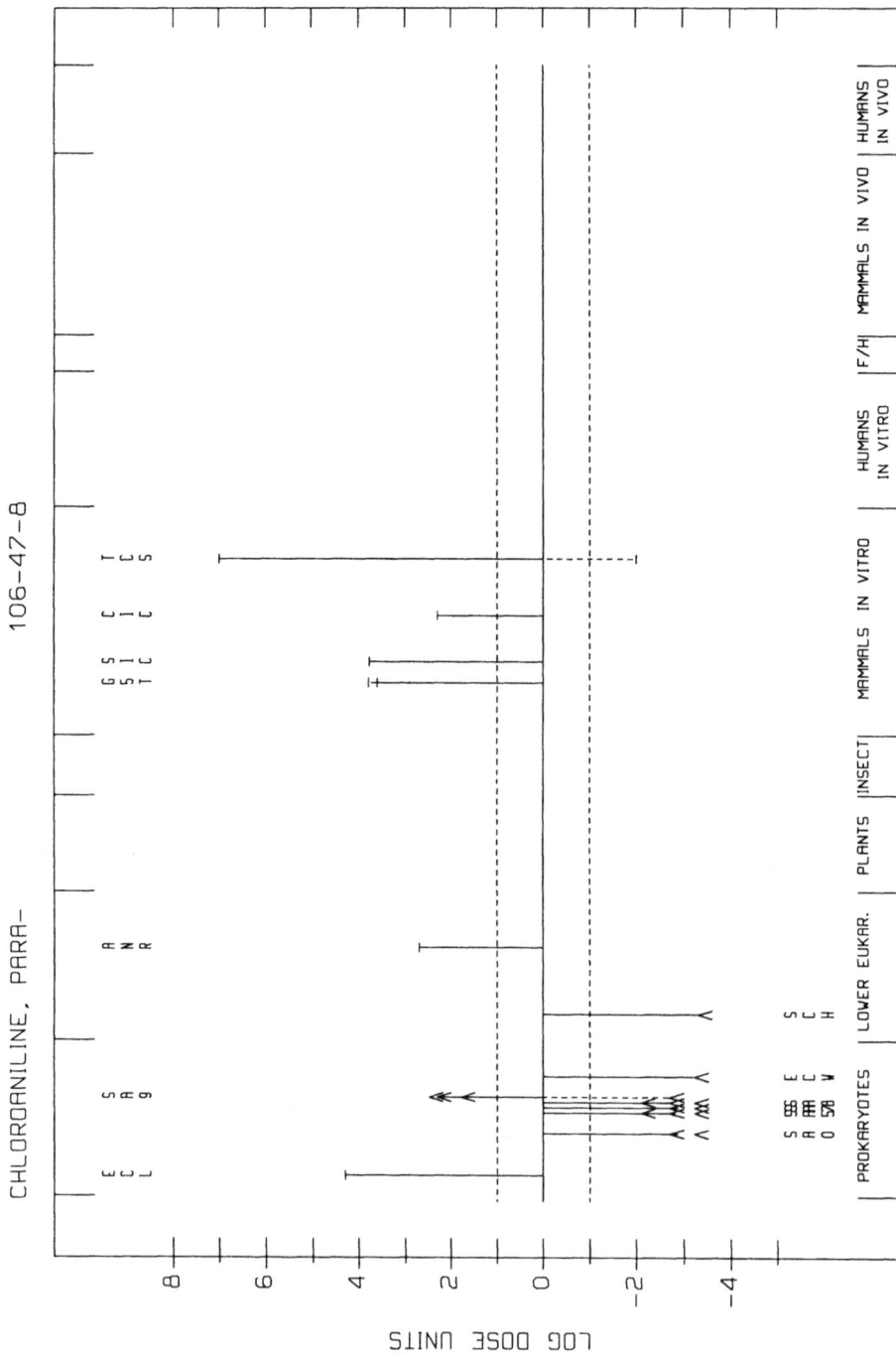

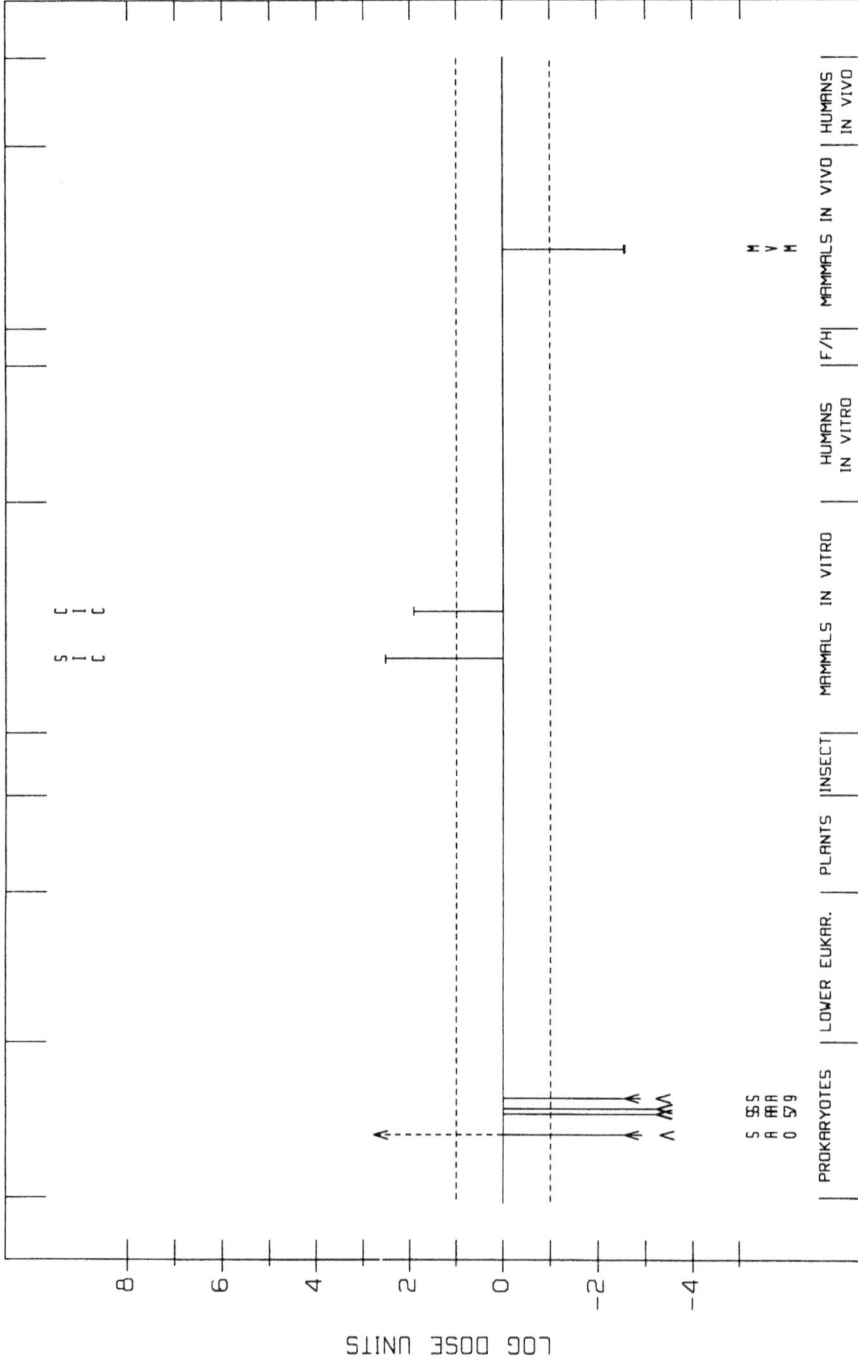

DIMETHYLANILINE, 2,6-

87-62-7

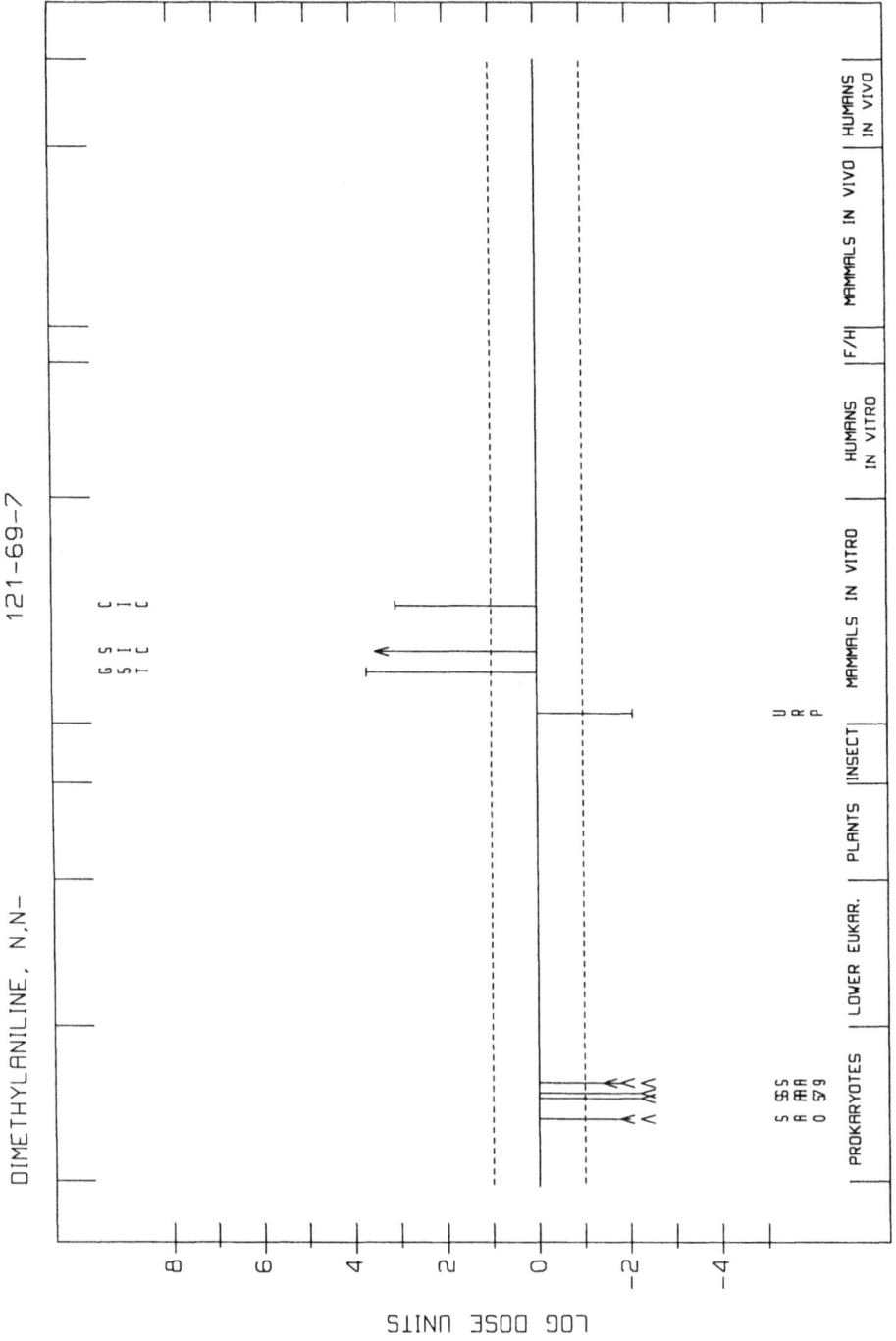

DIMETHYLANILINE, N,N-

121-69-7

LOG DOSE UNITS

SUPPLEMENTARY CORRIGENDA TO VOLUMES 1–56

Corrigenda to Volumes 1–41 are listed in Volume 42, pp. 251–264; additional corrigenda are given in Volume 43, p. 261, in Volume 45, p. 283, in Volume 46, p. 419, in Volume 47, p. 505, in Volume 50, p. 385, in Volume 51, p. 483 and in Volume 52, p. 513.

Volume 49	p. 640	*Delete* 100-00-2
	p. 642	*Delete* 100-00-1
	p. 644	*Delete* 100-00-5
	p. 646	*Delete* 100-00-4
	p. 648	*Delete* 100-00-3
Volume 51	p. 472	*Delete* 58-00-I
	p. 473	*Delete* 58-00-0B
	p. 474	*Delete* 58-00-D
	p. 476	*Delete* 58-00-1B
	p. 477	*Delete* 58-00-1G
	p. 478	*Delete* 58-00-1U
Volume 56	p. 554	*Add* 105650-23-5
	p. 565	*Replace* 999-99-9 *by* 116355-83-0
	p. 566	*Add* 116355-84-1

CUMULATIVE CROSS INDEX TO *IARC MONOGRAPHS ON THE EVALUATION OF CARCINOGENIC RISKS TO HUMANS*

The volume, page and year are given. References to corrigenda are given in parentheses.

A

A-α-C	40, 245 (1986); *Suppl. 7*, 56 (1987)
Acetaldehyde	36, 101 (1985) (*corr. 42, 263*); *Suppl. 7*, 77 (1987)
Acetaldehyde formylmethylhydrazone (*see* Gyromitrin)	
Acetamide	7, 197 (1974); *Suppl. 7*, 389 (1987)
Acetaminophen (*see* Paracetamol)	
Acridine orange	16, 145 (1978); *Suppl. 7*, 56 (1987)
Acriflavinium chloride	13, 31 (1977); *Suppl. 7, 56* (1987)
Acrolein	19, 479 (1979); 36,133 (1985); *Suppl. 7*, 78 (1987)
Acrylamide	39, 41 (1986); *Suppl. 7*, 56 (1987)
Acrylic acid	19, 47 (1979); *Suppl. 7*, 56 (1987)
Acrylic fibres	19, 86 (1979); *Suppl. 7*, 56 (1987)
Acrylonitrile	19, 73 (1979); *Suppl. 7*, 79 (1987)
Acrylonitrile–butadiene–styrene copolymers	19, 91 (1979); *Suppl. 7*, 56 (1987)
Actinolite (*see* Asbestos)	
Actinomycins	10, 29 (1976) (*corr. 42, 255*); *Suppl. 7*, 80 (1987)
Adriamycin	10, 43 (1976); *Suppl. 7*, 82 (1987)
AF-2	31, 47 (1983); *Suppl. 7*, 56 (1987)
Aflatoxins	1, 145 (1972) (*corr. 42, 251*); 10, 51 (1976); *Suppl. 7*, 83 (1987); 56, 245 (1993)
Aflatoxin B_1 (*see* Aflatoxins)	
Aflatoxin B_2 (*see* Aflatoxins)	
Aflatoxin G_1 (*see* Aflatoxins)	
Aflatoxin G_2 (*see* Aflatoxins)	
Aflatoxin M_1 (*see* Aflatoxins)	
Agaritine	31, 63 (1983); *Suppl. 7*, 56 (1987)
Alcohol drinking	44 (1988)
Aldicarb	53, 93 (1991)
Aldrin	5, 25 (1974); *Suppl. 7*, 88 (1987)
Allyl chloride	36, 39 (1985); *Suppl. 7*, 56 (1987)
Allyl isothiocyanate	36, 55 (1985); *Suppl. 7*, 56 (1987)
Allyl isovalerate	36, 69 (1985); *Suppl. 7*, 56 (1987)
Aluminium production	34, 37 (1984); *Suppl. 7*, 89 (1987)
Amaranth	8, 41 (1975); *Suppl. 7*, 56 (1987)

5-Aminoacenaphthene	*16*, 243 (1978); *Suppl. 7*, 56 (1987)
2-Aminoanthraquinone	*27*, 191 (1982); *Suppl. 7*, 56 (1987)
para-Aminoazobenzene	*8*, 53 (1975); *Suppl. 7*, 390 (1987)
ortho-Aminoazotoluene	*8*, 61 (1975) (*corr. 42*, 254);
	Suppl. 7, 56 (1987)
para-Aminobenzoic acid	*16*, 249 (1978); *Suppl. 7*, 56 (1987)
4-Aminobiphenyl	*1*, 74 (1972) (*corr. 42*, 251);
	Suppl. 7, 91 (1987)
2-Amino-3,4-dimethylimidazo[4,5-*f*]quinoline (*see* MeIQ)	
2-Amino-3,8-dimethylimidazo[4,5-*f*]quinoxaline (*see* MeIQx)	
3-Amino-1,4-dimethyl-5*H*-pyrido[4,3-*b*]indole (*see* Trp-P-1)	
2-Aminodipyrido[1,2-*a*:3′,2′-*d*]imidazole (*see* Glu-P-2)	
1-Amino-2-methylanthraquinone	*27*, 199 (1982); *Suppl. 7*, 57 (1987)
2-Amino-3-methylimidazo[4,5-*f*]quinoline (*see* IQ)	
2-Amino-6-methyldipyrido[1,2-*a*:3′,2′-*d*]imidazole (*see* Glu-P-1)	
2-Amino-1-methyl-6-phenylimidazo[4,5-*b*]pyridine (*see* PhIP)	
2-Amino-3-methyl-9*H*-pyrido[2,3-*b*]indole (*see* MeA-α-C)	
3-Amino-1-methyl-5*H*-pyrido[4,3-*b*]indole (*see* Trp-P-2)	
2-Amino-5-(5-nitro-2-furyl)-1,3,4-thiadiazole	*7*, 143 (1974); *Suppl. 7*, 57 (1987)
4-Amino-2-nitrophenol	*16*, 43 (1978); *Suppl. 7*, 57 (1987)
2-Amino-4-nitrophenol	*57*, 167 (1993)
2-Amino-5-nitrophenol	*57*, 177 (1993)
2-Amino-5-nitrothiazole	*31*, 71 (1983); *Suppl. 7*, 57 (1987)
2-Amino-9*H*-pyrido[2,3-*b*]indole (*see* A-α-C)	
11-Aminoundecanoic acid	*39*, 239 (1986); *Suppl. 7*, 57 (1987)
Amitrole	*7*, 31 (1974); *41*, 293 (1986) (*corr.*
	52, 513; *Suppl. 7*, 92 (1987)
Ammonium potassium selenide (*see* Selenium and selenium compounds)	
Amorphous silica (*see also* Silica)	*42*, 39 (1987); *Suppl. 7*, 341 (1987)
Amosite (*see* Asbestos)	
Ampicillin	*50*, 153 (1990)
Anabolic steroids (*see* Androgenic (anabolic) steroids)	
Anaesthetics, volatile	*11*, 285 (1976); *Suppl. 7*, 93 (1987)
Analgesic mixtures containing phenacetin (*see also* Phenacetin)	*Suppl. 7*, 310 (1987)
Androgenic (anabolic) steroids	*Suppl. 7*, 96 (1987)
Angelicin and some synthetic derivatives (*see also* Angelicins)	*40*, 291 (1986)
Angelicin plus ultraviolet radiation (*see also* Angelicin and some synthetic derivatives)	*Suppl. 7*, 57 (1987)
Angelicins	*Suppl. 7*, 57 (1987)
Aniline	*4*, 27 (1974) (*corr. 42*, 252);
	27, 39 (1982); *Suppl. 7*, 99 (1987)
ortho-Anisidine	*27*, 63 (1982); *Suppl. 7*, 57 (1987)
para-Anisidine	*27*, 65 (1982); *Suppl. 7*, 57 (1987)
Anthanthrene	*32*, 95 (1983); *Suppl. 7*, 57 (1987)
Anthophyllite (*see* Asbestos)	
Anthracene	*32*, 105 (1983); *Suppl. 7*, 57 (1987)
Anthranilic acid	*16*, 265 (1978); *Suppl. 7*, 57 (1987)
Antimony trioxide	*47*, 291 (1989)
Antimony trisulfide	*47*, 291 (1989)
ANTU (*see* 1-Naphthylthiourea)	
Apholate	*9*, 31 (1975); *Suppl. 7*, 57 (1987)
Aramite®	*5*, 39 (1974); *Suppl. 7*, 57 (1987)

B

Benzo[c]fluorene	32, 189 (1983); *Suppl.* 7, 58 (1987)
Benzo[ghi]perylene	32, 195 (1983); *Suppl.* 7, 58 (1987)
Benzo[c]phenanthrene	32, 205 (1983); *Suppl.* 7, 58 (1987)
Benzo[a]pyrene	3, 91 (1973); 32, 211 (1983);
	Suppl. 7, 58 (1987)
Benzo[e]pyrene	3, 137 (1973); 32, 225 (1983);
	Suppl. 7, 58 (1987)
para-Benzoquinone dioxime	29, 185 (1982); *Suppl.* 7, 58 (1987)
Benzotrichloride (*see also* α-Chlorinated toluenes)	29, 73 (1982); *Suppl.* 7, 148 (1987)
Benzoyl chloride	29, 83 (1982) (*corr.* 42, 261); *Suppl.* 7,
	126 (1987)
Benzoyl peroxide	36, 267 (1985); *Suppl.* 7, 58 (1987)
Benzyl acetate	40, 109 (1986); *Suppl.* 7, 58 (1987)
Benzyl chloride (*see also* α-Chlorinated toluenes)	11, 217 (1976) (*corr.* 42, 256); 29,
	49 (1982); *Suppl.* 7, 148 (1987)
Benzyl violet 4B	16, 153 (1978); *Suppl.* 7, 58 (1987)
Bertrandite (*see* Beryllium and beryllium compounds)	
Beryllium and beryllium compounds	1, 17 (1972); 23, 143 (1980) (*corr.* 42,
	260); *Suppl.* 7, 127 (1987)
Beryllium acetate (*see* Beryllium and beryllium compounds)	
Beryllium acetate, basic (*see* Beryllium and beryllium compounds)	
Beryllium–aluminium alloy (*see* Beryllium and beryllium compounds)	
Beryllium carbonate (*see* Beryllium and beryllium compounds)	
Beryllium chloride (*see* Beryllium and beryllium compounds)	
Beryllium–copper alloy (*see* Beryllium and beryllium compounds)	
Beryllium–copper–cobalt alloy (*see* Beryllium and beryllium compounds)	
Beryllium fluoride (*see* Beryllium and beryllium compounds)	
Beryllium hydroxide (*see* Beryllium and beryllium compounds)	
Beryllium–nickel alloy (*see* Beryllium and beryllium compounds)	
Beryllium oxide (*see* Beryllium and beryllium compounds)	
Beryllium phosphate (*see* Beryllium and beryllium compounds)	
Beryllium silicate (*see* Beryllium and beryllium compounds)	
Beryllium sulfate (*see* Beryllium and beryllium compounds)	
Beryl ore (*see* Beryllium and beryllium compounds)	
Betel quid	37, 141 (1985); *Suppl.* 7, 128 (1987)
Betel-quid chewing (*see* Betel quid)	
BHA (*see* Butylated hydroxyanisole)	
BHT (*see* Butylated hydroxytoluene)	
Bis(1-aziridinyl)morpholinophosphine sulfide	9, 55 (1975); *Suppl.* 7, 58 (1987)
Bis(2-chloroethyl)ether	9, 117 (1975); *Suppl.* 7, 58 (1987)
N,N-Bis(2-chloroethyl)-2-naphthylamine	4, 119 (1974) (*corr.* 42, 253);
	Suppl. 7, 130 (1987)
Bischloroethyl nitrosourea (*see also* Chloroethyl nitrosoureas)	26, 79 (1981); *Suppl.* 7, 150 (1987)
1,2-Bis(chloromethoxy)ethane	15, 31 (1977); *Suppl.* 7, 58 (1987)
1,4-Bis(chloromethoxymethyl)benzene	15, 37 (1977); *Suppl.* 7, 58 (1987)
Bis(chloromethyl)ether	4, 231 (1974) (*corr.* 42, 253);
	Suppl. 7, 131 (1987)
Bis(2-chloro-1-methylethyl)ether	41, 149 (1986); *Suppl.* 7, 59 (1987)
Bis(2,3-epoxycyclopentyl)ether	47, 231 (1989)
Bisphenol A diglycidyl ether (*see* Glycidyl ethers)	
Bisulfites (*see* Sulfur dioxide and some sulfites, bisulfites and metabisulfites)	
Bitumens	35, 39 (1985); *Suppl.* 7, 133 (1987)

C

Carrageenan — *10*, 181 (1976) (*corr. 42*, 255); *31*, 79 (1983); *Suppl. 7*, 59 (1987)

Catechol — *15*, 155 (1977); *Suppl. 7*, 59 (1987)

CCNU (*see* 1-(2-Chloroethyl)-3-cyclohexyl-1-nitrosourea)

Ceramic fibres (*see* Man-made mineral fibres)

Chemotherapy, combined, including alkylating agents (*see* MOPP and other combined chemotherapy including alkylating agents)

Chlorambucil — *9*, 125 (1975); *26*, 115 (1981); *Suppl. 7*, 144 (1987)

Chloramphenicol — *10*, 85 (1976); *Suppl. 7*, 145 (1987); *50*, 169 (1990)

Chlordane (*see also* Chlordane/Heptachlor) — *20*, 45 (1979) (*corr. 42*, 258)

Chlordane/Heptachlor — *Suppl. 7*, 146 (1987); *53*, 115 (1991)

Chlordecone — *20*, 67 (1979); *Suppl. 7*, 59 (1987)

Chlordimeform — *30*, 61 (1983); *Suppl. 7*, 59 (1987)

Chlorendic acid — *48*, 45 (1990)

Chlorinated dibenzodioxins (other than TCDD) — *15*, 41 (1977); *Suppl. 7*, 59 (1987)

Chlorinated drinking-water — *52*, 45 (1991)

Chlorinated paraffins — *48*, 55 (1990)

α-Chlorinated toluenes — *Suppl. 7*, 148 (1987)

Chlormadinone acetate (*see also* Progestins; Combined oral contraceptives) — *6*, 149 (1974); *21*, 365 (1979)

Chlornaphazine (*see N,N*-Bis(2-chloroethyl)-2-naphthylamine)

Chloroacetonitrile (*see* Halogenated acetonitriles)

para-Chloroaniline — *57*, 305 (1993)

Chlorobenzilate — *5*, 75 (1974); *30*, 73 (1983); *Suppl. 7*, 60 (1987)

Chlorodibromomethane — *52*, 243 (1991)

Chlorodifluoromethane — *41*, 237 (1986) (*corr. 51*, 483); *Suppl. 7*, 149 (1987)

Chloroethane — *52*, 315 (1991)

1-(2-Chloroethyl)-3-cyclohexyl-1-nitrosourea (*see also* Chloroethyl nitrosoureas) — *26*, 137 (1981) (*corr. 42*, 260); *Suppl. 7*, 150 (1987)

1-(2-Chloroethyl)-3-(4-methylcyclohexyl)-1-nitrosourea (*see also* Chloroethyl nitrosoureas) — *Suppl. 7*, 150 (1987)

Chloroethyl nitrosoureas — *Suppl. 7*, 150 (1987)

Chlorofluoromethane — *41*, 229 (1986); *Suppl. 7*, 60 (1987)

Chloroform — *1*, 61 (1972); *20*, 401 (1979); *Suppl. 7*, 152 (1987)

Chloromethyl methyl ether (technical-grade) (*see also* Bis(chloromethyl)ether) — *4*, 239 (1974); *Suppl. 7*, 131 (1987)

(4-Chloro-2-methylphenoxy)acetic acid (*see* MCPA)

Chlorophenols — *Suppl. 7*, 154 (1987)

Chlorophenols (occupational exposures to) — *41*, 319 (1986)

Chlorophenoxy herbicides — *Suppl. 7*, 156 (1987)

Chlorophenoxy herbicides (occupational exposures to) — *41*, 357 (1986)

4-Chloro-*ortho*-phenylenediamine — *27*, 81 (1982); *Suppl. 7*, 60 (1987)

4-Chloro-*meta*-phenylenediamine — *27*, 82 (1982); *Suppl. 7*, 60 (1987)

Chloroprene — *19*, 131 (1979); *Suppl. 7*, 160 (1987)

Chloropropham — *12*, 55 (1976); *Suppl. 7*, 60 (1987)

Chloroquine — *13*, 47 (1977); *Suppl. 7*, 60 (1987)

Chlorothalonil — *30*, 319 (1983); *Suppl. 7*, 60 (1987)

para-Chloro-*ortho*-toluidine and its strong acid salts	*16*, 277 (1978); *30*, 65 (1983);
(*see also* Chlordimeform)	*Suppl. 7*, 60 (1987); *48*, 123 (1990)
Chlorotrianisene (*see also* Nonsteroidal oestrogens)	*21*, 139 (1979)
2-Chloro-1,1,1-trifluoroethane	*41*, 253 (1986); *Suppl. 7*, 60 (1987)
Chlorozotocin	*50*, 65 (1990)
Cholesterol	*10*, 99 (1976); *31*, 95 (1983);
	Suppl. 7, 161 (1987)
Chromic acetate (*see* Chromium and chromium compounds)	
Chromic chloride (*see* Chromium and chromium compounds)	
Chromic oxide (*see* Chromium and chromium compounds)	
Chromic phosphate (*see* Chromium and chromium compounds)	
Chromite ore (*see* Chromium and chromium compounds)	
Chromium and chromium compounds	*2*, 100 (1973); *23*, 205 (1980);
	Suppl. 7, 165 (1987); *49*, 49 (1990)
	(*corr. 51*, 483)
Chromium carbonyl (*see* Chromium and chromium compounds)	
Chromium potassium sulfate (*see* Chromium and chromium compounds)	
Chromium sulfate (*see* Chromium and chromium compounds)	
Chromium trioxide (*see* Chromium and chromium compounds)	
Chrysazin (*see* Dantron)	
Chrysene	*3*, 159 (1973); *32*, 247 (1983);
	Suppl. 7, 60 (1987)
Chrysoidine	*8*, 91 (1975); *Suppl. 7*, 169 (1987)
Chrysotile (*see* Asbestos)	
CI Acid Orange 3	*57*, 121 (1993)
CI Acid Red 114	*57*, 247 (1993)
CI Basic Red 9	*57*, 215 (1993)
Ciclosporin	*50*, 77 (1990)
CI Direct Blue 15	*57*, 235 (1993)
CI Disperse Yellow 3 (*see* Disperse Yellow 3)	
Cimetidine	*50*, 235 (1990)
Cinnamyl anthranilate	*16*, 287 (1978); *31*, 133 (1983);
	Suppl. 7, 60 (1987)
CI Pigment Red 3	*57*, 259 (1993)
CI Pigment Red 53:1 (*see* D&C Red No. 9)	
Cisplatin	*26*, 151 (1981); *Suppl. 7*, 170 (1987)
Citrinin	*40*, 67 (1986); *Suppl. 7*, 60 (1987)
Citrus Red No. 2	*8*, 101 (1975) (*corr. 42*, 254);
	Suppl. 7, 60 (1987)
Clofibrate	*24*, 39 (1980); *Suppl. 7*, 171 (1987)
Clomiphene citrate	*21*, 551 (1979); *Suppl. 7*, 172 (1987)
Coal gasification	*34*, 65 (1984); *Suppl. 7*, 173 (1987)
Coal-tar pitches (*see also* Coal-tars)	*35*, 83 (1985); *Suppl. 7*, 174 (1987)
Coal-tars	*35*, 83 (1985); *Suppl. 7*, 175 (1987)
Cobalt[III] acetate (*see* Cobalt and cobalt compounds)	
Cobalt–aluminium–chromium spinel (*see* Cobalt and cobalt compounds)	
Cobalt and cobalt compounds	*52*, 363 (1991)
Cobalt[II] chloride (*see* Cobalt and cobalt compounds)	
Cobalt–chromium alloy (*see* Chromium and chromium compounds)	
Cobalt–chromium–molybdenum alloys (*see* Cobalt and cobalt compounds)	

Cobalt metal powder (*see* Cobalt and cobalt compounds)
Cobalt naphthenate (*see* Cobalt and cobalt compounds)
Cobalt[II] oxide (*see* Cobalt and cobalt compounds)
Cobalt[II,III] oxide (*see* Cobalt and cobalt compounds)
Cobalt[II] sulfide (*see* Cobalt and cobalt compounds)
Coffee   *51*, 41 (1991) (*corr. 52*, 513)
Coke production   *34*, 101 (1984); *Suppl. 7*, 176 (1987)
Combined oral contraceptives (*see also* Oestrogens, progestins   *Suppl. 7*, 297 (1987)
    and combinations)
Conjugated oestrogens (*see also* Steroidal oestrogens)   *21*, 147 (1979)
Contraceptives, oral (*see* Combined oral contraceptives;
    Sequential oral contraceptives)
Copper 8-hydroxyquinoline   *15*, 103 (1977); *Suppl. 7*, 61 (1987)
Coronene   *32*, 263 (1983); *Suppl. 7*, 61 (1987)
Coumarin   *10*, 113 (1976); *Suppl. 7*, 61 (1987)
Creosotes (*see also* Coal-tars)   *35*, 83 (1985); *Suppl. 7*, 177 (1987)
meta-Cresidine   *27*, 91 (1982); *Suppl. 7*, 61 (1987)
para-Cresidine   *27*, 92 (1982); *Suppl. 7*, 61 (1987)
Crocidolite (*see* Asbestos)
Crude oil   *45*, 119 (1989)
Crystalline silica (*see also* Silica)   *42*, 39 (1987); *Suppl. 7*, 341 (1987)
Cycasin   *1*, 157 (1972) (*corr. 42*, 251); *10*,
                                                          121 (1976); *Suppl. 7*, 61 (1987)
Cyclamates   *22*, 55 (1980); *Suppl. 7*, 178 (1987)
Cyclamic acid (*see* Cyclamates)
Cyclochlorotine   *10*, 139 (1976); *Suppl. 7*, 61 (1987)
Cyclohexanone   *47*, 157 (1989)
Cyclohexylamine (*see* Cyclamates)
Cyclopenta[*cd*]pyrene   *32*, 269 (1983); *Suppl. 7*, 61 (1987)
Cyclopropane (*see* Anaesthetics, volatile)
Cyclophosphamide   *9*, 135 (1975); *26*, 165 (1981);
                                                          Suppl. 7, 182 (1987)

D

2,4-D (*see also* Chlorophenoxy herbicides; Chlorophenoxy   *15*, 111 (1977)
    herbicides, occupational exposures to)
Dacarbazine   *26*, 203 (1981); *Suppl. 7*, 184 (1987)
Dantron   *50*, 265 (1990)
D&C Red No. 9   *8*, 107 (1975); *Suppl. 7*, 61 (1987);
                                                          57, 203 (1993)
Dapsone   *24*, 59 (1980); *Suppl. 7*, 185 (1987)
Daunomycin   *10*, 145 (1976); *Suppl. 7*, 61 (1987)
DDD (*see* DDT)
DDE (*see* DDT)
DDT   *5*, 83 (1974) (*corr. 42*, 253);
                                                          Suppl. 7, 186 (1987); *53*, 179 (1991)
Decabromodiphenyl oxide   *48*, 73 (1990)
Deltamethrin   *53*, 251 (1991)
Deoxynivalenol (*see* Toxins derived from *Fusarium graminearum,*
    F. culmorum and *F. crookwellense*)
Diacetylaminoazotoluene   *8*, 113 (1975); *Suppl. 7*, 61 (1987)

3,3'-Dichloro-4,4'-diaminodiphenyl ether   *16*, 309 (1978); *Suppl. 7*, 62 (1987)
1,2-Dichloroethane   *20*, 429 (1979); *Suppl. 7*, 62 (1987)
Dichloromethane   *20*, 449 (1979); *41*, 43 (1986);
     Suppl. 7, 194 (1987)

2,4-Dichlorophenol (*see* Chlorophenols; Chlorophenols,
     occupational exposures to)
(2,4-Dichlorophenoxy)acetic acid (*see* 2,4-D)
2,6-Dichloro-*para*-phenylenediamine   *39*, 325 (1986); *Suppl. 7*, 62 (1987)
1,2-Dichloropropane   *41*, 131 (1986); *Suppl. 7*, 62 (1987)
1,3-Dichloropropene (technical-grade)   *41*, 113 (1986); *Suppl. 7*, 195 (1987)
Dichlorvos   *20*, 97 (1979); *Suppl. 7*, 62 (1987);
     53, 267 (1991)
Dicofol   *30*, 87 (1983); *Suppl. 7*, 62 (1987)
Dicyclohexylamine (*see* Cyclamates)
Dieldrin   *5*, 125 (1974); *Suppl. 7*, 196 (1987)
Dienoestrol (*see also* Nonsteroidal oestrogens)   *21*, 161 (1979)
Diepoxybutane   *11*, 115 (1976) (*corr. 42*, 255); *Suppl. 7*,
     62 (1987)
Diesel and gasoline engine exhausts   *46*, 41 (1989)
Diesel fuels   *45*, 219 (1989) (*corr. 47*, 505)
Diethyl ether (*see* Anaesthetics, volatile)
Di(2-ethylhexyl)adipate   *29*, 257 (1982); *Suppl. 7*, 62 (1987)
Di(2-ethylhexyl)phthalate   *29*, 269 (1982) (*corr. 42*, 261); *Suppl. 7*,
     62 (1987)
1,2-Diethylhydrazine   *4*, 153 (1974); *Suppl. 7*, 62 (1987)
Diethylstilboestrol   *6*, 55 (1974); *21*, 173 (1979)
     (*corr. 42*, 259); *Suppl. 7*, 273 (1987)
Diethylstilboestrol dipropionate (*see* Diethylstilboestrol)
Diethyl sulfate   *4*, 277 (1974); *Suppl. 7*, 198 (1987);
     54, 213 (1992)
Diglycidyl resorcinol ether   *11*, 125 (1976); *36*, 181 (1985);
     Suppl. 7, 62 (1987)
Dihydrosafrole   *1*, 170 (1972); *10*, 233 (1976);
     Suppl. 7, 62 (1987)
1,8-Dihydroxyanthraquinone (*see* Dantron)
Dihydroxybenzenes (*see* Catechol; Hydroquinone; Resorcinol)
Dihydroxymethylfuratrizine   *24*, 77 (1980); *Suppl. 7*, 62 (1987)
Diisopropyl sulfate   *54*, 229 (1992)
Dimethisterone (*see also* Progestins; Sequential oral   *6*, 167 (1974); *21*, 377 (1979)
     contraceptives)
Dimethoxane   *15*, 177 (1977); *Suppl. 7*, 62 (1987)
3,3'-Dimethoxybenzidine   *4*, 41 (1974); *Suppl. 7*, 198 (1987)
3,3'-Dimethoxybenzidine-4,4'-diisocyanate   *39*, 279 (1986); *Suppl. 7*, 62 (1987)
para-Dimethylaminoazobenzene   *8*, 125 (1975); *Suppl. 7*, 62 (1987)
para-Dimethylaminoazobenzenediazo sodium sulfonate   *8*, 147 (1975); *Suppl. 7*, 62 (1987)
trans-2-[(Dimethylamino)methylimino]-5-[2-(5-nitro-2-furyl)-   *7*, 147 (1974) (*corr. 42*, 253); *Suppl. 7*,
     vinyl]-1,3,4-oxadiazole   62 (1987)
4,4'-Dimethylangelicin plus ultraviolet radiation (*see also*   *Suppl. 7*, 57 (1987)
     Angelicin and some synthetic derivatives)
4,5'-Dimethylangelicin plus ultraviolet radiation (*see also*   *Suppl. 7*, 57 (1987)
     Angelicin and some synthetic derivatives)
2,6-Dimethylaniline   *57*, 323 (1993)

Ethylene sulfide	*11*, 257 (1976); *Suppl. 7*, 63 (1987)
Ethylene thiourea	*7*, 45 (1974); *Suppl. 7*, 207 (1987)
Ethyl methanesulfonate	*7*, 245 (1974); *Suppl. 7*, 63 (1987)
N-Ethyl-*N*-nitrosourea	*1*, 135 (1972); *17*, 191 (1978);
	Suppl. 7, 63 (1987)
Ethyl selenac (*see also* Selenium and selenium compounds)	*12*, 107 (1976); *Suppl. 7*, 63 (1987)
Ethyl tellurac	*12*, 115 (1976); *Suppl. 7*, 63 (1987)
Ethynodiol diacetate (*see also* Progestins; Combined oral	*6*, 173 (1974); *21*, 387 (1979)
contraceptives)	
Eugenol	*36*, 75 (1985); *Suppl. 7*, 63 (1987)
Evans blue	*8*, 151 (1975); *Suppl. 7*, 63 (1987)

F

Fast Green FCF	*16*, 187 (1978); *Suppl. 7*, 63 (1987)
Fenvalerate	*53*, 309 (1991)
Ferbam	*12*, 121 (1976) (*corr. 42*, 256);
	Suppl. 7, 63 (1987)
Ferric oxide	*1*, 29 (1972); *Suppl. 7*, 216 (1987)
Ferrochromium (*see* Chromium and chromium compounds)	
Fluometuron	*30*, 245 (1983); *Suppl. 7*, 63 (1987)
Fluoranthene	*32*, 355 (1983); *Suppl. 7*, 63 (1987)
Fluorene	*32*, 365 (1983); *Suppl. 7*, 63 (1987)
Fluorescent lighting (exposure to) (*see* Ultraviolet radiation)	
Fluorides (inorganic, used in drinking-water)	*27*, 237 (1982); *Suppl. 7*, 208 (1987)
5-Fluorouracil	*26*, 217 (1981); *Suppl. 7*, 210 (1987)
Fluorspar (*see* Fluorides)	
Fluosilicic acid (*see* Fluorides)	
Fluroxene (*see* Anaesthetics, volatile)	
Formaldehyde	*29*, 345 (1982); *Suppl. 7*, 211 (1987)
2-(2-Formylhydrazino)-4-(5-nitro-2-furyl)thiazole	*7*, 151 (1974) (*corr. 42*, 253);
	Suppl. 7, 63 (1987)
Frusemide (*see* Furosemide)	
Fuel oils (heating oils)	*45*, 239 (1989) (*corr. 47*, 505)
Fumonisin B$_1$ (*see* Toxins derived from *Fusarium moniliforme*)	
Fumonisin B$_2$ (*see* Toxins derived from *Fusarium moniliforme*)	
Furazolidone	*31*, 141 (1983); *Suppl. 7*, 63 (1987)
Furniture and cabinet-making	*25*, 99 (1981); *Suppl. 7*, 380 (1987)
Furosemide	*50*, 277 (1990)
2-(2-Furyl)-3-(5-nitro-2-furyl)acrylamide (*see* AF-2)	
Fusarenon-X (*see* Toxins derived from *Fusarium graminearum*,	
F. culmorum and *F. crookwellense*)	
Fusarenone-X (*see* Toxins derived from *Fusarium graminearum*,	
F. culmorum and *F. crookwellense*)	
Fusarin C (see Toxins derived from *Fusarium moniliforme*)	

G

Gasoline	*45*, 159 (1989) (*corr. 47*, 505)
Gasoline engine exhaust (*see* Diesel and gasoline engine exhausts)	
Glass fibres (*see* Man-made mineral fibres)	
Glasswool (*see* Man-made mineral fibres)	

Glass filaments (*see* Man-made mineral fibres)
Glu-P-1 — *40*, 223 (1986); *Suppl. 7*, 64 (1987)
Glu-P-2 — *40*, 235 (1986); *Suppl. 7*, 64 (1987)
L-Glutamic acid, 5-[2-(4-hydroxymethyl)phenylhydrazide]
  (*see* Agaritine)
Glycidaldehyde — *11*, 175 (1976); *Suppl. 7*, 64 (1987)
Glycidyl ethers — *47*, 237 (1989)
Glycidyl oleate — *11*, 183 (1976); *Suppl. 7*, 64 (1987)
Glycidyl stearate — *11*, 187 (1976); *Suppl. 7*, 64 (1987)
Griseofulvin — *10*, 153 (1976); *Suppl. 7*, 391 (1987)
Guinea Green B — *16*, 199 (1978); *Suppl. 7*, 64 (1987)
Gyromitrin — *31*, 163 (1983); *Suppl. 7*, 391 (1987)

H

Haematite — *1*, 29 (1972); *Suppl. 7*, 216 (1987)
Haematite and ferric oxide — *Suppl. 7*, 216 (1987)
Haematite mining, underground, with exposure to radon — *1*, 29 (1972); *Suppl. 7*, 216 (1987)
Hairdressers and barbers (occupational exposure as) — *57*, 43 (1993)
Hair dyes, epidemiology of — *16*, 29 (1978); *27*, 307 (1982);
Halogenated acetonitriles — *52*, 269 (1991)
Halothane (*see* Anaesthetics, volatile)
HC Blue No. 1 — *57*, 129 (1993)
HC Blue No. 2 — *57*, 143 (1993)
α-HCH (*see* Hexachlorocyclohexanes)
β-HCH (*see* Hexachlorocyclohexanes)
γ-HCH (*see* Hexachlorocyclohexanes)
HC Red No. 3 — *57*, 153 (1993)
HC Yellow No. 4 — *57*, 159 (1993)
Heating oils (*see* Fuel oils)
Heptachlor (*see also* Chlordane/Heptachlor) — *5*, 173 (1974); *20*, 129 (1979)
Hexachlorobenzene — *20*, 155 (1979); *Suppl. 7*, 219 (1987)
Hexachlorobutadiene — *20*, 179 (1979); *Suppl. 7*, 64 (1987)
Hexachlorocyclohexanes — *5*, 47 (1974); *20*, 195 (1979) (*corr. 42*, 258); *Suppl. 7*, 220 (1987)

Hexachlorocyclohexane, technical-grade (*see* Hexachloro-
  cyclohexanes)
Hexachloroethane — *20*, 467 (1979); *Suppl. 7*, 64 (1987)
Hexachlorophene — *20*, 241 (1979); *Suppl. 7*, 64 (1987)
Hexamethylphosphoramide — *15*, 211 (1977); *Suppl. 7*, 64 (1987)
Hexoestrol (*see* Nonsteroidal oestrogens)
Hycanthone mesylate — *13*, 91 (1977); *Suppl. 7*, 64 (1987)
Hydralazine — *24*, 85 (1980); *Suppl. 7*, 222 (1987)
Hydrazine — *4*, 127 (1974); *Suppl. 7*, 223 (1987)
Hydrochloric acid — *54*, 189 (1992)
Hydrochlorothiazide — *50*, 293 (1990)
Hydrogen peroxide — *36*, 285 (1985); *Suppl. 7*, 64 (1987)
Hydroquinone — *15*, 155 (1977); *Suppl. 7*, 64 (1987)
4-Hydroxyazobenzene — *8*, 157 (1975); *Suppl. 7*, 64 (1987)
17α-Hydroxyprogesterone caproate (*see also* Progestins) — *21*, 399 (1979) (*corr. 42*, 259)
8-Hydroxyquinoline — *13*, 101 (1977); *Suppl. 7*, 64 (1987)
8-Hydroxysenkirkine — *10*, 265 (1976); *Suppl. 7*, 64 (1987)

Hypochlorite salts   *52*, 159 (1991)

I

Indeno[1,2,3-*cd*]pyrene   *3*, 229 (1973); *32*, 373 (1983);
                                                               Suppl. 7, 64 (1987)

Inorganic acids (*see* Sulfuric acid and other strong inorganic acids,
    occupational exposures to mists and vapours from)
Insecticides, occupational exposures in spraying and application of   *53*, 45 (1991)
IQ   *40*, 261 (1986); *Suppl. 7*, 64 (1987);
                                                               56, 165 (1993)
Iron and steel founding   *34*, 133 (1984); *Suppl. 7*, 224 (1987)
Iron-dextran complex   *2*, 161 (1973); *Suppl. 7*, 226 (1987)
Iron-dextrin complex   *2*, 161 (1973) (*corr. 42*, 252);
                                                               Suppl. 7, 64 (1987)

Iron oxide (*see* Ferric oxide)
Iron oxide, saccharated (*see* Saccharated iron oxide)
Iron sorbitol–citric acid complex   *2*, 161 (1973); *Suppl. 7*, 64 (1987)
Isatidine   *10*, 269 (1976); *Suppl. 7*, 65 (1987)
Isoflurane (*see* Anaesthetics, volatile)
Isoniazid (*see* Isonicotinic acid hydrazide)
Isonicotinic acid hydrazide   *4*, 159 (1974); *Suppl. 7*, 227 (1987)
Isophosphamide   *26*, 237 (1981); *Suppl. 7*, 65 (1987)
Isopropyl alcohol   *15*, 223 (1977); *Suppl. 7*, 229 (1987)
Isopropyl alcohol manufacture (strong-acid process)   *Suppl. 7*, 229 (1987)
    (*see also* Isopropyl alcohol; Sulfuric acid and other strong inorganic
    acids, occupational exposures to mists and vapours from)
Isopropyl oils   *15*, 223 (1977); *Suppl. 7*, 229 (1987)
Isosafrole   *1*, 169 (1972); *10*, 232 (1976);
                                                               Suppl. 7, 65 (1987)

J

Jacobine   *10*, 275 (1976); *Suppl. 7*, 65 (1987)
Jet fuel   *45*, 203 (1989)
Joinery (*see* Carpentry and joinery)

K

Kaempferol   *31*, 171 (1983); *Suppl. 7*, 65 (1987)
Kepone (*see* Chlordecone)

L

Lasiocarpine   *10*, 281 (1976); *Suppl. 7*, 65 (1987)
Lauroyl peroxide   *36*, 315 (1985); Suppl. 7, 65 (1987)
Lead acetate (*see* Lead and lead compounds)
Lead and lead compounds   *1*, 40 (1972) (*corr. 42*, 251); *2*, 52,
                                                               150 (1973); *12*, 131 (1976);
                                                               23, 40, 208, 209, 325 (1980);
                                                               Suppl. 7, 230 (1987)

Lead arsenate (*see* Arsenic and arsenic compounds)
Lead carbonate (*see* Lead and lead compounds)
Lead chloride (*see* Lead and lead compounds)
Lead chromate (*see* Chromium and chromium compounds)
Lead chromate oxide (*see* Chromium and chromium compounds)
Lead naphthenate (*see* Lead and lead compounds)
Lead nitrate (*see* Lead and lead compounds)
Lead oxide (*see* Lead and lead compounds)
Lead phosphate (*see* Lead and lead compounds)
Lead subacetate (*see* Lead and lead compounds)
Lead tetroxide (*see* Lead and lead compounds)
Leather goods manufacture   *25*, 279 (1981); *Suppl. 7*, 235 (1987)
Leather industries   *25*, 199 (1981); *Suppl. 7*, 232 (1987)
Leather tanning and processing   *25*, 201 (1981); *Suppl. 7*, 236 (1987)
Ledate (*see also* Lead and lead compounds) *12*, 131 (1976)
Light Green SF   *16*, 209 (1978); *Suppl. 7,* 65 (1987)
d-Limonene   *56*, 135 (1993)
Lindane (*see* Hexachlorocyclohexanes)
The lumber and sawmill industries (including logging)   *25*, 49 (1981); *Suppl. 7*, 383 (1987)
Luteoskyrin   *10*, 163 (1976); *Suppl. 7*, 65 (1987)
Lynoestrenol (*see also* Progestins; Combined oral contraceptives)   *21*, 407 (1979)

M

Magenta   *4*, 57 (1974) (*corr. 42*, 252);
                                             Suppl. 7, 238 (1987); *57*, 215 (1993)
Magenta, manufacture of (*see also* Magenta) *Suppl. 7,* 238 (1987)
Malathion   *30*, 103 (1983); *Suppl. 7*, 65 (1987)
Maleic hydrazide   *4*, 173 (1974) (*corr. 42*, 253);
                                             Suppl. 7, 65 (1987)
Malonaldehyde   *36*, 163 (1985); *Suppl. 7*, 65 (1987)
Maneb   *12*, 137 (1976); *Suppl. 7*, 65 (1987)
Man-made mineral fibres   *43*, 39 (1988)
Mannomustine   *9*, 157 (1975); *Suppl. 7*, 65 (1987)
Mate   *51*, 273 (1991)
MCPA (*see also* Chlorophenoxy herbicides; Chlorophenoxy   *30*, 255 (1983)
   herbicides, occupational exposures to)
MeA-α-C   *40*, 253 (1986); *Suppl. 7*, 65 (1987)
Medphalan   *9*, 168 (1975); *Suppl. 7*, 65 (1987)
Medroxyprogesterone acetate   *6*, 157 (1974); *21*, 417 (1979) (*corr. 42*,
                                             259); *Suppl. 7*, 289 (1987)
Megestrol acetate (*see* also Progestins; Combined oral
   contraceptives)
MeIQ   *40*, 275 (1986); *Suppl. 7*, 65 (1987);
                                             56, 197 (1993)
MeIQx   *40*, 283 (1986); *Suppl. 7*, 65 (1987)
                                             56, 211 (1993)
Melamine   *39*, 333 (1986); *Suppl. 7*, 65 (1987)
Melphalan   *9*, 167 (1975); *Suppl. 7*, 239 (1987)
6-Mercaptopurine   *26*, 249 (1981); *Suppl. 7*, 240 (1987)
Merphalan   *9*, 169 (1975); *Suppl. 7*, 65 (1987)

Mestranol (see also Steroidal oestrogens)   6, 87 (1974); 21, 257 (1979) (corr. 42, 259)

Metabisulfites (see Sulfur dioxide and some sulfites, bisulfites and metabisulfites)

Methanearsonic acid, disodium salt (see Arsenic and arsenic compounds)

Methanearsonic acid, monosodium salt (see Arsenic and arsenic compounds

Methotrexate   26, 267 (1981); Suppl. 7, 241 (1987)

Methoxsalen (see 8-Methoxypsoralen)

Methoxychlor   5, 193 (1974); 20, 259 (1979); Suppl. 7, 66 (1987)

Methoxyflurane (see Anaesthetics, volatile)

5-Methoxypsoralen   40, 327 (1986); Suppl. 7, 242 (1987)

8-Methoxypsoralen (see also 8-Methoxypsoralen plus ultraviolet radiation)   24, 101 (1980)

8-Methoxypsoralen plus ultraviolet radiation   Suppl. 7, 243 (1987)

Methyl acrylate   19, 52 (1979); 39, 99 (1986); Suppl. 7, 66 (1987)

5-Methylangelicin plus ultraviolet radiation (see also Angelicin and some synthetic derivatives)   Suppl. 7, 57 (1987)

2-Methylaziridine   9, 61 (1975); Suppl. 7, 66 (1987)

Methylazoxymethanol acetate   1, 164 (1972); 10, 131 (1976); Suppl. 7, 66 (1987)

Methyl bromide   41, 187 (1986) (corr. 45, 283); Suppl. 7, 245 (1987)

Methyl carbamate   12, 151 (1976); Suppl. 7, 66 (1987)

Methyl-CCNU [see 1-(2-Chloroethyl)-3-(4-methylcyclohexyl)-1-nitrosourea]

Methyl chloride   41, 161 (1986); Suppl. 7, 246 (1987)

1-, 2-, 3-, 4-, 5- and 6-Methylchrysenes   32, 379 (1983); Suppl. 7, 66 (1987)

N-Methyl-N,4-dinitrosoaniline   1, 141 (1972); Suppl. 7, 66 (1987)

4,4'-Methylene bis(2-chloroaniline)   4, 65 (1974) (corr. 42, 252); Suppl. 7, 246 (1987); 57, 271 (1993)

4,4'-Methylene bis(N,N-dimethyl)benzenamine   27, 119 (1982); Suppl. 7, 66 (1987)

4,4'-Methylene bis(2-methylaniline)   4, 73 (1974); Suppl. 7, 248 (1987)

4,4'-Methylenedianiline   4, 79 (1974) (corr. 42, 252); 39, 347 (1986); Suppl. 7, 66 (1987)

4,4'-Methylenediphenyl diisocyanate   19, 314 (1979); Suppl. 7, 66 (1987)

2-Methylfluoranthene   32, 399 (1983); Suppl. 7, 66 (1987)

3-Methylfluoranthene   32, 399 (1983); Suppl. 7, 66 (1987)

Methylglyoxal   51, 443 (1991)

Methyl iodide   15, 245 (1977); 41, 213 (1986); Suppl. 7, 66 (1987)

Methyl methacrylate   19, 187 (1979); Suppl. 7, 66 (1987)

Methyl methanesulfonate   7, 253 (1974); Suppl. 7, 66 (1987)

2-Methyl-1-nitroanthraquinone   27, 205 (1982); Suppl. 7, 66 (1987)

N-Methyl-N'-nitro-N-nitrosoguanidine   4, 183 (1974); Suppl. 7, 248 (1987)

3-Methylnitrosaminopropionaldehyde [see 3-(N-Nitrosomethylamino)-propionaldehyde]

3-Methylnitrosaminopropionitrile [see 3-(N-Nitrosomethylamino)-propionitrile]

4-(Methylnitrosamino)-4-(3-pyridyl)-1-butanal [*see* 4-(*N*-Nitrosomethyl-amino)-4-(3-pyridyl)-1-butanal]

4-(Methylnitrosamino)-1-(3-pyridyl)-1-butanone [*see* 4-(*N*-Nitrosomethyl-amino)-1-(3-pyridyl)-1-butanone]

N-Methyl-*N*-nitrosourea	*1*, 125 (1972); *17*, 227 (1978); *Suppl. 7*, 66 (1987)
N-Methyl-*N*-nitrosourethane	*4*, 211 (1974); *Suppl. 7*, 66 (1987)
Methyl parathion	*30*, 131 (1983); *Suppl. 7*, 392 (1987)
1-Methylphenanthrene	*32*, 405 (1983); *Suppl. 7*, 66 (1987)
7-Methylpyrido[3,4-*c*]psoralen	*40*, 349 (1986); *Suppl. 7*, 71 (1987)
Methyl red	*8*, 161 (1975); *Suppl. 7*, 66 (1987)
Methyl selenac (*see also* Selenium and selenium compounds)	*12*, 161 (1976); *Suppl. 7*, 66 (1987)
Methylthiouracil	*7*, 53 (1974); *Suppl. 7*, 66 (1987)
Metronidazole	*13*, 113 (1977); *Suppl. 7*, 250 (1987)
Mineral oils	*3*, 30 (1973); *33*, 87 (1984) (*corr. 42*, 262); *Suppl. 7*, 252 (1987)
Mirex	*5*, 203 (1974); *20*, 283 (1979) (*corr. 42*, 258); *Suppl. 7*, 66 (1987)
Mitomycin C	*10*, 171 (1976); *Suppl. 7*, 67 (1987)
MNNG [*see* *N*-Methyl-*N'*-nitro-*N*-nitrosoguanidine]	
MOCA [*see* 4,4'-Methylene bis(2-chloroaniline)]	
Modacrylic fibres	*19*, 86 (1979); *Suppl. 7*, 67 (1987)
Monocrotaline	*10*, 291 (1976); *Suppl. 7*, 67 (1987)
Monuron	*12*, 167 (1976); *Suppl. 7*, 67 (1987); *53*, 467 (1991)
MOPP and other combined chemotherapy including alkylating agents	*Suppl. 7*, 254 (1987)
Morpholine	*47*, 199 (1989)
5-(Morpholinomethyl)-3-[(5-nitrofurfurylidene)amino]-2-oxazolidinone	*7*, 161 (1974); *Suppl. 7*, 67 (1987)
Mustard gas	*9*, 181 (1975) (*corr. 42*, 254); *Suppl. 7*, 259 (1987)

Myleran (*see* 1,4-Butanediol dimethanesulfonate)

N

Nafenopin	*24*, 125 (1980); *Suppl. 7*, 67 (1987)
1,5-Naphthalenediamine	*27*, 127 (1982); *Suppl. 7*, 67 (1987)
1,5-Naphthalene diisocyanate	*19*, 311 (1979); *Suppl. 7*, 67 (1987)
1-Naphthylamine	*4*, 87 (1974) (*corr. 42*, 253); *Suppl. 7*, 260 (1987)
2-Naphthylamine	*4*, 97 (1974); *Suppl. 7*, 261 (1987)
1-Naphthylthiourea	*30*, 347 (1983); *Suppl. 7*, 263 (1987)
Nickel acetate (*see* Nickel and nickel compounds)	
Nickel ammonium sulfate (*see* Nickel and nickel compounds)	
Nickel and nickel compounds	*2*, 126 (1973) (*corr. 42*, 252); *11*, 75 (1976); *Suppl. 7*, 264 (1987) (*corr. 45*, 283); *49*, 257 (1990)

Nickel carbonate (*see* Nickel and nickel compounds)
Nickel carbonyl (*see* Nickel and nickel compounds)
Nickel chloride (*see* Nickel and nickel compounds)
Nickel–gallium alloy (*see* Nickel and nickel compounds)

Nickel hydroxide (*see* Nickel and nickel compounds)
Nickelocene (*see* Nickel and nickel compounds)
Nickel oxide (*see* Nickel and nickel compounds)
Nickel subsulfide (*see* Nickel and nickel compounds)
Nickel sulfate (*see* Nickel and nickel compounds)

Niridazole	*13*, 123 (1977); *Suppl. 7*, 67 (1987)
Nithiazide	*31*, 179 (1983); *Suppl. 7*, 67 (1987)
Nitrilotriacetic acid and its salts	*48*, 181 (1990)
5-Nitroacenaphthene	*16*, 319 (1978); *Suppl. 7*, 67 (1987)
5-Nitro-*ortho*-anisidine	*27*, 133 (1982); *Suppl. 7*, 67 (1987)
9-Nitroanthracene	*33*, 179 (1984); *Suppl. 7*, 67 (1987)
7-Nitrobenz[*a*]anthracene	*46*, 247 (1989)
6-Nitrobenzo[*a*]pyrene	*33*, 187 (1984); *Suppl. 7*, 67 (1987); *46*, 255 (1989)
4-Nitrobiphenyl	*4*, 113 (1974); *Suppl. 7*, 67 (1987)
6-Nitrochrysene	*33*, 195 (1984); *Suppl. 7*, 67 (1987); *46*, 267 (1989)
Nitrofen (technical-grade)	*30*, 271 (1983); *Suppl. 7*, 67 (1987)
3-Nitrofluoranthene	*33*, 201 (1984); *Suppl. 7*, 67 (1987)
2-Nitrofluorene	*46*, 277 (1989)
Nitrofural	*7*, 171 (1974); *Suppl. 7*, 67 (1987); *50*, 195 (1990)

5-Nitro-2-furaldehyde semicarbazone (*see* Nitrofural)

Nitrofurantoin	*50*, 211 (1990)

Nitrofurazone (*see* Nitrofural)

1-[(5-Nitrofurfurylidene)amino]-2-imidazolidinone	*7*, 181 (1974); *Suppl. 7*, 67 (1987)
N-[4-(5-Nitro-2-furyl)-2-thiazolyl]acetamide	*1*, 181 (1972); *7*, 185 (1974); *Suppl. 7*, 67 (1987)
Nitrogen mustard	*9*, 193 (1975); *Suppl. 7*, 269 (1987)
Nitrogen mustard *N*-oxide	*9*, 209 (1975); *Suppl. 7*, 67 (1987)
1-Nitronaphthalene	*46*, 291 (1989)
2-Nitronaphthalene	*46*, 303 (1989)
3-Nitroperylene	*46*, 313 (1989)

2-Nitro-*para*-phenylenediamine (*see* 1,4-Diamino-2-nitrobenzene)

2-Nitropropane	*29*, 331 (1982); *Suppl. 7*, 67 (1987)
1-Nitropyrene	*33*, 209 (1984); *Suppl. 7*, 67 (1987); *46*, 321 (1989)
2-Nitropyrene	*46*, 359 (1989)
4-Nitropyrene	*46*, 367 (1989)
N-Nitrosatable drugs	*24*, 297 (1980) (*corr. 42*, 260)
N-Nitrosatable pesticides	*30*, 359 (1983)
N'-Nitrosoanabasine	*37*, 225 (1985); *Suppl. 7*, 67 (1987)
N'-Nitrosoanatabine	*37*, 233 (1985); *Suppl. 7*, 67 (1987)
N-Nitrosodi-*n*-butylamine	*4*, 197 (1974); *17*, 51 (1978); *Suppl. 7*, 67 (1987)
N-Nitrosodiethanolamine	*17*, 77 (1978); *Suppl. 7*, 67 (1987)
N-Nitrosodiethylamine	*1*, 107 (1972) (*corr. 42*, 251); *17*, 83 (1978) (*corr. 42*, 257); *Suppl. 7*, 67 (1987)
N-Nitrosodimethylamine	*1*, 95 (1972); *17*, 125 (1978) (*corr. 42*, 257); *Suppl. 7*, 67 (1987)
N-Nitrosodiphenylamine	*27*, 213 (1982); *Suppl. 7*, 67 (1987)

O

Oestrogen–progestin combinations (*see* Oestrogens, progestins
  and combinations)
Oestrogen–progestin replacement therapy (*see also* Oestrogens,   *Suppl. 7*, 308 (1987)
  progestins and combinations)
Oestrogen replacement therapy (*see also* Oestrogens, progestins   *Suppl. 7*, 280 (1987)
  and combinations)
Oestrogens (*see* Oestrogens, progestins and combinations)
Oestrogens, conjugated (*see* Conjugated oestrogens)
Oestrogens, nonsteroidal (*see* Nonsteroidal oestrogens)
Oestrogens, progestins and combinations   *6* (1974); *21* (1979);
                                       Suppl. 7, 272 (1987)
Oestrogens, steroidal (*see* Steroidal oestrogens)
Oestrone (*see also* Steroidal oestrogens)   *6*, 123 (1974); *21*, 343 (1979)
                                       (*corr. 42*, 259)
Oestrone benzoate (*see* Oestrone)
Oil Orange SS   *8*, 165 (1975); *Suppl. 7*, 69 (1987)
Oral contraceptives, combined (*see* Combined oral contraceptives)
Oral contraceptives, investigational (*see* Combined oral
  contraceptives)
Oral contraceptives, sequential (*see* Sequential oral contraceptives)
Orange I   *8*, 173 (1975); *Suppl. 7*, 69 (1987)
Orange G   *8*, 181 (1975); *Suppl. 7*, 69 (1987)
Organolead compounds (*see also* Lead and lead compounds)   *Suppl. 7*, 230 (1987)
Oxazepam   *13*, 58 (1977); *Suppl. 7*, 69 (1987)
Oxymetholone [*see also* Androgenic (anabolic) steroids]   *13*, 131 (1977)
Oxyphenbutazone   *13*, 185 (1977); *Suppl. 7*, 69 (1987)

P

Paint manufacture and painting (occupational exposures in)   *47*, 329 (1989)
Panfuran S (*see also* Dihydroxymethylfuratrizine)   *24*, 77 (1980); *Suppl. 7*, 69 (1987)
Paper manufacture (*see* Pulp and paper manufacture)
Paracetamol   *50*, 307 (1990)
Parasorbic acid   *10*, 199 (1976) (*corr. 42*, 255);
                                       Suppl. 7, 69 (1987)
Parathion   *30*, 153 (1983); *Suppl. 7*, 69 (1987)
Patulin   *10*, 205 (1976); *40*, 83 (1986);
                                       Suppl. 7, 69 (1987)
Penicillic acid   *10*, 211 (1976); *Suppl. 7*, 69 (1987)
Pentachloroethane   *41*, 99 (1986); *Suppl. 7*, 69 (1987)
Pentachloronitrobenzene (*see* Quintozene)
Pentachlorophenol (*see also* Chlorophenols; Chlorophenols,   *20*, 303 (1979); *53*, 371 (1991)
  occupational exposures to)
Permethrin   *53*, 329 (1991)
Perylene   *32*, 411 (1983); *Suppl. 7*, 69 (1987)
Petasitenine   *31*, 207 (1983); *Suppl. 7*, 69 (1987)
Petasites japonicus (*see* Pyrrolizidine alkaloids)
Petroleum refining (occupational exposures in)   *45*, 39 (1989)
Some petroleum solvents   *47*, 43 (1989)
Phenacetin   *13*, 141 (1977); *24*, 135 (1980);
                                       Suppl. 7, 310 (1987)
Phenanthrene   *32*, 419 (1983); *Suppl. 7*, 69 (1987)

Prednimustine   *50*, 115 (1990)
Prednisone   *26*, 293 (1981); *Suppl. 7*, 326 (1987)
Procarbazine hydrochloride   *26*, 311 (1981); *Suppl. 7*, 327 (1987)
Proflavine salts   *24*, 195 (1980); *Suppl. 7*, 70 (1987)
Progesterone (*see also* Progestins; Combined oral contraceptives) *6*, 135 (1974); *21*, 491 (1979) (*corr. 42*, 259)

Progestins (*see also* Oestrogens, progestins and combinations)   *Suppl. 7*, 289 (1987)
Pronetalol hydrochloride   *13*, 227 (1977) (*corr. 42*, 256); *Suppl. 7*, 70 (1987)

1,3-Propane sultone   *4*, 253 (1974) (*corr. 42*, 253); *Suppl. 7*, 70 (1987)

Propham   *12*, 189 (1976); *Suppl. 7*, 70 (1987)
β-Propiolactone   *4*, 259 (1974) (*corr. 42*, 253); *Suppl. 7*, 70 (1987)

n-Propyl carbamate   *12*, 201 (1976); *Suppl. 7*, 70 (1987)
Propylene   *19*, 213 (1979); *Suppl. 7*, 71 (1987)
Propylene oxide   *11*, 191 (1976); *36*, 227 (1985) (*corr. 42*, 263); *Suppl. 7*, 328 (1987)
Propylthiouracil   *7*, 67 (1974); *Suppl. 7*, 329 (1987)
Ptaquiloside (*see also* Bracken fern)   *40*, 55 (1986); *Suppl. 7*, 71 (1987)
Pulp and paper manufacture   *25*, 157 (1981); *Suppl. 7*, 385 (1987)
Pyrene   *32*, 431 (1983); *Suppl. 7*, 71 (1987)
Pyrido[3,4-*c*]psoralen   *40*, 349 (1986); *Suppl. 7*, 71 (1987)
Pyrimethamine   *13*, 233 (1977); *Suppl. 7*, 71 (1987)
Pyrrolizidine alkaloids (*see* Hydroxysenkirkine; Isatidine; Jacobine; Lasiocarpine; Monocrotaline; Retrorsine; Riddelliine; Seneciphylline; Senkirkine)

Q

Quercetin (*see also* Bracken fern)   *31*, 213 (1983); *Suppl. 7*, 71 (1987)
para-Quinone   *15*, 255 (1977); *Suppl. 7*, 71 (1987)
Quintozene   *5*, 211 (1974); *Suppl. 7*, 71 (1987)

R

Radon   *43*, 173 (1988) (*corr. 45*, 283)
Reserpine   *10*, 217 (1976); *24*, 211 (1980) (*corr. 42*, 260); *Suppl. 7*, 330 (1987)
Resorcinol   *15*, 155 (1977); *Suppl. 7*, 71 (1987)
Retrorsine   *10*, 303 (1976); *Suppl. 7*, 71 (1987)
Rhodamine B   *16*, 221 (1978); *Suppl. 7*, 71 (1987)
Rhodamine 6G   *16*, 233 (1978); *Suppl. 7*, 71 (1987)
Riddelliine   *10*, 313 (1976); *Suppl. 7*, 71 (1987)
Rifampicin   *24*, 243 (1980); *Suppl. 7*, 71 (1987)
Rockwool (*see* Man-made mineral fibres)
The rubber industry   *28* (1982) (*corr. 42*, 261); *Suppl. 7*, 332 (1987)
Rugulosin   *40*, 99 (1986); *Suppl. 7*, 71 (1987)

S

Saccharated iron oxide   *2*, 161 (1973); *Suppl. 7*, 71 (1987)

Steel founding (*see* Iron and steel founding)

Sterigmatocystin — *1*, 175 (1972); *10*, 245 (1976); *Suppl. 7*, 72 (1987)

Steroidal oestrogens (*see also* Oestrogens, progestins and combinations) — *Suppl. 7*, 280 (1987)

Streptozotocin — *4*, 221 (1974); *17*, 337 (1978); *Suppl. 7*, 72 (1987)

Strobane® (*see* Terpene polychlorinates)

Strontium chromate (*see* Chromium and chromium compounds)

Styrene — *19*, 231 (1979) (*corr. 42*, 258); *Suppl. 7*, 345 (1987)

Styrene-acrylonitrile copolymers — *19*, 97 (1979); *Suppl. 7*, 72 (1987)

Styrene-butadiene copolymers — *19*, 252 (1979); *Suppl. 7*, 72 (1987)

Styrene oxide — *11*, 201 (1976); *19*, 275 (1979); *36*, 245 (1985); *Suppl. 7*, 72 (1987)

Succinic anhydride — *15*, 265 (1977); *Suppl. 7*, 72 (1987)

Sudan I — *8*, 225 (1975); *Suppl. 7*, 72 (1987)

Sudan II — *8*, 233 (1975); *Suppl. 7*, 72 (1987)

Sudan III — *8*, 241 (1975); *Suppl. 7*, 72 (1987)

Sudan Brown RR — *8*, 249 (1975); *Suppl. 7*, 72 (1987)

Sudan Red 7B — *8*, 253 (1975); *Suppl. 7*, 72 (1987)

Sulfafurazole — *24*, 275 (1980); *Suppl. 7*, 347 (1987)

Sulfallate — *30*, 283 (1983); *Suppl. 7*, 72 (1987)

Sulfamethoxazole — *24*, 285 (1980); *Suppl. 7*, 348 (1987)

Sulfites (*see* Sulfur dioxide and some sulfites, bisulfites and metabisulfites)

Sulfur dioxide and some sulfites, bisulfites and metabisulfites — *54*, 131 (1992)

Sulfur mustard (*see* Mustard gas)

Sulfuric acid and other strong inorganic acids, occupational exposures to mists and vapours from — *54*, 41 (1992)

Sulfur trioxide — *54*, 121 (1992)

Sulphisoxazole (*see* Sulfafurazole)

Sunset Yellow FCF — *8*, 257 (1975); *Suppl. 7*, 72 (1987)

Symphytine — *31*, 239 (1983); *Suppl. 7*, 72 (1987)

T

2,4,5-T (*see also* Chlorophenoxy herbicides; Chlorophenoxy herbicides, occupational exposures to) — *15*, 273 (1977)

Talc — *42*, 185 (1987); *Suppl. 7*, 349 (1987)

Tannic acid — *10*, 253 (1976) (*corr. 42*, 255); *Suppl. 7*, 72 (1987)

Tannins (*see also* Tannic acid) — *10*, 254 (1976); *Suppl. 7*, 72 (1987)

TCDD (*see* 2,3,7,8-Tetrachlorodibenzo-*para*-dioxin)

TDE (*see* DDT)

Tea — *51*, 207 (1991)

Terpene polychlorinates — *5*, 219 (1974); *Suppl. 7*, 72 (1987)

Testosterone (*see also* Androgenic (anabolic) steroids) — *6*, 209 (1974); *21*, 519 (1979)

Testosterone oenanthate (*see* Testosterone)

Testosterone propionate (*see* Testosterone)

2,2′,5,5′-Tetrachlorobenzidine — *27*, 141 (1982); *Suppl. 7*, 72 (1987)

2,3,7,8-Tetrachlorodibenzo-*para*-dioxin — *15*, 41 (1977); *Suppl. 7*, 350 (1987)

1,1,1,2-Tetrachloroethane — *41*, 87 (1986); *Suppl. 7*, 72 (1987)

1,1,2,2-Tetrachloroethane	*20*, 477 (1979); *Suppl. 7*, 354 (1987)
Tetrachloroethylene	*20*, 491 (1979); *Suppl. 7*, 355 (1987)
2,3,4,6-Tetrachlorophenol (*see* Chlorophenols; Chlorophenols, occupational exposures to)	
Tetrachlorvinphos	*30*, 197 (1983); *Suppl. 7*, 72 (1987)
Tetraethyllead (*see* Lead and lead compounds)	
Tetrafluoroethylene	*19*, 285 (1979); *Suppl. 7*, 72 (1987)
Tetrakis(hydroxymethyl) phosphonium salts	*48*, 95 (1990)
Tetramethyllead (*see* Lead and lead compounds)	
Textile manufacturing industry, exposures in	*48*, 215 (1990) (*corr. 51*, 483)
Theobromine	*51*, 421 (1991)
Theophylline	*51*, 391 (1991)
Thioacetamide	*7*, 77 (1974); *Suppl. 7*, 72 (1987)
4,4'-Thiodianiline	*16*, 343 (1978); *27*, 147 (1982); *Suppl. 7*, 72 (1987)
Thiotepa	*9*, 85 (1975); *Suppl. 7*, 368 (1987); *50*, 123 (1990)
Thiouracil	*7*, 85 (1974); *Suppl. 7*, 72 (1987)
Thiourea	*7*, 95 (1974); *Suppl. 7*, 72 (1987)
Thiram	*12*, 225 (1976); *Suppl. 7*, 72 (1987); *53*, 403 (1991)
Titanium dioxide	*47*, 307 (1989)
Tobacco habits other than smoking (*see* Tobacco products, smokeless)	
Tobacco products, smokeless	*37* (1985) (*corr. 42*, 263; *52*, 513); *Suppl. 7*, 357 (1987)
Tobacco smoke	*38* (1986) (*corr. 42*, 263); *Suppl. 7*, 357 (1987)
Tobacco smoking (*see* Tobacco smoke)	
ortho-Tolidine (*see* 3,3'-Dimethylbenzidine)	
2,4-Toluene diisocyanate (*see also* Toluene diisocyanates)	*19*, 303 (1979); *39*, 287 (1986)
2,6-Toluene diisocyanate (*see also* Toluene diisocyanates)	*19*, 303 (1979); *39*, 289 (1986)
Toluene	*47*, 79 (1989)
Toluene diisocyanates	*39*, 287 (1986) (*corr. 42*, 264); *Suppl. 7*, 72 (1987)
Toluenes, α-chlorinated (*see* α-Chlorinated toluenes)	
ortho-Toluenesulfonamide (*see* Saccharin)	
ortho-Toluidine	*16*, 349 (1978); *27*, 155 (1982); *Suppl. 7*, 362 (1987)
Toxaphene	*20*, 327 (1979); *Suppl. 7*, 72 (1987)
T-2 Toxin (*see* Toxins derived from *Fusarium sporotrichioides*)	
Toxins derived from *Fusarium graminearum*, *F. culmorum* and *F. crookwellense*	*11*, 169 (1976); *31*, 153, 279 (1983); *Suppl. 7*, 64, 74 (1987); *56*, 397 (1993)
Toxins derived from *Fusarium moniliforme*	*56*, 445 (1993)
Toxins derived from *Fusarium sporotrichioides*	*31*, 265 (1983); *Suppl. 7*, 73 (1987); *56*, 467 (1993)
Tremolite (*see* Asbestos)	
Treosulfan	*26*, 341 (1981); *Suppl. 7*, 363 (1987)
Triaziquone [*see* Tris(aziridinyl)-*para*-benzoquinone]	
Trichlorfon	*30*, 207 (1983); *Suppl. 7*, 73 (1987)
Trichlormethine	*9*, 229 (1975); *Suppl. 7*, 73 (1987); *50*, 143 (1990)

Trichloroacetonitrile (*see* Halogenated acetonitriles)
1,1,1-Trichloroethane   *20*, 515 (1979); *Suppl. 7*, 73 (1987)
1,1,2-Trichloroethane   *20*, 533 (1979); *Suppl. 7*, 73 (1987);
                                                                  52, 337 (1991)
Trichloroethylene   *11*, 263 (1976); *20*, 545 (1979);
                                                                  Suppl. 7, 364 (1987)
2,4,5-Trichlorophenol (*see also* Chlorophenols; Chlorophenols   *20*, 349 (1979)
    occupational exposures to)
2,4,6-Trichlorophenol (*see also* Chlorophenols; Chlorophenols,   *20*, 349 (1979)
    occupational exposures to)
(2,4,5-Trichlorophenoxy)acetic acid (*see* 2,4,5-T)
Trichlorotriethylamine hydrochloride (*see* Trichlormethine)
T$_2$-Trichothecene (*see* Toxins derived from *Fusarium sporotrichioides*)
Triethylene glycol diglycidyl ether   *11*, 209 (1976); *Suppl. 7*, 73 (1987)
Trifluralin   *53*, 515 (1991)
4,4′,6-Trimethylangelicin plus ultraviolet radiation (*see also*   *Suppl. 7*, 57 (1987)
    Angelicin and some synthetic derivatives)
2,4,5-Trimethylaniline   *27*, 177 (1982); *Suppl. 7*, 73 (1987)
2,4,6-Trimethylaniline   *27*, 178 (1982); *Suppl. 7*, 73 (1987)
4,5′,8-Trimethylpsoralen   *40*, 357 (1986); *Suppl. 7*, 366 (1987)
Trimustine hydrochloride (*see* Trichlormethine)
Triphenylene   *32*, 447 (1983); *Suppl. 7*, 73 (1987)
Tris(aziridinyl)-*para*-benzoquinone   *9*, 67 (1975); *Suppl. 7*, 367 (1987)
Tris(1-aziridinyl)phosphine oxide   *9*, 75 (1975); *Suppl. 7*, 73 (1987)
Tris(1-aziridinyl)phosphine sulphide (*see* Thiotepa)
2,4,6-Tris(1-aziridinyl)-*s*-triazine   *9*, 95 (1975); *Suppl. 7*, 73 (1987)
Tris(2-chloroethyl) phosphate   *48*, 109 (1990)
1,2,3-Tris(chloromethoxy)propane   *15*, 301 (1977); *Suppl. 7*, 73 (1987)
Tris(2,3-dibromopropyl)phosphate   *20*, 575 (1979); *Suppl. 7*, 369 (1987)
Tris(2-methyl-1-aziridinyl)phosphine oxide   *9*, 107 (1975); *Suppl. 7*, 73 (1987)
Trp-P-1   *31*, 247 (1983); *Suppl. 7*, 73 (1987)
Trp-P-2   *31*, 255 (1983); *Suppl. 7*, 73 (1987)
Trypan blue   *8*, 267 (1975); *Suppl. 7*, 73 (1987)
Tussilago farfara L. (*see* Pyrrolizidine alkaloids)

U

Ultraviolet radiation   *40*, 379 (1986); *55* (1992)
Underground haematite mining with exposure to radon   *1*, 29 (1972); *Suppl. 7*, 216 (1987)
Uracil mustard   *9*, 235 (1975); *Suppl. 7*, 370 (1987)
Urethane   *7*, 111 (1974); *Suppl. 7*, 73 (1987)

V

Vat Yellow 4   *48*, 161 (1990)
Vinblastine sulfate   *26*, 349 (1981) (*corr. 42*, 261);
                                                                  Suppl. 7, 371 (1987)
Vincristine sulfate   *26*, 365 (1981); *Suppl. 7*, 372 (1987)
Vinyl acetate   *19*, 341 (1979); *39*, 113 (1986);
                                                                  Suppl. 7, 73 (1987)
Vinyl bromide   *19*, 367 (1979); *39*, 133 (1986);
                                                                  Suppl. 7, 73 (1987)

PUBLICATIONS OF THE
INTERNATIONAL AGENCY FOR RESEARCH ON CANCER
Scientific Publications Series

(Available from Oxford University Press through local bookshops)

No. 1 Liver Cancer
1971; 176 pages (*out of print*)

No. 2 Oncogenesis and Herpesviruses
Edited by P.M. Biggs, G. de-Thé and L.N. Payne
1972; 515 pages (*out of print*)

No. 3 N-Nitroso Compounds: Analysis and Formation
Edited by P. Bogovski, R. Preussman and E.A. Walker
1972; 140 pages (*out of print*)

No. 4 Transplacental Carcinogenesis
Edited by L. Tomatis and U. Mohr
1973; 181 pages (*out of print*)

No. 5/6 Pathology of Tumours in Laboratory Animals, Volume 1, Tumours of the Rat
Edited by V.S. Turusov
1973/1976; 533 pages (*out of print*)

No. 7 Host Environment Interactions in the Etiology of Cancer in Man
Edited by R. Doll and I. Vodopija
1973; 464 pages (*out of print*)

No. 8 Biological Effects of Asbestos
Edited by P. Bogovski, J.C. Gilson, V. Timbrell and J.C. Wagner
1973; 346 pages (*out of print*)

No. 9 N-Nitroso Compounds in the Environment
Edited by P. Bogovski and E.A. Walker
1974; 243 pages (*out of print*)

No. 10 Chemical Carcinogenesis Essays
Edited by R. Montesano and L. Tomatis
1974; 230 pages (*out of print*)

No. 11 Oncogenesis and Herpesviruses II
Edited by G. de-Thé, M.A. Epstein and H. zur Hausen
1975; Part I: 511 pages
Part II: 403 pages (*out of print*)

No. 12 Screening Tests in Chemical Carcinogenesis
Edited by R. Montesano, H. Bartsch and L. Tomatis
1976; 666 pages (*out of print*)

No. 13 Environmental Pollution and Carcinogenic Risks
Edited by C. Rosenfeld and W. Davis
1975; 441 pages (*out of print*)

No. 14 Environmental N-Nitroso Compounds. Analysis and Formation
Edited by E.A. Walker, P. Bogovski and L. Griciute
1976; 512 pages (*out of print*)

No. 15 Cancer Incidence in Five Continents, Volume III
Edited by J.A.H. Waterhouse, C. Muir, P. Correa and J. Powell
1976; 584 pages (*out of print*)

No. 16 Air Pollution and Cancer in Man
Edited by U. Mohr, D. Schmähl and L. Tomatis
1977; 328 pages (*out of print*)

No. 17 Directory of On-going Research in Cancer Epidemiology 1977
Edited by C.S. Muir and G. Wagner
1977; 599 pages (*out of print*)

No. 18 Environmental Carcinogens. Selected Methods of Analysis. Volume 1: Analysis of Volatile Nitrosamines in Food
Editor-in-Chief: H. Egan
1978; 212 pages (*out of print*)

No. 19 Environmental Aspects of N-Nitroso Compounds
Edited by E.A. Walker, M. Castegnaro, L. Griciute and R.E. Lyle
1978; 561 pages (*out of print*)

No. 20 Nasopharyngeal Carcinoma: Etiology and Control
Edited by G. de-Thé and Y. Ito
1978; 606 pages (*out of print*)

No. 21 Cancer Registration and its Techniques
Edited by R. MacLennan, C. Muir, R. Steinitz and A. Winkler
1978; 235 pages (*out of print*)

No. 22 Environmental Carcinogens. Selected Methods of Analysis. Volume 2: Methods for the Measurement of Vinyl Chloride in Poly(vinyl chloride), Air, Water and Foodstuffs
Editor-in-Chief: H. Egan
1978; 142 pages (*out of print*)

No. 23 Pathology of Tumours in Laboratory Animals. Volume II: Tumours of the Mouse
Editor-in-Chief: V.S. Turusov
1979; 669 pages (*out of print*)

No. 24 Oncogenesis and Herpesviruses III
Edited by G. de-Thé, W. Henle and F. Rapp
1978; Part I: 580 pages, Part II: 512 pages (*out of print*)

List of IARC Publications

No. 25 Carcinogenic Risk. Strategies for Intervention
Edited by W. Davis and
C. Rosenfeld
1979; 280 pages (*out of print*)

No. 26 Directory of On-going Research in Cancer Epidemiology 1978
Edited by C.S. Muir and G. Wagner
1978; 550 pages (*out of print*)

No. 27 Molecular and Cellular Aspects of Carcinogen Screening Tests
Edited by R. Montesano,
H. Bartsch and L. Tomatis
1980; 372 pages £30.00

No. 28 Directory of On-going Research in Cancer Epidemiology 1979
Edited by C.S. Muir and G. Wagner
1979; 672 pages (*out of print*)

No. 29 Environmental Carcinogens. Selected Methods of Analysis. Volume 3: Analysis of Polycyclic Aromatic Hydrocarbons in Environmental Samples
Editor-in-Chief: H. Egan
1979; 240 pages (*out of print*)

No. 30 Biological Effects of Mineral Fibres
Editor-in-Chief: J.C. Wagner
1980; **Volume 1:** 494 pages **Volume 2:** 513 pages (*out of print*)

No. 31 N-Nitroso Compounds: Analysis, Formation and Occurrence
Edited by E.A. Walker, L. Griciute,
M. Castegnaro and M. Börzsönyi
1980; 835 pages (*out of print*)

No. 32 Statistical Methods in Cancer Research. Volume 1. The Analysis of Case-control Studies
By N.E. Breslow and N.E. Day
1980; 338 pages £18.00

No. 33 Handling Chemical Carcinogens in the Laboratory
Edited by R. Montesano *et al.*
1979; 32 pages (*out of print*)

No. 34 Pathology of Tumours in Laboratory Animals. Volume III. Tumours of the Hamster
Editor-in-Chief: V.S. Turusov
1982; 461 pages (*out of print*)

No. 35 Directory of On-going Research in Cancer Epidemiology 1980
Edited by C.S. Muir and G. Wagner
1980; 660 pages (*out of print*)

No. 36 Cancer Mortality by Occupation and Social Class 1851-1971
Edited by W.P.D. Logan
1982; 253 pages (*out of print*)

No. 37 Laboratory Decontamination and Destruction of Aflatoxins B_1, B_2, G_1, G_2 in Laboratory Wastes
Edited by M. Castegnaro *et al.*
1980; 56 pages (*out of print*)

No. 38 Directory of On-going Research in Cancer Epidemiology 1981
Edited by C.S. Muir and G. Wagner
1981; 696 pages (*out of print*)

No. 39 Host Factors in Human Carcinogenesis
Edited by H. Bartsch and
B. Armstrong
1982; 583 pages (*out of print*)

No. 40 Environmental Carcinogens. Selected Methods of Analysis. Volume 4: Some Aromatic Amines and Azo Dyes in the General and Industrial Environment
Edited by L. Fishbein,
M. Castegnaro, I.K. O'Neill and
H. Bartsch
1981; 347 pages (*out of print*)

No. 41 N-Nitroso Compounds: Occurrence and Biological Effects
Edited by H. Bartsch, I.K. O'Neill,
M. Castegnaro and M. Okada
1982; 755 pages £50.00

No. 42 Cancer Incidence in Five Continents, Volume IV
Edited by J. Waterhouse, C. Muir,
K. Shanmugaratnam and J. Powell
1982; 811 pages (*out of print*)

No. 43 Laboratory Decontamination and Destruction of Carcinogens in Laboratory Wastes: Some N-Nitrosamines
Edited by M. Castegnaro *et al.*
1982; 73 pages £7.50

No. 44 Environmental Carcinogens. Selected Methods of Analysis. Volume 5: Some Mycotoxins
Edited by L. Stoloff, M. Castegnaro,
P. Scott, I.K. O'Neill and H. Bartsch
1983; 455 pages £32.50

No. 45 Environmental Carcinogens. Selected Methods of Analysis. Volume 6: N-Nitroso Compounds
Edited by R. Preussmann, I.K.
O'Neill, G. Eisenbrand, B.
Spiegelhalder and H. Bartsch
1983; 508 pages £32.50

No. 46 Directory of On-going Research in Cancer Epidemiology 1982
Edited by C.S. Muir and G. Wagner
1982; 722 pages (*out of print*)

No. 47 Cancer Incidence in Singapore 1968–1977
Edited by K. Shanmugaratnam,
H.P. Lee and N.E. Day
1983; 171 pages (*out of print*)

No. 48 Cancer Incidence in the USSR (2nd Revised Edition)
Edited by N.P. Napalkov,
G.F. Tserkovny, V.M. Merabishvili,
D.M. Parkin, M. Smans and
C.S. Muir
1983; 75 pages (*out of print*)

No. 49 Laboratory Decontamination and Destruction of Carcinogens in Laboratory Wastes: Some Polycyclic Aromatic Hydrocarbons
Edited by M. Castegnaro *et al.*
1983; 87 pages (*out of print*)

No. 50 Directory of On-going Research in Cancer Epidemiology 1983
Edited by C.S. Muir and G. Wagner
1983; 731 pages (*out of print*)

No. 51 Modulators of Experimental Carcinogenesis
Edited by V. Turusov and R. Montesano
1983; 307 pages (*out of print*)

No. 52 **Second Cancers in Relation to Radiation Treatment for Cervical Cancer: Results of a Cancer Registry Collaboration**
Edited by N.E. Day and J.C. Boice, Jr
1984; 207 pages (*out of print*)

No. 53 **Nickel in the Human Environment**
Editor-in-Chief: F.W. Sunderman, Jr
1984; 529 pages (*out of print*)

No. 54 **Laboratory Decontamination and Destruction of Carcinogens in Laboratory Wastes: Some Hydrazines**
Edited by M. Castegnaro *et al.*
1983; 87 pages (*out of print*)

No. 55 **Laboratory Decontamination and Destruction of Carcinogens in Laboratory Wastes: Some N-Nitrosamides**
Edited by M. Castegnaro *et al.*
1984; 66 pages (*out of print*)

No. 56 **Models, Mechanisms and Etiology of Tumour Promotion**
Edited by M. Börzsönyi, N.E. Day, K. Lapis and H. Yamasaki
1984; 532 pages (*out of print*)

No. 57 **N-Nitroso Compounds: Occurrence, Biological Effects and Relevance to Human Cancer**
Edited by I.K. O'Neill, R.C. von Borstel, C.T. Miller, J. Long and H. Bartsch
1984; 1013 pages (*out of print*)

No. 58 **Age-related Factors in Carcinogenesis**
Edited by A. Likhachev, V. Anisimov and R. Montesano
1985; 288 pages (*out of print*)

No. 59 **Monitoring Human Exposure to Carcinogenic and Mutagenic Agents**
Edited by A. Berlin, M. Draper, K. Hemminki and H. Vainio
1984; 457 pages (*out of print*)

No. 60 **Burkitt's Lymphoma: A Human Cancer Model**
Edited by G. Lenoir, G. O'Conor and C.L.M. Olweny
1985; 484 pages (*out of print*)

No. 61 **Laboratory Decontamination and Destruction of Carcinogens in Laboratory Wastes: Some Haloethers**
Edited by M. Castegnaro *et al.*
1985; 55 pages (*out of print*)

No. 62 **Directory of On-going Research in Cancer Epidemiology 1984**
Edited by C.S. Muir and G. Wagner
1984; 717 pages (*out of print*)

No. 63 **Virus-associated Cancers in Africa**
Edited by A.O. Williams, G.T. O'Conor, G.B. de-Thé and C.A. Johnson
1984; 773 pages (*out of print*)

No. 64 **Laboratory Decontamination and Destruction of Carcinogens in Laboratory Wastes: Some Aromatic Amines and 4-Nitrobiphenyl**
Edited by M. Castegnaro *et al.*
1985; 84 pages (*out of print*)

No. 65 **Interpretation of Negative Epidemiological Evidence for Carcinogenicity**
Edited by N.J. Wald and R. Doll
1985; 232 pages (*out of print*)

No. 66 **The Role of the Registry in Cancer Control**
Edited by D.M. Parkin, G. Wagner and C.S. Muir
1985; 152 pages £10.00

No. 67 **Transformation Assay of Established Cell Lines: Mechanisms and Application**
Edited by T. Kakunaga and H. Yamasaki
1985; 225 pages (*out of print*)

No. 68 **Environmental Carcinogens. Selected Methods of Analysis. Volume 7. Some Volatile Halogenated Hydrocarbons**
Edited by L. Fishbein and I.K. O'Neill
1985; 479 pages (*out of print*)

No. 69 **Directory of On-going Research in Cancer Epidemiology 1985**
Edited by C.S. Muir and G. Wagner
1985; 745 pages (*out of print*)

No. 70 **The Role of Cyclic Nucleic Acid Adducts in Carcinogenesis and Mutagenesis**
Edited by B. Singer and H. Bartsch
1986; 467 pages (*out of print*)

No. 71 **Environmental Carcinogens. Selected Methods of Analysis. Volume 8: Some Metals: As, Be, Cd, Cr, Ni, Pb, Se, Zn**
Edited by I.K. O'Neill, P. Schuller and L. Fishbein
1986; 485 pages (*out of print*)

No. 72 **Atlas of Cancer in Scotland, 1975–1980. Incidence and Epidemiological Perspective**
Edited by I. Kemp, P. Boyle, M. Smans and C.S. Muir
1985; 285 pages (*out of print*)

No. 73 **Laboratory Decontamination and Destruction of Carcinogens in Laboratory Wastes: Some Antineoplastic Agents**
Edited by M. Castegnaro *et al.*
1985; 163 pages £12.50

No. 74 **Tobacco: A Major International Health Hazard**
Edited by D. Zaridze and R. Peto
1986; 324 pages £22.50

No. 75 **Cancer Occurrence in Developing Countries**
Edited by D.M. Parkin
1986; 339 pages £22.50

No. 76 **Screening for Cancer of the Uterine Cervix**
Edited by M. Hakama, A.B. Miller and N.E. Day
1986; 315 pages £30.00

No. 77 **Hexachlorobenzene: Proceedings of an International Symposium**
Edited by C.R. Morris and J.R.P. Cabral
1986; 668 pages (*out of print*)

No. 78 **Carcinogenicity of Alkylating Cytostatic Drugs**
Edited by D. Schmähl and J.M. Kaldor
1986; 337 pages (*out of print*)

No. 79 **Statistical Methods in Cancer Research. Volume III: The Design and Analysis of Long-term Animal Experiments**
By J.J. Gart, D. Krewski, P.N. Lee, R.E. Tarone and J. Wahrendorf
1986; 213 pages £22.00

No. 80 Directory of On-going Research in Cancer Epidemiology 1986
Edited by C.S. Muir and G. Wagner
1986; 805 pages (*out of print*)

No. 81 Environmental Carcinogens: Methods of Analysis and Exposure Measurement. Volume 9: Passive Smoking
Edited by I.K. O'Neill, K.D. Brunnemann, B. Dodet and D. Hoffmann
1987; 383 pages £35.00

No. 82 Statistical Methods in Cancer Research. Volume II: The Design and Analysis of Cohort Studies
By N.E. Breslow and N.E. Day
1987; 404 pages £35.00

No. 83 Long-term and Short-term Assays for Carcinogens: A Critical Appraisal
Edited by R. Montesano, H. Bartsch, H. Vainio, J. Wilbourn and H. Yamasaki
1986; 575 pages £35.00

No. 84 The Relevance of *N*-Nitroso Compounds to Human Cancer: Exposure and Mechanisms
Edited by H. Bartsch, I.K. O'Neill and R. Schulte-Hermann
1987; 671 pages (*out of print*)

No. 85 Environmental Carcinogens: Methods of Analysis and Exposure Measurement. Volume 10: Benzene and Alkylated Benzenes
Edited by L. Fishbein and I.K. O'Neill
1988; 327 pages £40.00

No. 86 Directory of On-going Research in Cancer Epidemiology 1987
Edited by D.M. Parkin and J. Wahrendorf
1987; 676 pages (*out of print*)

No. 87 International Incidence of Childhood Cancer
Edited by D.M. Parkin, C.A. Stiller, C.A. Bieber, G.J. Draper, B. Terracini and J.L. Young
1988; 401 pages £35.00

No. 88 Cancer Incidence in Five Continents Volume V
Edited by C. Muir, J. Waterhouse, T. Mack, J. Powell and S. Whelan
1987; 1004 pages £55.00

No. 89 Method for Detecting DNA Damaging Agents in Humans: Applications in Cancer Epidemiology and Prevention
Edited by H. Bartsch, K. Hemminki and I.K. O'Neill
1988; 518 pages £50.00

No. 90 Non-occupational Exposure to Mineral Fibres
Edited by J. Bignon, J. Peto and R. Saracci
1989; 500 pages £50.00

No. 91 Trends in Cancer Incidence in Singapore 1968–1982
Edited by H.P. Lee , N.E. Day and K. Shanmugaratnam
1988; 160 pages (*out of print*)

No. 92 Cell Differentiation, Genes and Cancer
Edited by T. Kakunaga, T. Sugimura, L. Tomatis and H. Yamasaki
1988; 204 pages £27.50

No. 93 Directory of On-going Research in Cancer Epidemiology 1988
Edited by M. Coleman and J. Wahrendorf
1988; 662 pages (*out of print*)

No. 94 Human Papillomavirus and Cervical Cancer
Edited by N. Muñoz, F.X. Bosch and O.M. Jensen
1989; 154 pages £22.50

No. 95 Cancer Registration: Principles and Methods
Edited by O.M. Jensen, D.M. Parkin, R. MacLennan, C.S. Muir and R. Skeet
1991; 288 pages £28.00

No. 96 Perinatal and Multigeneration Carcinogenesis
Edited by N.P. Napalkov, J.M. Rice, L. Tomatis and H. Yamasaki
1989; 436 pages £50.00

No. 97 Occupational Exposure to Silica and Cancer Risk
Edited by L. Simonato, A.C. Fletcher, R. Saracci and T. Thomas
1990; 124 pages £22.50

No. 98 Cancer Incidence in Jewish Migrants to Israel, 1961–1981
Edited by R. Steinitz, D.M. Parkin, J.L. Young, C.A. Bieber and L. Katz
1989; 320 pages £35.00

No. 99 Pathology of Tumours in Laboratory Animals, Second Edition, Volume 1, Tumours of the Rat
Edited by V.S. Turusov and U. Mohr
740 pages £85.00

No. 100 Cancer: Causes, Occurrence and Control
Editor-in-Chief L. Tomatis
1990; 352 pages £24.00

No. 101 Directory of On-going Research in Cancer Epidemiology 1989/90
Edited by M. Coleman and J. Wahrendorf
1989; 818 pages £36.00

No. 102 Patterns of Cancer in Five Continents
Edited by S.L. Whelan, D.M. Parkin & E. Masuyer
1990; 162 pages £25.00

No. 103 Evaluating Effectiveness of Primary Prevention of Cancer
Edited by M. Hakama, V. Beral, J.W. Cullen and D.M. Parkin
1990; 250 pages £32.00

No. 104 Complex Mixtures and. Cancer Risk
Edited by H. Vainio, M. Sorsa and A.J. McMichael
1990; 442 pages £38.00

No. 105 Relevance to Human Cancer of *N*-Nitroso Compounds, Tobacco Smoke and Mycotoxins
Edited by I.K. O'Neill, J. Chen and H. Bartsch
1991; 614 pages £70.00

No. 106 Atlas of Cancer Incidence in the Former German Democratic Republic
Edited by W.H. Mehnert, M. Smans, C.S. Muir, M. Möhner & D. Schön
1992; 384 pages £55.00

List of IARC Publications

No. 107 **Atlas of Cancer Mortality in the European Economic Community**
Edited by M. Smans, C.S. Muir and P. Boyle
1992; 280 pages £35.00

No. 108 **Environmental Carcinogens: Methods of Analysis and Exposure Measurement. Volume 11: Polychlorinated Dioxins and Dibenzofurans**
Edited by C. Rappe, H.R. Buser, B. Dodet and I.K. O'Neill
1991; 426 pages £45.00

No. 109 **Environmental Carcinogens: Methods of Analysis and Exposure Measurement. Volume 12: Indoor Air Contaminants**
Edited by B. Seifert, H. van de Wiel, B. Dodet and I.K. O'Neill
1993; 384 pages £45.00

No. 110 **Directory of On-going Research in Cancer Epidemiology 1991**
Edited by M. Coleman and J. Wahrendorf
1991; 753 pages £38.00

No. 111 **Pathology of Tumours in Laboratory Animals, Second Edition, Volume 2, Tumours of the Mouse**
Edited by V.S. Turusov and U. Mohr
Publ. due 1993; approx. 700 pages

No. 112 **Autopsy in Epidemiology and Medical Research**
Edited by E. Riboli and M. Delendi
1991; 288 pages £25.00

No. 113 **Laboratory Decontamination and Destruction of Carcinogens in Laboratory Wastes: Some Mycotoxins**
Edited by M. Castegnaro, J. Barek, J.-M. Frémy, M. Lafontaine, M. Miraglia, E.B. Sansone and G.M. Telling
1991; 64 pages £11.00

No. 114 **Laboratory Decontamination and Destruction of Carcinogens in Laboratory Wastes: Some Polycyclic Heterocyclic Hydrocarbons**
Edited by M. Castegnaro, J. Barek, J. Jacob, U. Kirso, M. Lafontaine, E.B. Sansone, G.M. Telling and T. Vu Duc
1991; 50 pages £8.00

No. 115 **Mycotoxins, Endemic Nephropathy and Urinary Tract Tumours**
Edited by M. Castegnaro, R. Plestina, G. Dirheimer, I.N. Chernozemsky and H Bartsch
1991; 340 pages £45.00

No. 116 **Mechanisms of Carcinogenesis in Risk Identification**
Edited by H. Vainio, P.N. Magee, D.B. McGregor & A.J. McMichael
1992; 616 pages £65.00

No. 117 **Directory of On-going Research in Cancer Epidemiology 1992**
Edited by M. Coleman, J. Wahrendorf & E. Démaret
1992; 773 pages £42.00

No. 118 **Cadmium in the Human Environment: Toxicity and Carcinogenicity**
Edited by G.F. Nordberg, R.F.M. Herber & L. Alessio
1992; 470 pages £60.00

No. 119 **The Epidemiology of Cervical Cancer and Human Papillomavirus**
Edited by N. Muñoz, F.X. Bosch, K.V. Shah & A. Meheus
1992; 288 pages £28.00

No. 120 **Cancer Incidence in Five Continents, Volume VI**
Edited by D.M. Parkin, C.S. Muir, S.L. Whelan, Y.T. Gao, J. Ferlay & J.Powell
1992; 1080 pages £120.00

No. 121 **Trends in Cancer Incidence and Mortality**
Edited by M. Coleman, J. Estève and P. Damiecki
1993; approx. 800 pages, approx £95.00

No. 122 **International Classification of Rodent Tumours. Part 1. The Rat**
Editor-in-Chief: U. Möhr
1992/93; 10 fascicles of 60–100 pages, £120.00

No. 123 **Cancer in Italian Migrant Populations**
Edited by M. Geddes, D.M. Parkin, M. Khlat, D. Balzi and E. Buiatti
1993; 292 pages, £40.00

No. 124 **Postlabelling Methods for Detection of DNA Adducts**
Edited by D.H. Phillips, M. Castegnaro and H. Bartsch
1993; 392 pages; £46.00

IARC MONOGRAPHS ON THE EVALUATION OF CARCINOGENIC RISKS TO HUMANS

(Available from booksellers through the network of WHO Sales Agents)

Volume 1 **Some Inorganic Substances, Chlorinated Hydrocarbons, Aromatic Amines, N-Nitroso Compounds, and Natural Products**
1972; 184 pages (*out of print*)

Volume 2 **Some Inorganic and Organometallic Compounds**
1973; 181 pages (*out of print*)

Volume 3 **Certain Polycyclic Aromatic Hydrocarbons and Heterocyclic Compounds**
1973; 271 pages (*out of print*)

Volume 4 **Some Aromatic Amines, Hydrazine and Related Substances, N-Nitroso Compounds and Miscellaneous Alkylating Agents**
1974; 286 pages Sw. fr. 18.-

Volume 5 **Some Organochlorine Pesticides**
1974; 241 pages (*out of print*)

Volume 6 **Sex Hormones**
1974; 243 pages (*out of print*)

Volume 7 **Some Anti-Thyroid and Related Substances, Nitrofurans and Industrial Chemicals**
1974; 326 pages (*out of print*)

Volume 8 **Some Aromatic Azo Compounds**
1975; 357 pages Sw. fr. 36.-

Volume 9 **Some Aziridines, N-, S- and O-Mustards and Selenium**
1975; 268 pages Sw.fr. 27.-

Volume 10 **Some Naturally Occurring Substances**
1976; 353 pages (*out of print*)

Volume 11 **Cadmium, Nickel, Some Epoxides, Miscellaneous Industrial Chemicals and General Considerations on Volatile Anaesthetics**
1976; 306 pages (*out of print*)

Volume 12 **Some Carbamates, Thiocarbamates and Carbazides**
1976; 282 pages Sw. fr. 34.-

Volume 13 **Some Miscellaneous Pharmaceutical Substances**
1977; 255 pages Sw. fr. 30.-

Volume 14 **Asbestos**
1977; 106 pages (*out of print*)

Volume 15 **Some Fumigants, The Herbicides 2,4-D and 2,4,5-T, Chlorinated Dibenzodioxins and Miscellaneous Industrial Chemicals**
1977; 354 pages Sw. fr. 50.-

Volume 16 **Some Aromatic Amines and Related Nitro Compounds - Hair Dyes, Colouring Agents and Miscellaneous Industrial Chemicals**
1978; 400 pages Sw. fr. 50.-

Volume 17 **Some N-Nitroso Compounds**
1978; 365 pages Sw. fr. 50.-

Volume 18 **Polychlorinated Biphenyls and Polybrominated Biphenyls**
1978; 140 pages Sw. fr. 20.-

Volume 19 **Some Monomers, Plastics and Synthetic Elastomers, and Acrolein**
1979; 513 pages (*out of print*)

Volume 20 **Some Halogenated Hydrocarbons**
1979; 609 pages (*out of print*)

Volume 21 **Sex Hormones (II)**
1979; 583 pages Sw. fr. 60.-

Volume 22 **Some Non-Nutritive Sweetening Agents**
1980; 208 pages Sw. fr. 25.-

Volume 23 **Some Metals and Metallic Compounds**
1980; 438 pages (*out of print*)

Volume 24 **Some Pharmaceutical Drugs**
1980; 337 pages Sw. fr. 40.-

Volume 25 **Wood, Leather and Some Associated Industries**
1981; 412 pages Sw. fr. 60.-

Volume 26 **Some Antineoplastic and Immunosuppressive Agents**
1981; 411 pages Sw. fr. 62.-

Volume 27 **Some Aromatic Amines, Anthraquinones and Nitroso Compounds, and Inorganic Fluorides Used in Drinking Water and Dental Preparations**
1982; 341 pages Sw. fr. 40.-

Volume 28 **The Rubber Industry**
1982; 486 pages Sw. fr. 70.-

Volume 29 **Some Industrial Chemicals and Dyestuffs**
1982; 416 pages Sw. fr. 60.-

Volume 30 **Miscellaneous Pesticides**
1983; 424 pages Sw. fr. 60.-

Volume 31 **Some Food Additives, Feed Additives and Naturally Occurring Substances**
1983; 314 pages Sw. fr. 60.-

Volume 32 **Polynuclear Aromatic Compounds, Part 1: Chemical, Environmental and Experimental Data**
1983; 477 pages Sw. fr. 60.-

Volume 33 **Polynuclear Aromatic Compounds, Part 2: Carbon Blacks, Mineral Oils and Some Nitroarenes**
1984; 245 pages Sw. fr. 50.-

Volume 34 **Polynuclear Aromatic Compounds, Part 3: Industrial Exposures in Aluminium Production, Coal Gasification, Coke Production, and Iron and Steel Founding**
1984; 219 pages Sw. fr. 48.-

Volume 35 **Polynuclear Aromatic Compounds, Part 4: Bitumens, Coal-tars and Derived Products, Shale-oils and Soots**
1985; 271 pages Sw. fr. 70.-

List of IARC Publications

Volume 36 **Allyl Compounds, Aldehydes, Epoxides and Peroxides**
1985; 369 pages Sw. fr. 70.-

Volume 37 **Tobacco Habits Other than Smoking: Betel-quid and Areca-nut Chewing; and some Related Nitrosamines**
1985; 291 pages Sw. fr. 70.-

Volume 38 **Tobacco Smoking**
1986; 421 pages Sw. fr. 75.-

Volume 39 **Some Chemicals Used in Plastics and Elastomers**
1986; 403 pages Sw. fr. 60.-

Volume 40 **Some Naturally Occurring and Synthetic Food Components, Furocoumarins and Ultraviolet Radiation**
1986; 444 pages Sw. fr. 65.-

Volume 41 **Some Halogenated Hydrocarbons and Pesticide Exposures**
1986; 434 pages Sw. fr. 65.-

Volume 42 **Silica and Some Silicates**
1987; 289 pages Sw. fr. 65.

Volume 43 **Man-Made Mineral Fibres and Radon**
1988; 300 pages Sw. fr. 65.-

Volume 44 **Alcohol Drinking**
1988; 416 pages Sw. fr. 65.

Volume 45 **Occupational Exposures in Petroleum Refining; Crude Oil and Major Petroleum Fuels**
1989; 322 pages Sw. fr. 65.-

Volume 46 **Diesel and Gasoline Engine Exhausts and Some Nitroarenes**
1989; 458 pages Sw. fr. 65.-

Volume 47 **Some Organic Solvents, Resin Monomers and Related Compounds, Pigments and Occupational Exposures in Paint Manufacture and Painting**
1989; 536 pages Sw. fr. 85.-

Volume 48 **Some Flame Retardants and Textile Chemicals, and Exposures in the Textile Manufacturing Industry**
1990; 345 pages Sw. fr. 65.-

Volume 49 **Chromium, Nickel and Welding**
1990; 677 pages Sw. fr. 95.-

Volume 50 **Pharmaceutical Drugs**
1990; 415 pages Sw. fr. 65.-

Volume 51 **Coffee, Tea, Mate, Methylxanthines and Methylglyoxal**
1991; 513 pages Sw. fr. 80.-

Volume 52 **Chlorinated Drinking-water; Chlorination By-products; Some Other Halogenated Compounds; Cobalt and Cobalt Compounds**
1991; 544 pages Sw. fr. 80.-

Volume 53 **Occupational Exposures in Insecticide Application and some Pesticides**
1991; 612 pages Sw. fr. 95.-

Volume 54 **Occupational Exposures to Mists and Vapours from Strong Inorganic Acids; and Other Industrial Chemicals**
1992; 336 pages Sw. fr. 65.-

Volume 55 **Solar and Ultraviolet Radiation**
1992; 316 pages Sw. fr. 65.-

Volume 56 Some Naturally Occurring Substances: Food Items and Constituents, Heterocyclic Aromatic Amines and Mycotoxins
1993; 600 pages Sw. fr. 95.-

Volume 56 Some Naturally Occurring Substances: Food Items and Constituents, Heterocyclic Aromatic Amines and Mycotoxins
1993; 600 pages Sw. fr. 95.-

Volume 57 **Occupational Exposures of Hairdressers and Barbers and Personal Use of Hair Colourants; Some Hair Dyes, Cosmetic Colourants, Industrial Dyestuffs and Aromatic Amines**
1993; 428 pages Sw. fr. 75.-

Supplement No. 1
Chemicals and Industrial Processes Associated with Cancer in Humans (IARC Monographs, Volumes 1 to 20)
1979; 71 pages (*out of print*)

Supplement No. 2
Long-term and Short-term Screening Assays for Carcinogens: A Critical Appraisal
1980; 426 pages Sw. fr. 40.-

Supplement No. 3
Cross Index of Synonyms and Trade Names in Volumes 1 to 26
1982; 199 pages (*out of print*)

Supplement No. 4
Chemicals, Industrial Processes and Industries Associated with Cancer in Humans (IARC Monographs, Volumes 1 to 29)
1982; 292 pages (*out of print*)

Supplement No. 5
Cross Index of Synonyms and Trade Names in Volumes 1 to 36
1985; 259 pages (*out of print*)

Supplement No. 6
Genetic and Related Effects: An Updating of Selected IARC Monographs from Volumes 1 to 42
1987; 729 pages Sw. fr. 80.-

Supplement No. 7
Overall Evaluations of Carcinogenicity: An Updating of IARC Monographs Volumes 1-42
1987; 440 pages Sw. fr. 65.-

Supplement No. 8
Cross Index of Synonyms and Trade Names in Volumes 1 to 46
1990; 346 pages Sw. fr. 60.-

IARC TECHNICAL REPORTS*

No. 1 **Cancer in Costa Rica**
Edited by R. Sierra,
R. Barrantes, G. Muñoz Leiva, D.M.
Parkin, C.A. Bieber and
N. Muñoz Calero
1988; 124 pages Sw. fr. 30.-

No. 2 **SEARCH: A Computer
Package to Assist the Statistical
Analysis of Case-control Studies**
Edited by G.J. Macfarlane,
P. Boyle and P. Maisonneuve
1991; 80 pages (out of print)

No. 3 **Cancer Registration in the
European Economic Community**
Edited by M.P. Coleman and
E. Démaret
1988; 188 pages Sw. fr. 30.-

No. 4 **Diet, Hormones and Cancer:
Methodological Issues for
Prospective Studies**
Edited by E. Riboli and
R. Saracci
1988; 156 pages Sw. fr. 30.-

No. 5 **Cancer in the Philippines**
Edited by A.V. Laudico,
D. Esteban and D.M. Parkin
1989; 186 pages Sw. fr. 30.-

No. 6 **La genèse du Centre
International de Recherche sur le
Cancer**
Par R. Sohier et A.G.B. Sutherland
1990; 104 pages Sw. fr. 30.-

No. 7 **Epidémiologie du cancer dans
les pays de langue latine**
1990; 310 pages Sw. fr. 30.-

No. 8 **Comparative Study of Anti-
smoking Legislation in Countries of
the European Economic Community**
Edited by A. Sasco, P. Dalla Vorgia
and P. Van der Elst
1992; 82 pages Sw. fr. 30.-

No. 9 **Epidemiologie du cancer dans
les pays de langue latine**
1991; 346 pages Sw. fr. 30.-

No. 11 **Nitroso Compounds:
Biological Mechanisms, Exposures
and Cancer Etiology**
Edited by I.K. O'Neill & H. Bartsch
1992; 149 pages Sw. fr. 30.-

No. 12 **Epidémiologie du cancer
dans les pays de langue latine**
1992; 375 pages Sw. fr. 30.-

No. 13 **Health, Solar UV Radiation
and Environmental Change**
Edited by A. Kricker, B.K.
Armstrong, M.E. Jones and R.C.
Burton
1993; 216 pages Sw.fr. 30.-

No. 14
**Epidémiologie du cancer dans les
pays de langue latine**
1993; 385 pages Sw. fr. 30.-

DIRECTORY OF AGENTS BEING TESTED FOR CARCINOGENICITY (Until Vol. 13 Information Bulletin on the Survey of Chemicals Being Tested for Carcinogenicity)*

No. 8 Edited by M.-J. Ghess,
H. Bartsch and L. Tomatis
1979; 604 pages Sw. fr. 40.-

No. 9 Edited by M.-J. Ghess,
J.D. Wilbourn, H. Bartsch and
L. Tomatis
1981; 294 pages Sw. fr. 41.-

No. 10 Edited by M.-J. Ghess,
J.D. Wilbourn and H. Bartsch
1982; 362 pages Sw. fr. 42.-

No. 11 Edited by M.-J. Ghess,
J.D. Wilbourn, H. Vainio and
H. Bartsch
1984; 362 pages Sw. fr. 50.-

No. 12 Edited by M.-J. Ghess,
J.D. Wilbourn, A. Tossavainen and
H. Vainio
1986; 385 pages Sw. fr. 50.-

No. 13 Edited by M.-J. Ghess,
J.D. Wilbourn and A. Aitio 1988;
404 pages Sw. fr. 43.-

No. 14 Edited by M.-J. Ghess,
J.D. Wilbourn and H. Vainio
1990; 370 pages Sw. fr. 45.-

No. 15 Edited by M.-J. Ghess, J.D.
Wilbourn and H. Vainio
1992; 318 pages Sw. fr. 45.-

NON-SERIAL PUBLICATIONS †

Alcool et Cancer
By A. Tuyns (in French only)
1978; 42 pages Fr. fr. 35.-

**Cancer Morbidity and Causes of
Death Among Danish Brewery
Workers**
By O.M. Jensen
1980; 143 pages Fr. fr. 75.-

**Directory of Computer Systems Used
in Cancer Registries**
By H.R. Menck and D.M. Parkin
1986; 236 pages Fr. fr. 50.-

* Available from booksellers through the network of WHO Sales agents.

† Available directly from IARC

www.ingramcontent.com/pod-product-compliance
Lightning Source LLC
Chambersburg PA
CBHW081759200326
41597CB00023B/4087